SIDNEY HURWITZ, M.D.

Associate Clinical Professor
Pediatrics and Dermatology
Yale University School of Medicine

CLINICAL PEDIATRIC DERMATOLOGY

A Textbook of Skin Disorders of Childhood and Adolescence

W. B. SAUNDERS COMPANY

Philadelphia   London   Toronto   Mexico City   Rio de Janeiro   Sydney   Tokyo

W. B. Saunders Company: West Washington Square
                            Philadelphia, PA   19105

                            1 St. Anne's Road
                            Eastbourne, East Sussex BN21 3UN, England

                            1 Goldthorne Avenue
                            Toronto, Ontario M8Z 5T9, Canada

                            Apartado 26370—Cedro 512
                            Mexico 4, D.F., Mexico

                            Rua Coronel Cabrita, 8
                            Sao Cristovao Caixa Postal 21176
                            Rio de Janeiro, Brazil

                            9 Waltham Street
                            Artarmon, N.S.W. 2064, Australia

                            Ichibancho, Central Bldg., 22-1 Ichibancho
                            Chiyoda-Ku, Tokyo 102, Japan

Library of Congress Cataloging in Publication Data

Hurwitz, Sidney.

Clinical pediatric dermatology.

1. Pediatric dermatology.   I. Title. [DNLM: 1. Skin
   diseases—In infancy and childhood. WS260 H967c]

RJ511.H87   618.92'5   80–5562

ISBN 0-7216-4872-X

Clinical Pediatric Dermatology   ISBN   0-7216-4872-X

Last digit is the print number: 9   8   7   6   5

Dedicated to
my wife
TEDDY
and my daughters
WENDY, LAURIE, and ALISON
Without whose patience, encouragement, understanding and sacrifice
this book could not have come to fruition.

PREFACE

Although 20 to 30 per cent of children and adolescents seen by pediatricians, family practitioners, and internists present problems related directly or indirectly to the skin, primary care physicians are often inadequately prepared in the knowledge of pathogenesis, diagnosis, and therapy of cutaneous disorders found in this age group. Throughout my fifteen years of busy private pediatric practice, I came to recognize the ever present need for a wider understanding of the skin diseases that affect children and adolescents. Ten years ago, my decision was to return to the Yale University School of Medicine to pursue a residency in dermatology, and subsequently to embark upon a career dedicated to the advancement of research, knowledge, and treatment of the skin in childhood and adolescence.

During the past decade there has been a rapidly growing interest in the field of pediatric dermatology. With this interest has surfaced the need for an up-to-date textbook on the various aspects of the skin in the pediatric patient. With the encouragement of my family and many colleagues in pediatrics and dermatology, this book has been written.

The text is designed to provide the clinician with information that will enable him to deal effectively with skin problems of the young. The new and exciting disorders as well as the commonly known diseases have been included. Histopathology has been described in an effort to help non-dermatologists to understand the signs and symptoms of cutaneous disease and as an aid to proper diagnosis and appropriate therapy. Emphasis in terminology is placed upon the simple, preferred terms for each disease, with references to other terms of historical significance. Focus is upon diagnosis and treatment; presentation is comprehensive yet concise. Cutaneous lesions are described in detail and extensively illustrated with more than 500 clinical photographs. Recent advances are stressed; more than 1,000 pertinent references with simple sentence summaries are included.

It is my feeling that in a textbook of this kind it is essential to reproduce skin disorders in color in an effort to portray variations in hue so valuable to accurate dermatological diagnosis. The cost of color reproduction is so great, however, that it is frequently impossible to utilize color plates and keep the price of the book within the range of practicality. In this book, the use of personal honoraria and the generosity of the following companies helped to underwrite the cost of reproduction of many color plates: Barnes Haind

Pharmaceuticals, Inc.; Dermik Laboratories, Inc.; E. R. Squibb & Sons, Inc.; Johnson & Johnson; Miles Pharmaceuticals, Division of Miles Laboratories, Inc.; Neutrogena Corporation; Reed & Carnrick Pharmaceuticals; Stiefel Laboratories, Inc.; Syntex Laboratories, Inc.; Syosset Laboratories; Texas Pharmacal Company; Upjohn Company; and Westwood Pharmaceuticals, Inc.

I am deeply indebted to numerous medical colleagues for encouragement and advice on the undertaking of this endeavor and in particular wish to express my sincere gratitude to Drs. Irwin M. Braverman, G. Martin Carter, James D. Cherry, Nancy B. Esterly, Maurice T. Fliegelman, Alvin H. Jacobs, Michael Jarratt, Guinter Kahn, James J. Leyden, Andrew M. Margileth, James J. Nordlund, Milton Orkin, and John S. Strauss, each of whom reviewed selected chapters during the preparation of this textbook. Appreciation is expressed to my office staff for their assistance and to Mrs. Marion Burgess for her work in the typing of the manuscript.

By far the most important persons concerned with the preparation of this book have been my wife Teddy and our three daughters, Wendy, Laurie, and Alison. In the beginning, my wife was the only one who recognized my dream of a career in pediatric dermatology. Without her enthusiasm and constant encouragement to forge ahead despite all obstacles, without her sacrifices during my second residency and in the early days of my new venture, and without her patience and devoted energy in reviewing my manuscripts, my dream would never have become a reality.

The writing of this textbook, which took six years of nights, weekends, and holidays, was done on "family time." The most important sacrifice in its execution was made by my wife and children who were forced to "wait in the wings" for the project to be completed. Without their sustained devotion and understanding, this textbook could never have come to fruition.

The research and writing of this text during a busy schedule of clinical practice, publishing, and lecturing has truly been a labor of love. My hope is that those who utilize this book will enjoy and benefit as much from the reading of it as I have from its research and writing.

SIDNEY HURWITZ, M.D.

CONTENTS

AN OVERVIEW OF DERMATOLOGIC DIAGNOSIS

Accurate diagnosis of cutaneous disease in infants and children, as in adults, is a systematic process that requires careful inspection, evaluation, and some knowledge of dermatologic terminology, morphology, and differential diagnosis. It must be recognized that disorders of the skin in infants and young children vary in many respects from occurrences of the same diseases in older children and adults and that the diagnosis and treatment may be confused by more sensitive reaction patterns, a tendency toward vesicle and bulla formation, and therapeutic dosages and regimens that frequently differ from those of adults.

The same basic principles applied to the detection of disorders of any other organ of the body are applicable to the study of cutaneous disease. It is desirable to perform a thorough physical examination, obtain an adequate history, and, whenever possible, verify the clinical impression by appropriate laboratory studies. The easy visibility of skin lesions all too frequently results in cursory examination and hasty diagnosis. This tendency must be overcome. The entire skin should be examined routinely and carefully, including the hair, scalp, nails, oral mucosa, anogenital regions, palms, and soles, as these often hold clues to the final diagnosis.

Examination should be conducted in a well-lighted room. Although natural daylight is the most effective type of illumination, fluorescent or incandescent lighting of adequate intensity may be satisfactory. A properly sequenced examination requires initial viewing of the patient at a distance in an effort to establish the overall status of the patient and his disorder. By this overall evaluation, distribution patterns and clues to the appropriate final diagnosis frequently can be recognized. This initial evaluation is followed by careful scrutiny of primary and subsequent secondary lesions in an effort to discern the characteristic feature of the disorder.

Although not always diagnostic, the morphology and configuration of cutaneous lesions are of considerable importance to the classification and diagnosis of cutaneous disease. Unfortunately, a lack of understanding of dermatologic terminology frequently poses a barrier to the description of cutaneous disorders by non-dermatologists. Accordingly, this review of dermatologic terms is included.

A GLOSSARY OF DERMATOLOGIC TERMS

Primary Lesions

The term primary refers to the most representative, but not necessarily the earliest, lesions; it does not refer to the cutaneous features brought about by secondary changes due to excoriation, eczematization, infection, or previous therapy.

Macules. Macules are flat circumscribed changes of the skin. They may be of any size, have no palpable manifestations, and are neither elevated nor depressed in reference to the surrounding skin. Macules may appear as areas of hyperpigmentation, hypopigmentation, or vascular abnormality. They are usually rounded, but may be oval or irregular, and may be distinct or may fade into the surrounding area. Examples include freckles, flat nevi, café au lait spots, areas of vitiligo or hypopigmentation, and flat vascular lesions such as telangiectases or capillary hemangiomas of the salmon patch or port-wine type.

Papules, nodules, plaques, and tumors. *Papules* are circumscribed elevated lesions of one to five millimeters in diameter. Examples include elevated nevi, verrucae, molluscum contagiosum, and individual lesions of lichen planus.

Nodules are circumscribed, elevated, usually solid lesions that measure roughly between 0.5

and 2 cm in diameter (some leeway in size is arbitrarily allowed here). They may be located only in the epidermis or may extend deeper into the dermis or subcutaneous tissue. Examples include fibromas, neurofibromas, xanthomas, intradermal or compound nevi, lesions of erythema nodosum, and various benign or malignant growths.

Plaques are elevated disc-shaped lesions that occupy a relatively larger area. They frequently are formed by a confluence of papules and may be seen in psoriasis, lichen simplex chronicus (neurodermatitis), or lesions of lichen planus.

Tumors are larger and deeper circumscribed solid lesions of the skin or subcutaneous tissue. They may be benign or malignant processes and include lesions such as lipomas, strawberry or cavernous hemangiomas, and various neoplastic growths.

Wheals. *Wheals* are a distinctive type of solid elevation formed by local, superficial, transient edema. White to pink or pale red in color, compressible, and evanescent, they often disappear within a period of hours. They vary in size and shape and may be seen in dermographism, insect bites, and various forms of urticaria.

Vesicles and bullae. *Vesicles* are sharply circumscribed, elevated fluid-containing lesions that measure 0.5 cm in diameter or less. Examples include lesions of herpes, dyshidrosis, pompholyx, varicella, and contact dermatitis.

Bullae are larger circumscribed, elevated fluid-containing lesions over 0.5 cm in diameter. They may be seen in burns, contact dermatitis, pemphigus, and epidermolysis bullosa.

Pustules. *Pustules* are circumscribed elevations that contain a purulent exudate. They may be bacterial in nature as in pyoderma (impetigo) or may be sterile as in pustular psoriasis, bromoderma, or smallpox.

Comedones. *Comedones* are plugged secretions of horny material retained within a pilosebaceous follicle. They may be flesh-colored closed comedones (white-heads) or slightly raised brown or black open comedones (blackheads). Closed comedones, in contrast to open comedones, may be difficult to visualize. They appear as pale, slightly elevated small papules without a clinically visible orifice. Since closed comedones are the precursors of the papules, pustules, cysts, or nodules of acne, they are of considerable clinical importance.

Burrows. *Burrows* are linear lesions produced by tunneling of an animal parasite in the stratum corneum. Burrows may be seen in scabies or cutaneous larva migrans (creeping eruption) and, when present, are highly characteristic and diagnostic of these disorders.

Telangiectasia. The term *telangiectasia* refers to a relatively permanent dilatation of superficial venules, capillaries, or arterioles of the skin. They may be seen in actinically damaged skin, rosacea, radiodermatitis, hereditary hemorrhagic telangiectasia (Osler-Rendu-Weber disease), essential telangiectasia, angiokeratomas, lesions of lupus erythematosus, lipomas, and basal cell epitheliomas, and when present in the cuticular region (cuticular telangiectasia) are a pathognomonic sign of connective tissue disease, such as lupus erythematosus, dermatomyositis, or scleroderma.

Secondary Lesions

Secondary lesions represent evolutionary changes that occur later on in the course of the cutaneous disorder. Although helpful in dermatologic diagnosis, they do not offer the same degree of diagnostic aid as that afforded by primary lesions of a cutaneous disorder.

Crusts and scales. *Crusts* are the result of dried remains of serum, blood, pus, or exudate overlying areas of lost or damaged epidermis. They may be seen in third-degree burns, in lesions of weeping eczematous dermatitis, or as dried honey-colored lesions of impetigo.

Scales are formed by an accumulation of compact desquamation layers of stratum corneum. A result of abnormal keratinization and exfoliation of cornified keratinocytes they may be greasy and yellowish in color (seborrheic dermatitis), silvery and mica-like (psoriasis), fine and barely visible (pityriasis alba or tinea versicolor), or large, adherent, and lamellar (in various forms of ichthyosis).

Fissures and erosions. A *fissure* is a dry or moist linear, often painful, cleavage in the cutaneous surface that results from marked drying and long-standing inflammation, thickening, and loss of elasticity of the integument. Fissures frequently appear in chronic dermatoses and calluses of the hands and feet.

Erosions are moist, slightly depressed vesicular lesions in which part or all of the epidermis has been lost or denuded. Since erosions do not extend into the underlying dermis or subcutaneous tissue, healing occurs without subsequent scar formation.

Excoriations and ulcerations. The term *excoriation* refers to a traumatized or abraded (usually self-induced) superficial loss of skin caused by scratching, rubbing, or scrubbing of the cutaneous surface. Excoriations are seen in pruritic disorders such as atopic dermatitis, neurotic excoriations, contact dermatitis, fiberglass dermatitis, prurigo nodularis, icterus, varicella, papular urticaria, dermatitis herpetiformis, scabies, pediculosis, and acne excoriée.

Cutaneous ulcers are the result of necrosis of the epidermis and part or all of the dermis and/or the underlying subcutaneous tissue. Ulcers may occur as the result of bacterial, parasitic, or fungal infection, tissue infarction, halogenoderma, scleroderma, ecthyma, frostbite, sickle cell disease, and benign or neoplastic necrosis of tissue (as in decubitus ulcers, basal cell epithelioma, or reticulum cell sarcoma).

Atrophy. *Atrophy* refers to cutaneous changes that result in depression of the epidermis, dermis, or both. Epidermal atrophy is characterized by thin, almost translucent epidermis, a loss of the normal skin markings, and wrinkling when subjected to lateral pressure or pinching of the affected area. In dermal atrophy there is a depression of the skin without change in color or skin markings.

Scars (cicatrices) and keloids. *Scars* are permanent fibrotic skin changes that develop following damage to the dermis. Initially pink or violaceous in color, as the color fades they remain as permanent white, shiny, sclerotic areas. Although fresh scars often tend to be hypertrophic, with passage of time (frequently six months to a year) they usually contract and become less apparent.

Hypertrophic scars must be differentiated from keloids, which represent an exaggerated connective tissue response to skin injury. Keloids are pink, smooth, and rubbery and often are traversed by telangiectatic vessels. They tend to increase in size long after healing has taken place and can be differentiated from hypertrophic scars by the fact that the surface of keloidal scars tends to proliferate beyond the area of the original wound.

Configuration of Lesions

Annular, circinate, or ring-shaped lesions. A number of dermatologic entities assume annular shapes and are interpreted as "ringworm" or superficial fungal infections. Although tinea is indeed one of the common annular dermatoses of childhood, other disorders that must be included in the differential diagnosis of ringed lesions include pityriasis rosea, seborrheic dermatitis, granuloma annulare, psoriasis, erythema multiforme, erythema annulare centrifugum, erythema chronicum migrans, secondary syphilis, sarcoidosis, urticaria, pityriasis alba, and tinea versicolor.

Arciform or arcuate lesions. The terms arciform and arcuate refer to lesions that assume arc-like configurations. Arciform lesions may be seen in erythema multiforme, urticaria, and pityriasis rosea.

Confluent lesions. Lesions that tend to join or run together are said to be confluent. Confluence of lesions is seen in childhood exanthems, rhus dermatitis, erythema multiforme, and urticaria.

Dermatomal lesions. Lesions localized into a dermatome supplied by one or more dorsal ganglia are said to be dermatomal in nature. Prominent examples of this type of distribution include lesions of herpes zoster and segmental vitiligo.

Discoid lesions. This term is used to describe lesions that are solid, moderately raised, and disc shaped. Although frequently utilized to differentiate cutaneous from systemic forms of lupus erythematosus, since one cannot determine from the clinical or histologic examination of a discoid lesion whether or not there is systemic involvement, a more appropriate term would be cutaneous rather than discoid.

Discrete lesions. Individual lesions that tend to remain separated and distinct are said to be discrete in nature. Discrete lesions appear in a variety of conditions and although perhaps of descriptive value, this term is neither characteristic nor diagnostic of any specific disorder.

Eczematoid or eczematous disorders. These terms are adjectives relating to eczema and suggest inflammation with a tendency to thickening, oozing, vesiculation, or crusting.

Grouping or clustering. Grouping and clustering are characteristic of vesicles of herpes simplex or herpes zoster, insect bites, lymphangioma circumscriptum, contact dermatitis, and bullous dermatosis of childhood.

Guttate lesions. Guttate or drop-like lesions are characteristic of flares of psoriasis in children and adolescents that follow an acute upper respiratory infection, usually, but not necessarily, streptococcal in nature.

Gyrate lesions. This term refers to twisted, coiled, or spiral-like lesions, such as may be seen in patients with urticaria and erythema annulare centrifugum.

Iris lesions. Iris or target-like lesions are concentric ringed lesions characteristic of erythema multiforme of both the regular and bullous (Stevens-Johnson) varieties.

Keratosis (keratotic). The term *keratosis* (*plural, keratoses*) refers to circumscribed patches of horny thickening, as seen in seborrheic or actinic (solar) keratoses, keratosis pilaris, and keratosis follicularis (Darier's disease). Keratotic is an adjective pertaining or relating to keratosis and frequently refers to the horny thickening of the skin seen in chronic dermatitis and callus formation.

Koebner phenomenon (isomorphic response). The Koebner phenomenon refers to an isomorphic response with the appearance of lesions along the site of injury. This phenomenon may be seen with warts, molluscum contagiosum, rhus dermatitis (poison ivy), psoriasis, lichen planus, lichen nitidus, pityriasis rubra pilaris, and keratosis follicularis (Darier's disease).

Linear disorders. Lesions in a linear or band-like configuration appear in the form of a line or stripe and may be seen in linear nevi (nevus unius lateris), linear morphea or scleroderma (the coupe de sabre deformity), or as lesions of lichen striatus.

Moniliform lesions. The term *moniliform* refers to a banded or necklace-like appearance. This is seen in monilethrix, a hair deformity characterized by beaded nodularities along the hair shaft.

Multiforme lesions. The term *multiforme* refers to disorders in which more than one variety or shape of cutaneous lesions occurs. The most common manifestation of this configuration is typified by the varied lesions seen in patients with erythema multiforme, early Henoch-Schönlein purpura, and polymorphous light eruption.

Polycyclic. The term *polycyclic* refers to oval lesions containing more than one ring. This frequently is seen in patients with urticaria.

Serpiginous. The term *serpiginous* describes the shape or spread of lesions in a serpentine or snake-like configuration. This term is used to describe lesions of cutaneous larva migrans (creeping eruption) and elastosis perforans serpiginosa.

Umbilicated lesions. The terms *umbilication* and *umbilicated* refer to lesions that are depressed or shaped like an umbilicus or navel. Examples include lesions of molluscum contagiosum, varicella, vaccinia, variola, herpes zoster, and Kaposi's varicelliform eruption.

Universal (universalis). The terms *universal* and *universalis* imply widespread disorders affecting the entire skin (as in alopecia universalis).

Zosteriform. The term *zosteriform* is a descriptive term that implies a linear arrangement along a nerve. This configuration is typified by lesions of herpes zoster and linear forms of keratosis follicularis (zosteriform Darier's disease).

REGIONAL DISTRIBUTION AND MORPHOLOGIC PATTERNS

The regional distribution and morphologic configuration of cutaneous lesions frequently are helpful in dermatologic diagnosis.

Acneform (acneiform) or acne-like distribution patterns. Acneform lesions are those appearing like or having the form of acne or lesions of acne. An acneform distribution refers to lesions primarily seen on the face, neck, chest, upper arms, shoulders, and back.

Atopic dermatitis. Sites of predilection include the face, trunk, and extremities in young children, the extremities (particularly the antecubital fossae and popliteal fossae) in older children and adults, and the face, neck, trunk, and antecubital fossae and popliteal fossae in adolescents and adults.

Erythema multiforme. Lesions of erythema multiforme may be widespread but have a distinct predilection for the hands and feet (particularly the palms and soles) and mucous membranes.

Herpes simplex. Lesions of herpes simplex may appear anywhere on the body but have a distinct predisposition for the areas about the lips, face, and genitalia. Herpes zoster generally has a dermatomal or nerve-like distribution and is usually but not necessarily unilateral. Over 75 per cent of cases occur between the second dorsal and second lumbar vertebrae, the fifth cranial nerve frequently is involved, and only rarely are lesions seen below the elbows or knees.

Lichen planus. Lesions of lichen planus frequently affect the limbs. Favorite sites include the lower extremities, the flexor surface of the wrists, the buccal mucosa, the trunk, and genitalia.

Lupus erythematosus. The favorite locations include the bridge of the nose and the malar eminences, scalp, ears, buccal mucosa, arms, legs, hands, fingers, back, chest, or abdomen. The patches tend to spread at the border and clear in the center, with atrophy, scarring, and telangiectases. It must be remembered that the malar or butterfly rash is neither specific for nor the most frequent sign of lupus erythematosus and that the presence of telangiectasia without the accompanying features of erythema, scaling, or atrophy is never a marker of this disorder.

Photodermatoses. Photodermatoses are cutaneous disorders caused or precipitated by exposure to light. Areas of predilection include the face, ears, upper chest, the dorsal aspect of the forearms and hands, and exposed areas of the legs, with sparing of the shaded regions of the upper eyelids, subnasal, and submental regions. The major photosensitivity disorders are lupus erythematosus, dermatomyositis, polymorphous light eruption, drug photosensitization, and porphyria.

Photosensitive reactions cannot be distinguished on a clinical basis from lesions of photocontact allergic conditions, may reflect internal as well as external photoallergens, and may simulate contact dermatitis from airborn sensitizers. Lupus erythematosus can be differentiated by the presence of atrophy, scarring, hyperpigmentation or hypopigmentation, and the presence of cuticular telangiectases. Dermatomyositis with swelling and erythema of the cheeks and eyelids should be differentiated from allergic contact dermatitis by the heliotrope hue and other associated changes, particularly those of the fingers (telangiectases of the cuticles, Gottron's papules, and subungual hyperkeratosis) when present.

Pityriasis rosea. This benign, exceedingly common eruption is observed most frequently in children and young adults but also may appear in infants. In 70 to 80 per cent of cases the generalized eruption starts with a solitary round or oval lesion known as the herald patch followed, after an interval of seven to ten days, by a generalized symmetrical eruption that involves mainly the trunk and proximal limbs, with the long axis of oval lesions parallel to the lines of cleavage in what has been termed a Christmas-tree pattern.

Psoriasis. Classic lesions of psoriasis consist of round, erythematous, well-marginated patches with a rich red hue covered by a characteristic grayish or silvery-white mica-like (micaceous) scale which, on removal, may result in pinpoint bleeding (Auspitz sign). Although exceptions occur, lesions generally are seen in a bilaterally symmetrical pattern with a predilection for the elbows, knees, scalp, lumbosacral, perianal, and genital regions. Nail involvement, a valuable diagnostic sign, is characterized by pitting of the nail plate, discoloration, separation of the nail from the nail bed (onycholysis), and an accumulation of subungual scale (subungual hyperkeratosis). A characteristic feature of this disorder is the Koebner or isomorphic response in which new lesions appear at sites of local injury.

Scabies. The diagnosis of scabies is best

made by a history of itching; a characteristic distribution of lesions on the wrists and hands (particularly the interdigital webs), forearms, genitalia, areolae, and buttocks; the recognition of primary lesions (particularly the pathognomonic burrow, when present; and the presence of disease among the patient's family or associates. In infants and young children the diagnosis is often overlooked because of a lower index of suspicion, an atypical distribution that includes the head, neck, palms, and soles, and obliteration of demonstrable primary lesions due to vigorous hygienic measures, excoriation, crusting, eczematization, and secondary infection.

Seborrheic dermatitis. Seborrheic dermatitis is an erythematous, scaly or crusting eruption that characteristically occurs on the scalp, face, postauricular, presternal, and intertriginous areas. The classic lesions are dull or pinkish yellow or salmon colored, with fairly sharp borders and overlying yellowish greasy scale. Morphologic and topographic variants occur in many combinations and with varying degrees of severity, from mild involvement of the scalp with occasional blepharitis to generalized and occasionally severe eczematous eruptions. The differential diagnosis includes atopic dermatitis, psoriasis, various forms of diaper dermatitis, Letterer-Siwe disease, scabies, pediculosis, tinea corporis or capitis, pityriasis rosea, pityriasis alba, contact dermatitis, Mucha-Habermann disease, Darier's disease, pityriasis rubra pilaris, and lupus erythematosus.

Warts. Warts are common viral cutaneous lesions characterized by the appearance of flesh-colored small papules of several morphologic types. They may be elevated or flat lesions and tend to appear in areas of trauma, particularly the dorsal surface of the face, hands, periungual areas, the elbows, knees, feet, and genital or perianal areas. Close examination may reveal capillaries appearing as punctate dots scattered over the surface.

Disorders associated with increased scaling. A large number of cutaneous diseases are associated with abnormalities of keratinization. These include the ichthyoses, keratosis pilaris, lichen spinulosis, palmar and plantar keratosis (keratoderma), pityriasis rubra pilaris, hypervitaminosis A (vitamin A intoxication), and keratosis follicularis (Darier's disease).

Variations in black skin and hair. The skin of black children varies in several ways from that of individuals of Caucasian and Oriental backgrounds. Among the black population, (1) genetic background, (2) relatively poor socio-economic status, and (3) mores and customs may at times alter the individual physician's therapeutic approach to cutaneous problems. Skin disorders more commonly seen are impetigo, papular urticaria, tinea capitis, sickle cell ulcers, and sarcoidosis. Tinea versicolor is very common in blacks because of a higher incidence in tropical climates and because of the easy visibility of

lesions in marked contrast to uninvolved surrounding skin. It has been noted that lichen nitidus is more apparent and possibly more common in black individuals; lichen planus is said to be more severe; and keloids are seen more frequently.

Erythema in black skin is difficult to see and frequently has a purplish tinge that can be confusing to unwary observers. In atopic dermatitis there is often a variation in pigmentary change (areas of hypopigmentation or hyperpigmentation are more extensive and more obvious) and lesions frequently have a follicular quality. Secondary syphilis often has a follicular quality and is papular and annular in nature. Psoriasis and pediculosis capitis are relatively uncommon and lupus erythematosus is seen only half as frequently in black individuals as it is in white individuals.

It should be noted that black skin tans on exposure to sunlight, and although slight erythema may develop after exposure to sun, sunburn and chronic sun-induced diseases such as actinic keratosis and actinically induced carcinomas of the skin (e.g., squamous cell carcinoma, keratoacanthoma, basal cell carcinoma, and malignant melanoma) have an extremely low incidence in blacks.

The hair of blacks varies from that of whites and orientals, as well. Black hair tends to tangle when dry and becomes matted when wet. As a result of its natural curly or spiral nature, pseudofolliculitis barbae is more common in blacks than whites. Frequent and liberal use of greasy lubricants and pomades produces a comedonal and papulopustular form of acne (pomade acne). Frequent use of picks for hair grooming, the use of hot pressing oils in hair straightening techniques, and tight braiding of the hair are common causes of traumatic alopecia.

Disorders of pigmentation. Various disorders of hyperpigmentation and hypopigmentation may become manifest in infancy and childhood. Disorders of hyperpigmentation include post-inflammatory hyperpigmentation, mongolian spots, various moles and nevi, café au lait spots, post-inflammatory hyperpigmentation, incontinentia pigmenti, fixed drug eruption, photodermatitis, phytophotodermatitis, chloasma, Riehl's melanosis, argyria, acanthosis nigricans, and Addison's disease. Yellowish discoloration of the skin is common in infants. This condition generally is related to the presence of carotene derived from excessive ingestion of foods, particularly yellow vegetables containing carotenoid pigments.

Disorders of depigmentation or hypopigmentation may be seen as vitiligo, post-inflammatory hypopigmentation, pityriasis alba, tinea versicolor, chemical depigmentation, halo nevi, achromic nevi, albinism and partial albinism (piebaldism), Waardenberg's syndrome, Vogt-Kayanagi syndrome, Tietz syndrome, Chediak-Higashi syndrome, tuberous sclerosis, incontinentia pigmenti achromians (hypomelanosis of Ito), and leprosy.

2

CUTANEOUS DISORDERS OF THE NEWBORN

NEONATAL SKIN

The skin of the infant differs from that of an adult in that it is thinner, less hairy, has weaker intercellular attachments, and produces fewer sweat and sebaceous gland secretions (Table 2–1). Although much has been published on the various disorders and phenomena peculiar to the integument of infants, it is unfortunate that to date actually very little is known about the physiologic variations and reactivity of the skin in the neonatal age group. As a result, the skin of the neonate presents a broad area for future research and investigation.

It has been held that newborn skin is more susceptible to external irritants. This concept remains controversial and requires further investigation. Percutaneous absorption is known to occur through two major pathways: via the cells of the stratum corneum and the epidermal malpighian layer (the transepidermal route) and via the hair follicle-sebaceous gland component (the transappendageal route). Although for years physicians have considered newborn skin to be more susceptible to the percutaneous absorption of potentially toxic substances, current data reveals that although the skin of the premature infant is indeed more permeable, undamaged skin of normal full-term newborns (except for the scrotal area) is no more susceptible to percutaneous absorption than that of older children or adults.[1, 2] The problem of percutaneous permeability and absorption in infancy, therefore, is one of a greater relative skin surface to body volume ratio in infants and small

Table 2-1 CHARACTERISTICS OF NEONATAL SKIN
IN COMPARISON WITH ADULT SKIN

Table 2-1 CHARACTERISTICS OF NEONATAL SKIN
IN COMPARISON WITH ADULT SKIN

1. Thinner, less hairy, weaker intercellular attachments
2. Fewer eccrine and sebaceous gland secretions
3. Increased susceptibility to external irritants
4. Increased susceptibility to micrococcal infection
5. Depressed contact allergen reactivity
6. Percutaneous permeability increased only in prematures, damaged, or scrotal skin

children (as compared to that of older children and adults). This results in the risk of higher blood level accumulations of potentially toxic substances in this age group.

SKIN CARE OF THE NEWBORN. The skin of the newborn is covered with a grayish-white greasy material termed vernix caseosa. The vernix represents a physiologic protective covering derived partially by secretion of the sebaceous glands and in part as a decomposition product of the infant's epidermis. Although its function is not as yet completely understood, most studies suggest that it be left on as a protective coating for the newborn skin and that it be allowed to come off by itself with successive changes of clothing (generally within the first few weeks of life).

The skin acts as a protective organ. Any break in its integrity, therefore, affords an opportunity for initiation of infection. Skin care of the newborn is complicated by the fact that the infant does not have protective skin flora at birth, has at least one, and possibly two, open surgical wounds (the umbilicus and circumcision site), and is exposed to fomites and personnel that potentially harbor a variety of infectious agents.[3]

Skin care should involve gentle cleansing with a non-toxic, non-abrasive neutral material. During the 1950's the use of hexachlorophene-containing compounds became routine for the skin care of newborn infants as prophylaxis against *Staphylococcus aureus* infection. In 1971 and 1972, however, the use of hexachlorophene preparations as skin cleansers for newborn infants was restricted because of studies demonstrating vacuolization in the central nervous system of infants and laboratory animals after prolonged application of these preparations. As a result, current recommendations for the management of skin care suggest gentle removal of blood from the face and head, and meconium from the perianal area, by careful water rinsing. The remainder of the skin is probably best left alone unless grossly soiled. Vernix caseosa should be removed from the face only, allowing that remaining on the rest of the body to come off by itself. For the remainder of the infant's stay in the hospital nursery, the buttocks and perianal regions should be cleansed with sterile water and cotton. A mild soap with water rinsing may also be used at diaper changes if desired.

There is no single method of umbilical cord care that has been proven to limit colonization and disease. Several methods include local application of alcohol, triple dye (an aqueous solution of brilliant green, proflavine, and crystal violet), and antimicrobial agents such as bacitracin, neosporin, or silver sulfadiazine cream.[3]

PHYSIOLOGIC DISORDERS OF THE NEWBORN

Neonatal dermatology, by definition, encompasses the spectrum of cutaneous disorders that arise during the first four weeks of life. Many such conditions are transient, appearing in the first few days to weeks of life, only to disappear shortly thereafter. The appreciation of normal phenomena and their differentiation from the more significant cutaneous disorders of the neonate is critical for the general physician, obstetrician, and pediatrician, as well as for the pediatric dermatologist.

At birth the skin of the full-term infant is normally soft, smooth, and velvety. Desquamation of neonatal skin generally takes place 24 to 36 hours after delivery and may not be complete until the third week of life. When seen at birth, this is an abnormal phenomenon and is indicative of postmaturity, intrauterine anoxia, or congenital ichthyosis.

The skin at birth has a purplish-red color that is most pronounced over the extremities. Except for the hands, feet, and lips, where the transition is gradual, this quickly changes to a pink hue. In a great number of infants a purplish discoloration of the hands, feet, and lips occurs during periods of crying, breathholding, or chilling. This normal phenomenon, termed *acrocyanosis*, appears to be associated with an increased tone of peripheral arterioles, which in turn creates vasospasm, secondary dilatation, and pooling of blood in the venous plexuses, which produce a cyanotic appearance to the involved areas of the skin. The intensity of cyanosis depends upon the degree of oxygen loss and the depth, size, and fullness of the involved venous plexus. Acrocyanosis, a normal physiologic phenomenon, should not be confused with true cyanosis.

Cutis Marmorata

Cutis marmorata is a normal reticulated bluish mottling of the skin seen on the trunk and extremities of infants and young children (Fig. 2–1). This phenomenon, a physiologic response to chilling, with resultant dilatation of capillaries and small venules, usually disappears as the infant is rewarmed. Although a tendency to cutis marmorata may persist for several weeks or months, this disorder bears no medical significance and treatment generally is unnecessary. In some children cutis marmorata may tend to recur until early childhood, and in patients with Down syndrome, trisomy 18, and the Cornelia de Lange syndrome, this reticulated marbling pattern may be persistent.[1] In some infants a white negative pattern of this phenomenon (*cutis marmorata alba*) may be

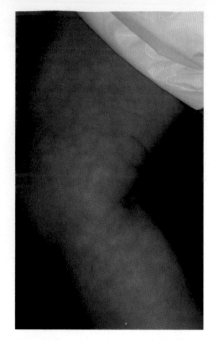

Figure 2–1 Cutis marmorata. A normal reticulated bluish pattern of the skin seen as a physiologic response to cool environmental temperatures in infants and, at times, young children.

created by a transient hypertonia of the deep vasculature. Cutis marmorata alba is also a transitory disorder and appears to have no clinical significance.

Harlequin Color Change

This condition, not to be confused with that of the harlequin fetus, is occasionally observed in full-term infants, but is usually seen in prematures. Seen in up to 10 per cent of infants, the harlequin color change occurs when the infant is lying on its side and consists of reddening of one half of the body with simultaneous blanching of the other half. Attacks develop suddenly and may persist for from 30 seconds to 20 minutes. The side lying uppermost is paler, and a clear line of demarcation runs along the midline of the body.

At times this line of demarcation may be incomplete, and when attacks are mild, areas of the face and genitalia may not be involved.

This phenomenon appears to be related to immaturity of hypothalamic centers that control the tone of peripheral blood vessels and has been observed in infants with severe intracranial injury as well as in infants who appear to be otherwise perfectly normal. Although the peak frequency of attacks of harlequin color change generally occurs between the second and fifth days of life, attacks may occur anywhere from the first few hours to as late as the second or third week of life.[4]

ABNORMALITIES OF SUBCUTANEOUS TISSUE

Skin turgor is generally normal during the first few hours of life. As normal physiologic dehydration occurs during the first three or four days of life (up to 10 per cent of birth weight), the skin generally becomes loose and wrinkled in appearance. Subcutaneous fat, normally quite adequate at birth, increases in amount until about nine months of age, thus accounting for the traditional chubby appearance of the healthy neonate. A decrease or absence of this normal panniculus is abnormal and suggests the possibility of prematurity, postmaturity, or placental insufficiency.

Sclerema neonatorum and subcutaneous fat necrosis appear to be clinical variants of the same disorder or closely allied abnormalities of subcutaneous tissue (Table 2–2). Although there is considerable confusion in the literature, recent evidence suggests that the biochemical abnormality in these two disorders may be identical.

Sclerema Neonatorum

Sclerema neonatorum is a diffuse, rapidly spreading, wax-like hardening of the skin and subcutaneous tissue that occurs in premature or debilitated infants during the first few weeks of life. The disorder, usually associated with a serious underlying condition such as sepsis or other infection, congenital heart disease, respiratory distress, diarrhea, or dehydration, is charac-

Table 2–2 CHARACTERISTIC DIFFERENCES BETWEEN SCLEREMA NEONATORUM AND SUBCUTANEOUS FAT NECROSIS

Sclerema Neonatorum	Subcutaneous Fat Necrosis
1. Serious underlying disease (sepsis, CHD, respiratory distress, diarrhea, or dehydration)	1. Healthy newborns
2. Wax-like hardening of skin and subcutaneous tissue in premature or debilitated infants	2. Circumscribed indurated and nodular areas of fat necrosis
3. Etiology: hypothermia, peripheral chilling with vascular collapse, defect in fatty acid mobilization?	3. Etiology: pressure on bony prominences during delivery, asphyxia, hypothermia, or diabetes in mother
4. Histopathology: edema and thickening of CT bands around fat lobules, needle-shaped clefts within fat cells	4. Histopathology: large fat lobules, inflammatory infiltrate in subcutaneous tissue, foreign body giant cells around crystals of fatty acid
5. Management: supportive care, heat, O₂, control of infection, IV fluids, systemic steroids	5. Management: aspiration of fluctuant lesions prn; most resolve spontaneously in 2–4 weeks.

terized by a diffuse non-pitting woody induration of the involved tissues. The process is symmetrical, usually starting on the legs and buttocks, and may progress to involve all areas except the palms, soles, and genitalia. As the disorder spreads, the skin becomes cold, yellowish-white, mottled, stony hard, and cadaver-like. The limbs become immobile, and the face acquires a fixed mask-like expression. The infants become sluggish, feed poorly, show clinical signs of shock, and in a high percentage of cases often go on to die.[5] Although the etiology of this disorder is unknown, it appears to represent a non-specific sign of grave prognostic significance rather than a primary disease.[1, 6] Infants with this disorder are characteristically small or premature, debilitated, weak, cyanotic, and lethargic. In 25 per cent of cases the mothers are ill at the time of delivery. Exposure to cold, hypothermia, peripheral chilling with vascular collapse, and an increase in the ratio of saturated to unsaturated fatty acids in the triglyceride fraction of the subcutaneous tissue (due to a defect in fatty acid mobilization) have been hypothesized, but lack confirmation, as possible causes for this disorder.[7, 8]

The histopathologic findings of sclerema neonatorum consist of edema and thickening of the connective tissue bands around the fat lobules. Although necrosis and crystallization of the subcutaneous tissue have been described, these findings are more characteristically seen in lesions of subcutaneous fat necrosis.

The prognosis of sclerema neonatorum is poor, and mortality occurs in from 50 to 75 per cent of affected infants. Death, when it occurs, generally is due to inanition, debilitation, and the associated underlying pathologic disorder. In those infants who survive, the cutaneous findings resolve without residual sequelae. As yet there is no specific therapy for sclerema neonatorum.

Supportive care with heat, oxygen, control of infection, management of the underlying disorder, and intravenous therapy for correction of fluid and electrolyte imbalance are essential. Although indications for their use are unclear and controlled studies fail to confirm their efficacy, in view of the fact that these infants are critically ill and the mortality rate continues to be high, the use of systemic corticosteroids in addition to antimicrobial agents has frequently been advocated for infants with this disorder.[9, 10, 11]

Subcutaneous Fat Necrosis

Subcutaneous fat necrosis is a benign self-limiting disease that affects apparently healthy full-term newborns and young infants. It is characterized by sharply circumscribed, indurated, and nodular areas of fat necrosis (Fig. 2–2). The etiology of this disorder remains unknown but appears to be related to trauma due to pressure on bony prominences during the time of delivery, asphyxia, hypothermia, and in some instances, diabetes mellitus in the mother.[12, 13, 14]

The onset of subcutaneous fat necrosis generally occurs during the first few days and weeks of life. Lesions appear as single or multiple localized, sharply circumscribed, usually painless areas of induration. At times, however, affected areas may be extremely tender and infants may be quite uncomfortable and may cry vigorously when they are handled. Lesions of subcutaneous fat necrosis vary in size from small nodules to large plaques and often reach a size of several centimeters in diameter. Although lesions may occur in any cutaneous area, sites of predilection include the cheeks, back, buttocks, arms, and thighs. Involved tissues are non-tender, of a reddish or violaceous hue, and of a non-pitting, stony consistency. Many lesions have an uneven lobulated surface with an elevated margin separating it from the surrounding normal tissue. Lesions of subcutaneous fat necrosis tend to have a good prognosis. Although they may develop extensive deposits of calcium, which may liquefy, drain, and heal with

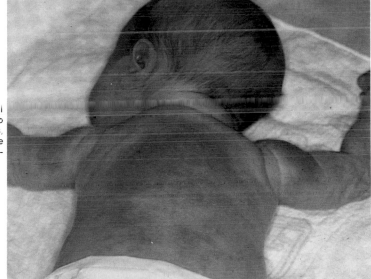

Figure 2–2. Subcutaneous fat necrosis of the newborn. Sharply circumscribed reddish to violaceous plaques or nodules on the cheeks, back, buttocks, arms, and thighs of otherwise apparently healthy newborns and young infants. (Courtesy of Richard Swint, M.D.)

scarring, most areas undergo spontaneous resolution within a period of several weeks.

Histologic examination of lesions of subcutaneous fat necrosis reveal larger than usual fat lobules and an extensive inflammatory infiltrate in the subcutaneous tissue consisting of lymphocytes, foreign body giant cells about crystals of fatty acid, and histiocytes.[12] Although many authors consider necrosis and crystallization of the subcutaneous fat to be part of the histopathology of sclerema neonatorum, needle-shaped clefts within fat cells with necrosis and crystallization of the subcutaneous fat are more characteristic of subcutaneous fat necrosis than sclerema of the newborn.

Most uncomplicated lesions of subcutaneous fat necrosis are self-limiting, resolve spontaneously within a period of two to four weeks (usually without atrophy or scarring), and require no specific therapy. Fluctuant lesions, however, should be aspirated with a small-gauge needle in an effort to prevent rupture, thus diminishing the possibility of or susceptibility to subsequent scarring. Rarely infants with associated hypercalcemia may require low calcium intake, restriction of vitamin D, and systemic corticosteroid therapy.[1]

MISCELLANEOUS CUTANEOUS DISORDERS

Miliaria

Differentiation of the epidermis and its appendages, particularly in the premature infant, is frequently incomplete at birth. As a result of this immaturity, a high incidence of sweat-retention phenomena may be seen in the newborn infant.[15] Miliaria, a common neonatal dermatosis caused by sweat retention, is characterized by a vesicular eruption with subsequent maceration and obstruction of the eccrine ducts. The pathophysiologic events that lead to this disorder are keratinous plugging of eccrine ducts and the escape of eccrine sweat into the skin below the level of obstruction (see Chapter 6).

Virtually all infants develop miliaria under appropriate conditions. In infants there are two principal forms of this disorder: miliaria crystallina (sudamina), which consists of clear superficial pinpoint vesicles without an inflammatory areola, and miliaria rubra (prickly heat), which is characterized by small discrete erythematous papules, vesicles, or papulovesicles (Fig. 2–3). The incidence of miliaria is greatest in the first few weeks of life owing to the relative immaturity of the eccrine ducts, which favors poral closure and sweat retention.

Therapy of miliaria is directed toward avoidance of excessive heat and humidity. Lightweight clothing, cool baths, and air conditioning are invaluable in the management of this disorder.

Milia

Milia commonly occur on the face of the newborn. Seen in 40 to 50 per cent of infants, they result from retention of keratin and sebaceous material within the pilosebaceous apparatus of the neonate. They appear as tiny one to two millimeter pearly white or yellow papules. Particularly prominent on the cheeks, nose, chin, and forehead, they may be few or numerous and are frequently grouped in the areas of involvement (see Figs. 6–17 and 8–34). Occasionally lesions may also be noted on the upper trunk, limbs, penis, or mucous membranes. Although milia of the newborn may persist into the second or third month, they usually disappear spontaneously during the first three or four weeks of life and, accordingly, require no therapy. Persistent milia in an unusual or widespread distribution, particularly when seen in association with other defects, may be seen as a manifestation of hereditary trichodysplasia (Marie Unna hypotrichosis) or the oral-facial-digital syndrome type I.[1]

Bohn's and Epstein's Pearls

Discrete, two to three millimeter round, pearly white or yellow, freely movable elevations at the gum margins or midline of the hard palate (termed Bohn's and Epstein's pearls, respectively) are seen in up to 85 per cent of newborn infants. Clinically and histologically the counterpart of facial milia, they disappear spontaneously, usually within a few weeks of life, and require no therapy.[1]

Sebaceous Gland Hyperplasia

Sebaceous gland hyperplasia represents a physiologic phenomenon of the newborn manifested by multiple yellow to flesh-colored tiny papules that occur on the nose, cheeks, and upper lips of full-term infants. A manifestation of maternal androgen stimulation, these represent a temporary

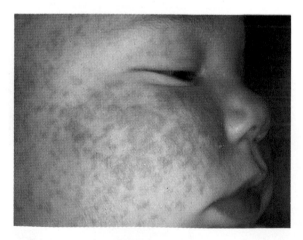

Figure 2–3 Miliaria rubra ("prickly heat"). Discrete erythematous papules, vesicles, and papulovesicles due to obstruction and rupture of epidermal sweat ducts.

disorder that resolves spontaneously, generally within the first few weeks of life.

Acne Neonatorum

Occasionally infants develop an eruption that resembles acne vulgaris as seen in adolescents (see Fig. 6–16). Although the etiology of this disorder is not clearly defined, it appears to develop as a result of hormonal stimulation of sebaceous glands that have not yet involuted to their childhood state of immaturity. In mild cases of acne neonatorum, therapy is often unnecessary; daily cleansing with soap and water may be all that is required. Occasionally mild keratolytic agents may be helpful (see Chapter 6).

Erythema Toxicum Neonatorum

Toxic erythema of the newborn (erythema toxicum neonatorum) represents a characteristic, asymptomatic, benign self-limiting cutaneous eruption of the neonatal period of unknown etiology. Composed of erythematous macules, papules, pustules, or a combination of these lesions, lesions of toxic erythema may occur anywhere on the body (except the palms and soles) and may vary in number from a few (two or three) to several hundred in number (Fig. 2–4). The fact that these lesions are not seen on the palms and soles is explained by the absence of pilosebaceous follicles in these regions.[16]

The eruption may first appear as a blotchy macular erythema that may develop into firm one to three millimeter pale yellow or white papules, pustules, or combination of these lesions on an erythematous base, the so-called "flea-bitten" rash of the newborn. The erythematous macules generally display an irregular or splotchy appearance, varying in size from a few millimeters to several centimeters in diameter. They may be seen in sharp contrast to the surrounding unaffected skin, may blend into a surrounding erythema, or may progress to present a confluent eruption.

Although erythema toxicum appears most frequently during the first three to four days of life, it has been seen at birth and may be noted as late as the tenth day of life.[16, 17, 18] Exacerbations and remissions may occur during the first two weeks of life. The duration of individual lesions varies from a few hours to sixteen days (the average duration is approximately two days).

The etiology of erythema toxicum remains obscure. Its reported incidence is variable, owing to the fleeting nature of the disorder and the disparity among reported observations on the part of clinicians. Some authors report an incidence as low as 4.5 per cent; others report incidences varying from 31 to 70 per cent of newborn infants.[19] No sexual or racial predisposition has been noted; discrepancies in racial incidence appear to be related to the difficulty of recognition of erythema on pigmented skin. The incidence does not differ significantly with respect to maternal history, condition at birth, or sex of the infant. It does, however, have a lower rate of incidence in prematures as contrasted with full-term infants, with an increase in incidence (from 0 to 59 per cent) as the gestational age increases (from 30 weeks or less to 42 weeks or more).[20]

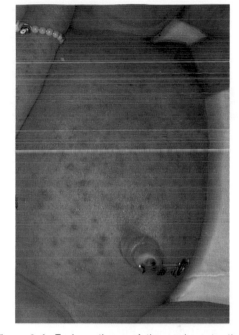

Figure 2–4 Toxic erythema of the newborn (erythema toxicum neonatorum) appears most frequently during the first three or four days of life. In this instance the disorder was present at birth.

The histopathologic picture of a papule of erythema toxicum reveals a characteristic accumulation of eosinophils about the pilosebaceous apparatus just below the dermal-epidermal junction of the skin; pustular lesions are the result of a perifollicular accumulation of these cells in a subcorneal or intradermal location.[16] Examination of the peripheral blood in affected infants has shown an eosinophilia in 7 to 15 per cent of cases. Although the eosinophilic response has led some observers to attribute the etiology of this disorder to a hypersensitivity reaction, specific allergens have never been implicated or confirmed. Studies of the acute inflammatory process in newborn infants reveal an eosinophilic response, suggesting that eosinophilia may be a normal newborn response to the stimulus of injury.[21] At present, therefore, the etiology of erythema toxicum remains obscure. Perhaps it represents a transient reaction of newborn skin to normal mechanical or thermal stimuli.[22]

Since erythema toxicum is a benign self-limiting asymptomatic disorder, no therapy is indicated. Occasionally, however, it may be confused with other eruptions of the neonatal period, namely transient neonatal pustular melanosis, milia of the newborn, miliaria, herpes simplex, or impetigo neonatorum. Of these herpes simplex neonatorum and impetigo are the most important because of the possibility of contagion or systemic involvement.

Toxic erythema can be rapidly differentiated by cytological examination of the contents of a pustule. A smear of intralesional contents of erythema toxicum prepared by Wright or Giemsa stain may reveal clusters of eosinophils and a relative absence of neutrophils. The presence of a predominance of neutrophils is suggestive of a bacterial infection; absence of bacteria on Gram stain and negative bacterial culture tend to rule out impetigo of the newborn.

Impetigo Neonatorum

Impetigo in newborns may occur as early as the second or third day, or as late as the second week of life. It usually presents as a superficial vesicular, pustular, or bullous lesion on an erythematous base. Vesicles and bullae are easily denuded, leaving a round, red, raw moist surface, usually without crust formation. Blisters are often wrinkled, contain some fluid, and are easily denuded without formation of crusts. Lesions tend to occur on moist or opposing surfaces of the skin, as in the diaper area, groin, axillae, and folds of the neck.

The term *"pemphigus neonatorum"* is an archaic misnomer occasionally applied to superficial bullous lesions of severe impetigo widely distributed over the surface of the body. The status of "pemphigus" neonatorum as a distinct nosologic entity is dubious. Fortunately, with improved neonatal care and appropriate antibiotic therapy, this severe form of neonatal pyoderma is rarely seen today.

Transient Neonatal Pustular Melanosis

Transient neonatal pustular melanosis is a recently recognized vesiculopustular and pigmented disorder of newborns first described in 1976. Seen in 4.4 per cent of black and 0.2 per cent of white newborns, it is characterized by superficial vesiculopustular lesions that rupture easily and evolve into evanescent pinhead-sized hyperpigmented macules.[23]

Lesions of transient neonatal pustular melanosis are usually present at birth. They generally begin as superficial vesiculopustular lesions that rupture easily during the first bathing and often leave a collarette of fine white scales around a pinhead-sized brown hyperpigmented macule that generally fades within a period of several weeks to months (Fig. 2–5). The lesions are most often seen in clusters under the chin, on the forehead, nape of the neck, lower back, and shins. Occasionally, lesions may also appear on the cheeks, trunk, and extremities. Rarely, blisters, which do not progress to pigmented macules, may be detected on the scalp, palms, and soles.

Lesions of transient neonatal pustular melanosis are sterile. Smears of vesicle fluid stained with Wright stain, in contrast to lesions of erythe-

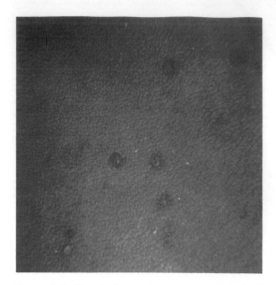

Figure 2–5 Transient neonatal pustular melanosis. Papulovesicles present at birth leave hyperpigmented macules surrounded by a collarette of fine scales. (Courtesy of Nancy B. Esterly, M.D.)

ma toxicum neonatorum, demonstrate variable numbers of neutrophils, few or no eosinophils, and cellular debris. Histopathologic examination of cutaneous biopsies of vesiculopustular lesions are characterized by hyperkeratosis of the stratum corneum and intracorneal and subcorneal separation with polymorphonuclear infiltration. Histopathologic examination of pigmented macular lesions reveals basket-weave hyperkeratosis and areas of focal basilar hyperpigmentation.

Transient neonatal pustular melanosis is a benign disorder, appears to have no associated systemic manifestations, and requires no treatment. Lesions are distinguishable from those of erythema toxicum and must be differentiated from pustulovesicles of staphylococcal or herpetic origin. Vesiculopustular lesions of transient neonatal pustular melanosis disappear in 24 to 48 hours, often leaving hyperpigmented pinhead-sized macules, which in turn generally regress within a period of three weeks to three months.

Seborrheic Dermatitis

Seborrheic dermatitis is a term that has been used to describe a self-limiting condition of the scalp, face, ears, trunk, and intertriginous areas characterized by greasy scaling associated with patchy redness, fissuring, and occasional weeping.

The cause of seborrheic dermatitis is not well understood. It appears to be an inflammatory disorder related to a dysfunction of the sebaceous glands and has a predilection for areas where the density of sebaceous glands is high.[15] Ostensibly under hormonal influence, this disorder first appears during the first few months of infancy when transplacental hormone levels are elevated. It frequently improves between 8 and 12 months of age

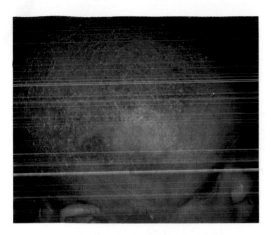

Figure 2–6 Seborrheic dermatitis of the scalp ("cradle cap").

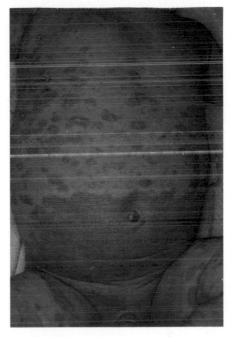

Figure 2–8 Greasy salmon-colored well-marginated scaly eruption of seborrheic dermatitis.

as these levels decline is less common during childhood, and reappears with elevation of hormone levels during adolescence. Whether seborrheic dermatitis of adolescence and adulthood is related to that of infancy remains unknown.

In newborns and infants seborrheic dermatitis often begins during the first 12 weeks of age, with a scaly dermatitis of the scalp termed "cradle cap" (Fig. 2–6). This disorder may spread over the face, including the forehead, ears, eyebrows, nose, and back of the head, and often clears spontaneously by 8 to 12 months of age (Fig. 2–7). Erythematous greasy salmon-colored, and sharply marginated oval scaly lesions may involve other parts of the

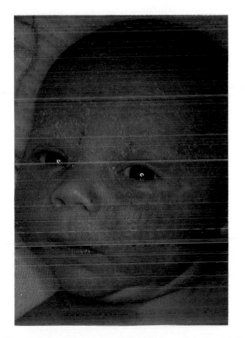

Figure 2–7 Seborrheic dermatitis on the face. Infantile seborrheic dermatitis may be differentiated from atopic dermatitis by its very early onset, a lack of pruritus and personal or family history of atopy, and the absence of vesiculation and lichenification.

body, particularly the intertriginous and flexural areas, the postauricular regions, the trunk, umbilicus, anogenital areas, and groin (Fig. 2–8). Infants with these lesions usually lack stigmata of atopy (itching, dry skin, follicular keratosis) and personal or family history of atopic disease.

The histologic picture of seborrheic dermatitis is not specific and has features of both psoriasis and chronic dermatitis. Parakeratosis is well marked, and the epidermis shows slight to moderate acanthosis with some elongation of the rete ridges, slight intracellular edema, and spongiosis. The dermis reveals a mild non-specific chronic inflammatory infiltrate. Spongiosis, although seen in seborrheic dermatitis, is not present in psoriasis and is a helpful differentiating feature between these two disorders.

The prognosis of infantile seborrheic dermatitis is good. Some patients clear within three to four weeks, even without treatment, and most cases clear spontaneously by eight to twelve months of age. The diagnostic features include its early onset, the characteristic greasy nature of the eruption with its predilection for the scalp and intertriginous areas, and a general lack of associated pruritus. Occasionally seborrheic dermatitis may be followed by typical atopic dermatitis. Whether this represents a chance occurrence or perhaps a specific constitutional predisposition is still controversial.

Infantile seborrheic dermatitis may be differentiated from atopic dermatitis by its early onset, a lack of pruritus and personal or family history of atopy, and the absence of vesiculation and lichenification. Although seborrheic dermatitis can at times be mistaken for Letterer-Siwe disease, the presence of discrete one to three millimeter yellowish to reddish-brown infiltrated papules at the periphery of the eruption, purpuric lesions, hepatosplenomegaly, adenopathy, fever, anemia, thrombocytopenia, and skeletal tumors can help differentiate the latter disorder. When the diagnosis remains in doubt, a cutaneous punch biopsy may help differentiate the two conditions.

TREATMENT. Treatment of seborrheic dermatitis of the scalp is best managed by frequent shampooing, preferably with one of the commercially available antiseborrheic shampoos (those containing sulfur and salicylic acid are generally satisfactory). If the scales are thick and adherent, removal can be facilitated by the use of slightly warmed mineral oil or petrolatum. In stubborn or persistent cases, wrapping the scalp in a warm damp towel before shampooing may assist removal of thick scales and crusts, or the use of "P&S" liquid, a specially prepared mixture of liquid paraffin oil, sodium chloride, and phenol, or "P&S" ointment, a mixture of sodium chloride and phenol in petrolatum (Chester A. Baker Laboratories), may be helpful.

When the scalp is shampooed, mothers should be instructed that gentle scrubbing of the scalp is safe and often necessary in order to facilitate removal of the thick adherent scales. Antiseborrheic agents should be left on for an appropriate period of time (long enough to soften and loosen the scales properly). Failure to allow the agent to stay on for the recommended period and inadequate scrubbing of the scales are common causes for failure of otherwise adequate antiseborrheic therapy. For stubborn or persistent lesions, a topical corticosteroid lotion, alone or in combination with three to five per cent sulfur precipitate or salicyclic acid or both, is frequently effective. This preparation may be used three times a day initially and its frequency reduced or discontinued as the eruption improves.

Leiner's Disease

Leiner's disease is a rare disorder of infancy characterized by generalized seborrheic dermati-

tis; intractable, severe diarrhea; marked wasting and dystrophy; and recurrent local and systemic infections, usually of gram-negative etiology. Many authors now consider this disorder, which was described primarily during the preantibiotic era, to be an extensive form of seborrheic dermatitis of unknown etiology. This disorder may occur during the first week of life, but generally begins suddenly in infants between two and four months of age. Girls are affected more frequently than boys, and the proportion of breast-fed babies affected is said to be high.[15]

The dermatosis is described as one of universal erythema and loosening of the epidermis with scale and crust formation (Fig. 2–9). Generally considered to be a severe exfoliative variant of seborrheic dermatitis, it commonly begins as a progressive increase in severity of seborrheic dermatitis of the scalp or flexures, or by the sudden development of intense erythema of the entire skin surface with profuse desquamation of fine, branny scales on the face; heavy crusting of the scalp and eyebrows; and a thick, profound exfoliation of the trunk and extremities. The scalp is often covered with thick, greasy, yellow crusts, as seen in severe seborrheic dermatitis, and a patchy or total alopecia may be noted. A protracted severe diarrhea resistant to usual therapeutic measures is frequently seen. Although the course may be relatively benign in some infants, dehydration, fever, inanition, and death are not infrequent sequelae in patients with severe resistant forms of this disorder.

The small number of recently reported cases of Leiner's disease makes assessment of mortality difficult. It now appears that most cases of Leiner's disease that progressed to diarrhea and death occurred in the preantibiotic era, and today there appear to be few reports of death in infants with this disorder.

Familial Leiner's Disease with C_5 Dysfunction

Recent descriptions of familial cases of infants with severe forms of Leiner's disease, associated with generalized exfoliative dermatitis within a

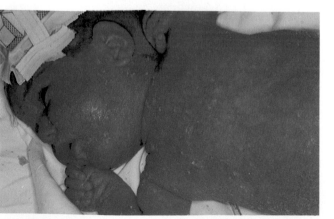

Figure 2–9 Leiner's disease. Generalized exfoliative seborrheic dermatitis with erythema, desquamation, and crusting.

week or two of birth, severe diarrhea, recurrent gram-negative infections, wasting and death (similar to those originally described by Leiner) report finding a defect in function of the fifth component of complement (C_5). This dysfunction of C_5 resulted in decreased phagocytosis (opsonic activity) of the patient's serum and resulted in failure to thrive and recurrent sepsis with an ominous prognosis. Whether or not infants with C_5 dysfunction syndrome represent true cases of Leiner's disease remains controversial.[24]

In patients found to have C_5 dysfunction, vigorous antibiotic therapy combined with infusions of fresh plasma or whole blood may be life saving. It should be noted, however, that a diagnosis of severe seborrheic dermatitis does not warrant a diagnosis of Leiner's disease and that therapy with fresh frozen plasma should be restricted to only those children with severe dermatitis, systemic manifestations, and laboratory evidence of C_5 dysfunction.[25, 26]

DEVELOPMENTAL ABNORMALITIES OF THE NEONATE

Congenital Hemihypertrophy

Hemihypertrophy is a developmental defect in which one side of the body is larger than the other. Although differences in symmetry are often detectable during the newborn period, they usually become more striking with growth of the child. The cutaneous findings most often associated with hemihypertrophy are pigmentation, telangiectasia, abnormal nail growth, and hypertrichosis (Fig. 2–10). Body temperature and sweating differences

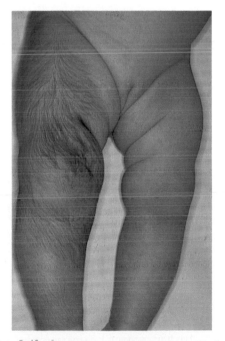

Figure 2-10 Congenital hemihypertrophy with hypertrichosis (Hurwitz S, Klaus S: Arch. Dermatol. 103:98–100, 1971).

have also been reported in patients with this disorder.[27]

Of particular significance is the fact that about 50 per cent of persons with hemihypertrophy have associated anomalies. Significant malformations include Wilms' tumor, aniridia, cataracts, ear deformities, internal hemangiomas, genitourinary tract anomalies, adrenocortical neoplasms, and brain tumors. Patients who exhibit congenital hemihypertrophy, therefore, should be evaluated for the tumors and congenital malformations often associated with this disorder. During infancy and early childhood, these patients should be examined at regular intervals for possible development of liver, adrenocortical, or renal neoplasms.

Aplasia Cutis Congenita

Aplasia cutis congenita is a congenital defect of the integument characterized by localized absence of the epidermis, dermis, and, at times, subcutaneous tissues. The defect is present at birth, and although it generally occurs on the scalp, may also involve the skin of the face, trunk, and extremities.[28, 29]

The disorder usually presents as solitary or multiple sharply demarcated weeping or granulating oval, circular, elongated, stellate, or triangular defects ranging in size from one to three centimeters in diameter. In 70 per cent of cases the ulceration is singular, in 20 per cent it is double, and in 8 per cent of patients three or more cutaneous defects may be noted.[28] In 60 per cent of patients aplasia cutis congenita occurs on the scalp, usually near the sagittal suture of the vertex or over adjacent parietal regions. In more than 50 per cent of reported cases the defect is located in the midline of the scalp, and in 30 per cent of patients it is seen in an area adjacent to this position.[15] Although aplasia cutis congenita may also affect the occiput, the postauricular areas, and the face, involvement of these areas appears to be relatively rare.

At birth the cutaneous defect may vary from a denuded ulceration with a red weeping or granulating base to an area of erosion covered with a thin friable membrane. Histologic examination reveals an absence of epidermis, absence or paucity of appendageal structures, a variable decrease in dermal elastic tissue, and, in deeper lesions, a complete deficit of all layers of the skin and subcutaneous tissues. As healing takes place the defect is replaced by smooth, gray, hairless parchment-like scar tissue (Fig. 2–11). After the lesions heal, the total absence of epidermal appendages in the area of the defect and the presence of rudimentary or malformed appendages in histologic examination of the surrounding edge is highly characteristic.

Other developmental abnormalities reported in association with aplasia cutis include cleft lip and palate, syndactyly, hydrocephalus, defects of the underlying skull, malformations of the brain, transverse defects at variable levels of the limbs

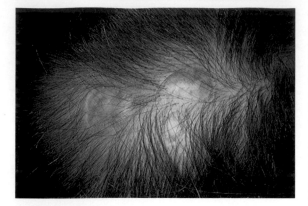

Figure 2–11   Parchment-like scars of the scalp (aplasia cutis congenita).

manifested as hemimelia and aphalangia, colobomas, meningomyelocele, anencephaly, microphthalmus, congenital heart disease, tracheoesophageal fistula, and vascular anomalies.[29, 30]

The etiology of aplasia cutis congenita remains unknown. Although most instances of this disorder are sporadic, familial cases are suggestive of autosomal dominant inheritance with reduced penetrance.[31, 32] Incomplete closure of the neural tube or an embryologic arrest of skin development has been suggested as an explanation of midline lesions.[33] This hypothesis, however, fails to account for lesions of the trunk and limbs. In such instances, vascular abnormality of the placenta, with a degenerative rather than aplastic or traumatic origin has been postulated as the cause of cutaneous defects.[34]

Recognition of aplasia cutis congenita and differentiation of it from forceps or other birth injury will help prevent possible medicolegal complications occasionally seen with this disorder. Except for residual scarring and defects that overlie the sagittal suture where fatal hemorrhage from the sagittal sinus has been reported, the prognosis of aplasia cutis generally is good. With conservative therapy designed to prevent further trauma and secondary infection, most small defects of the scalp heal well during the first few weeks to months of life. Defects of lytic lesions of the skull generally heal spontaneously by five to seven months.[32] As the child matures, most scars become relatively inconspicuous and require no correction. Those that are large and obvious, however, generally respond to multiple punch graft transplants or surgical excision followed by plastic repair.

Bitemporal Aplasia Cutis Congenita with Other Cutaneous Abnormalities

In 1963 Setleis and others described five children of three families, all of Puerto Rican ancestry, who presented unique characteristic clinical defects confined to the face. Termed "congenital ectodermal dysplasia of the face," features

of the affected children were an aged leonine appearance; absent eyelashes from either eyelid or multiple rows of lashes on the upper lids with absence of those of the lower lids; eyebrows that slanted sharply upward and laterally; scar-like defects on each temple; puckered skin about the eyes; a scar-like median ridge of the chin; and a nose and chin that seemed rubbery when palpated.[35]

Rudolph et al. subsequently described an 8-year-old Puerto Rican girl with a peculiar "old lady" facies with a prominent jaw; mild frontal bossing; flattened bridge of the nose; narrowed palpebral fissure; stenotic nares with shiny atrophic skin at the margins; low-set small and abnormally shaped ears; missing lateral eyebrows; flesh-colored hyperkeratotic papules on the arms, thighs, and back; bilaterally symmetrical, slightly hyperpigmented, depressed oval areas on the temples covered with smooth shiny skin with an apparent lack of underlying subcutaneous tissue; and small irregularities of the underlying skull.[30]

Although this entity was described as an example of "bitemporal aplasia cutis congenita with other cutaneous abnormalities," it appears that the patient had a defect similar to that described fourteen years earlier by Setleis and associates as "congenital ectodermal dysplasia of the face". It appears that all six patients demonstrate a similar clinical syndrome.[30, 36]

Congenital Sinus Defects

A congenital dermal sinus is a developmental epithelium-lined tract that extends inward from the surface of the skin. Since midline fusion of ectodermal and neuroectodermal tissue occurs at the cephalic and caudal ends of the neural tube, the majority of such defects are seen in the suboccipital and lumbosacral regions.

Dermal sinus openings may be difficult to visualize, particularly in the occipital region where they may be hidden by hair.[15] A localized thickening of the scalp, hypertrichosis, dimpling, or vascular nevi in the midline of the neck or back should alert the physician to the possibility of such an anomaly. These sinuses are of clinical importance as portals for infections that may give rise to abscesses, osteomyelitis, or meningitis. X-rays of suspicious areas should be performed to rule out the possibility of associated spina bifida or other bony abnormality.

Most authorities agree that dermal sinuses occurring above the lumbosacral area should be excised during the newborn period; controversy, however, exists as to the management of congenital defects in the lumbosacral and coccygeal regions. Available evidence at this time suggests that asymptomatic infants with lumbosacral, sacral, or coccygeal sinuses can be followed for a four to six-month period providing the parents have been instructed to contact a physician immediately if there is any evidence of inflammation, discharge of fluid, poor bladder or bowel control, or abnormality of the lower extremities. Sinography and probing are contraindicated because of the possibility of introducing infection. If infection develops, surgery should be undertaken as soon as the infection is brought under control. If abnormal neurologic signs develop or if after a four to six-month period the bottom of a presumed sinus is not clearly visible, surgical exploration is advisable.[37]

Congenital Fistulas of the Lower Lip

Congenital fistulas of the lower lip (congenital lip pits) may be unilateral or bilateral and may be seen alone or in association with other anomalies of the face and extremities.[15, 31] They are characterized by single or paired circular or slit-like depressions on either side of the midline of the lower lip at the edge of the vermilion border. Also known as labial fistulae or congenital pits of the lips, these depressions represent blind sinuses that extend inwards through the orbicularis oris muscle to a depth of 0.5 to 2.5 cm. At times lip pits may also be seen to communicate with underlying salivary glands.

Congenital lip pits may be inherited as an autosomal dominant disorder with penetrance estimated at 80 per cent. They may be seen alone, or, in 70 per cent of patients, in association with cleft lip or cleft palate. Other associated anomalies include clubfoot, talipes equinovarus, syndactyly, and the popliteal pterygium syndrome (an autosomal dominant disorder with cleft lip with or without cleft palate, filiform adhesions between the eyelids, pterygium of the leg, limiting its mobility, and anomalies of the genitourinary system, and congenital heart disease.).[38, 39]

Other than recognition of possible associated defects, most patients with congenital lip pits require no specific therapy. When communication with underlying mucous glands results in secretion of mucus onto the lip surface, surgical excision of the sinus tract and its glandular tissue, or transposition of the sinus tract onto a buccal surface, may be indicated.[15]

CONGENITAL INFECTIONS OF THE FETUS

Viral, bacterial, and parasitic infections during pregnancy are frequently associated with widespread systemic involvement, serious permanent sequelae, and, at times, a variety of cutaneous manifestations. Of these, congenital rubella infection, herpes neonatorum, congenital syphilis, cytomegalic inclusion disease, and congenital toxoplasmosis are perhaps the most significant.

Congenital Rubella Infection

Ever since the work of Gregg in 1941, physicians have been aware of the teratogenic effects of rubella contracted during pregnancy. Congenital rubella occurs following maternal rubella infection during the first 20 weeks of pregnancy. At least 15 to 20 per cent of offspring of women who contract this disorder during the first trimester of pregnancy are afflicted with one or more serious congenital malformations. If infants are followed for a period of years, however, an additional 15 per cent may be added to this figure.

At present, an estimated 14 to 16 per cent of women between 14 and 40 years of age are seronegative for rubella antibody and accordingly remain susceptible to risk of infection during the child-bearing period. The earlier in pregnancy that maternal rubella occurs, the greater the risk to the fetus. Thus, 50 per cent or more of children born to women who contract rubella during the first four weeks of pregnancy may have gross congenital anomalies; by the third or fourth month of gestation this incidence falls to 2 to 6 per cent; and by 18 to 20 months the risk is practically nil.[40]

CLINICAL MANIFESTATIONS. The clinical manifestations of congenital rubella are varied. Investigations of the consequences of the 1963–1965 rubella epidemic have shown that infants of mothers with rubella infection during early pregnancy may develop systemic involvement in addition to the classic triad of congenital cataracts, deafness, and congenital malformations of the heart. Infected infants are usually born at term, but with low birth weight. They may show only a few manifestations at birth or may be asymptomatic, with consequences of fetal rubella only apparent in subsequent months, or may have a wide systemic involvement characterized by growth retardation, thrombocytopenic purpura, hyperbilirubinemia, hepatosplenomegaly, pneumonia, cardiac defects, eye disorders, deafness, osseous defects, and meningoencephalitis.

Purpura. The most prominent cutaneous feature of congenital rubella is purpura. In a study of 200 infants with congenital rubella infection, thrombocytopenic purpura was detected in 70 (35 per cent). Of these, 86 per cent demonstrated platelet levels of 90,000/mm³ or less. Of interest is the fact that the duration of thrombocytopenia was not affected by corticosteroid therapy and platelet levels generally (but not always) returned to normal within a period of one to four months.[38]

"Blueberry Muffin" Lesions. Another prominent cutaneous feature of congenital rubella infection may be seen as bluish red infiltrated macules measuring two to eight millimeters in diameter, the so-called "blueberry muffin" lesions (Fig. 2–12). Blueberry muffin lesions are usually noted at birth or within the first 24 hours. New lesions rarely appear after two days of age. Lesions may be few or numerous and generally appear on the head, neck, trunk, or extremities. Many of the larger lesions tend to be raised (approximately one to two millimeters above the surrounding skin surface). They generally are circular in configuration and vary from a dark blue to a purplish-red (magenta) color. Smaller infiltrated macules are flat, oval, or circular

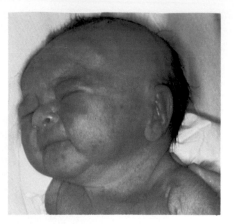

Figure 2–12 Congenital rubella syndrome with petechiae and blueberry muffin lesions. (Courtesy of Louis Gluck, M.D.)

in configuration and less violaceous, varying in color from dark red to pale grayish-purple or copper brown. Blueberry muffin lesions usually disappear within a period of three to six weeks (the larger lesions regressing more slowly than the smaller flat macules in this disorder).[39]

Histologic studies of blueberry muffin lesions reveal discrete dermal aggregates of relatively large nucleated cells and non-nucleated erythrocytes. A result of dermal erythropoiesis (rather than true hemorrhage), these infiltrated lesions, characteristic of viral infection of the fetus, are not unique to infants with congenital rubella, but may also be seen in patients with congenital toxoplasmosis and cytomegalic virus inclusion disease.[41]

Other cutaneous manifestations of congenital rubella infection include hyperpigmentation of the naval, forehead, cheeks, and sites of previous trauma; seborrhea of the cheeks, forehead, and body; eczema; and recurrent urticaria. Vasomotor instability, manifested by poor peripheral circulation, with generalized mottling of the face and acral areas, cyanosis of dependent extremities, and vivid flushing of the ears, cheeks, fingertips, and toes upon elevation of the affected infant's surrounding environmental temperature, may also be seen in association with this disorder.[42]

DIAGNOSIS. Congenital rubella syndrome should be suspected in infants with intrauterine growth retardation, congenital manifestations such as glaucoma, cataracts, deafness, thrombocytopenic purpura, blueberry muffin lesions, hepatosplenomegaly, cardiac defects, pneumonia, meningoencephalitis, or osseous defects. Bony abnormalities are seen in up to 80 per cent of affected infants at or near birth and include a large anterior fontanel and characteristic small longitudinal areas of translucency in the metaphyses of long bones (especially the distal femur and proximal tibia) during the first two or three months of life.[43] It must be noted, however, that these bony abnormalities resemble those of other fetal viral infections, such as cytomegalic inclusion disease, and are not pathognomonic of the disorder.

The diagnosis of congenital rubella may be confirmed by isolation of rubella virus from the nose, pharyngeal secretions, cerebrospinal fluid, or other secretions of tissues obtained at biopsy; by identification of specific rubella neutralizing antibody in the IgM fraction of the neonate; or by the presence of hemagglutinating antibody (HI) in the sera of suspected infants beyond the age of five or six months.[44, 45, 46]

MANAGEMENT. Infants with neonatal rubella thrive poorly, and approximately 20 to 30 per cent die within the first year of life. There is no specific treatment for the rubella-infected child apart from supportive therapy and recognition of potential disabilites. Because of the high incidence of ophthalmic complications, careful evaluation of the eyes is important and ophthalmologic consultation should be obtained for all affected infants. Although purpura and petechiae secondary to thrombocytopenia may be severe, true hemorrhagic difficulties do not appear to present a major problem, and corticosteroid therapy does not appear to be indicated for infants with this complication.[44]

It must be remembered that over 80 per cent of infants with congenital rubella shed virus during the first month of life, some continue to shed virus for periods of six to nine months, and in severely affected infants (5 to 10 per cent) the virus may be detected for periods as long as 12 months. After two years the risk of viral shedding is extremely small.[47] Affected infants should be isolated and handled only by personnel not considered at risk (those known to be seropositive for rubella with HI antibody titers of 1 to 8 or greater). Following discharge from the hospital no special precautions are necessary other than prevention of potential risk to pregnant visitors.[48]

With currently available live attenuated rubella vaccine and present recommendations for vaccination of all children between one year old and puberty, congenital rubella should be a preventable disease. It should be noted, however, that vaccination should not be administered to infants less than 15 months of age, since the possible persistence of maternal antibody might interfere with an adequate immunologic response. In view of the fact that infection with attenuated virus presents a potential risk to the fetus, rubella vaccine should not be administered to pregnant women or to those who might become pregnant within a period of two months.[42]

Susceptible women who are exposed to rubella during the first trimester of pregnancy pose a difficult problem of management. Ideally, all pregnant women should have blood drawn for rubella serology at their first obstetric visit. Serum antibody to rubella of 1 to 16 or greater is indicative of immunity. If no rubella titer is detectable, or if the antibody titer is one to eight or less, any women thought to be exposed to rubella should have a second serum specimen examination two or three weeks after the suspected or possible infection. For those without available serum antibody information, an immediate rubella antibody (HI) titer should be determined and repeated two or three weeks later. If a rise in titer occurs, or if the presence of rubella IgM is noted, it is highly likely that congenital infection has occurred and the woman should be counseled.

Because of the high risk of fetal damage, women known to have contracted maternal rubella during the early months of pregnancy may consider the option of therapeutic abortion. This decision, however, must be based upon the age of the mother, the expectancy of other children, the gestational time of infection, and the patient's personal feeling regarding therapeutic abortion.

The use of immune serum globulin for the prevention of rubella in pregnant women exposed to rubella remains controversial. Since available evidence indicates that immune globulin may suppress clinical infection without preventing viremia, it is difficult to justify its routine use as prophylaxis for women exposed during the first trimester of pregnancy. Some studies, however, suggest that immune globulin might lessen the likelihood of infection and fetal damage. The use of immune globulin, accordingly, may be justified for exposed susceptible women who, for reasons of religion or otherwise, prefer not to undergo therapeutic abortion.[48]

Congenital Varicella-Zoster Virus Infection

Although congenital varicella or zoster infection may be life-threatening to the fetus, relatively few cases have been reported to date (as of 1977 only 40 such cases had been reported in the literature).[49] Effects on the fetus induced by varicella-zoster represent a spectrum ranging from moderate or no residual problems to very severe, crippling, or life-threatening complications.[50]

Most infants born to mothers with varicella infection early in pregnancy appear to be normal. Current evidence, however, reveals that congenital varicella infection may be extremely severe and, at times, life-threatening.[51, 52] Since 5 to 16 per cent of women of child-bearing age are susceptible to chickenpox, the fact that so few cases have been recognized to date may be related to the fact that not all women who develop varicella while pregnant are infected early in pregnacy, that some infants infected in fetal life may have infection without sequelae, and that the varicella-zoster virus does not cross the placenta as readily as other viruses.[50]

Although congenital varicella syndrome, when it occurs, is usually seen in infants whose mothers had varicella or disseminated zoster infection early in pregnancy (during the first trimester or early in the second),[50, 51] skin ulcers have recently been described in an infant whose mother had varicella as late as the third trimester of pregnancy.[52] Manifestations of this disorder include low birth weight for gestational age, eye defects, (microphthalmia, cataracts, and chorioretinitis), encephalomyelitis (often with severe brain

damage), hypoplastic limbs with flexion-contractures, cutaneous cicatricial scars, micrognathia, pneumonitis, and increased susceptibility to infection.[49-51, 53]

The diagnosis of congenital varicella syndrome is confirmed by a rise in varicella-zoster antibody titers measured by complement fixation, fluorescent antibody to membrane antigen (FAMA), immune adherence hemagglutination (IAHA), or passive hemagglutination (PHA). Most state laboratories will perform one or more of these tests, or they may be obtained through the Center for Disease Control in Atlanta, Georgia.

Herpes Neonatorum

Disseminated herpes virus hominis simplex infection in the newborn infant is generally thought to be associated with a grave prognosis in terms of mortality and severe neurologic sequelae among survivors. Current evidence, however, reveals that herpes simplex infection in young infants may result in a broad spectrum of illness, ranging from death or recovery with severe central nervous system or ocular damage to mild or asymptomatic infection with apparent complete recovery.[54]

It is agreed that most neonatal herpes infections are due to type 2 (genital) herpes virus hominis, acquired either by ascending infection from the mother's genital area to the intrauterine infant after premature rupture of membranes, or by spread to the infant during delivery through the birth canal of an infected mother. Recent reports, however, suggest that infection of the newborn may also be acquired by intrauterine infection due to maternal viremia with transplacental spread or by postnatal hospital or household contact with other infants or persons with oral herpes infection.[55, 56]

Neonatal herpetic infection may be categorized as disseminated, local, or asymptomatic.[57] The relative frequency of the various forms of neonatal infection is still unknown. Similarly, the prognosis for each form is not completely elucidated. The disseminated form of neonatal herpes affects the visceral organs, chiefly the liver and adrenal glands; it may also involve the central nervous system and other organs and appears to be associated with the highest mortality. More than half the newborns with herpes simplex neonatorum have skin manifestations, and about one half of infected infants, if untreated, will die or suffer serious neurologic or ocular sequelae.[57]

Intrauterine herpes simplex infection may be termed early or late, depending upon the time of infection.[55] Early intrauterine infection with resulting disturbance of embryogenesis occurs during the first eight weeks of gestation. Although evidence of early infection is limited, it may result in abortion or severe congenital malformation (intrauterine growth retardation, diffuse brain damage, intracranial calcification, microcephaly, microphthalmia, chorioretinitis, retinal dysplasia,

poor prognosis. The most common clinical manifestations are anemia, fever, wasting, hepatosplenomegaly, lymphadenopathy, rhinitis (usually known as "snuffles"), mucocutaneous eruptions, and pseudoparalysis.

Rhinitis or "Snuffles." Rhinitis (snuffles) is generally the first sign of congenital syphilis and is rarely absent in the infant with clinically manifest disease. It usually appears between the second and sixth weeks of life and is the result of an ulcerous lesion of the nasal mucosa. It begins with swelling and obstruction of the nasal mucosa with a profuse mucopurulent nasal discharge. With ulceration of the nasal mucous membranes and erosion of small blood vessels this discharge often becomes serosanguineous. When ulceration is deep enough to involve the cartilage of the nasal bone, the normal architecture is destroyed, thus giving rise to the classic saddle nose deformity characteristically seen in this disorder.

Cutaneous Manifestations. Cutaneous lesions of congenital syphilis may be seen in one third to one half of infants affected by this disorder. They may be quite varied in character but must commonly appear as large round or oval maculopapular or papulosquamous lesions (Fig. 2–16) comparable to those seen in secondary syphilis of the adolescent or adult.[1, 67, 68] The eruption may appear on any part of the body, but usually is most pronounced on the face, dorsal surface of the trunk and legs, the diaper area, and, at times, the palms and soles. The eruption generally develops slowly, is bright pink or red in color, and gradually fades to a coppery-brown color. It disappears spontaneously over a period of one to three months, often leaving a residual area of hyper- or hypopigmentation. Vesicobullous hemorrhagic lesions are relatively rare but, especially when seen on the palms and soles, are highly diagnostic of this disorder.[1] The palms and soles may be fissured, erythematous, and, as a result of subcutaneous edema, indurated with a dull red, shiny, almost polished appearance. Concomitant with these changes, desquamation of the skin in large

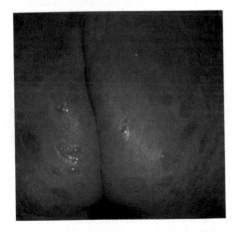

Figure 2–16 Eroded papular lesions of congenital syphilis. (Courtesy of Dr. Gabriela Lowy, Rio de Janeiro, Brazil)

dry flakes may occur over the entire body. Even when not present elsewhere, this desquamation may still be detected around the nails of the fingers and toes of affected infants.[1, 68]

Mucous membrane patches, seen in approximately one-third of infants, are among the most characteristic and most infectious of the early lesions seen in congenital syphilis. Although they may occur on any mucous surface, they generally appear in the mouth and on the lips. They are round, small, flat, slightly raised, pale and moist, and, when numerous, may fuse to cover large areas of the mucous membranes. At mucocutaneous junctions they tend to weep and may cause fissures, which often extend out from the lips in a radiating fashion over the surrounding skin. When deep these may leave residual scars (rhagades) in the adjacent circumoral region.

Raised, flat moist wart-like lesions (condylomata lata) commonly appear in any of the moist areas of the body surface of infants with congenital syphilis. Also extremely infectious, they are most commonly seen in the anogenital regions, about the nares, and at the angles of the mouth.

Visceral Involvement. Hepatomegaly may be seen in 50 to 75 per cent of affected infants. It is frequently associated with icterus and, at times, ascites, splenomegaly, and generalized enlargement of the lymph nodes. Palpable epitrochlear nodes, although not pathognomonic, are highly suggestive of congenital syphilis. The jaundice, together with the anemia, edema, and cutaneous changes seen after the eruption has faded, produces a peculiar dirty, whitish-brown (café au lait) appearance to the skin. Damage to the hematopoietic system with hemolytic anemia, and at times thrombocytopenia, is an almost constant feature of early congenital syphilis. When seen with hepatosplenomegaly, jaundice, and large numbers of nucleated erythrocytes in the peripheral circulation, an erroneous diagnosis of erythroblastosis fetalis may be made.

Osseous Manifestations. Although only 15 per cent of infants with congenital syphilis show clinical signs of osteochondritis, 90 per cent of infants will show radiologic evidence of osteochondritis and periostitis after the first month of life. Syphilitic osteochondritis may occur in any bone but is found most frequently in the long bones of the extremities. X-ray findings consist of increased widening of the epiphyseal line with increased density of the shafts, spotty areas of translucency, and a resultant moth-eaten appearance. In most cases the bony lesions are asymptomatic. In some infants, however, severe involvement may lead to subepiphyseal fracture with epiphyseal dislocation and extremely painful pseudoparalysis of one or more extremity (the so-called pseudoparalysis of Parrot).

Dactylitis is a rare form of osteochondritis of the small bones of the hands and feet that usually appears between six months and two years of age. Commonly found in the metatarsals, metacarpals, and proximal phalanges of the hands, its presence can frequently be detected by a cylindrical swelling of the affected bone with reddening of the overlying skin and relatively little pain or discomfort of the involved area.[68]

Periosteal lesions, unlike those of osteochondritis, are seldom present at birth. Periostitis of the frontal bones of the skull, when severe, is at least partially responsible for the flat overhanging forehead that persists as a stigma of children severely infected in infancy. The radiologic changes of periostitis are usually most pronounced during the second to sixth months of life and rarely persist beyond the age of two years. Lesions are usually diffuse (in contrast to the localized involvement characteristic of lesions of osteochondritis) and frequently extend the entire length of the involved bone. First seen as a thin, even line of calcification outside the cortex of the involved bone, the lesions progress and additional layers of opaque tissue are laid down, with the resulting "onion-peel" appearance of advanced periostitis. This eventually produces calcification and thickening of the cortex and, when severe, a permanent deformity. In the tibia, this results in an anterior bowing referred to as sabre-shins. In the skull it is seen (in 30 to 60 per cent of patients) as frontal or parietal bossing. Although anterior tibial bowing was formerly a frequent occurrence in congenital syphilis, it probably represented vitamin D deficiency in combination with syphilitic osteoperiostitis. Since vitamin D deficiency is currently a clinical rarity, periosteal bossing and sabre-shins are relatively uncommon clinical features of congenital syphilis today.

Central Nervous System Involvement. Even though clinical evidence of central nervous system involvement is a relatively uncommon finding, cerebrospinal fluid abnormalities may be detected in 40 to 50 per cent of infants with congenital syphilis.[60, 61] This is demonstrated by increased protein, mononuclear pleocytosis of up to 200 or 300 cells per cubic millimeter, or by a positive cerebrospinal fluid VDRL. Clinical evidence of meningitis with bulging of the fontanel, opisthotonos, and, at times, convulsions, generally portends a poor prognosis. Low grade syphilitic meningitis may result in a mild degree of hydrocephalus, and children with central nervous system involvement continuing beyond the period of infancy may go on to demonstrate marked residua with varying degrees of physical and mental retardation. Those with meningovascular involvement frequently are mentally retarded and prone to convulsions, transient hemiplegia, and spastic paralysis. Although juvenile forms of general paresis and tabes dorsalis may occur, these findings are extremely rare.[69]

Late Congenital Syphilis. Late congenital syphilis is that form of congenital syphilis which persists beyond two years of age. It also includes varying signs and stigmata of congenital syphilis in individuals in whom the diagnosis was overlooked or in those patients who were inadequately treated early in the course of the disease. The stigmata most suggestive of congenital syphilis are interstitial keratitis, Hutchinson's incisors, mulberry (or moon) molars, and eighth nerve deafness.

Interstitial Keratitis. Seen in 20 to 50 per cent of affected children, interstitial keratitis is perhaps the most common late manifestation of congenital syphilis, appearing between six and 14 years of age. It generally begins in one eye, eventually becomes bilateral, and is characterized by a steamy bloodshot opacity of the cornea associated with pain, photophobia, lacrimation, and impaired vision. Early diagnosis and prompt treatment frequently result in rapid recovery without residual defect. At times, however, the second eye also may become involved, even after therapy has been initiated, and scarring of the cornea and deep corneal vascularization may persist after the process has healed.

Dental Changes. Perhaps the most pathognomonic signs of this disorder are the dental changes of late congenital syphilis. Although the result of infection at an early age, their appearance at the time of eruption of the permanent teeth merits their inclusion among the manifestations of late congenital syphilis.

The deciduous teeth of children with early congenital syphilis are prone to caries but show no specific abnormalities characteristic of this disorder. The term *Hutchinson teeth* is applied to deformities of the permanent upper central incisors characterized by central notching of the biting edges with tapering of the lateral side of the teeth toward the biting edge (so-called screwdriver teeth). The simultaneous appearance of interstitial keratitis, Hutchinson teeth, and eighth nerve deafness is termed Hutchinson's triad. Although described as a time-honored sign of congenital syphilis, owing to the relative infrequency of eighth nerve deafness, this triad is actually extremely uncommon and rarely seen.

The *mulberry* or *Moon molar* (named after the English surgeon who first described it) is a malformation of the lower first six-year molar. The mulberry appearance is created by poorly developed cusps crowded together on the crown. Since these teeth are subject to rapid decay, mulberry molars are rarely seen past puberty. When present, however, they are pathognomonic of congenital syphilis. Carabelli's tubercle is the name given to an accessory cusp that develops on the inner aspect of the upper first molar. This deformity occurs with equal frequency in non-syphilitic as well as congenital syphilitic patients. The presence of Carabelli's tubercle should not be regarded as a sign of congenital syphilis.[69]

Gummas. Also occurring as a late manifestation of congenital syphilis and considered to be the result of a hypersensitivity phenomenon, gummas may appear in the bones of the skull (or in the tibias) where they may erode the bone and go on to involve the subcutaneous tissue and cutaneous surface. As they progress to become necrotic, ulcerations with thick indurated borders generally are seen. Although gummas usually respond dramatically to antibiotic therapy, those affecting the nasal septum or palate frequently result in a residual saddle-nose or cleft palate deformity.

Higoumenakis' Sign. Unilateral thickening of the inner third or the clavicle (Higouménakis' sign) is frequently described as a manifestation of late congenital syphilis. Since fracture of the middle third of the clavicle is the most common fracture occurring at birth, consequent healing and thickening of the involved bone often produces a clinical picture similar to that seen with Higouménakis' abnormality. This finding should therefore not be considered a reliable stigma of late congenital syphilis.[70]

Syphilitic Arthritis. Arthritis may affect any of the larger joints (particularly the knees). Painless effusion into one or both knees may be known as *Clutton's joints.* Clutton's joints generally become apparent between the eighth and fifteenth years of life, are not accompanied by fever, respond well to therapy or may involute spontaneously over a period of several months or years, and leave no residual effects.

Paroxysmal Cold Hemoglobinuria. Characterized by shaking chills and voiding of dark urine within a period of eight hours following exposure to cold, paroxysmal cold hemoglobinuria may also occur as a manifestation of late congenital syphilis. This disorder is the result of autohemolysis following exposure to cold and generally is seen in patients with late congenital syphilis who did not receive treatment. Paroxysmal cold hemoglobinuria, in the absence of other definitive signs, although not pathognomonic, is highly suggestive of late congenital or untreated acquired syphilis.

Ocular changes. Choroiditis, retinitis, and optic atrophy may also be seen as late manifestations of congenital syphilis. Optic atrophy, when present, is usually seen in conjunction with neurosyphilis.

DIAGNOSIS. Early manifestations of congenital syphilis generally are so typical that the diagnosis of an infant with florid infection, once suspected, is usually not difficult. Unfortunately, the vast majority of infants frequently have minimal or no clinical evidence of infection. In such cases, early diagnosis often depends upon the physician's index of suspicion and awareness of the possibility of the disorder.

Placental changes (consisting of focal villositis, endovascular and perivascular proliferation in villous vessels, and relative immaturity of villi) often assist in early diagnosis of congenital syphilis. Diagnosis may be confirmed by positive darkfield examination from the umbilical vein or from moist lesions of the skin or mucous membranes, by characteristic bone changes on x-ray, and by positive serologic tests for syphilis. Serologic tests, however, in the newborn must be interpreted with caution since their results may be due to passive transfer of reaginic and IgG treponemal antibodies from the mother. The presence of these antibodies in the serum of the neonate merely indicates that the mother has or has had syphilis. A serologic titer in the neonate higher than that of the mother, however, is diagnostic. If no other indications of active infection are evident, with serologic titers equal to or lower than the maternal titer, infants should be followed closely (without treatment) with repeated titers taken at appropriate intervals. In cases of passive transfer of antibody, the neonatal titer should not exceed that of the mother and should revert to negative by the time the infant has reached three to four months of age.

An IgM fluorescent treponema antibody absorption test for the detection of congenital syphilis (the FTA-ABS-IgM test) is based upon the fact that IgM antibodies are too large to cross the placental barrier and so generally are absent in the newborn. The presence of IgM antibody against *Treponema pallidum,* therefore, in the neonatal period establishes the presence of active infection in the infant.[71] In cases in which the mother is infected late in pregnancy, both mother and child may be nonreactive at delivery. In such infants, clinical signs and rising titers during the ensuing weeks will confirm the diagnosis.

TREATMENT. Penicillin is the treatment of choice for all forms of congenital as well as acquired syphilis. Recent studies have demonstrated that 25 per cent of fetuses infected in utero die before birth and 30 per cent of infants with congenital syphilis, if not treated, will die shortly after delivery.[69] Once there is evidence of disease, treatment should be instituted immediately. Infants without central nervous system involvement should be treated by procaine penicillin G in a dosage of 50,000 units per kilogram once daily for at least 10 days. If daily injections cannot be administered, a single intramuscular injection of benzathine penicillin G (50,000 units per kilogram) may be satisfactory.

Infants with evidence of central nervous system involvement should receive crystalline penicillin G daily (30,000 to 50,000 units per kilogram in two or three doses) or procaine penicillin G (50,000 units per kilogram in one daily dose) for a minimum of two weeks and preferably for a total of three weeks. Since studies with benzathine penicillin suggest inadequate penetration of the central nervous system of neonates when serum penicillin levels are low, the use of benzathine penicillin G for congenital syphilis with central nervous system involvement is probably inadequate and should not be recommended.[72]

Cytomegalic Inclusion Disease

Cytomegalic inclusion disease in the neonate is a generalized infection caused by the cytomegalovirus, a DNA virus of the herpes virus group. Endemic in nature, cytomegalovirus may occur in 3.5 to 6.0 per cent of pregnant women in the United States. Of these, cytomegalovirus (CMV) excretion is found in only 0.5 to 2.0 per cent of newborns and only 1 in 3000 develops the classic syndrome of cytomegalic inclusion disease.[73]

CLINICAL MANIFESTATIONS. Approximately 90 per cent of congenital cytomegalovirus infections are asymptomatic. The remaining 10 per cent may have mild to severe, and occasionally fatal, cytomegalic inclusion disease.[74] Infection in infants is generally transmitted from a pregnant mother with inapparent infection across the placenta to the fetus late in gestation. Most of the reported cases are in premature infants or in those below average for their gestational age. Since most infections are asymptomatic, diagnosis is only made in the full-blown syndrome, one generally manifested by icterus, hepatosplenomegaly, and hemorrhagic diatheses.[74]

Typical clinical findings include lethargy, the appearance of jaundice within the first 24 hours of life, hepatosplenomegaly, abdominal distension, anemia, thrombocytopenia, respiratory distress, protracted interstitial pneumonia, central nervous system depression, convulsions, and chorioretinitis. Cerebral calcifications (often paraventricular in location) may be noted on skull x-ray. Cutaneous manifestations include petechiae and purpura, a generalized maculopapular eruption, and, in some instances, a generalized papulonodular eruption with blueberry muffin lesions similar to those seen in infants with congenital rubella and neonatal toxoplasmosis.[75]

Until recently, clinically apparent disease due to acquired rather than congenital cytomegalovirus infection had not been recognized except in patients with primary or iatrogenic immune deficiency. It is now recognized, however, that in previously healthy older children and adults, CMV infection may result in a variety of abnormalities, including an infectious mononucleosis-like illness (cytomegalovirus mononucleosis), infectious polyneuritis, hepatomegaly with abnormal liver function tests, and particularly in those with a deficiency of cellular immunity, pneumonitis.[76]

Most symptomatic cases of congenital cytomegalic inclusion disease are fatal within the first two months of life. Those who survive frequently manifest severe neurologic defects, namely microcephaly, mental retardation, deafness, spastic diplegia, convulsive disorders, optic atrophy, and blindness.[77, 78]

DIAGNOSIS. Diagnosis of cytomegalic inclusion disease may be established by the finding of distinctive large cells containing intranuclear and cytoplasmic inclusions from the urine, liver biopsies, gastric washings, or cerebrospinal fluid, or by direct isolation of the cytomegalovirus from the pharynx, urine, or fibroblasts of cell cultures from affected infants. Since bacterial growth may interfere with viral cultures, efforts to prevent bacterial contamination must be made. Only urine specimens collected by a clean catch technique or by aseptic suprapubic puncture should be utilized, and the specimens should be treated with antibiotics. When the diagnosis remains in doubt, persistent or rising complement-fixation titers may provide confirmatory evidence. Since IgM does not cross the placental barrier, specific fluorescence of cytomegalovirus IgM antibody in the newborn is useful in the diagnosis of active congenital cytomegalovirus inclusion disease.

MANAGEMENT. To date there is no effective therapy for cytomegalic inclusion disease, and prognosis for the patient with severe involvement is poor.[68] Although cytosine and adenosine arabinoside have been used experimentally, to date there is no evidence that they have any lasting effect on the prognosis of this disorder. Infants excreting CMV virus should be isolated during their hospital stay and female personnel who are or may soon become pregnant should not be involved with the care of these infants. Although presence of the disorder in subsequent pregnancies has been noted, this is unusual and the prognosis for future pregnancies is generally good.[79]

Congenital Toxoplasmosis

Toxoplasmosis is a parasitic disorder that may affect infants and children as well as adults. Caused by *Toxoplasma gondii*, a tiny intracellular protozoan that may invade any tissue (with the exception of erythrocytes) of all mammals, many birds, and some reptiles, toxoplasmosis generally occurs as a clinically silent infection of the gravid woman. It is transmitted to the fetus by invasion of the blood stream during a stage of maternal parasitemia, and may result in a wide spectrum of clinical signs and symptoms. Acquired toxoplasmosis is a disorder of older children or adults accidentally infected either by ingestion of raw meat contaminated by toxoplasma cysts or by contact with soil containing resistant oocysts from the excreta of infected cats, dogs, or chickens.[80]

CLINICAL MANIFESTATIONS. In congenital toxoplasmosis the fetus may be stillborn, born prematurely, or born at full term. Illness apparent at birth or during the first few weeks of life may be characterized by malaise, vomiting, diarrhea, fever, a maculopapular rash, icterus, lymphadenopathy, hepatomegaly, splenomegaly, hydrocephaly, microcephaly, microphthalmus, or convulsions. Chorioretinitis in the region of the macula, seen in 80 to 90 per cent of infants with congenital toxoplasmosis, is highly characteristic but not diagnostic of this disorder. Laboratory findings in patients with congenital toxoplasmosis reveal anemia, eosinophilia, thrombocytopenia, and, at times, severe leukopenia. The cerebrospinal fluid may be xanthochromic and may contain leukocytes, erythrocytes, and an elevated level of protein. Skull films of affected infants frequently reveal diffuse punctate comma-shaped intracranial calcifications.

The cutaneous manifestations of congenital or acquired toxoplasmosis may consist of a generalized rubella-like maculopapular eruption that may be ecchymotic or purpuric and generally spares the face, palms, and soles. There may be a scarlatiniform eruption or subcutaneous nodules scattered over the trunk and extremities. Annular, urticarial pinkish papules, or very rarely a vesicular rash or a micropapular typhus-like rash that spares the palms, soles, face, and scalp may also occur at times. In most severe cases, the rash develops during the first weeks of illness, persists for one to six days (rarely more than one or two weeks), and may be followed by desquamation or hyperpigmentation. Like congenital rubella and cytomegalic inclusion disease, congenital toxoplasmosis may be associated with dermal erythropoiesis, which presents clinically as localized or generalized bluish, hemorrhagic, infiltrated macules or as papular blueberry muffin lesions, similar to those seen in congenital rubella and cytomegalic inclusion disease.[81]

DIAGNOSIS. The diagnosis of congenital toxoplasmosis is made on the basis of clinical evidence supported by demonstration of the organism in biopsy specimens of lymph node, liver, or spleen, or in Wright or Giemsa-stained smears of centrifuged cerebrospinal or ventricular fluid. Isolation of the parasite in laboratory-reared animals (mice, hamsters, or rabbits proven toxoplasma-free prior to use) inoculated with blood, bone marrow, cerebrospinal fluid, saliva, or fresh suspensions of lymph node or other suspected tissue from biopsy or autopsy specimens is confirmatory.

The Sabin-Feldman dye test is positive 10 to 14 days after the initial infection and attains its maximum titer in four to five weeks. It tends to persist indefinitely at lower levels and is valuable for the detection of neutralizing antibody in the serum. In this test, after incubation with normal serum at 37° C, *T. gondii* organisms obtained from peritoneal exudate become swollen and stain with alkaline methylene blue added to the suspension. In the presence of serum from a patient with elevated antibody titers to toxoplasmosis the parasite remains unstained. Titers of 1:1000 to 1:16,000 are usual for at least some months in the sera of mothers and infants or young children with congenital disease.

Since dye test antibodies cross the maternal placenta, this test remains of limited value in the early diagnosis of congenital toxoplasmosis.[82] If the Sabin-Feldman dye test remains positive beyond a period of three or four months, it generally indicates active infection of the fetus. Since IgM does not cross the placental barrier, a more rapid and specific diagnosis can be established (as in cytomegalic inclusion disease) on a single infant serum by demonstration that infant's antibodies are in the IgM fraction and, therefore, not of maternal origin. Here again, a fluorescent antibody test for the detection of fetal IgM antibody to the toxoplasma organism is valuable as a rapid confirmatory test. Other tests include a complement fixation test and indirect hemagglutination.

Dye test antibodies (Sabin-Feldman), hemagglutinating antibodies (the Jacobs-Lunde hemagglutination test), and fluorescent antibodies rise early and persist. Complement-fixation antibodies are the last to increase and disappear sooner. The tuberculin-type skin test is of little value in infants and young children, since a positive reaction does not appear until 9 to 12 months after the onset of infection. Spurious results in some surveys have led to doubts as to the reliability of this test. The tuberculin-type skin test, therefore, should never be relied upon as a sole criterion for the diagnosis of this disorder.

MANAGEMENT. Most cases of toxoplasmosis are subclinical or are associated with mild symptomatology. Although congenital infections may vary in their severity, chorioretinitis, residual brain damage, and fatalities are not uncommon. In the face of an extremely high mortality rate in infants with fulminating infection, and because of the serious sequelae that may develop even in asymptomatic infants, once a diagnosis of congenital toxoplasmosis is established the patient should receive specific therapy whether or not the infection is clinically apparent or the patient asymptomatic.[83, 84]

For severe congenital infection, sulfadiazine, 150 to 200 mg/kg/day in four divided doses, in combination with pyrimethamine (Daraprim, Burroughs Wellcome) in dosages of 1 to 2 mg/kg/day in two divided doses for periods of 30 days or more, appears to be the most effective approach.[84] It must be remembered, however, that both pyrimethamine and sulfonamides are potentially toxic. Most physicians are familiar with the untoward effects of sulfonamides (crystalluria, hematuria, and hypersensitivity). Pyrimethamine is a folic acid antagonist that produces reversible and usually gradual depression of the bone marrow. All patients treated with pyrimethamine, therefore, should have a peripheral blood cell and platelet count twice a week while on this therapy. Folinic acid (in the form of leucovorin calcium) has been used to facilitate return of circulating platelets to normal. Available as Calcium Leucovorin Injection (Lederle), this substance may be ingested and, in contrast to folic acid (which has been recommended by some authorities), does not appear to inhibit the therapeutic action of pyrimethamine.[84]

The prognosis for infants with toxoplasmosis manifested at birth, particularly when it involves the liver and bone marrow predominantly, is poor. Although infants who become asymptomatic after a few weeks and who have predominantly central nervous system involvement often survive, their ultimate prognosis is poor. Many suffer from chorioretinitis and subsequent blindness, may become microcephalic, or hydrocephalic, and mentally defective. Infants with severe forms of congenital toxoplasmosis, accordingly, often require corticosteroids (prednisone in dosages of 1 or 2 mg/kg/day or its equivalent) until evidence of inflammatory processes such as chorioretinitis and high cerebrospinal fluid protein has subsided.[84]

DIAPER DERMATITIS

Diaper dermatitis (diaper rash) is perhaps the most common cutaneous disorder of infancy and early childhood. Seen most frequently in infants and children less than two years of age, diaper dermatoses usually begin between the first and second months of life and, if not properly controlled, may recur at intervals until the child no longer wears diapers.

The term "diaper rash" is used all too frequently in a diagnostic sense, as though the diverse dermatoses that may affect the anogenital region of infants and young children constitute a single, specific clinical entity.[85] In actuality, diaper dermatitis is not a specific diagnosis and is best viewed as a variable symptom complex, a family of disorders initiated by a combination of factors, the most significant being prolonged contact with or irritation by the urine and feces, maceration engendered by wet diapers and impervious diaper coverings, and, in a high percentage of cases, secondary infection with *Candida albicans*.[86]

Although frequently no more than a disagreeable nuisance, eruptions in this area may progress to secondary infection and ulceration, become complicated by other superimposed cutaneous disorders, or may be a source of confusion when a dermatologic disease of entirely different etiology arises in the anogenital region.[87] The term diaper dermatitis reflects a variety of inflammatory disorders of the skin that occur on the lower aspect of the abdomen, genitalia, buttocks, and upper portions of the thighs in infants, young children, and incontinent or paralyzed individuals.

For years ammonia caused by bacterial breakdown of urea in the child's urine was thought to be a major factor in the etiology of diaper rash.[88] In 1921, when Cooke demonstrated that an aerobic gram-positive bacillus *(Bacillus ammoniagenes)* was capable of liberating ammonia from urea, this organism was seized upon as the etiologic agent of most diaper dermatoses.[89] Recent studies, however, refute the role of ammonia and urea-splitting bacteria in the etiology of this disorder and incriminate a combination of wetness, impervious diaper coverings, and *Candida albicans* as the primary factor in the initiation of most diaper eruptions in infants and small children.[86, 90]

In some instances diaper dermatitis may be complicated by other superimposed conditions, and occasionally it may present as the first sign of a more severe or systemic disorder. In the absence of precise etiologic diagnosis, treatment based primarily upon topographic distribution alone may fail to achieve satisfactory therapeutic results. All diaper eruptions, therefore, should be subjected to critical analysis prior to the initiation of definitive therapy.

CLINICAL MANIFESTATIONS

Friction Dermatitis. The most prevalent form of diaper dermatitis is the chafing or friction dermatitis that affects most infants at some time. Generally present on areas where friction is the most pronounced (the inner surfaces of the thighs, the genitals, buttocks, and the abdomen), the eruption tends to wax and wane quickly, is frequently aggravated by the use of harsh talcum preparations, consists of a mild erythema with a shiny glazed surface and occasional papules, and responds quickly to frequent diaper changes, avoidance of diapers whenever possible, and simple drying measures.[86]

Irritant Dermatitis. Irritant or contact diaper dermatitis is usually confined to the convex surfaces of the buttocks, perineal area, the lower abdomen and proximal thighs, with sparing of the intertriginous creases (Fig. 2–17). The disorder may be attributable to contact with proteolytic enzymes and irritant chemicals, such as harsh soaps, detergents, and topical medications. Other significant factors appear to be excessive heat, moisture, and sweat retention associated with the warm subtropical environment produced by impervious diaper coverings.

Allergic Dermatitis. Diaper dermatitis based on an allergic reaction, when present, may complicate an irritant diaper dermatitis or may arise de novo. It is frequently localized to the convex areas exposed to the contactants, with sparing of the intertriginous areas. True sensitization reactions, although relatively uncommon in infants, are generally attributable to detergent soap preparations,

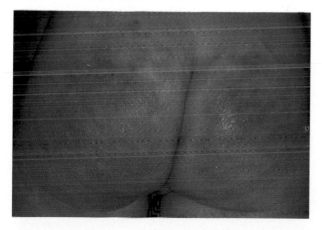

Figure 2–17 Contact-type diaper dermatitis. The eruption is localized to convex surfaces with sparing of the intertriginous areas.

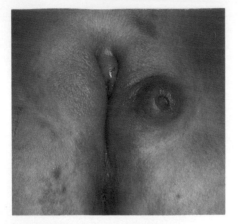

Figure 2–18 Papulo-erosive eruption with crater-like appearance (Jacquet's dermatitis) on the labia majora.

topical antibiotics, or topical medications aggravating a pre-existing diaper dermatitis.

In mild diaper eruptions the skin may be diffusely reddened, with papules, vesicles, edema, and scaling of the involved areas. With beginning resolution a shiny, wrinkled parchment paper-like appearance may be noted. In more severe cases, papules, vesicles, psoriasiform lesions, annular plaques, secondary erosions, ulcerations, and infiltrated nodules may occur.

Jacquet's Dermatitis. The term *Jacquet's dermatitis* is often used to describe a severe papulo-erosive eruption with umbilicated or crater-like appearance (Fig. 2–18). In male infants, ulceration and crusting of the glans penis and urinary meatus may create difficulty or discomfort on micturition.

Intertrigo. Intertrigo is a common type of skin eruption in the diaper area, particularly in hot weather or when infants are overdressed. Usually well demarcated with maceration and oozing, intertrigo generally involves the inguinal region, the intergluteal area, and the fleshy folds of the thigh. Miliaria, caused by heat and sweat retention, is characteristic and often seen in association with intertrigo of the diaper area.

Seborrheic Dermatitis. Diagnosis of seborrheic dermatitis of the diaper area may be simplified by recognition of a characteristic salmon-colored greasy lesion with a yellowish scale and a predilection for intertriginous areas (Fig. 2–19). Coincident involvement of the scalp, face, neck, postauricular and flexural areas helps establish the true nature of this eruption. Atopic dermatitis in the diaper area is not diagnostic in itself. When seen in association with typical lesions on the cheeks, antecubital or popliteal fossae and a family history of atopy, however, the correct diagnosis can generally be established.

Cutaneous Candidiasis. Candidal (monilial) diaper dermatitis is a commonly overlooked disorder and should be suspected whenever a diaper rash fails to respond to usual therapeutic measures. Cutaneous candidiasis is a common sequela to systemic antibiotic therapy and should be considered in any diaper dermatitis that develops during or shortly following antibiotic administration.

The typical candidal diaper rash presents as a more or less widespread erythema on the buttocks, lower abdomen, and inner aspects of the thighs. It is characterized by a vivid beefy red color, which develops as the result of specific irritant toxins elaborated by candida organisms. The eruption is characterized by a raised edge, sharp marginization with white scales at the border of lesions, and pinpoint pustulo-vesicular satellite lesions (the diagnostic markers of this disorder) (Fig. 2–20). Although cutaneous candidiasis frequently occurs in association with oral thrush (Fig. 2–21) commonly the mouth is bypassed and the infection is frequently confined exclusively to the diaper area. Infants harbor candida albicans organisms in the lower intestine, and it is from this focus that infected feces present the primary source for monilial diaper eruptions.[85]

Occasionally the diagnosis of candidal diaper dermatitis may be verified by microscopic examination of skin scrapings with potassium hydroxide or by Gram stain or PAS (periodic acid-Schiff) stain (Fig. 2–22). Although egg-shaped budding yeasts and hyphae or pseudohyphae may, at times,

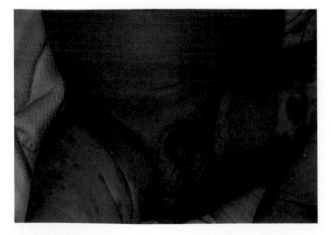

Figure 2–19 Seborrheic diaper dermatitis. Salmon-colored greasy lesions with a yellowish scale and predilection for intertriginous areas.

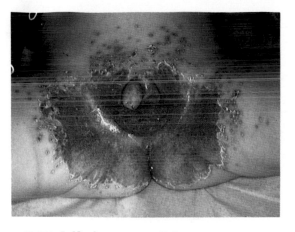

Figure 2-20 Candidal (monilial) diaper dermatitis with characteristic vivid red color, sharp margination, and pustulovesicular satellite lesions.

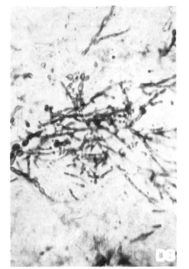

Figure 2-22 Budding yeasts with hyphae and pseudo-hyphae on microscopic examination of a cutaneous scraping (Courtesy of Alfred Kopf, M.D., New York University School of Medicine).

be identified by this relatively simple technique, a characteristic growth of white mucoid colonies on Sabouraud's or Nickerson's medium can confirm the diagnosis more consistently, usually within a mere 48 to 72 hour period (Fig. 2-23).

Psoriasis. Psoriasis of the diaper area, although not particularly common, must also be considered in persistent diaper eruptions that fail to respond to otherwise seemingly adequate therapy (see Fig. 5-2). The dark ruby-red, well marginated plaques with silvery mica-like scales are often associated with involvement of the trunk, face, or scalp. Family history may help confirm this diagnosis. The Koebner reaction, due to an isomorphic response, may be the cause of psoriasis when it occurs in the diaper area. Here lesions of psoriasis tend to erupt in areas of epidermal injury.

Congenital Syphilis. Congenital syphilis, once one of the most common severe disorders of infancy, fortunately is relatively uncommon today. When this condition occurs, it usually begins between two and six weeks of age, with macules, papules and bullous lesions of the anogenital re-

gion and an associated involvement of the palms and soles. Condylomata lata (large moist hypertrophic papules and flat nodules) may be seen about the anus, buttocks, other folds of the body, and angles of the mouth of infected infants. The infant is usually premature, marasmic, fretful, and dehydrated. "Snuffles," a severe form of rhinitis, often with blood-stained mucous and copious discharge, is frequently present. The color of the skin is often yellow or café au lait, hepatosplenomegaly is common, and there may be an associated anemia. The papular eruption in this disorder resembles that seen in acquired secondary syphilis, except that in the congenital disease lesions are usually larger, reddish-brown in color, and more infiltrated. The diagnosis can be confirmed by radiological changes (osteochondritis in the epiphyses of long bones), by demonstration of *Treponema pallidum*

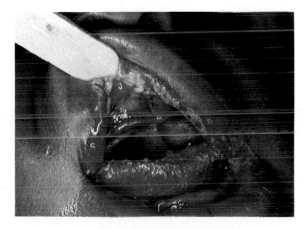

Figure 2-21 Oral candidiasis (thrush). Grayish-white, often confluent, friable cheesy patches or plaques on the surface of the buccal mucosa, tongue, and gingiva.

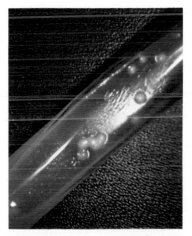

Figure 2-23 White mucoid colonies of *Candida albicans* on Sabouraud's medium.

from the skin or mucous membranes, and by serological investigation.

Letterer-Siwe Disease. Letterer-Siwe disease (histiocytosis) may also have a characteristic predilection for the diaper area. The eruption (often seborrhea-like) is most frequently seen in the groin, axillae, and retro-auricular areas. Characteristic lesions of this disorder consist of clusters of yellowish to reddish-brown infiltrated papules, often with hemorrhagic or purpuric qualities. A hemorrhagic seborrhea-like eruption with chronic genito-crural ulceration should suggest the diagnosis of Letterer-Siwe disease (Fig. 2–24). Histiocytic infiltrate on cutaneous biopsy is diagnostic of this disorder.

Acrodermatitis. Acrodermatitis enteropathica is an uncommon, although serious disorder with cutaneous lesions in the diaper area. The eruption often mimics monilial diaper dermatitis, with erythematous plaques suggesting severe candidiasis or psoriasis. *Candida albicans* has been isolated from the skin and mucosal lesions in 20 per cent of cases; this association does not represent a primary etiologic factor, but rather a secondary infection in these areas. Vesiculo-bullous eruptions of the periorificial areas, fingers, and toes; cachexia; alopecia; and diarrhea help differentiate this disorder.

TREATMENT. The management of diaper dermatitis is directed at keeping the area clean and dry and limiting irritation and maceration by avoidance of rubber diaper coverings. Frequent diaper changes, especially at night, thorough cleansing, with a mild or antibacterial soap, and the judicious use of topical therapy may be sufficient to keep the patient free from this disorder. Dusting powders help reduce moisture and irritation to this area. Those with antibacterial and antimonilial effects (Caldesene Medicated Powder, Pharmacraft, or ZeaSorb Medicated Powder, Stiefel) are particularly helpful in this respect. Talcum powder, although used for generations, can be irritating and may aggravate the friction and maceration so frequently seen in association with this disorder.

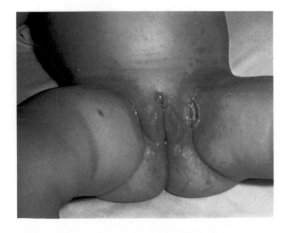

Figure 2–24 Histiocytosis-X (Letterer-Siwe disease) in the diaper area (Courtesy of Irwin M. Braverman: Skin Signs of Systemic Disease, W. B. Saunders Co., Philadelphia, 1970).

Severe and secondarily infected dermatitis should be treated systemically with appropriate antibiotics. Candidal infection requires the topical application of a potent antimonilial agent: iodochlorhydroxyquin (Vioform Cream 3 per cent, Ciba); nystatin, available as Nilstat Cream (Lederle), Mycostatin or Mycolog Cream or Ointment (Squibb); miconazole (Micatin Cream or Lotion, Johnson and Johnson); clotrimazole, available as Lotrimin (Delbay); or Mycelex (Dome) cream or solutions, or amphotericin B (Fungizone Cream, Lotion, or Ointment, Squibb). Severe cases often benefit from open wet compresses of tap water or a 1:20 or 1:40 solution of aluminum acetate. This concentration can be prepared by the use of Domeboro Packets or Tablets (Dome Laboratories); one packet or tablet in a pint of water will make a 1:40 solution of aluminum acetate. Topical corticosteroids applied lightly in a thin film are effective in inflammatory or contact dermatitis and will hasten recovery of damaged skin. If candida is resistant to topical therapy, or if there is evidence of monilia in the mouth as well as the perianal area, topical therapy may be supplemented by oral nystatin, available as Nilstat Oral Suspension, Lederle (200,000 units four times a day) or Mycostatin Suspension, Squibb (100,000 units four times a day) for a period of 6 to 12 days. For recurrent diaper dermatitis, preparations such as 1–2–3 ointment (Rosen's ointment), made up of Burow's solution 10.0, Aquaphor 20.0, zinc oxide paste, plain, q.s. ad 60, are particularly useful. To this prescription one may add 1.0 cc of Zephiran concentrate (12.8 per cent), 5 per cent Chloromycetin, 5 per cent Bacitracin, Vioform, or Nystatin (100,000 units per gram).

GRANULOMA GLUTEALE INFANTUM

Granuloma gluteale infantum is a benign disorder of infancy characterized by reddish-purple granulomatous nodules that measure anywhere from 0.5 to 4.0 cm in diameter and occur in the groin, on the buttocks, lower aspect of the abdomen, penis, and intertriginous areas of the axillae and neck (Fig. 2–25). Although the ominous appearance of these lesions may suggest a lymphomatous or sarcomatous process, the disorder appears to represent a unique cutaneous response to local inflammation, maceration, and secondary infection (usually *Candida albicans*).[91] Since lesions of granuloma gluteale infantum may resemble early lesions of Kaposi sarcoma and may involve areas other than those of the diaper region, other names suggested for this disorder include Kaposi sarcoma-like granuloma and granuloma intertriginosum infantum.[92, 93]

Granulomas may arise in a variety of infections, such as tuberculosis, syphilis, and deep fungal infection; as allergic reactions to zirconium; in foreign body reactions; and in response to irritation, maceration, and infection in the intertriginous and diaper areas of infants and young children.

Although nodular lesions of granuloma glu-

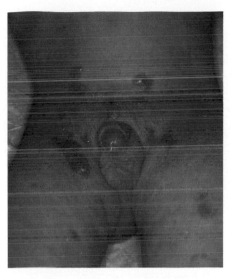

Figure 2-25 Granuloma gluteale infantum. Reddish-purple granulomatous nodules in the diaper area.

teale infantum may at times suggest sarcomatous or lymphomatous processes, they can be differentiated on the basis of clinical and histopathologic features. Light and electron microscopic examination of the nodular lesions of granuloma gluteale infantum reveal a hyperplastic epidermis with inflammatory cells (mainly neutrophils), a parakeratotic stratum corneum, and a dense inflammatory infiltrate throughout the depth of the cutis, with hemorrhage, neutrophils, lymphocytes, histiocytes, plasma cells, eosinophils, newly formed capillaries, and giant cells (Fig. 2–26).[94]

Lymphomatous lesions of the skin reveal large masses of patchy accumulations of lymphoma cells, or an inflammatory infiltrate mixed with lymphoma cells. Lesions of granuloma gluteale infantum lack the fibrous proliferative features, spindle cell formations, and mitoses which assist in the differentiation of this disorder from the more severe granulomatous processes.

Occasionally Kaposi sarcoma may occur on various parts of the body of infants and children as well as adults. This condition generally appears on the hands and feet of adults of central European or African origin. Rarely a disease of American or European children, Kaposi sarcoma in African children infrequently affects the skin and usually occurs in the lymph nodes, salivary glands, and ocular glands. When seen in Bantu children of Africa, massive involvement of the lymph nodes (especially the cervical nodes), salivary glands, eyelids, and conjunctivae generally precedes the appearance of skin lesions.

Lesions of granuloma gluteale infantum resolve completely and spontaneously within a period of several months after treatment of the initiating inflammatory process with its associated maceration and secondary infection. Although the use of intralesional steroid or impregnated flurandrenolide tape (Cordran tape, Dista Products) may hasten resolution of lesions, such therapy is unnecessary and not recommended.[95]

ACRODERMATITIS ENTEROPATHICA

Acrodermatitis enteropathica is a hereditary disorder that appears in early infancy and is characterized by acral and periorificial vesicobullous, pustular, and eczematoid skin lesions; alopecia; nail dystrophy; diarrhea; glossitis; stomatitis; and frequent secondary infection due to bacterial or candidal organisms.[96, 97] Although the clinical characteristics of this disease were originally described by Danbolt and Closs in 1930, it was not until 1942 that they defined the disorder as a specific entity and, because of the acral distribution of skin lesions and associated gastrointestinal abnormalities, designated it by its present name.[98] The inheritance pattern of acrodermatitis enteropathica is believed to be autosomal recessive with nearly equal incidence in male and female patients. Involvement in siblings, but not in parents, and a history of familial occurrence in 65 per cent of patients conforms to this suggested hypothesis of a recessive mode of transmission.[96, 98]

CLINICAL MANIFESTATIONS. The triad of dermatitis, diarrhea, and alopecia classically appears at the time of weaning from breast to cow's milk. Although some patients are never diagnosed

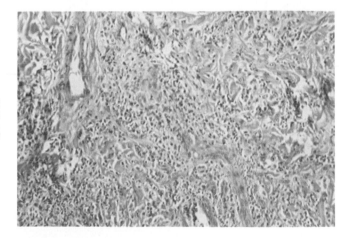

Figure 2-26 Dense inflammatory infiltrate of granuloma gluteale infantum (light micrograph). A lack of proliferative features, spindle cell formation, and mitoses assist in the differentiation of this disorder from sarcomatous and lymphomatous processes.

until adulthood, it appears that these individuals actually had their disease in a mild form during childhood. The onset of symptoms, therefore, usually begins early in life, generally between the age of one or two weeks to 20 months, with an average age of onset at nine months.

Typically infants with acrodermatitis enteropathica are listless, anoretic, and apathetic. Tissue wasting is present with an associated failure to thrive. During periods of exacerbation, frothy, bulky, foul-smelling diarrheal stools, typical of those in patients with celiac syndrome, are seen. Other findings include conjunctivitis, photophobia, stomatitis, perlèche, recurring monilial or bacterial infection, and alopecia of the scalp, eyelashes or eyebrows or both. Children suffering from this disorder exhibit a striking uniformity of appearance, mainly because of the alopecia and periorificial lesions.

The syndrome usually begins with small moist erythematous lesions localized around the body orifices (mouth, nose, ears, eyes, and perineum) and symmetrically located on the buttocks and extensor surface of major joints (elbows, knees, hands, and feet), the scalp, and the fingers and toes (the acral aspect of this disorder) (Fig. 2–27). The cutaneous lesions are similar to those of severe moniliasis or pustular psoriasis, depending upon the areas that are affected.

Drooling and change of hair color to red are additional findings seen during the active phase of the disease.[99] Other features include growth retardation in 80 per cent and mental changes in the form of schizoid features, with frequent crying, irritability, and restlessness during periods of exacerbation in 40 per cent of patients.[96, 100]

The basic cutaneous lesion of acrodermatitis enteropathica is a vesicobullous eruption that arises from an erythematous base. The blisters quickly collapse, begin to dry and crust, and sharply marginated lichenified or psoriasiform plaques develop at these sites. On the face, the eroded and crusted peribuccal plaques may appear impetiginized, and secondary infection with *Candida albicans* is common. When the fingers

and toes are involved there is marked erythema and swelling of the paronychial tissues, often with subsequent nail deformity. If unrecognized or untreated, acrodermatitis enteropathica follows an intermittent but relentlessly progressive course and, as a consequence of general disability, infection, or both, frequently ends in fatality.[96]

Prior to the description and naming of acrodermatitis enteropathica by Danbolt and Closs in 1942, the disease was first described by Wendt in 1902 as a variant of epidermolysis bullosa of the dystrophic or letalis type.[97] Since that time numerous pathogenetic mechanisms have been hypothesized. These included an abnormality of tryptophan metabolism; intestinal abnormalities with absorption of a dietary protein rendered toxic by incomplete digestion; infections with bacteria, yeasts, or parasites; a variation of cystic fibrosis; a defect in the interconversion of unsaturated fatty acids in the synthesis of essential fatty acids; and various unsubstantiated theories based upon findings in patients with lactose intolerance.[101-105]

MANAGEMENT. Although the etiology of this disorder remained enigmatic, the course and prognosis were improved dramatically by the introduction of treatment by the oral administration of diiodohydroxyquinolin in 1953.[100] Until recently, diiodohydroxyquinolin (Diodoquin, Searle), with or without breast milk, was the mainstay of therapy. Although successful in dosages of 200 to 2000 mg per day, serious side effects, especially optic neuritis, optic atrophy, and peripheral neuropathy, have been reported in patients following prolonged high dosage therapy. Other reported side effects include hair loss, furunculosis (iodine sensitivity), agranulocytosis, chills, fever, headache, abdominal discomfort, and thyroid hypertrophy with elevated serum levels of protein-bound iodine.

Iodochlorhydroxyquin (Entero-Vioform, Ciba), a congener of Diodoquin, has also been implicated as the cause of thousands of cases of a neurological syndrome of subacute myelo-optic neuropathy (SMON) in Japan during the years that this drug was available without prescription.[106] Although empirical treatment of patients with acrodermatitis enteropathica with diiodohydroxyquinolin was eminently successful and lifesaving in many instances, complete remissions were rare, and the potential toxicity associated with this preparation suggests that therapy with Diodoquin no longer be recommended in the management of patients with this disorder.

The etiology of acrodermatitis enteropathica remained controversial until 1973 when Moynahan first demonstrated low serum zinc levels and a rapid response to the administration of zinc sulfate in patients with this disorder.[108] Although many questions regarding the precise pathogenesis of zinc deficiency remain unanswered, the basic defect appears to be related to a gastrointestinal malabsorption of zinc.[107-110]

Recent investigations of the monocyte system suggest suppression of cellular chemotaxis of

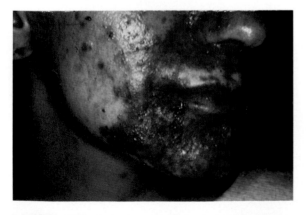

Figure 2–27 Periorificial eruption of acrodermatitis enteropathica (Courtesy of Irwin M. Braverman: Skin Signs of Systemic Disease. W. B. Saunders Co., Philadelphia, 1970).

monocytes and neutrophils in patients with acrodermatitis enteropathica. Since patients with this disorder suffer from frequent and persistent bacterial and monilial infection, it has been theorized that a zinc-dependent defect in chemotaxis may contribute to this susceptibility. These findings, therefore, suggest an important role for zinc in neutrophil and monocyte chemotaxis and a correctable immune defect in patients with this disorder.[111]

Until the role of zinc in the etiology of this disorder was recognized, diagnosis was made on the basis of the characteristic eruption, gastrointestinal disturbances (with exacerbations and remissions), the peculiar mental state during periods of exacerbation, and the associated alopecia. Skin biopsy is not diagnostic and shows a variable picture dependent upon the age and clinical appearance of the lesions. There may be hyperkeratotis, parakeratosis, intraepidermal pustules, spongiosis, acanthosis with downward projection of the rete pegs, and a mild polymorphic infiltrate in the upper region of the dermis.[96] Today, however, a decrease in zinc levels in plasma, red blood cells, hair, and urine may be considered diagnostic (serum zinc levels of 70–110 micrograms/100 ml are considered normal, and levels of 50 micrograms/100 ml or lower, appear to be diagnostic of this disorder.)[112] It should be noted, however, that there may be sources of error caused by zinc contamination of glass tubes and rubber stoppers. Blood samples, therefore, should be collected in acid-washed sterile plastic tubes with the use of acid-washed plastic syringes.

Blood zinc determinations should always be done prior to treatment in order to determine that the patient actually has acrodermatitis enteropathica. Diiodohydroxyquin is no longer considered the treatment of choice for this disorder. It now is apparent that zinc gluconate or sulfate, without diiodohydroxyquin or breast milk, is highly effective in dosages of 5 mg/kg/day given two or three times a day. Available in tablets containing up to 15 mg of elemental zinc, zinc sulfate or gluconate may be given in fruit juice, is well tolerated by patients, and provides a safe and inexpensive form of therapy for this formerly severe disorder of infancy and childhood.

References

1. Solomon LM, Esterly NB: Transient cutaneous lesions. In Neonatal Dermatology. W. B. Saunders Co., Philadelphia, 1973.

   A monograph on the cutaneous disorders of infants and neonates.

2. Nachman RL, Esterly NB: Increased skin permeability in preterm infants. J. Pediatr. 79:628–632, 1971.

   Topical applications of 10 per cent Neo-Synephrine reveal rapid cutaneous blanching in premature infants of 28 to 34 weeks gestation, a less dramatic response in infants 35 to 37 weeks, and generally no response in those of 38 to 42 weeks gestation.

3. Committee on Fetus and Newborn: Skin care of the newly born infant. In Standards and Recommendations for Hospital Care of Newborn Infants, Sixth Edition. American Academy of Pediatrics, Evanston, Illinois, 1977, 120–122.

   Concern related to bathing newborn infants with hexachlorophene leads to a redefinition of appropriate skin care in hospital nurseries.

4. Pearson HA, Cone TE Jr: Harlequin color change in young infants with tricuspid atresia. J. Pediatr. 50:609–612, 1957.

   Improvement of harlequin color change in a 3 1/2-month-old infant with tricuspid atresia corrected by aorta-pulmonary artery anastomosis suggests unsaturation of arterial oxygen as a triggering mechanism for this phenomenon.

5. Hughes WE, Hammond ML: Sclerema neonatorum. J. Pediatr. 32:676–692, 1948.

   A review of the clinical findings of 28 infants with sclerema neonatorum.

6. Warwick WJ, Ruttenberg HD, Quie PG: Sclerema neonatorum — a sign not a disease. JAMA 184:680–683, 1963.

   The clinical course of 18 infants with sclerema suggests this disorder to be a sign of potentially fatal underlying disease.

7. Kellum RE, Ray TL, Brown GR: Sclerema neonatorum. Report of case analysis of subcutaneous and epidermal-dermal lipids by chromatographic methods. Arch. Dermatol. 97:372–380, 1968.

   Increase in the saturated-unsaturated ratio of fatty acids in subcutaneous triglycerides of a patient with sclerema neonatorum suggests defective fatty acid mobilization as the cause of this disorder.

8. Horsefield GI, Yardley HJ: Sclerema neonatorum. J. Invest. Dermatol. 44:326–332, 1965.

   Increased ratio of saturated to unsaturated fatty acids may be related to poorly developed enzyme systems in newborns with sclerema.

9. Kendall N, Ledis S: Sclerema neonatorum successfully treated with corticotropin (ACTH). Am. J. Dis. Child. 83:52–53, 1952.

   Apparent successful treatment of sclerema suggests further trial of corticotropin for infants with this disorder.

10. Wickes IG: Sclerema neonatorum: recovery with cortisone. Arch. Dis. Child. 31:419–421, 1956.

    Apparent success of steroid therapy in sclerema neonatorum appears to justify its use for infants with this potentially fatal disorder.

11. Levin SE, Bakst CM, Isserow L: Sclerema neonatorum treated with corticosteroids. Br. Med. J. 2:1533–1536, 1961.

    In a study of 25 infants with sclerema, corticosteroids did not appear to influence the course of this disorder.

12. Marks MD: Subcutaneous adipose derangements of the newborn. Am. J. Dis. Child. 104:122–130, 1962.

    An attempt to clarify the terminology and differentiation of various subcutaneous adipose tissue disorders in the neonate.

13. Blake HA, Goyette EM, Lytes CS, et al.: Subcutaneous fat necrosis complicating hypothermia. J. Pediatr. 46:78–80, 1965.

    Subcutaneous fat necrosis follows the use of hypothermia in cardiac surgery.

14. Duhn R, Schoen EJ, Siu M: Subcutaneous fat necrosis with extensive calcification after hypothermia in two newborn infants. Pediatrics 41:661–664, 1968.

    Hypothermia as therapy for neonatal asphyxia appeared to cause subcutaneous fat necrosis.

15. Beare JM, Rook A: The Newborn. In Rook A, Wilkinson DS, Ebling FJG: Textbook of Dermatology, 2nd ed. Blackwell Scientific Publications, Oxford, 1972, 168–194.

A comprehensive review of the anatomy, physiology, and disorders of the neonatal integument.

16. Lüders D: Histologic observations in erythema toxicum neonatorum. Pediatrics 26:219–224, 1960.

The first histologic description of erythema toxicum neonatorum.

17. Levy HL, Cothran F: Erythema toxicum neonatorum present at birth. Am. J. Dis. Child. 103:617–619, 1962.

Erythema toxicum noted at the time of delivery.

18. Marino LJ: Toxic erythema present at birth. Arch. Dermatol. 92:402–403, 1965.

An additional report of erythema toxicum noted at birth supports the concept that this disorder may occur in utero.

19. Taylor WB, Bondurant CP: Erythema neonatorum allergicum — a study of the incidence in two hundred newborn infants and a review of the literature. Arch. Dermatol. 76:591–594, 1957.

The reported incidence of erythema toxicum varies because of the fleeting nature of this disorder and a disparity of clinical observations on the part of clinicians.

20. Carr JA, Hodgman JD, Freeman RI, et al.: Relationship between toxic erythema and infant maturity. Am. J. Dis. Child. 112:129–134, 1966.

The incidence of erythema toxicum appears to increase with gestational age.

21. Eitzman DV, Smith RT: The non-specific inflammatory cycle in the neonatal infant. Am. J. Dis. Child. 97:326–334, 1959.

Eosinophilia appears to be a normal newborn response to injury.

22. Keitel HG, Yadav V: Etiology of toxic erythema. Am. J. Dis. Child. 106:306–309, 1963.

Toxic erythema: a transient reaction of newborn skin to mechanical or thermal stimulation?

23. Ramamurthy RS, Riveri M, Esterly NB, et al.: Transient neonatal pustular melanosis. J. Pediatr. 88:831–835, 1976.

A previously undescribed skin eruption of newborns consisting of transient vesiculopustules and pigmented macules.

24. Esterly NB: Leiner's disease. In Demis DJ, Dobson RL, McGuire J: Clinical Dermatology, Vol. 1. Harper and Row, Hagerstown, Md., 1979, 1–7.

A review of Leiner's disease and familial Leiner's disease with C₅ dysfunction.

25. Jacobs JC, Miller ME: Fatal familial Leiner's disease: a deficiency of the opsonic activity of serum complement. Pediatrics 49:225–232, 1972.

Two patients with a deficiency of phagocytosis enhancement (opsonization) related to dysfunction of the fifth component of serum complement (C₅). Whether these patients actually represented true cases of Leiner's disease or a specific disorder with C₅ dysfunction is uncertain.

26. Miller ME, Koblenzer PJ: Leiner's disease and deficiency of C₅. J. Pediatr. 80:879–880, 1972.

Children with a deficiency of opsonic activity of the fifth component of serum complement (C₅) and a clinical course similar to that of Leiner's disease improved dramatically following infusion with fresh frozen plasma.

27. Hurwitz S, Klaus SN: Congenital hemihypertrophy with hypertrichosis. Arch. Dermatol. 103:98–100, 1971.

Since approximately 50 per cent of individuals with hemihypertrophy have associated anomalies, affected individuals should be carefully evaluated for other congenital malformations and neoplasms of liver, adrenal cortex, and kidneys.

28. Peer LA, Duyn JV: Congenital defect of the scalp. Plast. Reconstr. Surg. 3:722–726, 1948.

An infant with aplasia cutis with a large scalp defect (2.5 × 6 × 10 cm) died at 12 weeks of age as a result of necrosis, inflammation, and ulceration of the involved area, with hemorrhage due to rupture of the sagittal sinus.

29. Resnick SS, Koblenzer PJ, Pitts FW: Congenital absence of the scalp with associated vascular anomaly. Clin. Pediatr. 4:322–324, 1965.

A 4-day-old with aplasia cutis in association with an anomalous superficial scalp vein. Ligation of the vessel was carried out to prevent hemorrhage and facilitate early closure of the defect.

30. Rudolph RI, Schwartz W, Leyden JJ: Bitemporal aplasia cutis congenita. Occurrence with other abnormalities. Arch. Dermatol. 110:615–618, 1974.

A report of bilateral aplasia cutis of the temples in an 8-year-old with peculiar facies and findings similar to those seen in "congenital ectodermal dysplasia of the face."

31. Fisher M, Schneider R: Aplasia cutis congenita in three successive generations. Arch. Dermatol. 108:252–253, 1973.

Three cases of aplasia cutis congenita in three successive generations of one family suggest an autosomal dominant mode of inheritance.

32. Hodgman JE, Mathies AW, Levan NE: Congenital scalp defects in twin sisters. Am. J. Dis. Child. 110:293–294, 1965.

Identical congenital scalp defects in twin girls with lytic lesions of the underlying bone suggests a defect in the embryologic development of the scalp and underlying skull.

33. Mannino FL, Jones KL, Bernischke K: Congenital skin defects and fetus papyraceus. J. Pediatr. 9:559–564, 1977.

Two unrelated infants with cutaneous defects of the trunk and limbs, each with an associated monozygotic twin fetus papyraceus (a mummified twin fetus), indicate a specific pattern of malformation distinct from aplasia cutis.

34. Levin DL, Nolan KS, Esterly NB: Congenital absence of the skin. J. Am. Dermatol. 2:203–206, 1980.

Report of a 5-day-old girl with a single placental artery, infarction of the placenta, and congenital absence of the skin provides evidence for a degenerative rather than an aplastic or traumatic origin of congenital aplasia cutis.

35. Setleis H, Kramer B, Valcarel M, et al.: Congenital ectodermal dysplasia of the face. Pediatr. 32:540–548, 1963.

A review of 5 children of 3 families with clinical defects confined to the face, believed to be due to the multiple effects of a single gene.

36. Rudolph RI, Schwartz W, Leyden JJ: Amendation to "bitemporal aplasia cutis congenita." Arch. Dermatol. 110:636, 1974.

"Bitemporal aplasia cutis congenita" and "congenital ectodermal dysplasia of the face" appear to be one and the same.

37. Powell KR, Cherry JD, Hougen TJ, et al.: A prospective search for congenital dermal abnormalities of the craniospinal axis. J. Pediatr. 87:744–750, 1975.

A study of 1997 consecutive term newborns revealed one or more abnormalities of the craniospinal axis in three per cent of neonates.

38. Gorlin RJ, Pindborg JJ, Cohen MM Jr: Cleft lip-palate and congenital lip fistulas. In Syndromes of the Head and Neck, 2nd ed. McGraw-Hill Book Company, New York, 1976, 115–117.

Lip pits may be associated with cleft lip, cleft palate, and various skeletal disorders.

39. Pauli RM, Hall JG: Lip pits, cleft lip and/or palate, and

congenital heart disease. Am. J. Dis. Child. *134*:293–295, 1980.

Three infants with lip pits and cleft lip, cleft palate, or both, in association with congenital heart disease.

40. Cooper LZ, Green RH, Krugman S, et al.: Neonatal thrombocytopenic purpura and other manifestations of rubella contracted in utero. Am. J. Dis. Child. *110*:416–427, 1965.

A study of 200 infants with congenital rubella syndrome reveals a broad spectrum of associated abnormalities.

41. Brough AJ, Jones D, Page RH, et al.: Dermal erythropoiesis in neonatal infants: a manifestation of intrauterine viral disease. Pediatrics *40*:627–635, 1967.

Six infants with extramedullary dermal erythropoiesis as a manifestation of congenital viral infection.

42. Desmond MM, Wilson GS, Melnick JL, et al.: Congenital rubella encephalitis. Course and early sequelae. J. Pediatr. *71*:311–331, 1967.

A review of neurologic abnormalities and cutaneous manifestations in 100 infants with congenital rubella infection.

43. Rudolph AJ, Yow MD, Phillips A, et al.: Transplacental rubella infection in newly born infants. JAMA *191*:843–845, 1965.

Manifestations of 25 infants with congenital rubella syndrome: encephalomyelitis, hepatosplenomegaly, osseous defects, and generalized purpura with thrombocytopenia.

44. Cooper LZ, Krugman S: Diagnosis and management: congenital rubella. Pediatrics *37*:335–338, 1966.

Studies on the natural history and course of congenital rubella serve to clarify many aspects of diagnosis and management of this disorder.

45. Stewart GL, Parkman PD, Hopps HE, et al.: Rubella-virus hemagglutination-inhibition test. N. Engl. J. Med. *276*:554–557, 1967.

The hemagglutination-inhibition test (HI test) for rubella marks an advance in the detection and management of the congenital rubella syndrome.

46. Sever JL, Fuccillo DA, Gilnick GL, et al.: Rubella antibody determinations. Pediatrics *40*:789–797, 1967.

Comparison of four methods for detection of rubella antibody: hemagglutination inhibition, neutralization, fluorescence, and complement fixation.

47. Horstmann DM, Banatvala JE, Riordan JT, et al.: Maternal rubella and the rubella syndrome in infants. Epidemiologic, clinical, and virologic observations. Am. J. Dis. Child. *110*:408–415, 1965.

Clinical observations on 36 infants with the rubella syndrome reveal a relatively high proportion to have a petechial and/or purpuric eruption, thrombocytopenia, hepatosplenomegaly, and a gradual decline in virus excretion over a period of months.

48. Cherry JD: Rubella (German measles) and congenital rubella. *In* Gellis SS, Kagan BM: Current Pediatric Therapy, 8. W. B. Saunders Co., Philadelphia, 1978, 613–616

Current aspects of the management of rubella and the congenital rubella syndrome.

49. Schaffer AJ, Avery ME: Viral infections of the fetus. *In* Diseases of the Newborn, 4th ed. W. B. Saunders Co., Philadelphia, 1977, 806–819.

A review of recognized congenital viral infections of the newborn, their clinical signs and sequelae.

50. Frey HM, Bialkin G, Gershon AA: Congenital varicella: case report of a serologically proved long-term survivor. Pediatrics *59*:110–112, 1977.

Report of a female infant with chorioretinitis and cicatricial cutaneous scars attributed to varicella infection of the mother in the second trimester of pregnancy.

51. Freud P: Congenital varicella. Am. J. Dis. Child. *96*:730–733, 1958.

Varicella in an infant of a mother who had chickenpox eight days prior to delivery was manifested by fever and a characteristic eruption that developed 48 hours after birth.

52. Asha Bai PV, John TJ: Congenital skin ulcers following varicella in late pregnancy. J. Pediatr. *94*:65–67, 1979.

Skin ulcers in an infant born to a mother who had varicella in the third trimester of pregnancy suggests that the spectrum of disease in the affected fetus is related to the time that varicella was acquired in utero.

53. Srabstein JC, Morris N, Larke RPB, et al.: Is there a congenital varicella syndrome? J. Pediatr. *84*:239–243, 1974.

A report of an infant with multiple congenital anomalies (microphthalmia, cataracts, chorioretinitis, micrognathia, encephalomyelitis, pneumonitis, hypotrophic leg with flexion contractures, and cutaneous scars) ascribed to maternal varicella infection early in pregnancy.

54. Torphy DE, Ray CG, McAlister R, et al.: Herpes simplex virus infection in infants; a spectrum of disease. J. Pediatr. *76*:405–408, 1970.

Five infants with disseminated herpes virus infection present a broad spectrum of illness ranging from death or severe central nervous system damage to apparent complete recovery.

55. Komorous JM, Wheeler CE, Briggaman RA, et al.: Intrauterine herpes simplex infections. Arch. Dermatol. *113*:918–922, 1977.

A report of two infants with documented herpes simplex infection *in utero* and associated congenital malformations.

56. Francis DP, Hermann KL, McMahon JR, et al.: Nosocomial and maternally acquired herpesvirus hominis infections. A report of four fatal cases in neonates. Am. J. Dis. Child. *129*:889–893, 1975.

Of four fatal cases of infantile herpes simplex infection, three infants appeared to have been infected in utero or at delivery; the fourth infant did not develop signs of illness until age six weeks, suggesting possible infection by indirect contact with one of the other three infants.

57. Nahmias AJ, Josey WE, Naib Z: Significance of herpes simplex virus infection during pregnancy. Clin. Obstet. Gynecol. *15*:929–938, 1972.

A review of herpes virus hominis infection during pregnancy, its sequelae, and management.

58. Montgomery JR, Flanders RW, Yow MD: Congenital anomalies and herpes virus infection. Am. J. Dis. Child. *126*:364–366, 1973.

Report of an infant with early intrauterine type 2 herpes infection manifested by chorioretinopathy, psychomotor retardation, intrauterine growth retardation, cardiac abnormalities, short digits, and cutaneous findings.

59. Hovig DE, Hodgman JE, Mathies AW, et al.: Herpesvirus hominis (simplex) infection in the newborn. Am. J. Dis. Child. *115*:438–444, 1968.

A report of three infants with nonvesicular cutaneous lesions at birth.

60. Kahn G: Diseases of the skin of the newborn. *In* Modern problems in Pediatrics, Pediatric Dermatology, Vol. 17. S. Karger, Basel, 1975, 95–100.

Review of the common cutaneous disorders of the neonate presented at the 1st International Symposium of Pediatric Dermatology in Mexico City in 1973.

61. Music SI, Fine EM, Yasushi T: Zoster like disease in the newborn due to herpes-simplex virus. N. Engl. J. Med. *284*:24–26, 1971.

On the basis of this report, viral cultures of lesions in the newborn must be obtained before any etiologic factor can be ascribed to a zoster-like distribution of vesicles in the neonate.

62. Hodgman JE, Freedman RI, Levan NE: Neonatal dermatology, transplacental infections. Pediatr. Clin. North Am. *18*:747–756, 1971.

A review of neonatal infections in a symposium on pediatric dermatology.

63. Gerson AA: Herpes simplex infections. *In* Gellis SS, Kagan BM (Eds.): Current Pediatric Therapy, 8. W. B. Saunders Co., Philadelphia, 1978, 623–625.

Current approach to the problem of herpes simplex infection in infants.

64. Chi'en LT, Whitley RJ, Nahmias AJ et al.: Antiviral chemotherapy and neonatal herpes simplex virus infection; a pilot study — experience with adenine arabinoside (ARA-A). Pediatrics *55*:678–685, 1975.

Study of 13 infants suggests that Ara-A, when used within its non-toxic range, may be efficacious in the treatment of neonatal herpes simplex virus infection.

65. Wilkinson RH, Heller RM: Congenital syphilis: resurgence of an old problem. Pediatrics *47*:27–30, 1971.

Current increase in incidence of venereal disease suggests increased awareness for this temporarily forgotten disorder.

66. Harter CA, Benirschke K: Fetal syphilis in the first trimester. Am. J. Obstet. Gynecol. *124*:705–711, 1976.

Examinations of 9 and 10-week-old fetuses disprove the concept that *T. pallidum* does not cross the placenta before the fourth month of pregnancy.

67. Lee RV, Risser WL: A case of fatal, congenital syphilis in Connecticut. Conn. Med. *41*:470–472, 1977.

A case of neonatal death from congenital syphilis prompts review of the problems of diagnosis and management of this disorder.

68. Hardy PH Jr: Spirochetal infections. *In* Cooke RE: The Biologic Basis of Pediatric Practice. McGraw-Hill Book Co., New York, 1968, 781–790.

A comprehensive review of syphilis as manifested in infants and children.

69. Saxoni F, Lapatsanis P, Pantelakis SN: Congenital syphilis: a description of 18 cases and re-examination of an old but ever-present disease. Clin. Pediatr. *6*:687–691, 1967.

Although syphilis is again a public health problem, detection early in pregnancy plus adequate treatment can prevent transmission of the disease to the fetus.

70. Robinson RCV: Review article: Congenital syphilis. Arch. Dermatol. *99*:599–610, 1969.

A timely review of the many stigmata of congenital syphilis.

71. Mamunes P, Cave VG, Budell JW, et al.: Early diagnosis of neonatal syphilis. Evaluation of a gamma M fluorescent treponemal antibody test. Am. J. Dis. Child. *120*:17–21, 1970.

IgM measurements and gamma M-fluorescent treponemal antibody tests performed on the cord sera of 43 seroactive neonates prove the gamma M-FTA test to be an accurate additional way to diagnose congenital syphilis in the neonatal period.

72. Kaplan JM, McCracken GH: Clinical pharmacology of benzathine penicillin G in neonate — with regard to its recommended use in congenital syphilis. J. Pediatr. *82*:1069–1072, 1973.

Failure to detect penicillin activity in cerebrospinal fluid of 3 or 4 infants may indicate inadequate penetration of the central nervous system of neonates when serum levels are low.

73. Milunsky A: Causes of abnormalities in newborns. *In* Schaffer AJ, Avery ME (Eds.): Diseases of the Newborn, 4th ed. W. B. Saunders Co., Philadelphia, 1977, 71–88.

Up to 10 per cent of cases of microcephaly and mental retardation may be associated with cytomegalovirus infection during pregnancy.

74. Montgomery R, Youngblood L, Medearis DN Jr: Recovery of cytomegalovirus from the cervix in pregnancy. Pediatrics *49*:524–531, 1972.

In a study of 71 pregnant Navajo women and 125 women in Pittsburgh, although cytomegalovirus was recovered from 11 per cent of the mothers, none was recovered from their newborn infants.

75. Medearis DN Jr: Cytomegalic inclusion disease: An analysis of the clinical features based on the literature and six additional cases. Pediatrics *19*:467–480, 1957.

Clinical and pathologic characteristics of 42 infants who died of neonatal cytomegalic inclusion disease.

76. Hanshaw JB: Cytomegalovirus infections. *In* Gellis SS, Kagan BM (Eds.): Current Pediatric Therapy, 8. W. B. Saunders Co., Philadelphia, 1978, 630–631.

Since congenital cytomegalic inclusion disease may result in spastic quadriplegia, mental retardation, and obstructive hydrocephalus, long-range measures must be planned on an individual basis.

77. Berenberg W, Nankervis G: Long-term follow-up of cytomegalic disease of infancy. Pediatrics *46*:403–410, 1970.

Infants with symptoms of cytomegalic inclusion disease early in life have a poor prognosis in terms of psychomotor development.

78. Hanshaw JB, Scheiner AP, Morley AW, et al.: School failure and deafness after "silent" congenital cytomegalovirus infection. N. Engl. J. Med. *295*:468–470, 1976.

Low intelligence quotients and bilateral hearing losses are noted in children with inapparent cytomegalic infection that occurred during the neonatal period.

79. Embil JA, Ozere RL, Haldane EV: Congenital cytomegalovirus infection in two siblings from consecutive pregnancies. J. Pediatr. *77*:417–421, 1970.

Although evidence suggests that infants generally receive their infection from mothers who have their first contact with cytomegalovirus during their pregnancy, this report suggests that subsequent pregnancies also can result in neonatal cytomegalic inclusion disease.

80. Kean BH, Kimball AC, Christenson WN: Epidemic acute toxoplasmosis. JAMA *208*:1002–1004, 1969.

Five medical students acquire acute adult lymphadenitic toxoplasmosis following ingestion of inadequately cooked hamburgers.

81. Andreev VC, Angelov N, Zlatkov NB: Skin manifestations in toxoplasmosis. Arch. Dermatol. *100*:196–199, 1969.

Bizarre recurrent eruptions in a patient with acquired toxoplasmosis — an autoimmune disorder with histiolymphocytic and histiomonocytic infiltrate around dermal vessels?

82. Kean BH, Kimball AC: The complement fixation test in the diagnosis of congenital toxoplasmosis. Am. J. Dis. Child. *131*:21–28, 1977.

Since dye test antibodies cross the placenta, the Sabin-Feldman dye test is of limited value in the early diagnosis of congenital toxoplasmosis.

83. Saxon SA, Knight W, Reynolds DW, et al.: Intellectual deficits in children born with subclinical toxoplasmosis: preliminary report. J. Pediatr. *82*:792–797, 1973.

Varying degrees of intellectual impairment in eight children born with subclinical toxoplasmosis suggest justification for early vigorous treatment of this disorder.

84. Remington JS: Toxoplasmosis. *In* Gellis SS, Kagan BM (Eds.): Current Pediatric Therapy, 8. W. B. Saunders Co., Philadelphia, 1978, 664–665.

An updated review of the management of childhood toxoplasmosis.

85. Kozinn PJ, Taschdjian CL, Burchall JJ: "Diaper rash," a diagnostic anachronism. J. Pediatr. 59:75–80, 1961.

As a result of constant irritation and maceration, the diaper area is a fertile soil for a variety of dermatoses.

86. Leyden JJ, Kligman AM: The role of microorganisms in diaper dermatitis. Arch. Dermatol. 114:56–59, 1978.

Studies on forty infants with no history of diaper dermatitis and 100 infants with diaper rash refute the concept that microorganisms and ammonia play a central role in the pathogenesis of this disorder.

87. Swift S: Diaper dermatitis. Pediatr. Clin. North Am. 3:759–769, 1956.

A review of previously held concepts of etiology and therapy of diaper dermatitis.

88. Zahorsky J: The ammoniacal diaper in infants and young children. Am. J. Dis. Child. 10:436–440, 1915.

In the early 1900's physicians came to view urinary ammonia as an important etiologic factor in diaper dermatitis.

89. Cooke JV: The etiology and treatment of ammonia dermatitis of the gluteal region of infants. Am. J. Dis. Child. 22:481–492, 1921.

Isolation of a gram-positive urea-splitting organism from stools of a number of infants led to the assumption that an etiological relationship existed between this organism, the presence of ammonia in the diaper, and diaper dermatitis.

90. Leyden JJ, Katz S, Stewart R, et al.: Urinary ammonia and ammonia-producing organisms in infants with and without diaper dermatitis. Arch. Dermatol. 113:1678–1680, 1977.

Microbiological and experimental studies reveal Candida albicans (not ammonia liberated by micro-organisms) as a primary factor in the initiation of diaper dermatitis.

91. Tappeiner J, Pfleger L: Granuloma glutaeale infantum. Hautarzt 22:383–388, 1971.

Report of a previously undescribed nodular eruption in six infants.

92. Uyeda K, Nakayasu K, Takaishi Y, et al.: Kaposi sarcoma-like granuloma on diaper dermatitis — a report of five cases. Arch. Dermatol. 107:605–607, 1973.

Since lesions on five infants resembled early lesions of Kaposi sarcoma, "Kaposi sarcoma-like granuloma" is suggested as the name for this disorder.

93. Hamada T: Letters to the editor: Granuloma intertriginosum infantum (Granuloma glutaele infantum). Arch. Dermatol. 111:1072–1073, 1975.

Due to its association with irritation and monilial infection of the intertriginous regions of the neck and genitocrural region in a 3-month-old girl, granuloma intertriginosum infantum is suggested as the name for this eruption.

94. Uyeda K, Nakayasu K, Takaishi Y, et al.: Electron microscopic observations of the so-called granuloma glutaeale infantum. J. Cutan. Pathol. 1:26–32, 1974.

Electron microscopic examination of lesions revealed three types of giant cells: in the first type, the cells had widely enlarged endoplasmic reticulum, in the second they phagocytized erythrocytes, in the third they had vesicles and granules and were similar to histiocytes.

95. Kikuchi I, Jono M: Letters to the editor: Flurandrenolide-impregnated tape for granuloma glutaeale infantum. Arch. Dermatol. 112:564, 1976.

Two cases of granuloma glutaeale infantum showed early resolution of lesions following topical application of flurandrenolide-impregnated tape; one patient developed an associated steroid-induced atrophy.

96. Wells BT, Winkelmann RK: Acrodermatitis enteropathica — report of 6 cases. Arch. Dermatol. 84:90–102, 1961.

Review of acrodermatitis enteropathica based upon a compilation of 58 cases in the world literature and six additional cases that had previously been labeled with other diagnoses.

97. Neldner KH, Hagler L, Wise WR, et al.: Acrodermatitis enteropathica — a clinical and biochemical survey. Arch. Dermatol. 110:711–721, 1974.

A review of etiologic theories of acrodermatitis enteropathica and reasons for the efficacy of diiodohydroxyquin (Diodoquin) therapy in a 21-year-old woman with this disorder.

98. Danbolt N, Closs K: Acrodermatitis enteropathica. Acta Derm. Venereol. 23:127–169, 1942.

The original description of acrodermatitis based on a study of 2 children.

99. Hirsh FS, Michel B, and Strain WH: Gluconate zinc in acrodermatitis enteropathica. Arch. Dermatol. 112:475–478, 1976.

Two children with acrodermatitis enteropathica successfully treated with zinc gluconate.

100. Dillaha CJ, Lorincz AL, and Aavik OR: Acrodermatitis enteropathica — review of the literature and a report on a case successfully treated with diodoquin. JAMA 152:509–512, 1953.

The serendipitous use of diiodohydroxyquin (Diodoquin) resulted in the use of this agent in the therapy of acrodermatitis enteropathica for many years.

101. Hansson O: Acrodermatitis enteropathica. Acta Derm. Venerol. 43:465–471, 1963.

A recently disproved theory suggesting abnormal tryptophan metabolism, producing a metabolite with a toxic effect on the cutaneous and intestinal epithelium as the etiology of acrodermatitis enteropathica.

102. Cash R, Berger CK: Acrodermatitis enteropathica: defective metabolism of unsaturated fatty acids. J. Pediatr. 74:717–729, 1969.

Studies of a patient with acrodermatitis enteropathica who responded dramatically to the parenteral administration of linoleic acid suggested defective interconversions of unsaturated fatty acids as the etiology of this disorder.

103. Moynahan EJ, Johnson FR, McMinn RMH: Acrodermatitis enteropathica: demonstration of possible enzyme defect. Proc. R. Soc. Med. 56:300–301, 1963.

Duodenal and jejunal biopsies suggest an enzyme defect in the intestinal mucosa with resulting absorption of a toxic substance as the etiology of skin lesions and clinical manifestations of acrodermatitis enteropathica.

104. Lynch WS, Roenigk HH Jr: Acrodermatitis enteropathica — successful zinc therapy. Arch. Dermatol. 112:1304–1307, 1976.

A review of acrodermatitis enteropathica and report of successful treatment of a 21-year-old woman who had suffered with this disorder since the age of 3 months.

105. Milla PJ: Acrodermatitis enteropathica with lactose intolerance. Proc. R. Soc. Med. 85:16–17, 1972.

Lactose intolerance suggested as the etiology in three patients with acrodermatitis enteropathica from ethnic groups where beta-galactosidase deficiency is common.

106. Fleisher DI, Hepler RS, Landau JW: Blindness during diiodohydroxyquin (Diodoquin) therapy: a case report. Pediatrics 54:106–108, 1974.

The third report of optic neuritis: a 2-year-old boy who developed major loss of visual acuity and degenerative changes in his optic nerves and retinas during long-term high dosages of Diodoquin therapy.

107. Moynahan EJ, Barnes PM: Zinc deficiency and a synthetic diet for lactose intolerance. Lancet 1:676–677, 1973.

A patient with lactose intolerance and acrodermatitis enteropathica who improved only after the addition of zinc to his diet led to the discovery of zinc deficiency and its role in the etiology of acrodermatitis enteropathica.

108. Moynahan EJ: Acrodermatitis enteropathica: a lethal inherited human zinc-deficiency disorder. Lancet 2:399–400, 1974.

Nine children and one infant with acrodermatitis entero-pathica became completely symptom free and could eat a normal diet after they started receiving zinc supplements.

109. Neldner KH, Hambidge KM: Zinc therapy of acrodermatitis enteropathica. N. Engl. J. Med. 292:879–882, 1975.

Oral zinc sulfate (200 mg a day) results in rapid resolution of acrodermatitis enteropathica in a 23-year-old woman with a history of this disorder present since the age of 6 months.

110. Michaelssohn G: Zinc therapy in acrodermatitis entero-pathica. Acta Derm. Venereol. 54:377–381, 1974.

An 18-year-old male with widespread skin changes of acrodermatitis enteropathica and incipient optic atrophy probably due to chlorquinaldol therapy improved on oral zinc in dosages of 45 mg three times daily.

111. Weston WL, Huff JC, Humbert JR, et al.: Zinc correction of defective chemotaxis in acrodermatitis enteropathica. Arch. Dermatol. 113:422–425, 1977.

Investigation of monocyte system in three patients with acrodermatitis enteropathica revealed a zinc-correctable suppressed cellular chemotaxis of monocytes during zinc deficiency.

112. Hambidge KM, Walravens PA: Acrodermatitis enteropathica. Int. J. Dermatol. 17:380–387, 1978.

A current discussion of acrodermatitis enteropathica, its clinical features, diagnosis, and management.

ECZEMATOUS ERUPTIONS IN CHILDHOOD

Atopic dermatitis, one of the most common skin disorders seen in infants and children, is a source of frustration to parents and presents a challenge to immunologists, pediatricians, and dermatologists alike. Affecting about 3 per cent of the childhood population, this disorder is confusing from several aspects.[1] Confusion frequently exists because the terms *dermatitis* and *eczema* are often used synonymously and interchangeably. To the pediatrician the term eczema generally denotes a chronic fluctuating skin eruption occurring in atopic individuals. To the dermatologist eczema refers not to a disease but to a symptom complex consisting of an acute form of inflammatory eruption characterized by itching, redness, papules, vesicles, edema, serous discharge, and crusts. In this context it fails to cover the chronic, thickened, leathery hyperpigmented forms. He therefore adds a modifying adjective to the term dermatitis to specify the particular form of eruption under consideration, hence the terms contact dermatitis, seborrheic dermatitis, nummular dermatitis, and atopic dermatitis.

Atopic Dermatitis

Atopic dermatitis is the most common cause of eczema in children. Any discussion of the etiology of this disorder presents obvious difficulties, stemming in part from the complexity of the disorder and our ignorance of many of the basic mechanisms of the disease. In view of the conflicting data, therefore, it would be premature to attempt to develop an etiologic hypothesis to account for the multiple abnormalities characteristic of this disorder.

The concept of "atopy" (the word is derived from the Greek *atopia*, meaning "different" or "out of place") was originated by Coca, an allergist at Columbia, in 1923.[2] He first described it as a form of hypersensitivity based upon a hereditary influence. Although he placed only asthma and hay fever in this category, he felt that eventually eczema, too, would be included. Shortly thereafter, in 1933, Wise and Sulzberger coined the term atopic dermatitis as it is used today.[3] This term is useful since it can be used to include the subacute and chronic, as well as the acute, forms of this disorder. By this designation a predisposition to asthma and hay fever is also implied, for as we know, 30 to 50 per cent of children with atopic dermatitis (infantile eczema) will go on to develop one of these forms of atopy. This is in contrast to the normal population in which the incidence of atopy is only 10 per cent of individuals. It must be remembered, however, that the term "atopic der-

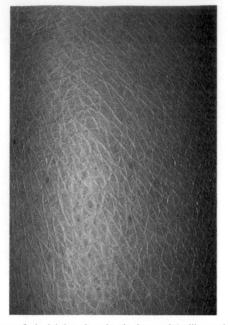

Figure 3–1 Ichthyosis vulgaris, large plate-like scales on the pretibial aspect of the lower leg. About 50 per cent of individuals with autosomal dominant ichthyosis vulgaris show one or more atopic manifestations.

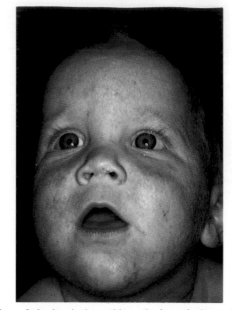

Figure 3–2 Atopic dermatitis on the face of a 6-month-old infant. Note the atopic pleats, long luxuriant eyelashes, and the pallor of the paranasal and buccal areas.

matitis" does not necessarily imply that the skin lesions of this disorder are caused by a union of antigen and antibody.

STIGMATA ASSOCIATED WITH ATOPIC DERMATITIS. Although the cause of atopic dermatitis is not known, it has become evident that patients with this disorder have many systemic and cutaneous abnormalities besides their chronic pruritus and skin eruptions. Common associated findings include a tendency toward dry skin, a lower threshold to pruritic stimuli, keratosis pilaris, increased palmar markings, and atopic pleats.

Dryness and Itching. Atopic skin has an increased tendency to dryness and a peculiar itching response often referred to as a "spreading itch." Cutaneous dryness and itching are the outstanding symptoms of atopic dermatitis and appear to

hold a key to the pathogenesis of this disorder. This tendency to dry skin is particularly noticeable on the extensor surfaces of the arms and legs, and in many patients, ichthyosis vulgaris is seen in association with this disorder (Fig. 3–1). Although more than 50 per cent of atopic patients have dry skin, the true frequency of ichthyosis is unknown because of the varied incidence with which the ichthyotic component has been diagnosed.[4]

Characteristically the skin of patients with atopic dermatitis is worse during the winter months, owing to a low relative humidity aggravated by heating of the home and frequent bathing. The water-binding properties of stratum corneum appear to be due to hygroscopic water-soluble lipoprotein complexes. If these lipid materials are removed by solvents, the stratum corneum loses its capacity to act as a water barrier. Excessive bathing seems to remove lipoprotein complexes that hold water in the stratum corneum and seems to aggravate this loss of moisture. Transepidermal

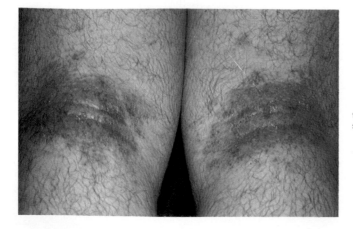

Figure 3–3 Atopic dermatitis. Oozing eczematous lesions in the popliteal fossae, a characteristic site of predilection.

water loss has been demonstrated to be greater in patients with atopic dermatitis than in controls and might contribute to the inability of many individuals with atopic dermatitis to maintain soft and pliable skin and may explain the cutaneous dryness common to many patients with atopic dermatitis. Such skin is easily chapped and split, particularly when the relative humidity of the atmosphere falls below 50 per cent.[5]

Damage consequent to rubbing or scratching of this highly sensitive skin is particularly aggravating, triggers the pruritic cycle, and initiates rubbing and scratching, which results in the characteristic eczematoid reaction seen in patients with this disorder. This pruritus can be self-perpetuating by means of the "itch-scratch-itch" cycle (a phenomenon wherein pruritus stimulates a bout of scratching) resulting in renewed irritation and further pruritus.[6] In susceptible persons a phenomenon of sweat retention also complicates the picture and may precipitate the itch-scratch-itch cycle.

Sites of Predilection. The sites of predilection are perhaps the best known peculiarity of the patient with atopic dermatitis. The face is favored in young infants (Fig. 3–2), extensor surfaces of the arms and legs in the crawling ages of eight to ten months, and the antecubital and popliteal fossae (Fig. 3–3), face, and neck in older children, adolescents, and adults (Fig. 3–4).

Keratosis Pilaris. Another associated finding is the follicular hyperkeratosis or chicken-skin appearance known as keratosis pilaris (Fig. 3–5). These lesions, most prominent on the trunk, buttocks, and outer aspects of the arms and legs, represent large cornified plugs in the upper part of the hair follicles. This cornification with a state of contraction of the erector pili muscles gives the skin a stippled appearance resembling gooseflesh or plucked chicken skin. Keratosis pilaris is not seen at birth, is very common from early child-

Figure 3–5 Keratosis pilaris. Fine keratotic papules most prominently seen on the trunk, buttocks, and lateral aspects of the upper arms and thighs. An early and often persistent manifestation of ichthyosis vulgaris and atopic dermatitis.

hood onward, and is an early and often persistent manifestation of ichthyosis vulgaris and atopic dermatitis.

Accentuated Palmar Creases. Many atopic patients exhibit an increased number of fine lines and accentuated markings of the palms (Fig. 3–6),

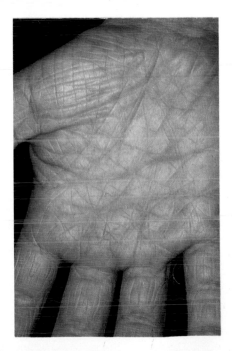

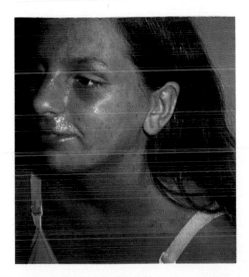

Figure 3–4 Excoriated infected atopic dermatitis on the face, neck, and chest; common areas of involvement in older children, adolescents, and adults.

Figure 3–6 Accentuated palmar creases—usually present at birth and persisting throughout life—a common stigma of atopic dermatitis.

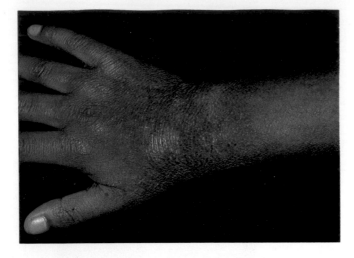

Figure 3–7 Lichenification. A hyperpigmented thickened leathery reaction to persistent rubbing and scratching, characteristically seen in patients with chronic atopic dermatitis.

which are usually present at birth and persist throughout life. Partially due to xerosis, they may result from thickening of the skin and may convey a poor prognosis as to the duration and severity of the disorder.

Lichenification. Also seen is the characteristic thickened, leathery, hyperpigmented lichenification, which is pathognomonic of chronic atopic dermatitis when it occurs on the wrists, ankles, and popliteal and antecubital fossae of atopic children and adolescents (Fig. 3–7).

Atopic Pleats. Atopic individuals also have a distinct tendency toward an extra line or groove of the lower eyelid, the so-called atopic pleat (Fig. 3–8). The atopic pleat, seen just below the lower lid of both eyes, is present at birth, or shortly thereafter, and is retained throughout life.[7] I consider this groove (frequently referred to as Morgan's fold, Dennie's pleat, or a Mongolian line) as an interesting finding, possibly related to edema of the lower eyelids. I do not consider it a hallmark, but rather a suggestive feature of the atopic diathesis.

Personality Disorders. Children with atopic dermatitis have been found to have characteristic personality traits. They are noted to be active,

restless, irritable, and aggressive individuals, frequently precocious and bright, with a forceful, driving personality. In individuals where the dermatitis becomes worse and uncontrolled, the affected children often become selfish, dominating and spoiled (Fig. 3–9). Such patients tend to lose their leadership qualities, often become frustrated or depressed, and occasionally go on to develop deep-rooted emotional disturbances.[8] Today, with our better understanding of the nature of the disorder and more effective therapeutics, it is gratifying to see that this reaction is less common than it was in the past.

Pallor. The patient with atopic dermatitis also has various unexplained physiologic abnormalities and paradoxical responses to various stimuli. They are prone to cold hands and generalized pallor, particularly about the nose, mouth, and ears (Fig. 3–10). This phenomenon, formerly considered to be a manifestation of vasoconstriction, is now thought to be caused by capillary dilation and an increased vascular permeability, resulting in edema and blanching of the surrounding tissues.

White Dermographism. When the skin of most normal individuals (those without atopic

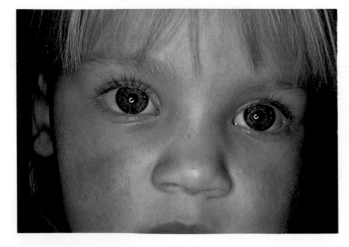

Figure 3–8 Atopic pleats (Morgan's folds, Dennie's lines). Accentuated lines or grooves below the margin of the lower eyelids of both eyes.

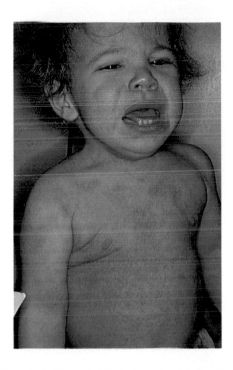

Figure 3-9 Characteristic facies of an infant with atopic dermatitis.

normal

dermatitis) is stroked firmly with a pointed but not sharp instrument, the triple response of Lewis and Grant (sometimes termed "the triple response of Lewis") follows. This response is characterized by a red line, flare, and wheal reaction. A red line develops within fifteen seconds at the exact site of stroking. This is followed, generally within 15 to 45 seconds, by an erythematous flare (due to an axon-reflex vasodilatation of arterioles) The response finally eventuates in a wheal (due to trans-

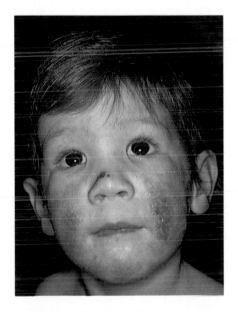

Figure 3-10 Atopic dermatitis. Note paranasal and periorbital pallor.

udation of fluid from the injured capillaries in the original stoke line) one to three minutes later.   *abnorm*

Individuals with atopic dermatitis, however, demonstrate a paradoxical blanching of the skin termed "white dermographism." The initial red line develops but is replaced, generally within a period of ten seconds, by a white line without an associated wheal, hence the term white dermographism. This reaction also may occur in non-atopic individuals with allergic contact dermatitis. Although this phenomenon is not pathognomonic of either disorder, it is highly characteristic and frequently helpful in the diagnosis of atopic dermatitis.[9]

Delayed Blanching. Another unusual reaction frequently associated with atopic dermatitis is known as the delayed blanching phenomenon. In this phenomenon the normal red flare occurs, only to be followed by an abnormal white blanching of the skin after acetylcholine injection. The delayed blanch phenomenon is seen in the skin of 70 per cent of patients with atopic dermatitis. Although uncommon in normal adults, this response is seen in newborn infants, patients with contact dermatitis, and young children who appear to be normal, but it too is non-specific and therefore not diagnostic of atopic dermatitis.[9, 10]

Cataracts and Keratoconus. A peculiar association of atopic dermatitis is the tendency toward early development of cataracts reportedly seen in 4 to 12 per cent of patients with this disorder.[11] These cataracts appear at a much earlier period of life than senile cataracts. They mature rapidly, are usually bilateral, central, shield-shaped, and involve the posterior or the anterior superficial cortex, or both, rather than the peripheral and medullar areas as seen in individuals with senile cataracts.[12] Usually asymptomatic, they are generally seen only by slit lamp examination. Although the development of cataracts can be associated with long-term use of potent topical and systemic steroids, atopic cataracts were described long before 1952 when compound F was released, and recent studies have shown that the long-term use of potent corticosteroids is not the cause of this phenomenon in patients with atopic dermatitis.[13, 14]

Keratoconus (elongation of the corneal surface), although uncommon, has been reported in about 1 per cent of patients with atopic dermatitis and seems to develop independently of cataracts. Keratoconus has been considered to be the result of continuous rubbing of the eyes or as a degenerative change in the cornea. Onset is in childhood. After a period of some years the disease is arrested, and contact lenses are frequently beneficial.

Altered Cell-Mediated Immunity. Patients with atopic dermatitis have evidence of altered cell-mediated immunity. Perhaps the most obvious result of this is the susceptibility to unusual cutaneous infections, especially viral, such as disseminated vaccinia (eczema vaccinatum) and herpes simplex (eczema herpeticum). Atopic individuals may also have an increased susceptibility to warts, molluscum contagiosum, and fungi (*Trichophyton rubrum*).[15] Other studies have indicated a lowered incidence of allergic contact dermatitis in patients. Whereas Rhus (poison ivy) sensitivity is noted in 61 per cent of controls, studies reveal an incidence of sensitivity in only 15 per cent of individuals with atopic dermatitis.[16]

Other Physiologic Abnormalities. Other recognizable physiologic abnormalities seen in a high percentage of individuals with atopic dermatitis include a tendency toward abnormally flat glucose tolerance curves, an increased predisposition to hypotension, and a hyperactive cold pressor reaction. The latter phenomenon, an abnormal blood pressure elevation induced by immersion of a hand in ice water, is probably associated with vasoconstriction of the peripheral vascular system.

PATHOGENESIS. Although the cause of atopic dermatitis remains unknown, evidence suggests that the underlying basis is a constitutional predisposition to develop pruritus. The itching leads to scratching, skin trauma, and the chronic cutaneous changes characteristic of this disorder. The skin is more easily irritated than normal integument, and when pruritus occurs it initiates a "spreading" itch, thus producing more irritation, further pruritus, and the so-called itch-scratch-itch cycle. Although the pathogenesis remains unclear, the pruritus may be related to the inherent tendency toward dryness of the skin and various unexplained paradoxical physiologic responses to pharmacological stimuli seen in individuals with this disorder.

The role of specific allergens in the pathogenesis of atopic dermatitis remains controversial. Although atopic eczema may indeed have an allergic component in infants, the antigen-antibody union is probably not directly responsible for the rash that develops in this condition. Allergic reactions may induce urticaria and itching, but the skin lesions themselves appear to develop in response to the rubbing and scratching induced by this reaction.[17, 18]

As yet there is no satisfactory inclusive theory of atopy, one that could explain its peculiar immunologic features as well as the abnormal responses to pharmacological agents. An interesting hypothesis is based on the beta-adrenergic theory of atopy first suggested by Szentivanyi in 1968.[19] When applied to the skin, the theory of beta-adrenergic blockade relates the peculiar irritability of the skin to an imbalance in the autonomic nervous system. It is postulated that in atopy there is reduced function of the beta-adrenergic system. This autonomic imbalance induces a reduction in activity or blockade of the beta-adrenergic receptor (adenyl cyclase), or perhaps an increase in activity of alpha-receptors, with a resultant dysfunction of cyclic AMP. As a result of this phenomenon there is an increased release of the pharmacological mediators (histamine, bradykinin, and slow reacting substance — SRSA). These media-

tors produce vasodilatation, increased vascular permeability, edema and urticaria, which in turn may be responsible for the pruritus and inflammatory cutaneous changes characteristic of atopic dermatitis. This theory may also explain the mechanism whereby psychic stimuli, infection, mechanical injury, and immunological reactions play a role in the exaggerated skin irritability of these individuals.

Although Szentivanyi theorized that the biochemical abnormality represented a deficiency or abnormality of the enzyme adenyl cyclase, recent studies have shown no reduction in the adenyl cyclase activity of the cells in individuals with atopic dermatitis. This does not disprove the theory. It merely suggests a need for further investigation of adenyl cyclase and its related pathways.[20]

The role of hypersensitivity in atopic dermatitis remains controversial. Ishizaka's discovery of immunoglobulin E, the reaginic antibody, in 1966, however, adds credibility to Szentivanyi's theory.[21, 22] The union of antibody and antigen appears to precipitate mast cell release of pharmacologic mediators (histamine, bradykinin, and slow reacting substance); this induces the itching, rubbing, and scratching that lead to the cutaneous lesions characteristic of this disorder. Juhlin and Johannsen have demonstrated elevated serum IgE levels in 82 per cent of patients with atopic dermatitis,[23] and Ogawa and others subsequently demonstrated a relationship between IgE levels and the severity of the dermatitis,[24] thus adding further credibility to this theory.

Pediatricians and dermatologists frequently disagree on the relationship between allergy to food protein and atopic dermatitis in children. Whereas dermatologists usually minimize the role of diet in this disorder, pediatricians often suggest a close association between food ingestion (namely egg white, wheat, milk, and citruses) and atopic dermatitis, particularly in children under one year of age. It is feasible that these foods may indeed act as allergens and that the reactions to food in atopic dermatitis could be due to the release of physiologic mediators with resultant vasodilation and possibly to effects on sweat secretion and, after puberty, on the pilosebaceous apparatus. Pruritus, therefore, may well be the primary connecting link between foods and the symptoms and cutaneous manifestations of atopic dermatitis.

This controversy may be due to the fact that most children seen by the dermatologist are those who have not responded to treatment initiated by the allergy-oriented pediatrician. A high percentage of eczematous skin eruptions in infants and children, however, are not caused by ingestants, nor are they cured by the removal of certain foods from the diet. It is probably just as much an error, therefore, to overlook the possible role of allergy in this age group as it is to attribute all manifestations of the disease to foods and ingested allergens.

CLINICAL MANIFESTATIONS. Atopic dermatitis may be divided into three phases based upon the age of the patient and the distribution of lesions. These arbitrary divisions may be referred to as the infantile, childhood, and adult forms of this disorder.[25]

#1 The infantile form of atopic dermatitis usually begins between the period of two and six months of age and, in 50 per cent of patients, clears by two to three years of age (see Figs. 3–2, 3–9, 3–10). It is characterized by intense itching, erythema, papules, vesicles, oozing, and crusting. In infants, it usually begins on the cheeks, forehead, or scalp and then extends to the trunk or extremities in scattered, often symmetrical, patches. Although scaling and crusting of the scalp may suggest a diagnosis of seborrheic dermatitis, the severe itching, a personal or family history of atopy, and the character and distribution of lesions help differentiate the two disorders. In children one year of age or older, lesions often take on the appearance of nummular eczema, with sharply defined oval scaly eruptions on the face, trunk, and extremities.

#2 The childhood phase of atopic dermatitis may follow the infantile stage without interruption and usually occurs during the period from 4 to 10 years of age. Affected individuals in this age group are less likely to have exudative and crusted lesions and have a greater tendency toward chronicity and lichenification. Eruptions are characteristically more dry and papular in appearance and often occur as circumscribed scaly patches. The classic areas of involvement in this group are the wrists, ankles, and antecubital and popliteal regions (Fig. 3–11). Pruritus is frequently severe, and infection and irritation from scratching often modify the lesions. Again, remission may occur at any time before the prepubertal age, or the eruption may go on to merge into the succeeding adolescent and adult phase of this disorder.

#3 The adolescent and adult stage of atopic dermatitis begins at the age of 12 and frequently continues onward into the early twenties. Predominant areas of involvement include the flexor folds, the face and neck, the upper arms and back, and the dorsa of the hands, feet, fingers, and toes. The eruption is characterized by dry and thick lesions, confluent papules, and the formation of large lichenified plaques. Weeping, crusting, and exudation may occur, but they are usually the result of superimposed external irritation or infection.

Seventy-five per cent of individuals with atopic dermatitis improve by 10 to 14 years of age, and 25 per cent of patients continue to have difficulty during their adult life. Cases persisting or beginning after the middle twenties are the most difficult to manage and usually have little tendency to spontaneous cure. Fortunately, these are relatively rare.[26]

DIAGNOSIS. The diagnosis of atopic dermatitis is based upon the evaluation of the aggregate of signs, symptoms, stigmata, course, and associated familial findings. Typical cases may be recognized easily. Atypical ones, however, may require long study and a careful differential diagnosis.[26]

The disease is characterized by severe spas-

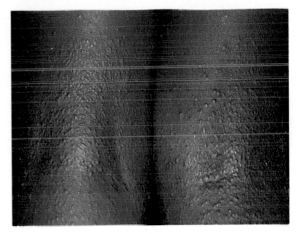

Figure 3–11 Papular atopic dermatitis, particularly common in the antecubital and popliteal areas of black individuals.

modic itching and its consequences. Clinically, it is recognized as a pruritic, erythematous, papular and vesicular eruption, with edema, serous discharge, and crusting. An important diagnostic feature is the fact that the borders of lesions of atopic dermatitis tend to gradually merge into the surrounding skin (Fig. 3–12) and, except in chronic cases of lichen simplex chronicus (neurodermatitis), are generally not well marginated.

Sites of predilection, a well-recognized peculiarity of the patient with atopic dermatitis, frequently are helpful and can aid in determining the true nature of the eruption. In chronic forms of this disorder, scaling, lichenification, hyperpigmentation, thickening, and fissuring are characteristic and at times pathognomonic (see Fig. 3–7).

When the diagnosis remains in doubt, histopathologic examination of cutaneous lesions will at times help to ascertain the true nature of the eruption. Acute lesions of infantile atopic dermatitis reveal hyperkeratosis, parakeratosis, and hyperplasia of the epidermis, with an absence or diminution of the granular cell layer. Essential

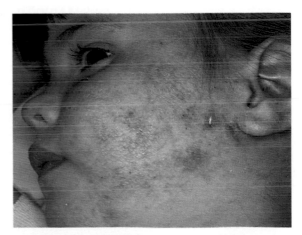

Figure 3–12 Atopic dermatitis. Eczematoid lesions merging into the surrounding skin.

diagnostic features include increased intercellular and intracellular accumulation of fluid (spongiosis), with migration of leukocytes (exocytosis) through the epidermis.

Chronic lesions of atopic dermatitis are characterized by increased hyperkeratosis with areas of parakeratosis and papillomatosis (upward proliferation of dermal papillae). Although these chronic changes may at times resemble those of psoriasis, the fact that there is more edema and a lack of clubbing of the rete ridges in lesions of atopic dermatitis helps differentiate these two disorders.

DIFFERENTIAL DIAGNOSIS. Atopic dermatitis is a chronic fluctuating disease. The distribution and morphology of lesions vary with age, but itching remains as the cardinal symptom of this disorder. Although many skin conditions may occasionally resemble atopic dermatitis, certain characteristics assist in their differentiation.

Seborrheic dermatitis is characterized by a greasy yellow or salmon-colored scaly eruption that may involve the scalp, cheeks, trunk, extremities, and diaper area (see Figs. 2–6, 2–7, 2–8, and 2–19). The major differentiating features include a tendency toward earlier onset, characteristic greasy yellowish or salmon-colored lesions with a predisposition for intertriginous areas (Figs. 3–13, 3–14), a generally well-circumscribed eruption, and a relative absence of pruritus.

Contact dermatitis can be divided into irritant contact dermatitis and allergic contact dermatitis. *Primary irritant dermatitis* is frequently seen in infants and young children. In this disorder the site of eruption varies with the etiologic agent. It commonly is seen on the cheeks and the chin (owing to salivary secretion and associated rubbing of the involved areas), the extensor surfaces of the extremities (as a result of harsh soaps, detergents, or rough sheets), and the diaper area (from urine, feces, soaps, detergents, and the irritation associated with harsh talcum powder preparations). Primary irritant dermatitis is generally milder, less pruritic, and not as eczematoid in

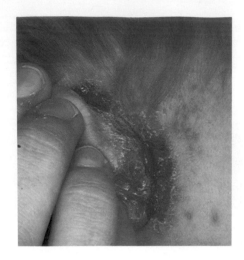

Figure 3–14 Infected postauricular seborrheic dermatitis.

appearance as the eruptions seen in association with atopic dermatitis.

Allergic contact dermatitis, although relatively uncommon in the first few months of life, can mimic almost any type of eczematous eruption and is characterized by a well-circumscribed pruritic, erythematous papular and vesicular eruption. Although such eruptions involute spontaneously upon identification and removal of the cause, this disorder often requires a carefully detailed history and prolonged observation before the true causative agent is identified.

Nummular dermatitis (derived from the Latin, meaning coin-like) is a distinctive disorder characterized by coin-shaped lesions. Measuring one to several centimeters in diameter, lesions of nummular dermatitis develop on dry skin (especially during winter months in heated homes with low humidity). The eruption begins with minute vesicles and papules that enlarge by confluence or peripheral extension, thus forming the discrete erythematous coin-like lesions studded with papules and vesicles characteristic of this disorder (Fig. 3–15). Although in the past nummular eczema has been thought by many to be a manifestation of atopic dermatitis, recent studies of IgE levels in patients with this disorder suggest nummular eczema to be a manifestation of dry skin (xerosis) and ichthyosis rather than a characteristic of atopy and atopic dermatitis.[27]

Psoriasis, another common skin disease of children as well as adults, must also be included in the differential diagnosis of infants and children with atopic dermatitis. The fully developed lesion of psoriasis has a full rich red hue and a loosely adherent silvery micaceous ("mica-like") scale. Psoriatic lesions are usually well defined, with a sharply delineated edge and have a predilection for the extensor surfaces (particularly the elbows and knees), the scalp, and the genital regions. Lesions may at times merge to form gyrate or annular configurations. The acute guttate (droplike) form of psoriasis often appears as an explo-

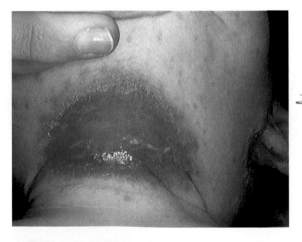

Figure 3–13 Intertrigo of the neck in an infant with seborrheic dermatitis.

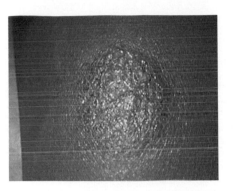

Figure 3–15 Nummular eczema. A well-circumscribed papulovesicular coin-shaped lesion on the pretibial area in a patient with ichthyosis vulgaris.

sive eruption of small, teardrop-like lesions that are predominantly seen over the trunk. Guttate flares of psoriasis are often seen in children following an upper respiratory infection, particularly those of streptococcal etiology.

A valuable clue in the diagnosis of psoriasis is the frequent presence of nail involvement. Seen in 25 to 50 per cent of patients, pitting or small punctate dimpling of the nail plate is the most common nail finding and results from an intermittent psoriatic defect in the matrix as the nail is formed. Although pitted nails may also be seen in atopic dermatitis and alopecia areata, the nail pits seen in atopic dermatitis (due to cutaneous eczematous changes in the areas of the nail matrix) are usually larger and more irregular in shape. Nail pits seen in association with alopecia areata frequently are grid-like and less deep than those seen in patients with psoriasis.

Scabies in infants and children is commonly complicated by eczematous changes due to scratching and rubbing of involved areas or topical therapeutic agents. The diagnosis of scabies is best made by the history of itching, a characteristic distribution of lesions, the recognition of primary lesions (particularly the pathognomonic burow when present), positive identification of the mite on microscopic examination of skin scrapings, and the presence of infestation among the patient's family or associates (see Chapter 14).

Letterer-Siwe disease, seen at the severe fulminating end of the histiocytosis spectrum, usually occurs during the first year of life and is almost exclusively limited to children up to three years of age (see Chapter 18). In this disorder the skin eruption generally begins with a scaly, erythematous seborrhea-like eruption on the scalp, behind the ears, and in the intertriginous regions. On close inspection the presence of reddish-brown or purpuric papules or vesicular or crusted papules (in infants) is characteristic. When the diagnosis is indeterminate, cutaneous biopsy may confirm the true nature of the eruption.

Acrodermatitis enteropathica is a hereditary disorder characterized by vesiculobullous eczematoid lesions of the acral and periorificial areas, failure to thrive, diarrhea, alopecia, nail dys-

trophy, and frequent secondary bacterial or monilial infection. The characteristic distribution of lesions, accompanied by listlessness, diarrhea, and failure to thrive, helps differentiate lesions of acrodermatitis enteropathica from those of atopic dermatitis.

Wiskott-Aldrich syndrome, an X-linked recessive disorder seen in male infants, is characterized by a triad of severe eczematous dermatitis, thrombocytopenic purpura, and increased susceptibility to infection. These infants have recurrent pyogenic infection, bloody diarrhea, purpuric lesions, and defects in cellular and humoral immunity (isohemagglutinins are absent from the blood, the serum gamma M-globulin is usually decreased, and the serum gamma A-globulin is often markedly increased).[28]

Phenylketonuria is a hereditary disorder characterized by mental retardation, seizures, diffuse hypopigmentation, blond hair, eczema, and photosensitivity. Caused by a defect in the enzyme phenylalanine hydroxylase, the disorder can usually be detected soon after birth by appropriate screening studies. An elevated blood phenylalanine concentration of 15 mg per 100 ml is usually accepted as presumptive evidence of this disorder (see Chapter 7).

COMPLICATIONS. *Secondary infection* is the most common complication seen in atopic dermatitis. Usually associated with group A beta-hemolytic streptococci and, even more frequently, staphylococcus organisms, studies suggest that the skin of patients with atopic dermatitis may be inherently favorable for *Staphylococcus aureus* colonization.[29] Whether this is related to chronic excoriation, depressed phagocytic function, or T-cell abnormality is as yet undetermined, but studies reveal a staphylococcus carrier rate of 93 per cent in lesions of atopic dermatitis, 76 per cent in uninvolved (normal) skin, and 79 per cent from the anterior nares.[30] Pyoderma associated with atopic dermatitis is usually manifested by erythema with exudation and crusting, greasy moist scales, and small pustules in the advancing edge (Fig. 3–16). This complication must be considered whenever a flare of chronic atopic dermatitis develops or fails to respond to appropriate therapy.

There is strong evidence endorsing the practice of adding an antibiotic, either topical if the dermatitis is localized or systemic if the dermatitis is widespread or unresponsive to other conventional therapy.[20] Penicillin G is the drug of choice in the treatment of known group A streptococcal skin infections. When the cause is not known immediately and when *Staphylococcus aureus* is a distinct consideration, erythromycin or a semisynthetic penicillin, such as nafcillin, oxacillin, or dicloxacillin, should be used. If the secondary infection is due to group A beta-hemolytic streptococcus, treatment should be continued for at least 10 days. Although systemic antibiotics may be valuable in the elimination of cutaneous streptococci, they do not appear to prevent glomerulonephritis due to streptococcal cutaneous infection.

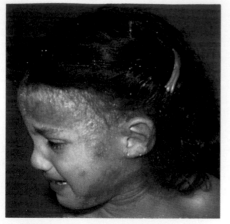

Figure 3–16 Infected atopic dermatitis.

In areas in which nephritogenic M strains of streptococci are endemic, urinalysis should be performed and patients should be watched for signs of glomerulonephritis for at least seven weeks after treatment.[31]

Kaposi's varicelliform eruption is another, even more severe, complication of atopic dermatitis. It is caused by the virus of herpes simplex or vaccinia and may be referred to as eczema herpeticum or eczema vaccination. Heretofore eczema vaccinatum occasionally followed smallpox vaccination of an eczematoid child, but was more frequently contracted by accidental contact with a recently vaccinated individual. Now that vaccination is no longer compulsory and vaccinia appears to have been eliminated (even in endemic areas of the world), it is hoped that eczema vaccinatum will no longer be a problem for individuals with atopic dermatitis.

The explosive development of a vesicular eruption in an atopic individual should raise the possibility of Kaposi's varicelliform eruption. Umbilication of the vesicles is characteristic (Fig. 3–17), and the diagnosis can be verified by the Tzanck test. In this test a cytologic examination is made of scraped vesicles with a search for multinuclear virus "giant cells," balloon cells, and, on rare occasion, intranuclear inclusions on Giemsa-stained smear (see Fig. 2–14).

The treatment of eczema herpeticum is symptomatic, requires maintenance of adequate hydration, control of fever, and prevention of secondary bacterial infection, and generally runs its course within a period of two to three weeks. For severe cases adenine arabinoside (Ara-A), administered in a dosage of 10 to 15 mg/kg/day by continuous 12-hour intravenous drip for 10 to 15 days, appears to be effective.

For patients with eczema vaccinatum, the use of passively administered antibodies in the form of vaccinia immune gamma globulin (VIG, Hyland Laboratories), 0.6 to 1.0 ml/kg administered once or twice intramuscularly, has been helpful. For severe cases, the investigational drug N-methylisatin beta-thiosemicarbazone (Marboran, Burroughs Wellcome), 200 mg/kg orally followed by 50 mg/kg every six hours for three days, has been recommended. After a three-day rest period, an additional three-day course may be given.

MANAGEMENT

Reduction of Dryness and Pruritus. The treatment of atopic dermatitis is dependent upon the management of dry and itching skin. The problem is particularly troublesome in winter when it is aggravated by heat in the house and low humidity. Patients should be instructed to limit bathing and to use lubricants that help moisten and rehydrate the skin. This diminishes the tendency toward dryness and pruritus that seems to be critically involved in the pathogenesis of this condition. A mild soap (such as Dove or Neutragena) may be used, and when lubricant is applied, it is best administered over slightly moistened skin. This seals in the moisture, rehydrates, lubricates, and moisturizes the skin, and thus diminishes the inherent dryness and itchiness that appear to trigger the eczematoid eruptions seen in patients with atopic dermatitis.

Cetaphil lotion, which contains cetyl alcohol, steryl alcohol, and propylene glycol, may be used as a cleansing and lubricating agent for individuals with dry skin. This lipid-free hydrophilic lotion may be applied liberally and rubbed gently over the skin once or twice a day (without water) until a light foaming occurs. Following removal by light wiping with a soft cotton cloth, diaper, or cleansing tissue, a protective film of stearyl alcohol and propylene glycol remains.

Bubble baths are contraindicated. When bath-

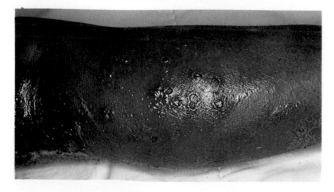

Figure 3–17 Eczema herpeticum (Kaposi's varicelliform eruption) with umbilicated vesiculopustular lesions.

ing is allowed, it is recommended that water be tepid or at room temperature (hot water stimulates vasodilatation and subsequent pruritus). Bath oils are only slightly beneficial and since they tend to make the tub slippery, should be used sparingly and cautiously, if at all, particularly with children.

Attention to clothing is also important. Soft cotton clothing is recommended rather than wool or other harsh materials, which tend to precipitate itching and scratching. Fuzzy toys, stuffed animals, and pets such as cats and dogs should also be avoided because of their potential allergenicity and the inherent predisposition of these patients to other atopic disorders such as hay fever and asthma.

Reduction of perspiration is helpful since many patients have considerable difficulty adjusting to hot and humid weather owing to eccrine sweating and sweat retention. Air conditioning is sometimes helpful during summer months, and frequent airing of the bedroom and humidification helps to relieve the adverse effects of excessive skin dryness during winter months.

Wet Compresses. Topical therapy of the acute stage of atopic dermatitis is aided by open wet compresses. When properly applied, open wet compresses have a soothing, antipruritic, and cleansing action on acutely inflamed skin. They tend to dry weeping or oozing lesions, clean crusts, assist in the rehydration of dry skin, and, through evaporation of water, afford cooling to inflamed and irritated tissue. Aluminum acetate (as in Burow's solution, 1:20 or 1:40) is germicidal and, by precipitation of protein, suppresses the weeping and oozing of acutely inflamed lesions. Burow's solution, 1:40, is prepared by dissolving one packet or effervescent tablet (Domeboro effervescent tablets or packets, Dome Laboratories) in a pint of cool or tepid tap water.

For the best results, wet dressings are applied during the acute stage of the disorder for a period of up to five days with a soft cloth such as a man's handkerchief, a thin diaper, or strips of bed sheeting. Gauze squares are contraindicated because of their tendency to adhere to skin and cause irritation. Washcloths and heavy toweling interfere with evaporation and therefore are not as effective as soft cloth for this purpose.

Solutions should be tepid, lukewarm, or at body temperature. If too hot, vasodilatation occurs with resulting weeping and pruritus; if too cold, vasoconstriction occurs. This may relieve warmth and pruritus temporarily, but secondary vasodilatation soon develops, thus reversing the process. Compresses should be moderately wet, not dripping, and should be remoistened at intervals. Following the compress, a topical steroid may be applied and, in severe cases, the topical steroid may be applied both before and after the compress. The hydration by the wet compress relieves the dryness of the skin, breaks the skin surface barrier, and facilitates the penetration and action of the applied steroid preparation.

Dietary Restrictions. Although benefit from dietary restrictions may be interpreted with skepticism, many physicians advocate the elimination of specific foods in the management of atopic dermatitis during the first year or two of life. It is important to realize that in some instances specific foods may indeed produce a visible or clinically imperceptible urticarial reaction, vasodilatation, and possible effects on sweat secretion that may initiate pruritus and an associated exacerbation of a pre-existing dermatitis.[4, 18] For such infants, milk, wheat, eggs, tomatoes, citruses, chocolate, wheat products, spiced foods, fish, and nuts or peanut butter may be eliminated until the disorder is controlled by limiting baths and using mild soaps, frequent lubrication, topical corticosteroids, and appropriate antipruritic agents.

As the child grows older, food reactivity diminishes and the importance of inhalant allergens increases. In the older child, therefore, although food elimination is less often of value, a careful dietary history will occasionally reveal important information. Effective therapy requires a careful history, observation of ingestants that might trigger an exacerbation, particularly during the first year or two of life, at least a temporary elimination of suspected food allergens, and, of primary consideration, judicious management of the dry and itching skin characteristic of this disorder.

Skin Tests and Hyposensitization. These are of little value and rarely necessary in the management of children with atopic dermatitis. While patients with atopic dermatitis often demonstrate reactions to a variety of allergens, there is no proof that hyposensitization is beneficial. Although skin tests may occasionally provide clues to the cause of persistent or recurrent eruptions not responsive to the usual rational therapy, in general there seems to be little relationship between positive skin tests and the causation of flares.

Standards for patch testing in young children are poor, irritant reactions are frequent, and in children under eight years of age, false-negative and false-positive reactions are common.[32] When hyposensitization for respiratory allergies is carried out in a child with atopic dermatitis, care must be exercised to avoid flares of the dermatitis, which occasionally occur as the dose of extract is increased.[33]

As an alternative to skin tests, an in vitro test, the radioallergosorbent test (RAST) for serum IgE specific antigen, is currently commercially available. RAST may be more sensitive than prick or scratch skin tests but is less sensitive than intradermal testing and is substantially more expensive. Another test, the radioimmunosorbent technique (RIST), has also become available. Although raised total IgE levels can be determined by the RIST, and circulating reagins can be detected by the RAST, the value of these tests in the management of atopic dermatitis requires further investigation.

Topical Steroids. Potent steroid preparations are most effective in the treatment of atopic dermatitis. There is a science, however, to their use. It involves the selection of the correct strength corticosteroid in the proper formulation for the particular disease process and specific areas of involvement.[34]

The potency of topical steroids is related to their vehicle as well as to their chemical formulation.

In general, gels appear to penetrate more effectively, are somewhat more drying, are well accepted in hairy areas such as the scalp, and are particularly effective in the management of acute weeping or vesicular lesions. Steroid ointments afford the advantage of occlusion, more effective penetration, and greater efficacy than equivalent cream or lotion formulations. They are particularly effective in the management of dry, lichenified, or plaque-like areas of dermatitis. Ointment formulations, however, tend to occlude eccrine pores, may induce sweat retention and pruritus, and accordingly are not as well tolerated during the summer months when heat, perspiration, and high humidity are significant. Creams and lotions are somewhat less potent than gel and ointment formulations. They, however, afford the advantages of greater convenience and acceptability during hot weather and in intertriginous or hairy areas. It should be remembered that gels and lotions are drying and, except for wet or oozing lesions, are generally not indicated in the management of atopic dermatitis.

The use of steroid-impregnated polyethylene film, available as Cordran tape (Dista Products Company), or the occlusion of treated areas with polyethylene film, such as Saran wrap, appears to enhance the penetration of corticosteroids up to 100-fold. This mode of therapy is particularly effective for short periods of time (eight to twelve hours a day on successive days) for patients with chronic lichenified or recalcitrant plaques of dermatitic skin. Occlusive techniques, however, are contraindicated for prolonged periods of time, are not recommended in acute infected or intertriginous areas, and occasionally may result in local infection, miliaria, folliculitis, and, with prolonged use, in an increased incidence of atrophy and striae. Occlusive steroid dressings, accordingly, should be used for relatively short periods of time, with appropriate admonition regarding overuse and potential adverse reactions.

Many practitioners erroneously associate fluorination of glucocorticosteroids with biological potency. However, hydrocortisone butyrate (Locoid, Brocades, England; not available in the United States), a valerate derivative of hydrocortisone (Westcort cream, Westwood Pharmaceuticals) is a potent hydrocortisone preparation. Conversely, certain fluorinated agents, such as betamethasone alcohol, fluocinolone alcohol, and dexamethasone, are less effective than some of the more highly potent topical formulations. In Table 3–1 a summary of topical steroid potency based upon vasoconstrictor assays is presented in order to familiarize physicians with the relative potency of various steroid preparations. In this table, group I is the most potent and group VI is the least

Table 3–1 ORDER OF POTENCY OF TOPICAL STEROIDS
(From most to least potent)

I. Diprosone ointment 0.05%
Florone ointment 0.05%
Halog cream 0.1%
Lidex cream 0.05%
Lidex ointment 0.05%
Topicort ointment 0.25%
Topsyn gel 0.05%

II. Aristocort cream 0.5%
Diprosone cream 0.05%
Florone cream 0.05%
Flurobate gel 0.025%
 (Benisone gel)
Topicort cream 0.25%
Valisone lotion 0.1%
Valisone ointment 0.1%

III. Aristocort ointment 0.1%
Cordran ointment 0.05%
Kenalog ointment 0.1%
Synalar cream (HP) 0.2%
Synalar ointment 0.025%

IV. Cordran cream 0.05%
Kenalog cream 0.1%
Kenalog lotion 0.025%
Synalar cream 0.025%
Valisone cream 0.1%
Westcort cream 0.2%

V. Desonide cream 0.05%
Locorten cream 0.03%

VI. Topicals with hydrocortisone, Alphaderm, dexamethasone, flumethalone, prednisolone, methyl prednisolone.

From Stoughton RB: A perspective on topical corticosteroid therapy. In Farber EM, Cox AJ: Psoriasis, Proceedings of the Second International Symposium Yorke Medical Books. New York, 1976, p. 224. Updated by personal communication with Dr. Stoughton.

potent, with no significant difference between agents in any given group.[34]

Considering the wide use of topical corticosteroids, there have been relatively few reports of adverse reaction due to their absorption. When applied over large areas of dermatitic skin, or when used under occlusion, the possibility of systemic absorption, however, must be considered, particularly in infants and small children, and suppression of the pituitary-adrenal axis, although relatively uncommon, has been documented.[4, 35-39]

Other potential side effects of potent topical steroids, particularly when used under occlusion or for long periods of time, include cutaneous atrophy, steroid rosacea, striae (Fig. 3–18), and telangiectasia.[34] Potent topical steroids, however, may be used in small areas for short periods of time with little risk of absorption. Once the disorder is under control, it is advisable to taper the therapy to a moderately potent topical corticosteroid and, as the disorder continues to improve, to one of the milder potency hydrocortisone formulations. This gradual reduction of topical steroid potency over a period of weeks is advisable in an effort to avoid a rebound phenomenon that tends to occur with too rapid discontinuation of topical steroids. Following this gradual reduction of topical steroids, the disorder can frequently be rela-

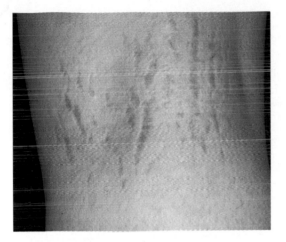

Figure 3–18 Atrophic striae. Shallow linear depressed lesions in the popliteal fossae due to prolonged use of potent topical corticosteroids.

tively well maintained by a regimen of limited baths, frequent lubrication, and antipruritics (as needed) in an effort to minimize the dryness and itchiness inherent in this disorder.

Tar Preparations. Although tar preparations have been replaced to a certain degree by topical corticosteroids, they are still effective in the management of subacute, chronic, and lichenified forms of dermatitis. The mechanism by which tar formulations act upon abnormal skin is not known, but they appear to have vasoconstrictive, astringent, disinfectant, and antipruritic properties, and help correct abnormal keratinization by a decrease in epidermal proliferation and dermal infiltration. Heretofore, many patients found tar formulations to be cosmetically objectionable. Newer, cosmetically acceptable preparations, however, have recently been made available. Of these, Estar gel (Westwood) and Psorigel (Owen Laboratories) appear to be well tolerated and effective. Prolonged use of tar preparations, however, may be associated with the production of folliculitis and, since tars tend to promote photosensitivity, they should be used with some degree of caution in sun-exposed areas. The incidence of this reaction, however, has probably been overstated; it is extremely uncommon.

Urea Formulations. Urea-containing preparations tend to produce a softening, hydrophilic, antibacterial, and anesthetic effect on the stratum corneum and occasionally appear to provide a therapeutic effect on dry skin, atopic dermatitis, and the pruritus associated with these disorders. Because of an occasional tendency toward stinging, 10 per cent rather than 20 per cent urea concentrations are frequently advisable in young children, particularly in those with acute or fissured dermatoses.[40, 41]

Urea may be formulated with topical corticosteroids or with emollient creams or lotions. Some of the presently available urea preparations include Aquacare-HP cream or lotion (Herbert La-

boratories), Nutraplus cream or lotion (Owen Laboratories), and Carmol-20 cream (Syntex).

Antihistamines. For proper management of the eczematous eruptions in atopic dermatitis, it is imperative that pruritus be controlled. Although various antihistamines have been used, their mode of action appears to be related to their sedative action as well as to their antihistaminic qualities. Hydroxyzine (Atarax or Vistaril) has excellent antihistaminic and antipruritic qualities, with less of a tendency to sedation. Benadryl or Phenergan is valuable when sedation is desirable.

Sedatives. For patients unable to sleep despite appropriate topical and antipruritic therapy, chloral hydrate is a valuable sedative and soporific. For children and infants it is available as a syrup (Noctec, Squibb), which contains 500 mg per teaspoonful, or as rectal suppositories containing 0.65 or 1.3 gm. The sedative dose of chloral hydrate for children is 10 to 20 mg/kg/dose, repeated, if necessary, at intervals of six to eight hours.

Systemic Steroids. Appropriate antibiotics are important in the treatment of secondary infection. Systemic steroids, however, should be reserved for only those few extremely severe cases that cannot be controlled by other means. Long-term steroid administration is seldom justified and frequently results in severe side effects.[38] An added problem following the use of systemic steroids is the difficulty in weaning patients from this form of therapy without severe and recurrent exacerbations. Therapy with lubrication, effective antipruritics, and potent topical steroids seldom makes this form of therapy necessary. Proper management, therefore, can usually control atopic dermatitis, even in the most severe cases, without necessitating the use of systemic steroids with their serious side effects, associated difficulties, and complications.

Pityriasis Alba

Pityriasis alba is a common cutaneous disorder characterized by discrete asymptomatic hypopigmented patches on the face, neck, upper trunk, and proximal extremities of children and young adults. Individual lesions vary from one to several centimeters in diameter and have sharply delineated margins and a fine branny scale (Fig. 3–19).

The cause is unknown, but this disorder appears to represent a non-specific dermatitis (possibly a form of atopic dermatitis). Most cases appear following sun exposure and result from a disturbance in pigmentation of the affected areas. This lack of pigment, formerly attributed to a screening effect by the thickened stratum corneum, appears to be related to interference in melanization of the epidermal cells.

Differential diagnosis includes tinea corporis, tinea versicolor, vitiligo, the white macules seen in association with tuberous sclerosis, and post-inflammatory hypopigmentation secondary to

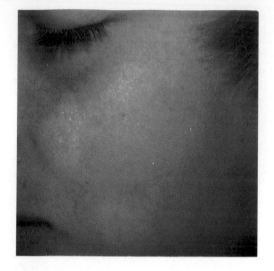

Figure 3-19 Pityriasis alba. Circumscribed scaly hypopigmented lesions on the cheek.

atopic dermatitis, psoriasis, or pityriasis rosea. Topical corticosteroids and lubrication followed by sun exposure appear to diminish the dry skin and fine scaling, allowing repigmentation of involved areas, generally within a period of several weeks.

Hyperimmunoglobulin E (Hyper IgE) Syndrome

In recent years a syndrome consisting of extremely high immunoglobulin E levels, repeated cutaneous infections, and chronic dermatitis was described.[42] Termed the hyperimmunoglobulin E syndrome, this disorder appears to have four main features. One is a tendency toward recurrent skin infections (usually staphylococcal but occasionally streptococcal) that usually begin in infancy and include superficial pustules, excoriated crusted plaques, cellulitis, suppurative lymphadenitis, and abscesses, and, in some individuals, candidiasis. Other features include extreme elevation of serum IgE (usually 10 times, often 100 times, that of normal values), defective neutrophil chemotaxis, peripheral blood eosinophilia in some individuals, and a personal or family history of atopy (often with an eczematoid eruption similar to that seen in atopic dermatitis).[43]

The term *Job's syndrome* refers to a subgroup of patients with the hyperimmunoglobulin E syndrome. Individuals with the Job syndrome are women who, in addition to displaying the major features of the hyper IgE syndrome, may have red hair, hyperextensible joints, and a tendency to develop huge cold, chronic, and recurrent staphylococcal abscesses that deform and distort the body contour. In such patients the elevated serum IgE does not appear to interfere with neutrophil or monocyte chemotaxis, but the impaired chemotaxis may be due to an intrinsic neutrophil defect.

A defective erythema response may explain the lack of redness, heat, or pain ordinarily associated with abscesses (hence the term "cold") in such patients.[44]

Other abnormalities seen with atopic dermatitis include an increased incidence of vitiligo, alopecia areata, and an increased susceptibility to warts, molluscum contagiosum, and tinea infection. Although the etiology of these phenomena remains uncertain, human infection with the papilloma virus and the subsequent appearance of warts is common and may be due in part to a defective immunologic mechanism. Present evidence suggests that patients with atopic dermatitis may have an associated defect in cell-mediated immunity that may impair host defense and account for recurrent warts or chronic molluscum contagiosum infection.[45]

Wiskott-Aldrich Syndrome

The Wiskott-Aldrich syndrome is an X-linked recessive disorder characterized by a triad of severe recalcitrant dermatitis, thrombocytopenia with bleeding, and recurrent pyogenic infection.[46] In this disorder male infants have defects in cell-mediated and humoral immunity, with low or absent antibodies to blood group antigens A and B (isohemagglutinins), deficient IgM levels (with compensatory increases in levels of IgA and IgE), impaired delayed hypersensitivity, and impaired or absent antibody response to virus infections and bacterial antigens.

This rare syndrome, confined to male infants, has its onset from the time of birth to four months of age. The clinical features of this disorder include an eczematoid eruption that usually begins on the scalp, face, buttocks, and antecubital and popliteal fossae shortly after birth (frequently during the second or third month of life). Affected infants are susceptible to a variety of bacterial, fungal, and virus infections, of which otitis media is the most prominent.

As the disease progresses the eczema becomes extensive, often purpuric, and a generalized exfoliative dermatitis frequently develops.

When exfoliative erythroderma occurs, it is refractory to therapy and usually persists until the death of the patient. Until recently, death usually occurred early in life, and almost always before the age of five to seven years, from overwhelming infection or hemorrhage or both. The oldest known survivor recorded to date is a 15-year-old[28] and, as in other immunoglobulin deficiency states, there is a high incidence of lymphoreticular malignancy in children who survive early childhood.

Treatment of the Wiskott-Aldrich syndrome consists of genetic counseling, appropriate topical therapy for the eczematoid eruption, antibiotics, periodic plasma transfusions in order to supplement the child's immunologic system, and the recently introduced use of transfer factor. Vigorous antibiotic therapy and the recent introduction of transfer factor appear to offer a more optimistic outlook for this severe and previously unresponsive disorder.

Lichen Simplex Chronicus

Lichen simplex chronicus (circumscribed neurodermatitis) is a localized, chronic pruritic disorder characterized by patches of dermatitis that result from repeated itching, scratching, and rubbing of the involved area. Although the etiology of this disorder is unknown, lesions are produced and perpetuated by rubbing and scratching. The pruritus may begin in an area of normal-appearing skin or may be initiated in a pre-existing lesion of atopic, seborrheic, or contact dermatitis, lichen planus, or psoriasis.

Lesions of lichen simplex chronicus, rarely seen in young children, generally occur in adolescents or adults (particularly women), with a peak incidence in adults between 30 and 50 years of age. The disorder may develop at any location on the body, but the most common areas of involvement are those that are easily reached and may be scratched unobtrusively (particularly during periods of tension and concentration). These include the nape or sides of the neck, the wrists, ankles, and pretibial areas (Fig. 3–20). Other common sites of involvement include the inner aspects of the thighs, the vulva, scrotum, and perianal areas.

The clinical features of lichen simplex chronicus include single or multiple oval plaques with a long axis measuring anywhere from five to 15 centimeters in diameter. During the early stages the skin is reddened and slightly edematous and normal markings are somewhat exaggerated. Older lesions are characterized by well-circumscribed patches of dry, thickened, scaly, pruritic hyper- or hypopigmented plaques. At times flat-topped confluent excoriated papules may be seen in the center of lesions.

The diagnosis of lichen simplex chronicus is dependent on the presence of pruritic lichenified plaques in the characteristic sites of predilection. Lesions of tinea corporis may be differentiated by a lack of lichenification, by the presence of a vesicular or scaly border (often with clearing in the center), demonstration of hyphae on microscopic examination of skin scrapings, and by fungal culture. Psoriatic plaques generally may be differentiated by a characteristic thick, adherent white or silvery scale, their underlying deep red hue, and characteristic areas of involvement. Lesions of atopic dermatitis may be differentiated by history, the presence of atopic stigmata, and a tendency toward involvement in antecubital and popliteal areas.

The histopathologic appearance of lesions of lichen simplex chronicus is that of a chronic dermatitis. It is characterized by hyperkeratosis, areas of parakeratosis, acanthosis, and elongation of the rete ridges. Spongiosis may be present, but vesiculation does not occur. Dermal papillae are broad and elongated, and there is a chronic perivascular inflammatory infiltrate accompanied by fibroblasts and fibrosis in the dermis.

The successful management of lichen simplex chronicus depends upon an appreciation of the itch-scratch-itch cycle and the associated scratching and rubbing that accompany and perpetuate this disorder. Topical application of potent corticosteroids, under occlusion if necessary, and the administration of systemic antipruritics (antihistamine or hydroxyzine) will usually induce remission of the pruritus and the eruption within a period of several weeks. Open wet compresses with tepid tap water or Burow's solution will hasten resolution of chronic as well as acutely inflamed lesions. In particularly stubborn lesions, occlusive dressings and the use of an intralesional steroid (triamcinolone acetonide diluted with isotonic saline or lidocaine to a concentration of 5 mg per ml) may be necessary.

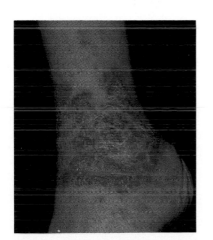

Figure 3–20 Infected lichen simplex chronicus (neurodermatitis).

Seborrheic Dermatitis

Seborrheic dermatitis is a term used to refer to an erythematous, scaly or crusting eruption that occurs primarily in the so-called "seborrheic" areas (those with a highest concentration of sebaceous glands), namely the scalp, face, postauricular, presternal, and intertriginous areas. Although the specific etiology of seborrheic dermatitis remains unknown, it appears to be related to an inflammatory reaction of the skin in constitutionally predisposed individuals. Many attempts have been made to relate infection with bacteria or *Pityrosporum ovale* to the etiology of this disorder. Although seborrheic dermatitis frequently has been associated with increased susceptibility to pyogenic infection, there is no evidence that these organisms play any role as primary pathogens of this disorder.

PATHOGENESIS. Seborrheic dermatitis is most commonly seen in infants and adolescents. It appears in infancy between the second and tenth weeks of life (usually the third or fourth) and, although it may continue throughout life, it usually clears spontaneously by eight to twelve months and generally does not recur until the onset of puberty. Infantile seborrheic dermatitis often begins with a non-eczematous erythematous scaly dermatitis of the scalp (termed "cradle cap") or the diaper area and is manifested by thin dry scales or sharply defined round or oval patches covered by thick, yellowish-brown greasy crusts (Figs. 2–6, 2–8). Although infantile seborrheic dermatitis has many features in common with seborrheic dermatitis of adolescence and adult life, it lacks the presence of follicular lesions and clinically evident seborrhea normally seen in association with seborrheic dermatitis as seen in older individuals.[47]

DIAGNOSIS. The disorder commonly begins and may be confined to the scalp in infants, but may progress and spread downward over the forehead, ears, eyebrows, nose, and back of the head. Erythematous greasy salmon-colored scaly lesions may involve other parts of the body, particularly the intertriginous and flexural areas of the body (see Fig. 3–13), the postauricular areas (see Fig. 3–14), the trunk, umbilicus, anogenital areas, and groin (see Fig. 2–19). Pruritus is slight or absent, and the disorder usually lacks the stigmata generally associated with atopic dermatitis. The prognosis of seborrheic dermatitis, even without treatment, is usually good and most cases clear spontaneously, usually within a period of several weeks or months. Although infantile seborrheic dermatitis may at times be succeeded by atopic dermatitis such cases may result from a chance occurrence. To date there is no evidence that these two disorders are constitutionally or genetically related.

The diagnostic features of infantile seborrheic dermatitis are its early onset, lack of pruritus and stigmata of atopy, a greasy yellowish or salmon-colored scale, the generally well-circumscribed nature of the lesions, and its predisposition for the scalp and intertriginous regions. Differentiation of this disorder from Letterer-Siwe disease is predicated upon the lack of purpura, hepatosplenomegaly, lymphadenopathy, anemia, thrombocytopenia, and osseous lesions, and, if the diagnosis remains in doubt, histopathologic examination of cutaneous lesions.

The histopathologic picture of seborrheic dermatitis is not diagnostic. The pathologic findings are those of a low-grade inflammatory process, with parakeratosis, moderate acanthosis, some elongation of the rete ridges, and slight intracellular edema and spongiosis. Although the histologic picture has features of both psoriasis and chronic dermatitis, the presence of spongiosis generally is lacking in lesions of psoriasis, thus helping in the histopathologic differentiation of these two disorders.

In infants, when the erythema and scaling of seborrheic dermatitis becomes severe, generalized, and exfoliative, the diagnosis of *Leiner's disease* must be considered. Previously this disease was considered to be a variant of seborrheic dermatitis, but this relationship has never been proven. Infantile seborrheic dermatitis may be differentiated from Leiner's disease by a lack of constitutional findings (diarrhea, fever, inanition), alopecia, a lack of associated infections, and the relatively benign nature of seborrheic dermatitis (see Leiner's Disease, Chapter 2 and Fig. 2–9).

Between puberty and middle age, seborrheic dermatitis may appear on the scalp as a dry fine flaky desquamation commonly known as pityriasis sicca or dandruff. This disorder is an extreme form of normal desquamation in which scales of the scalp become abundant and visible. Erythema and scaling of various degrees may also involve the supraorbital areas between the eyebrows and above the bridge of the nose, the nasolabial crease, lips, pinna, retroauricular areas and the aural canal.

Occasionally a patient may have an eruption that has clinical features of both seborrheic dermatitis and psoriasis. Such eruptions may be termed *seborrhiasis* or *sebopsoriasis*. Lesions of seborrheic dermatitis can be differentiated from those of psoriasis by a lack of the characteristic vivid red hue, micaceous scale, a predisposition toward flexural rather than extensor aspects of the extremities, and the fact that lesions of seborrhea generally tend to remain within the confines of the hairline. Lesions of psoriasis (or seborrhiasis) frequently extend beyond the hairline and, in general, are more resistant to standard antiseborrheic therapy.

Blepharitis is a form of seborrheic dermatitis in which the eyelid margins are red and covered with small white scales. Seborrheic dermatitis may also involve the sideburns, beard, and mustache areas, with diffuse redness, greasy scaling, and pustulation. The severity and course of seborrheic eruptions of the eyelids and bearded areas are variable and have a tendency to chronicity and recurrence.

TREATMENT. The therapy of seborrheic dermatitis depends on the nature, severity, and location of the disorder. If one concentrates on clearing the scalp lesions in infantile seborrheic dermatitis, the remainder of the eruption usually responds rapidly to topical corticosteroid preparations, alone or in combination with iodochlorhydroxyquin, (Vioform or Vioform-HC, Ciba, or Vytone cream, Dermik Laboratories). The scalp should be treated with an antiseborrheic shampoo. Those containing sulfur or salicylic acid, or both, are generally satisfactory. If the scale is extremely thick and adherent, it can be loosened by warmed mineral oil massaged into the scalp or by the use of "P&S" liquid (Chester A. Baker Laboratories). When used, "P&S" liquid should be allowed to remain on the scalp for a period of eight to twelve hours, followed by scrubbing with the fingers or a soft brush in an effort to loosen the scales prior to an appropriate shampoo. In stubborn cases, a

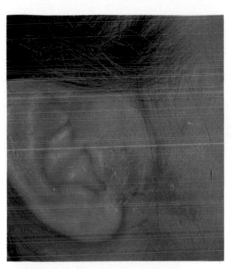

Figure 3–21 Infectious eczematoid dermatitis of the pre-auricular area. The clinical picture is that of impetigo associated with and spreading beyond the preceding eczematous or seborrheic lesions.

topical corticosteroid lotion, with or without 3 to 5 per cent sulfur precipitate or salicylic acid, or both, may be used on the infant's scalp one to three times daily.

Adolescents with seborrhea of the scalp may use similar antiseborrheic shampoos. Those with more stubborn involvement may use shampoos containing pyrithione, hydroxyquinolin, tars, or selenium sulfide. For patients with associated erythema or pruritus, topical steroid lotions or sprays may be utilized.

Lesions of seborrheic dermatitis on other areas of the body respond rapidly to topical corticosteroid creams. Since it is advisable to avoid high-potency fluorinated steroids on the face, topical preparations such as desonide (Tridesilon, Dome) or hydrocortisone cream in a 1.0 per cent concentration may be utilized. Blepharitis may be managed by gentle warm water compresses followed by topical sulfacetamide ointment (Sulamyd) or sulfacetamide with 0.5 per cent prednisolone (Metimyd, Schering). Corticosteroids on the eyelids must be used with caution.

COMPLICATIONS. Seborrheic dermatitis of the intertriginous or diaper areas occasionally may be complicated by secondary monilial or bacterial infection. Iodochlorhydroxyquin cream, available as Vioform or Vioform-HC (Ciba), Vytone (Dermik), or preparations containing anticandidal or antibacterial agents or both generally are helpful. For patients refractory to topical treatment or for those with extensive secondary bacterial infection (*infectious eczematoid dermatitis* (Fig. 3–21), bacterial cultures and appropriate systemic antibiotics are frequently necessary.

Intertrigo

Intertrigo is a superficial inflammatory dermatitis that occurs in areas where the skin is in apposition (Figs. 3–13 and 3–14). As a result of friction, heat, and moisture, the affected areas become erythematous, macerated, and secondarily infected by bacteria or fungi.

Treatment is directed toward elimination of the macerated skin. Open wet compresses, dusting powders (ZeaSorb), topical steroid lotions, and, when indicated, appropriate antibiotics or fungicidal agents may be used.

Pompholyx

Pompholyx (dyshidrotic eczema) is a term used to describe a non-specific acute recurrent or chronic eczematous eruption of the palms, soles, and lateral aspects of the fingers. Of unknown etiology, it is characterized by deep-seated vesicles in various inflammatory stages, hyperhidrosis, and, at times, an associated burning or itching. The distribution of lesions generally is bilateral and somewhat symmetrical. Attacks usually last a few weeks but, because of frequent relapses, may persist for longer periods of time.

Although the cause of dyshidrotic eczema is unknown, it occurs chiefly in nervous individuals and, in many instances, emotional stress appears to be a provocative factor. Attacks of pompholyx are characterized by the sudden appearance of crops of clear "sago-grain"-like vesicles. The contents are commonly clear or colorless; occasionally they may become straw-colored or purulent. Vesicles rapidly become confluent and, at times, may present as large bullae.

When unilateral or only affecting one area of the hands, pompholyx may be confused with contact dermatitis. "Id" reactions, pustular psoriasis, and primary fungal infections must be considered in the differential diagnosis of this disorder. The true diagnosis can be differentiated, however, on the basis of fungal culture and histopathologic examination of lesions. Histologic examination of biopsied lesions reveals intra-epidermal vesicles with balloon cells, usually little or no inflammatory changes, and varying degrees of spongiosis.

The natural course of pompholyx is one of frequent recurrence (often several times a year). Although not a disorder of eccrine glands, per se, the use of 20 per cent topical aluminum chloride, available as Drysol (Person & Covey) is at times helpful in the control of this disorder. Open wet compresses tend to macerate and open the vesicles, and applications of topical corticosteroid creams, although not curative, help to relieve the manifestations of this disorder. When stress or nervousness appears to be a factor, sedative or mild tranquilizing agents may be helpful and, when infection is present, antibiotics may be administered topically or systemically.

Lichen Striatus

Lichen striatus is a self-limiting, usually unilateral, linear dermatitis of unknown origin that usually occurs in children. It consists of discrete and confluent, minute, slightly raised lichenoid papules that evolve suddenly, usually on an extremity, but occasionally may involve the face, neck, trunk, or buttocks. It may occur early in infancy, generally affects children between the ages of 5 and 10 years, and, on occasion, has been reported in older individuals.

Girls appear to be infected two to three times as frequently as males. The eruption is asymptomatic, reaches its maximum extent within several days to a few weeks, and generally regresses spontaneously within a period of six months to a year. The involved area varies from several millimeters to one or two centimeters in width and is characterized by a linear band of small flat-topped pink or flesh-colored papules, occasionally surmounted by a fine silvery scale (Fig. 3–22). In dark-skinned or tanned individuals the eruption may appear as a scaly or papular band-like area of hypopigmentation (Fig. 3–23). Although the band is usually continuous, it may occasionally be interrupted or interspersed by coalescent plaques several centimeters in diameter along the area of linear configuration.

The differential diagnosis of lichen striatus is not difficult if the disorder is kept in mind. It may be recognized by its highly characteristic linear appearance. The differential diagnosis includes nevus unius lateris, linear lichen planus, psoriasis, tinea corporis, and verruca plana. When the diagnosis remains in doubt, histopathologic examination of a cutaneous biopsy will help exclude other possible linear eruptions.

The histologic changes of lichen striatus are similar to those of a chronic dermatitis. The prima-

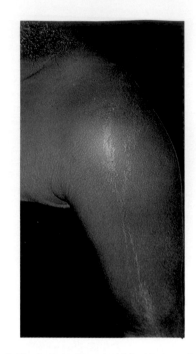

Figure 3–23 A dark-skinned child with hypopigmented linear papular lesions of lichen striatus.

ry feature of this disorder is a dense, usually perivascular, but occasionally band-like, lymphohistiocytic infiltrate of the dermis.[48] The epidermis may show slight invasion by lymphocytes, with focal areas of acanthosis, parakeratosis, and spongiosis, and occasionally dyskeratotic cells resembling the grains and corps ronds of Darier's disease may be seen in the granular layer.

Lichen striatus is an asymptomatic self-limiting disorder of relatively short duration. Although therapy is not necessary, for those who for cosmetic reasons or otherwise prefer treatment, topical corticosteroids, steroids under occlusion, or intralesional steroids may hasten resolution of lesions.

Frictional Lichenoid Dermatitis

Frictional lichenoid dermatitis (frictional lichenoid eruption, juvenile papular dermatitis, recurrent summertime pityriasis of the elbows and knees) is a recurring cutaneous disorder affecting children, especially boys, between 4 and 12 years of age. Most cases are seen in the spring and summer months when outdoor activities are common and many cases are associated with playing in sand-boxes (sand-box dermatitis).

The eruption is characterized by aggregates of discrete lichnoid papules, one or two millimeters in diameter, which occur primarily on the elbows, knees, and backs of the hands of children in whom such areas are subject to minor frictional trauma without protection of clothing (Fig. 3–24). Lesions may be hypopigmented, pruritus is occasionally but not necessarily present, and it is my impres-

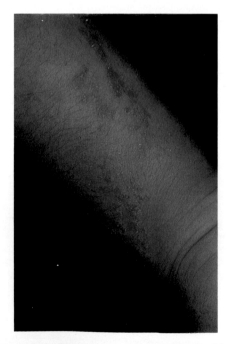

Figure 3–22 Lichen striatus. A self-limiting, usually unilateral linear dermatitis generally seen on the extremities of children.

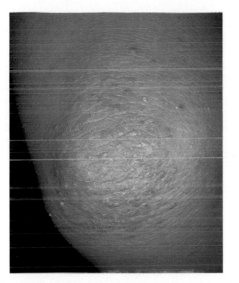

Figure 3–24 Frictional lichenoid dermatitis. Aggregates of lichenoid papules occur primarily on the elbows, knees, knuckles, and backs of the hands of children.

sion that many children with this disorder have a predisposition to atopy.

Histopathologic changes are non-specific and include hyperkeratosis, a moderate degree of acanthosis, and areas of lymphocytic infiltration in the upper dermis. The differential diagnosis of this disorder includes psoriasis and the Gianotti-Crosti syndrome (a disorder of young children characterized by clustered flesh-colored lichenoid papules, one to five millimeters in diameter, on the legs, thighs, buttocks, extensor aspects of the arms and, finally, the face, of undetermined, possibly viral, etiology, which generally resolves spontaneously within a period of six weeks) (Fig. 3–25).

The management of frictional lichenoid dermatitis includes avoidance of frictional trauma to the involved areas (as might occur with leaning on elbows and knees) and the use of topical cortico-steroids and lubricating creams, with or without the addition of 10 to 20 per cent urea.[49, 50]

Nummular Eczema

Nummular eczema is a cutaneous eruption characterized by discoid or coin-shaped plaques of eczema. The name is derived from the Latin word "nummulus," which refers to its coin-like size and configuration.

Lesions of nummular eczema are composed of minute papules and vesicles, which enlarge by peripheral extension to form discrete, round or oval erythematous, often lichenfied and hyperpigmented plaques varying in size from one to several centimeters in diameter (see Fig. 3–15). They usually occur on the extensor surfaces of the hands, arms, and legs, as single or multiple lesions, on dry or asteatotic skin. Pruritus is variable. Occasionally the face and trunk may be involved.

The specific etiology of this disorder is unknown; however, it seems to appear in a cold or dry environment and is aggravated by excessive bathing and local irritants such as wool or harsh or drying soaps. There have been conflicting reports in the literature regarding the association of nummular eczema with atopic dermatitis. This relationship has been refuted by a lack of increase in the incidence of atopy and relatively normal IgE levels in patients with this eruption. Nummular eczema is a scaly dermatosis that appears related to dry skin rather than to atopy.[27] Since pathogenic staphylococci have been cultured from lesions of nummular eczema and since, at times, the disease appears to improve with antibiotic administration, it has been suggested that micro-organisms may contribute to the pathogenesis and persistence of this disorder.

Nummular eczema must be differentiated from allergic contact dermatitis, atopic dermatitis, psoriasis, and superficial dermatophyte infections of the skin. This disorder is characterized by pinpoint vesicles and generally shows the histologic picture of a subacute dermatitis with

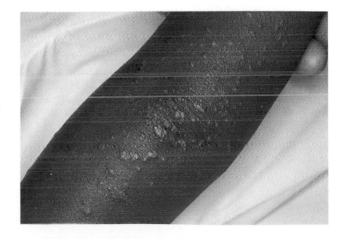

Figure 3–25 Gianotti-Crosti disease (infantile lichenoid acrodermatitis).

acanthosis and scattered intradermal vesicles at various levels of the epidermis surrounded by spongiosis.

Effective therapy depends upon limited baths, frequent lubrication, and potent topical steroids, preferably in an ointment base or under occlusion (assuming, of course, that associated secondary infection is controlled).

Winter Eczema

Winter eczema (eczema hiemalis), also known as asteatotic eczema, eczema craquelée, or xerotic eczema, is a subacute eczematous dermatitis characterized by pruritic scaly erythematous patches, usually associated with dryness and dehydration (asteatosis) of the epidermis. Generally seen on the extremities, occasionally the trunk, these changes are most frequent during wintertime when the humidity is low, particularly in older individuals and adolescents who bathe or shower frequently with harsh or drying soaps. Frequent bathing with incomplete drying and resultant evaporation of moisture causes dehydration of the epidermis, with redness, scaling, and fine cracking that may resemble cracked porcelain (hence the term eczema craquelée).

The diagnosis of eczema hiemalis is established by the characteristic eczematous, occasionally fissured, patches of dermatitis overlying dry (xerotic) skin in individuals with a history of frequent bathing or showering and exposure to low temperatures and low humidity.

The treatment of winter eczema is centered around the maintenance of proper hydration of the stratum corneum and is dependent upon the routine use of emollients or lubricating creams or lotions, limitation of bathing (with mild soaps such as Dove or Neutragena), the use of humidifiers where feasible, and topical corticosteroids (preferably those in an ointment base) for individual lesions.

Infectious Eczematoid Dermatitis

Infectious eczematoid dermatitis is a term used to describe a distinct clinical form of dermatitis in which secondary bacterial infection is superimposed upon lesions of atopic, nummular, or seborrheic dermatitis (see Fig. 3–21). In this disorder the dermatitis extends from preceding lesions and is characterized by circumscribed eczematous plaques, with vesicles, pustules, exudation and/or crusting on an erythematous base. Coagulase-positive *Staphylococcus aureus* is the organism most frequently associated with this disorder.

Infectious eczematoid dermatitis is best managed by appropriate systemic antibiotics based upon bacterial culture and sensitivities, open wet dressings, and topical application of corticosteroids. In cases that are not severe, topical antibiotics and topical corticosteroids without systemic antibiotics may be adequate. When systemic antibiotics are used, the concomitant use of topical antibiotics generally is not necessary.

Fixed Drug Eruption

Fixed drug eruption is a term used to describe a sharply localized, circumscribed round or oval dermatitis that characteristically recurs in the same site or sites each time the offending drug is administered. Lesions are solitary at first, but with repeated attacks, new lesions usually appear and existing lesions may tend to increase in size. The lesions tend to be erythematous and dusky at their onset with well-defined borders. At times they may become bullous, with subsequent desquamation or crusting and a residual hyperpigmentation that may persist for months.

The mechanism of the production of fixed drug eruptions remains unknown. Phenolphthalein is the most common of the long list of drugs capable of causing this disorder. Other causative preparations include barbiturates, penicillin, streptomycin, sulfonamides, antipyrine, quinine and its derivatives, salicylates, potassium iodide, atabrine, emetine (Ipecac), gold, phenylbutazone, chlordiazepoxide (Librium), and diphenylhydantoin (Dilantin).[51]

In the early stages of fixed drug eruption, histopathologic examination of lesions may reveal subepidermal bullae with degeneration of the detached portion of the epidermis (not unlike the picture seen in erythema multiforme). In the late stages, melanin may be seen within macrophages in the upper dermis, and there is an increase in the amount of melanin in the basal layers of the epidermis.

Contact Dermatitis

Contact dermatitis may be defined as an eczematous eruption produced either by local exposure to a primary irritating substance or by an acquired allergic response to a sensitizing substance (Fig. 3–26). When the dermatitis is due to a non-allergic reaction of the skin, it is termed an *irritant contact dermatitis;* when a manifestation of delayed hypersensitivity to a contact allergen, it is termed *allergic contact dermatitis.* An eczematous allergen is defined as a substance that is not primarily irritating on a first exposure, but with repeated exposure, causes an allergic sensitization of the delayed type. A primary eczematous irritant, on the other hand, may be defined as a substance that produces an eczematous response on the basis of irritation rather than by immunologic means.[52]

PRIMARY IRRITANT DERMATITIS. The skin in infancy is thin and highly vascularized, reddens quickly when irritated, and appears to be more resistant to contact sensitization than that of older children and adults. Common substances that produce primary irritant dermatitis include harsh soaps, bleaches, detergents, solvents, acids

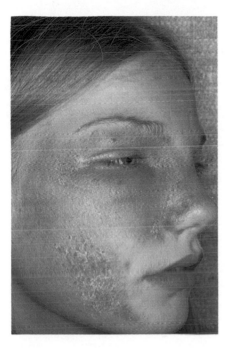

Figure 3–26 Contact dermatitis. Poison ivy (rhus) dermatitis.

(Fig. 3–27), alkalis, fiberglass particles, baby oils containing antiseptics such as oxyquinoline sulfate, bubble baths, certain foods, saliva, talcum particles, urine, feces, and intestinal secretions. The only variation in the severity of the dermatitis from person to person, or from time to time in the same person, is a result of the condition of the skin at the time of exposure, the strength of the irritant, the location of the eruption, the cumulative effect of repeated exposures to the irritating substance, and local factors such as perspiration, maceration, and occlusion.[53]

ALLERGIC CONTACT DERMATITIS. The incidence of allergic contact dermatitis in children is far less (approximately one eighth) than seen in adults, with figures of 1.5 per cent in the former as compared to 13 per cent in older age groups.[54] The

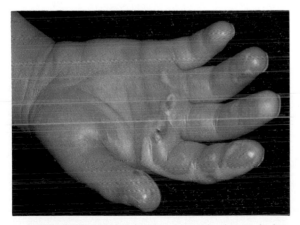

Figure 3–27 Primary irritant dermatitis due to hydrochloric acid, with blistering.

process responsible for contact sensitization appears to be deficient at birth and matures more slowly than other processes of resistance and immunity such as phagocytosis and circulating antibody formation.

Infants below the age of one year have a markedly depressed ability to react to allergens; children between one and three have an intermediate ability; and children between three and eight years are readily sensitized and show a depth of sensitivity and intensity of reaction comparable to that seen in adults.[55, 56] The decreased reactivity of infant skin to potential allergens, although not completely understood, appears to be related to the decreased exposure of infants and young children to potential sensitizing allergens and a decreased function of cell-mediated immune mechanisms in this age group.

The capacity to become sensitized is probably under genetic control. The mechanism of sensitization is not well understood, but it appears to be a classic example of type IV (delayed) hypersensitivity (see Chapter 19). The presence of antibodies in allergic contact dermatitis remains unproven, but evidence suggests an antibody-like reaction associated with sensitized tissue lymphocytes as the mediators of these responses. The allergen may be the contactant itself or a derivative of the contactant metabolized within the skin. The eczematous reaction is elicited by the contact of the specific circulating cells with localized antigen, which in turn causes the development of an inflammatory process.[57]

Allergic contact dermatitis may develop within seven to ten days following initial exposure to a sensitizing substance, or exposure may continue for months or even years before manifestations of allergy develop. Once the area has become sensitized, however, re-exposure to the offending allergen may result in an acute dermatitis within a relatively brief period (generally eight to twelve hours following exposure to the sensitizing allergen).

The diagnosis of allergic contact dermatitis is made on the appearance and distribution of skin lesions, aided, when possible, by a history of contact with an appropriate allergen. Acute eczematous lesions are characterized by an intense erythema accompanied by edema, papules, vesiculation (sometimes bullae), oozing, and a sharp line of demarcation between the involved and normal skin (Fig. 3–28). In the subacute phase, vesiculation is less pronounced and is mixed with crusting, scaling, and thickening of the skin. Chronic lesions, conversely, are characterized by lichenification, fissuring, scaling, and little or no vesiculation.[58]

Clinically, the distribution of lesions is characterized by the mode of sensitization. In the infant and young child, circumoral dermatitis may appear as a response to a primary irritant, or as an allergic contact dermatitis from foods such as tomatoes, oranges, carrots, or spinach. Here the dermatitis is caused by direct contact with the

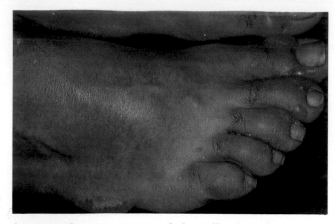

Figure 3–28 Contact dermatitis due to the dye in a sandal made of the hide of the water buffalo (water-buffalo sandal dermatitis).

skin, not from ingestion of the offending food substances. This may be aggravated by regurgitation of food particles, dribbling of saliva, and rubbing of the involved areas.

The histopathologic picture of eczematous allergic contact dermatitis generally is not pathognomonic of this condition and seldom permits differentiation from other forms of eczema. The histologic description for acute, subacute, and chronic dermatitis, therefore, applies in general to contact dermatitis.

Patch Testing. The patch test, a valuable aid in the diagnosis of contact skin sensitivity in older children and adults, is frequently unreliable in children below the age of one year and (as a consequence of the fact that normal adult reactivity is not reached until seven to eight years of age) often difficult to interpret in children under the age of eight years.

When patch testing is used, patches should be placed on grossly normal, non-hairy skin. Patch testing should be deferred in the presence of extensive active dermatitis, at which time the entire skin may be irritable, false-positive reactions may be obtained, and a strongly positive patch-test reaction may cause acute exacerbation of the dermatitis. The systemic administration of corticosteroids is not a contraindication to patch testing and, although patch testing of patients while they are on corticosteroid therapy might tend to mask weak patch test responses (which are of little clinical significance), it generally will not mask or alter significant reactions to allergens applied in standard concentrations.

Patch tests generally should be kept in place for 48 hours, and a reading can be made after an interval of 20 to 60 minutes following removal of the patch. This brief time interval is required in order to allow the skin to recover from the effects of pressure, which may produce mild transient erythema or a temporary blanching effect, resulting in false reactions. Doubtful reactions should be read again after a period of 24 hours. Unless testing for weak sensitizers (such as fabrics or cosmetics), a 1 plus (1+) reaction (simple erythema) is usually of no clinical significance. Erythema and papules indicate a 2 plus (2+) reaction; erythema, papules, and vesicles are read as 3 plus

(3+); and marked edema and vesicles indicate four plus reactions (4+).[53]

It must be remembered that occasionally positive reactions may have no clinical significance. Similarly, the offending material may not give rise to a positive reaction at the site of the test, but may show a positive test if carried out on an area of skin closer to the point of the previously existing dermatitis. The value of patch tests is corroborative and should be used only as a guide in an attempt to confirm a suspected allergen. Furthermore, scratch and intracutaneous tests are not indicated in contact dermatitis, since this condition is neither mediated by nor associated with skin sensitizing antibodies.[57]

Poison Ivy (Rhus Dermatitis). In the United States, poison ivy, poison oak, and poison sumac produce more cases of allergic contact dermatitis than all other contactants combined.[53, 58] The plants causing poison ivy dermatitis are included under the botanical term Rhus. Poison ivy and poison oak are the principal causes of Rhus dermatitis in the United States.

The poison ivy plant, with its characteristic three leaflets more or less notched at the edge, grows luxuriantly as a shrub or woody rope-like vine in vacant lots, among grasses, and on trees or fences throughout all sections of the United States except the extreme southwest. Poison sumac grows as a shrub or tree, never as a vine. It has 7 to 13 leaflets (arranged in pairs along a central stem) with a single leaflet at the end, is relatively uncommon, grows less abundantly, and is found only in woody or swampy areas primarily east of the Mississippi River. Poison oak, conversely, grows as an upright shrub, is most prominent on the west coast, and is not a problem in the eastern United States. Although Rhus dermatitis is more common in the summertime, the eruption may occur at any time of year by direct contact with the sensitising allergen from the leaves, roots, or twigs of plants.

No matter which of the rhus plants produces the eruption there is no difference in the antigen or clinical appearance of the dermatitis. Furthermore, since the Rhus group belongs to the family of plants known as Anacardiacae, cross reactions may occur with chemicals and nuts from related plants, namely furniture lacquer derived from the Japanese lacquer tree, oil from the shell of the cashew nut, the fruit pulp of the gingko tree (a large ornamental tree of China and Japan), the rind of the mango, and the marking nut tree of India, from which a black "ink" used to mark wearing apparel is produced. The allergic contact dermatitis to this ink is termed "dhobi itch."[53]

Pathogenesis. The eruption produced by poison ivy and related plants is a delayed contact hypersensitivity reaction to an oleoresin (uroshiol) of which the active sensitizing ingredient is pentadecylcatechol. It is characterized by itching, redness, papules, vesicles, and bullae (see Fig. 3–26). A linear distribution, the Koebner reaction, with an irregular spotty distribution is highly characteristic of the eruption (Fig. 3–29). When contact is indirect, such as from a pet that has the oleoresin on its fur, the dermatitis is often diffuse, thus making the diagnosis more difficult unless the true nature of exposure is suspected. In the fall, when brush and leaves are burned, it must be remembered that the sensitizing oil may be vaporized and transmitted by smoke to exposed cutaneous surfaces.

Rhus dermatitis usually appears, in susceptible individuals, within one to three days after contact with the sensitizing oleoresin; in highly sensitive individuals it may occur within eight hours of exposure. Such temporal differences are probably due to the degree of exposure, individual susceptibility, and regional variation in cutaneous reactivity.

About 70 per cent of the population of the United States would acquire Rhus dermatitis if exposed to the plants or the sensitizing oleoresin contained in its leaves, stems, and roots. The result is an acute eczematous eruption, which, barring complications or re-exposure to the offending allergen, persists for a variable period of one to three weeks.

Management. The best prophylaxis, as with any type of allergic contact dermatitis, is complete avoidance of the offending allergen. Patients should be instructed in how to recognize and avoid members of the poison Rhus group. Unfortunately, no topical measure is effective in the prevention of poison ivy dermatitis. When poison ivy is present in the garden or children's play areas, chemical destruction or physical removal is indicated.

In an effort to minimize the degree of dermatitis, individuals with known exposure should wash thoroughly as rapidly as possible so that removal of the oil is accomplished, preferably within five to ten minutes of exposure. If the oleoresin is not carefully removed shortly after exposure, the allergen may be transmitted by the fingers to other parts of the body (particularly the face, forearms, or male genitalia). Contrary to popular belief, however, the fluid content of vesicles and bullae is not contagious and does not produce new lesions. Thus, unless the sensitizing antigen is still on the skin, the disorder is neither autoinocuous nor contagious from one person to another.

Complete change of clothing is advisable and, whenever possible, contaminated clothing should be washed with soap and water. Harsh soaps and vigorous scrubbing offer no advantage over simple soaking and cool water. Thorough washing does not prevent a severe dermatitis in highly sensitive persons. It may, however, reduce the reaction and prevent spread of the oleoresin. When early washing is not feasible, it is worthwhile to wash at the first opportunity in an effort to remove any oleoresin remaining on the skin or clothing and thereby prevent its transfer to other parts of the body.

In the management of mild Rhus dermatitis, treatment with an antipruritic "shake" lotion such as calamine lotion is helpful. Topical preparations containing potential sensitizers such as antihistamines or benzocaine and zirconium, however, should be avoided. As in other acute eczematous eruptions, cool compresses with plain tap water or Burow's solution are soothing, help remove crusts, and relieve pruritus. Administration of potent topical corticosteroids and the systemic use of antihistamines and antipruritic agents are helpful. Topical steroids, however, are only partially effective in the acute stages of Rhus dermatitis. They are helpful in suppressing the pruritic manifestations and give temporary relief, but do little to hasten involution of individual lesions. Aerosol-type sprays, gels, or lotions are often helpful. Because they cover the acutely involved areas more easily and have a drying tendency, they appear to be beneficial in the management of acute weeping and bullous lesions. Aseptic aspiration of large vesicles or bullae is frequently helpful and assists in the relief of discomforting symptoms associated with such lesions.

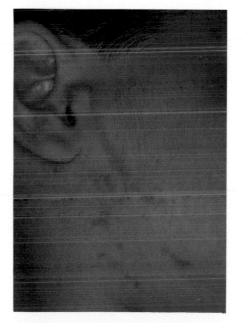

Figure 3–29 Characteristic linear distribution (Koebner reaction) in poison ivy (rhus) dermatitis.

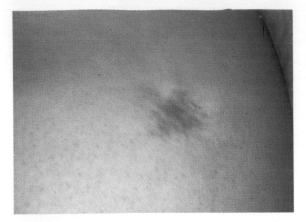

Figure 3–30 Local atrophy of buttock due to intralesional steroid injection (most cases fortunately resolve spontaneously, generally within a period of six to fourteen months).

In severe and incapacitating cases of Rhus dermatitis, short-term systemic corticosteroid treatment may be indicated. Systemic steroid therapy may be initiated with dosages in the range of 20 to 30 mg of prednisone or its equivalent, with gradually tapering dosages over a period of two to three weeks. Premature termination of systemic steroids may result in a rapid rebound, with return of the dermatitis to its original intensity. The use of systemic steroids in injectable form should be discouraged, however, since the dosage can be neither modified nor terminated in the event of adverse reaction or need for change in therapy (Fig. 3–30).

Desensitization to the oleoresin of poison ivy by the systemic administration of Rhus antigen remains controversial at this time. Standardization of material is difficult, and systemic reactions are not uncommon with the use of hyposensitization procedures. For those cases where hyposensitization is deemed advisable, a reliable active oleoresin is supplied by Hollister-Stier Laboratories. Hyposensitization consists of daily ingestion of small but increasing amounts of poison ivy oleoresin. This program appears to be beneficial in some individuals, provided enough oleoresin is administered, but effective doses often produce uncomfortable side effects, such as pruritus ani, dermatitis, urticaria, and dyshidrosis. Desensitization for poison ivy, therefore, is frequently disappointing and should be reserved only for extremely sensitive patients who cannot avoid repeated exposure to the antigen.

House Plant and Flower Dermatitis. Common flowers and house plants present a common source for contact dermatitis in adults as well as children. Of the many flowers that are capable of causing dermatitis, chrysanthemums, asters, and various types of daisies appear to be among the most frequent offenders. Prolonged and repeated contact, however, is necessary, and florists, horticulturists, and gardeners rather than children appear to be the most frequently affected by this form of sensitization.

Among the common house plants, philodendrons, geraniums, and poinsettias are frequent causes of contact dermatitis. In this form of contact dermatitis the hands and arms are involved (since exposure to the plant generally takes place when the patient washes, oils, or plucks the leaves). Diffenbachia, another common house plant closely related to philodendron, may be a cause of dermatitis in exposed sensitized individuals.

Contact dermatitis may also be caused by handling other plants and flowers, namely the daffodil, buttercup, foxglove, lilac, lady slipper, magnolia, and bulbs of tulip and narcissus plants. Treatment of all plant dermatitides is similar to that outlined for poison ivy dermatitis.[53]

Pollen Dermatitis. Dermatitis caused by plant pollens, particularly ragweed, is a fairly common cause of contact dermatitis in children as well as adults. The ragweed pollens contain two antigens, an aqueous protein fraction that may produce asthma, hay fever, and occasionally an atopic-type dermatitis, and an oleoresin capable of producing sensitization and eczematous contact dermatitis.

Air-borne pollen dermatitis generally involves the exposed surfaces of the face, neck, arms, legs, and V area of the chest. Although pollen dermatitis may at times resemble a photosensitivity dermatitis due to plants, drugs, or topical preparations, the lines of demarcation produced by pollen contact dermatitis are not as sharp as those seen in eruptions due to photosensitivity. This lack of sharp delineation in pollen dermatitis is due to the fact that pollen grains often get inside the clothing, thus extending the area of dermatitis to include the upper chest, shoulders, and upper back.

Clothing Dermatitis. Although non-specific irritation from fabrics, rubber, dyes, and cleaning solutions is not uncommon, eczematoid contact dermatitis due to true sensitization to fabrics is rarely seen in childhood. Dermatitis from cotton is virtually non-existent (except for the fact that the sizing used in cotton to stiffen or glaze the material occasionally may sensitize the skin and produce a dermatitis).[59] Silk is an occasional sensitizer, and wool is usually a primary irritant rather than a true contact sensitizer. In recent years, primarily as a result of formaldehyde or formaldehyde resins used in their manufacture, "drip-dry" and crease-resistant fabrics have been responsible for many cases of contact dermatitis. This type of dermatitis is more likely to occur in individuals whose clothes are tight-fitting and close to the skin. The inner thighs and popliteal fossae are particularly susceptible to formaldehyde contact sensitivity.

Instances of irritation or dermatitis attributable to dyes in wearing apparel are remarkably few. The incidence of dermatitis from a dye is generally increased, however, if the dye "bleeds" readily from the fabric. Certain individuals tolerate light colors in clothing but may, on occasion, acquire a dermatitis from dark clothing, particularly that dyed black or dark blue (since the concentration of dyes in dark clothing is much higher than that of dyes in light-colored clothing, dark colors tend to "bleed" more readily than dyes of lighter hue). Whenever washable garments are suspected of causing dermatitis, such clothes should be washed before they are worn again. This frequently will result in removal of irritants and sensitizers, thus occasionally allowing them to be worn without further difficulty.[53]

Spandex is a non-rubber stretchable polyurethane fiber used in girdles, brassieres, and support hose. Although not a problem in spandex manufactures in the United States, allergic contact dermatitis has been reported in foreign-made spandex girdles and brassieres (owing to the presence of the potent sensitizer mercaptobenzothiazole).

Shoe Dermatitis. Shoe dermatitis is an extremely common form of contact dermatitis in childhood. This dermatosis, all too frequently misdiagnosed as tinea pedis (a disorder extremely uncommon in children prior to puberty), usually begins over the dorsal surface of the base of the great toe, may remain localized to that area indefinitely, and spreads by extension to the dorsal surfaces of the feet and other toes (Fig. 3–31). There is erythema, lichenification, and in severe cases, weeping and crusting. A valuable diagnostic feature of shoe dermatitis is the fact that the interdigital spaces, except in severe cases, remain relatively normal in appearance. This is in contrast to the maceration, scaling, and occasional vesiculation of the interdigital webs, particularly those between the fourth and fifth, and, at times the third and fourth toes of either or both feet, usually associated with tinea pedis. The thick skin of the plantar surfaces is generally more resistant, but may at times demonstrate a keratotic dermatitis over the distal areas, the instep, or at times the entire plantar surface.

Pathogenesis. A variety of factors play a role in the pathogenesis of shoe dermatitis. The occlusive effect of hosiery and shoes inhibits the evaporation of moisture, which tends to "leach" out the

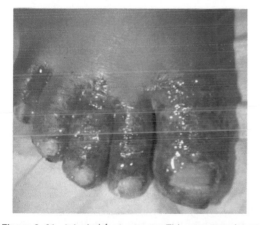

Figure 3–31 Infected foot eczema. This common dermatosis should not be confused with tinea pedis, a disorder that is extremely uncommon in prepuberal children.

chemicals in shoes and increase the percutaneous penetration of potentially irritating and sensitizing agents contained therein. Particularly in children, the dermatitis may become sharply localized to the dorsal aspect of the toes as a result of friction and irritation from ill-fitting shoes rather than from allergic sensitization to agents contained in shoes or sneakers.

The most common causes of shoe dermatitis are rubber, adhesives and cements, tanning agents, and dyes. Seventy-five per cent of cases of shoe dermatitis are due to rubber that contains accelerators (mercaptobenzothiazole and tetramethylthiuram monosulfide) or rubber antioxidants (monobenzyl ether of hydroquinone). Adhesive agents are also common sources for sensitization. Here, rubber, ether, plasticizers, esters that improve the plasticity of rubber, and phenolic resins may be implicated. Tanning agents toughen collagen in leather and allow it to resist wear, water, putrefaction, and changes due to heat.

Of the various agents used in the manufacture of shoes, the dichromates appear to be the most frequently implicated as sources of shoe dermatitis. Leather dyeing is usually done with azo-aniline dyes. These dyes are well "fixed" to the leather, rarely leach out, and accordingly are relatively uncommon causative factors in the pathogenesis of shoe dermatitis.[53]

Management. Patients with shoe sensitivity should avoid shoes whenever possible, and the control of hyperhidrosis of the feet will frequently aid in the management of individuals with this disorder. Open sandals should be worn, if tolerated, and children should be encouraged to change their socks frequently and remove their shoes whenever possible. Practical shoe substitutes include canvas-topped tennis sneakers, unlined moccasins, or shoes with Celastic box toes (since rubber box toes are a frequent source of sensitivity).

Patients with shoe allergy can now choose from a wide selection of attractive all-vinyl shoes. Although polyvinyl shoes tend to increase the tendency to perspiration, they frequently lack many of the potential sensitizers seen in regular shoes. Bass Weejuns loafers, shoes that contain no rubber accelerators, are suitable for both casual and dress wear, and vinyl tennis shoes such as those made by Converse (Naut-1, Fast Break, or Official Cub) are frequently acceptable substitutes. Since the inner sole is a frequent source of contact sensitization, removal and replacement with cork insoles, Dr. Scholl's Air Foam Pads or Johnson's Odor-Eaters, held in place with a non-rubber adhesive such as Elmer's glue is frequently helpful.

The management of active shoe dermatitis, as in other eczematous disorders, is aided by the use of open wet compresses, topical corticosteroids, and antipruritic agents. Since hyperhidrosis is usually responsible for the "leaching" out of potential sensitizing agents, utilization of measures that minimize excessive perspiration of the feet is advisable. The topical use of aluminum chloride, available as Drysol (Person and Covey) or tannic acid soaks (2 tea bags in a quart of water), once or twice weekly will frequently assist in the control of hyperhidrosis, and non-caking agents such as Zea-Sorb powder (Steifel) dusted freely into shoes and hosiery not only tend to lessen perspiration but may also act as a mechanical barrier, thereby limiting contact with potential allergens and irritants.

Metal and Metal Salt Dermatitis. The most common forms of contact dermatitis to metals are those caused by sensitivity to nickel, chromates, and mercury. Most objects containing metal or metal salts are combinations of several metals, some of which may have been used to plate the surface, thus enhancing its attractiveness, tensile strength, or durability.

Since we all are constantly exposed to nickel, nickel dermatitis is one of the most common causes of metal contact sensitivity (Fig. 3–32). Whereas in previous years nickel dermatitis was seen almost exclusively in workers in the nickel industry, today nickel reactions appear with greater frequency. In teen-age girls and women wearing earrings, ear lobe dermatitis is a cardinal sign of nickel dermatitis. Many consumers and even jewelers do not realize that most metal alloys, including those of gold and silver, contain nickel. Although stainless steel contains nickel and chrome (two common allergens), the elements in stainless steel are firmly bound and seldom result in contact sensitivity reactions.

Patch testing for nickel sensitivity can be performed with a five cent coin, provided that World War II nickels made up of silver, copper, and manganese are not used and that non-specific pressure effects are not confused with true allergic eczematous eruptions. If a substance is suspected of containing free nickel, application of a test solution of dimethylglyoxine in a 10 per cent aqueous solution of ammonia to the suspected item will cause the suspected metal to turn pink. Since

piercing of ears is responsible for sensitization to nickel and nickel products, ear piercing should be done with a stainless steel needle, and persons undergoing this procedure should be advised to wear only stainless steel earrings until the earlobes are completely healed.

Once the presence of hypersensitivity to nickel has been established, the hypersensitivity usually lasts for years. Patients, therefore, must be taught how to avoid contact with nickel objects through the use of proper substitutes. Periodic coating of the offending metal with clear nail polish, or the use of topical aerosol dexamethasone (Decadron) spray on both the skin of the individual and that portion of the nickel-plated object that comes into contact with the skin, at times may be helpful for those who prefer to continue to wear potentially allergenic jewelry. The combination of dexamethasone and the film formed by the isopropyl myristate is necessary for successful prophylaxis, since corticosteroid alone or isopropyl myristate alone does not protect nickel-sensitive patients. Both the skin and the nickel-plated object should be sprayed twice at five-minute intervals, and in warm weather and for patients who perspire profusely (since perspiration tends to release the bound nickel), dexamethasone spray may have to be repeated after a period of six hours.[60]

Cosmetic Dermatitis. The most common cosmetic agents causing allergic contact dermatitis are hair dyes, lipsticks, antiperspirants, paraphenylenediamine (a popular oxidation-type hair dye), nail lacquers, and sunscreening agents. In many instances, the eyelids are affected not only by cosmetics applied to the lids and lashes, but also by preparations applied to the scalp, face, and nails. In most instances, cutaneous allergic reactions take on the form of an eczematous dermatitis. However, antiperspirants and poison-ivy preparations containing zirconium may produce allergic granulomatous reactions. Although the incidence of lanolin (wool wax, wool grease, and wool fat) sensitivity obtained from the fleece of sheep is very low, lanolin and its derivatives may be present under many different names and guises. Should patients be found to have allergic sensitivity to lanolin, the manufacturers of "hypoallergenic" cosmetics can furnish lanolin-free products.

In the United States, parabens (compounds containing p-hydroxybenzoic acid) are frequently added in low concentrations to creams, lotions, and cosmetics in an attempt to retard microbial growth. Since the concentration of paraben in topical preparations is too low (below 0.5 per cent) to produce a positive patch test to the medications, patch tests for paraben sensitivity should be performed with a five per cent concentration of paraben in petrolatum.

Neomycin, a topical antibiotic incorporated into many topical preparations, is reported to have a high incidence of allergenicity. The majority of contact allergies to this agent, however, are seen in older individuals, particularly those with chronically inflamed skin. In view of the frequent topical

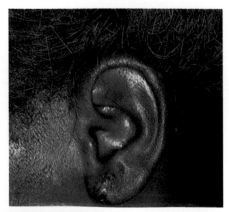

Figure 3–32 Ear lobe dermatitis. A cardinal sign of nickel dermatitis.

use of neomycin in children (without evidence of sensitization), when adults and individuals with chronic dermatoses are excluded, the incidence of neomycin sensitivity appears to be appreciably lower, approximately one in 100,000 uses rather than the frequently cited 3.0 to 6.0 per cent.[61] When neomycin sensitivity is considered, patch testing requires the use of appropriate material (20 per cent concentrations in aqueous solution or petrolatum, rather than the lower levels seen in most proprietary formulations).

Ethylenediamine, a compound stabilizer seen in various topical preparations, cross-reacts with antihistamines and aminophylline and is a potent sensitizer capable of producing an eczematous contact-type dermatitis. Adequate patch testing requires a 1 per cent concentration, approximately five times that found in commercial products. This sensitizer joins neomycin and the parabens as an agent that may cause dermatitis but yet may produce a negative patch test response when the commercially available topical preparation is used in patch testing. Antihistamines that are ethylenediamine derivatives are particularly active topical sensitizers and may produce systemic eczematous contact dermatitis when administered to individuals previously sensitized by topical application of ethylenediamine.[53]

Adhesive Tape Dermatitis. Although most cutaneous reactions related to the wearing of adhesive tape are of a mechanical rather than contact sensitivity type, allergic reactions may be due to the rubber compounds (rubber accelerators or antioxidants) that have been incorporated into the adhesive or the vinyl backing of the adhesive. Dermicel (Johnson and Johnson), Steri-strips or Microspore surgical tape (3 M Company), and non-rubber "acrylate" are helpful for those individuals allergic to or irritated by ordinary adhesive tapes.

Fiberglas Dermatitis

Fiberglas particles frequently cause intense pruritus owing to the fact that the fine glass fiber particles from Fiberglas insulation panels or drapes can penetrate the skin and cause an eruption consisting of small erythematous follicular papules. At times clothes washed in a washing machine in which fiberglas materials have been washed are also capable of inducing this cutaneous reaction.

Fiberglas dermatitis clinically appears to represent a patchy folliculitis or subacute dermatitis. Microscopic examination of skin scrapings of involved areas or suspected articles of clothing may reveal pale greenish, granular rod-like fibers approximately one to two times the width of a hair.

Patients with Fiberglas dermatitis respond to removal of exposure to the offending agents, topical corticosteroids, systemic antipruritics, and, when necessary, epidermal stripping to facilitate removal of embedded particles.[62]

Autosensitization Dermatitis

Autosensitization is a term used to describe a clinical disorder created by sensitization of the body by circulating antibody or by specifically activated lymphocytes (delayed hypersensitivity) to constituents of its own tissues.[63] Frequently referred to as an "id" reaction, the disorder is characterized by an acute papulovesicular eruption that appears on the forearms, flexor aspects of the upper arms, the extensor aspects of the upper arms and thighs, and, less commonly, the face and trunk. The disorder usually appears acutely over a few days and nearly always is preceded by an exacerbation of the pre-existing dermatitis by infection, rubbing, or inappropriate therapy. The eruption is nearly always symmetrical, but may demonstrate an isomorphic response (the Koebner phenomenon) or light sensitivity. Lesions begin as discrete edematous papules or papulovesicles and are generally associated with a moderate to severe degree of pruritus.

The acute eruption may subside spontaneously in a few weeks, if the primary dermatitis is controlled. Relapses, however, are common, particularly when the initial local lesion flares and is followed by a further disseminated eruption.

The diagnosis of autosensitization dermatitis (autoeczematization) is made clinically on the basis of a generalized papulovesicular eruption that develops in the wake of a pre-existing eczematoid dermatitis. Treatment depends upon open wet compresses, antihistamines, and the use of topical corticosteroid preparations. Control of the primary lesion is important in order to prevent further or recurrent antigenic stimulation. Although seldom indicated, a two to three-week course of systemic corticosteroids may at times be necessary in cases that are unresponsive to more conservative therapy.

References

1. Walker RB, Warin RP: The incidence of eczema in early childhood. Br. J. Dermatol. 68:182–183, 1956.

   A review of 1024 children revealed the incidence of eczema or atopic dermatitis in early childhood to be approximately 3 per cent.

2. Coco AF, Cooke RA: On the classification of the phenomenon of hypersensitiveness. J. Immunol. 8:163 182, 1923.

   A discussion of hypersensitivity and its classification into normal and abnormal groups.

3. Wise F, Sulzberger MB: Yearbook of Dermatology and Syphilology. Yearbook Publishers, Inc., Chicago, 1933, 59.

   The term "atopic dermatitis" permits inclusion of the eruption from its acute eczematous form to the chronic lichenified lesions that technically fail to merit the term "eczema."

4. Rajka G: Atopic dermatitis. W.B. Saunders Co., Philadelphia, 1975.

   An inclusive review of the etiology and clinical aspects of atopic dermatitis.

5. Lobitz WC, Dobson RL: Physical and physiological clues for diagnosing eczema. JAMA 161:1226–1229, 1956.

Cutaneous findings as an aid in the diagnosis of atopic dermatitis.

6. Cormia FE: The basis of itching (discussion). J. Pediatr. 66:207–209, 1965.

Itching is a modified form of pain carried on slow afferent fibers, the intensity varying with the number of free nerve endings in the affected area.

7. Morgan DB: A suggestive sign of allergy. Arch. Dermat. & Syph. 57:1050, 1948.

The terms "Morgan's fold" and "Dennie's pleat" are used to describe a definite wrinkle that appears just beneath the margin of the lower eyelids (originally described by Dr. Charles C. Dennie, who first called the attention of students to the sign, which he felt rather pathognomonic for patients with allergy).

8. Kierland RR: Certain stigmata associated with atopic dermatitis. *In* Baer RJ (Ed.): Atopic Dermatitis. New York University Press, New York, 1955, 43–45.

A classic description of cutaneous findings helpful in the diagnosis of atopic dermatitis.

9. Uehara M, Ofugi S: Abnormal vascular reactions in atopic dermatitis. Arch. Dermatol. 113:627–629, 1977.

White dermographism, nicotinic acid blanching, and delayed blanching with metacholine occur in atopic dermatitis and in non-atopic patients with allergic contact dermatitis.

10. Norins AL: Atopic dermatitis. Pediatr. Clin. North Am. 18:801–838, 1971.

A thorough review of the pathogenesis, natural course, clinical findings, and management of atopic dermatitis.

11. Roth HL, Kierland RR: The natural history of atopic dermatitis. Arch. Dermatol. 89:209–214, 1964.

A clinical survey with a 20-year follow-up of approximately 500 cases of atopic dermatitis.

12. Brunsting L, Reed WB, Bair HL: Occurrence of cataracts and keratoconus with atopic dermatitis. Arch. Dermatol. 72:237–241, 1955.

A distinctive form of cataract appears as a complication of atopic dermatitis during adolescence and early adult life.

13. Dunand P, Chai H, Weltman D, et al.: Posterior polar cataracts and steroid therapy in children. J. Allergy Clin. Immunol. 55:123, 1975.

Slit-lamp studies of 92 children on long-term steroid therapy revealed 10 children (10.8 per cent) with evidence of cataracts.

14. Sevel D, Weinberg MB, Van Niekirk CH: Lenticular complications of long-term steroid therapy in children with asthma and eczema. J. Allergy Clin. Immunol. 60:215–217, 1977.

Of forty-two children with chronic asthma (including ten with associated eczema) on long-term oral steroids, only one was found to have cataracts commensurate with corticosteroid therapy, but the authors emphasize that children on long-term steroid therapy be examined for possible posterior capsular cataracts.

15. Hanifin JM, Lobitz WC Jr: Newer concepts of atopic dermatitis. Arch. Dermatol. 113:663–670, 1977.

A review of present concepts of etiology and immunologic association in patients with atopic dermatitis.

16. Jones HE, Lewis CW, McMarlin SL: Allergic contact sensitivity in atopic dermatitis. Arch. Dermatol. 107:217–222, 1973.

Comparison studies of poison ivy sensitivity revealed an incidence of 15 per cent reactivity in patients with atopic dermatitis as compared with 61 per cent in the control group.

17. Strauss JS: Atopic allergy and atopic dermatitis — a discussion of their relationship. NY State J. Med. 59:53–58, 1959.

Specific protein antigens may cause exacerbations of atopic dermatitis.

18. Strauss JS, Kligman AM: The relationship of atopic allergy and dermatitis. Arch. Dermatol. 75:806–811, 1957.

Inhalant and ingested allergens probably are secondary rather than primary factors in the causation of dermatitic flares.

19. Szentivanyi A: The beta-adrenergic theory of the atopic abnormality in bronchial asthma. J. Allergy 42:203–232, 1968.

A theory of atopy based upon a cellular control system mediated through adenyl cyclase and cyclic AMP.

20. Mier PD, Urselmann E: The adenyl cyclase of skin. II. Adenyl cyclase levels in atopic dermatitis. Br. J. Dermatol. 83:360–364, 1970.

Skin biopsy specimens from lesions of atopic dermatitis, from atopic "uninvolved" skin, and from the skin of healthy individuals reveal no decrease in adenyl cyclase activity in atopics.

21. Ishizaka K, Ishizaka T: Physicochemical properties of reaginic antibody. 1. Association of reaginic activity with an immunoglobulin other than gamma A or gamma G-globulin. J. Allergy 37:169–185, 1966.

Sera from atopic patients fractionated by chromatography reveal a unique immunoglobulin (IgE) capable of passive sensitization of normal skin.

22. Ishizaka K, Ishizaka T: Identification of gamma E-antibodies as a carrier of reaginic activity. J. Immunol. 99:1187–1198, 1967.

Evidence supports the concept that gamma E-globulin is the reaginic antibody against antigen E.

23. Juhlin C, Johannsen SGO: Immunoglobulin E. Arch. Dermatol. 100:12–16, 1969.

Elevated serum levels of IgE detected in 82 per cent of patients with atopic dermatitis.

24. Ogawa M, Berger PA, McIntyre OR, et al.: IgE in atopic dermatitis. Arch. Dermatol. 103:575–580, 1971.

The mean serum IgE levels in atopic dermatitis are higher than those of control groups; a strong correlation exists between this level and the severity of dermatitis.

25. Sulzberger MB: Atopic dermatitis: its clinical and histologic picture. American Practitioner and Digest of Treatment 6:1079–1088, 1955.

A classic description of atopic dermatitis.

26. Sulzberger MB: Atopic dermatitis — Part III. *In* Fitzpatrick TB, et al.: Dermatology in General Medicine. McGraw-Hill Inc., New York, 1971, 687–694.

A comprehensive review of atopic dermatitis, its clinical manifestations, and therapy.

27. Kreuger GG, Kahn G, Weston WL, et al.: IgE levels in nummular eczema and ichthyosis. Arch. Dermatol. 107:56–58, 1973.

Significantly lower IgE levels in 26 patients with nummular eczema suggest that nummular eczema is not a manifestation of atopic dermatitis.

28. Jorgensen HP: Nonfatal Wiskott-Aldrich syndrome in a 15-year-old boy. Arch. Dermatol. 106:541–542, 1972.

The oldest known survivor of a disorder in which affected individuals have a short life expectancy, with death usually occurring in infancy or within the first few years of life.

29. Leyden JJ, Marples RR, Kligman AM: *Staphylococcus aureus* in the lesions of atopic dermatitis. Br. J. Dermatol. 90:525–530, 1974.

Staphylococcus aureus was isolated from 90 per cent of 50 patients with chronic atopic dermatitis.

30. Aly R, Maibach HI, Shinefield HR: Microbial flora of atopic dermatitis. Arch. Dermatol. 113:780–782, 1977.

Studies of the skin and anterior nares of 39 patients with atopic dermatitis reveal a 93 per cent incidence of *Staphylo-*

coccus aureus carriage in cutaneous lesions, a 76 per cent incidence in non-involved skin, and a 79 per cent carriage rate in the anterior nares.

31. Lasch EE, Frankel V, Pardy PA, et al.: Epidemic glomerulonephritis in Israel. J. Infect. Dis. *124*:141–147, 1971.

Early treatment of streptococcal infection does not appear to prevent the development of acute nephritis.

32. Rostenberg A Jr, Sulzberger MB: Some results of patch tests: compilation and discussion of cutaneous reactions to about 500 substances as elicited by over 10,000 tests in 1,000 patients. Arch. Dermatol. & Syph. 35:433–454, 1937.

In a review of a large series of patch tests, patients with atopic dermatitis were shown to have a low incidence of positive reactions.

33. Derbes VJ, Caro MR: Localized eczema induced by housedust extract injections. Arch. Dermatol. 75:804–805, 1957.

Patches of eczema appearing at sites of housedust vaccine injections in an asthmatic patient add support to the concept that the skin of atopics may react to desensitization and inhalant allergens by the development of eczematoid exacerbations.

34. Stoughton RB: A perspective of topical corticosteroid therapy. *In* Farber EM, Cox AJ: Psoriasis, Proceedings of the Second International Symposium. Yorke Medical Books, New York, 1976, 219–226.

A review of topical corticosteroid formulations, their use, and relative efficacy.

35. Hill CJH, Rostenberg A Jr: Adverse effects from topical steroids. Cutis *21*:624–628, 1978.

A review of the local and systemic disorders that may occur following administration of topical corticosteroids.

36. Feiwel M: Percutaneous absorption of topical steroids in children. Br. J. Dermatol. *81*:113–116, 1969.

Potent topical steroids may be used judiciously in infantile eczema for short periods of time.

37. Taylor DS, Malinson FD, Gak C: Pituitary-adrenal function following topical triamcinolone and occlusion. Arch. Dermatol. 92:174–177, 1965.

A study of six adult patients demonstrates that topical application of potent steroids under occlusion can affect pituitary-adrenal function.

38. Feiwel M, James VH, Barnett ES: Effect of potent topical steroids on plasma-cortisol levels of infants and children with eczema. Lancet *1*:485–487, 1969.

A drop in plasma cortisol levels in children on long-term potent topical corticosteroids alerts physicians to the possible systemic effects of the routine use of topical glucocorticosteroids.

39. Kezckes K, Frain-Bell W, Honeyman AC, et al.: The effect on adrenal function of treatment of eczema and psoriasis with triamcinolone acetonide. Br. J. Dermatol. 79:475–486, 1967.

Topical corticosteroids used under polyethylene occlusion or on large or denuded areas over long periods of time can result in pituitary-adrenal suppression.

40. Hindson TC: Urea in the topical treatment of atopic eczema. Arch. Dermatol. *104*:284–285, 1971.

The addition of 10 per cent urea to a commercially available steroid cream gave better results in the treatment of subacute and chronic atopic eczema than the steroid cream alone.

41. Roth HL, Gellin GA: Atopic dermatitis: treatment with a urea-corticosteroid cream. Cutis *11*:237–239, 1973.

In a study of 70 patients with atopic dermatitis, the addition of 10 per cent urea to a 1 per cent hydrocortisone cream produced a statistically significant greater degree of improvement in a shorter period of time.

42. Buckley RH, Wray BB, Belnaker EZ: Extreme hyperimmun-

oglobulinemia E and undue susceptibility to infection. Pediatrics 49:59–70, 1972.

Clinical and immunologic features of two adolescent boys with recurrent pyogenic infections are judged to constitute a new syndrome characterized by recurrent bacterial and fungal infections, impaired cell-mediated immunity, and exceptionally high serum IgE concentrations.

43. Stanley J, Perez D, Gigli I, et al.: Hyperimmunoglobulin E syndrome. Arch. Dermatol. *114*:765–767, 1978.

The clinical spectrum of hyperimmunoglobulin E syndrome may include atopic dermatitis, mucocutaneous candidiasis, systemic infections, and/or the features of Job's syndrome.

44. Paslin D, Norman ME: Atopic dermatitis and impaired neutrophil chemotaxis in Job's syndrome. Arch. Dermatol. *113*:801–805, 1977.

Defective erythema responses to histamine, methyl niacinate, and metocholine (mecholyl) chloride may explain the lack of redness, heat, or pain in cold abscesses seen in patients with Job's syndrome.

45. Pauly CR, Artis WM, Jones HE: Atopic dermatitis, impaired cellular immunity, and molluscum contagiosum. Arch. Dermatol. *114*:391–393, 1978.

A substantial elevation in IgE level and depressed cell-mediated immunity are demonstrated in a young man with chronic molluscum contagiosum and atopic dermatitis.

46. Aldrich RA, Steinberg AG, Campbell DD: Pedigree demonstrating a sex-linked recessive condition characterized by draining ears, eczematoid dermatitis and bloody diarrhea. Pediatrics *13*:133–139, 1954.

A severe recalcitrant dermatitis, thrombocytopenia, and sex-linked recessivity are seen as part of a disorder initially described by Wiskott in 1937.

47. Beare JM, Rook A: Infantile seborrheic dermatitis. *In* Rook A, Wilkinson DS, Ebling FJG (Eds.): Textbook of Dermatology, 2nd ed. Blackwell Scientific Publications, Oxford, 1972, 177–179.

Infantile seborrheic dermatitis is a distinctive self-limiting non-eczematous erythematosquamous eruption with many features of seborrheic dermatitis of adolescents and adults.

48. Reed RJ, Meek T, Ichinose H: Lichen striatus: a model for the histologic spectrum of lichenoid reactions. J. Cutan. Path. 2:1–18, 1975.

Lichen striatus is characterized by a primary lymphohistiocytic infiltrate that involves a portion of the papillary dermis and the contiguous epidermis.

49. Waisman M, Sutton RL: Frictional lichenoid eruption in children: recurrent pityriasis of the elbows and knees. Arch. Dermatol. 94:592–593, 1966.

A distinctive scaly lichenoid eruption of the extremities, particularly the elbows and knees, in children four to twelve years of age.

50. Goldman L, Kitzmiller KW, Ritchfield DF: Summer lichenoid dermatitis of the elbows in children. Cutis *13*:836–838, 1974.

In seven children a pruritic eruption of the elbows and knees during the summertime seemed to clear with the advent of cool weather.

51. Savin J A: Current causes of fixed drug eruptions. Br. J. Dermatol. 83:546–549, 1970.

A review of medications usually implicated as the cause of fixed drug eruption.

52. Rostenberg A Jr: Primary irritant and allergic eczematous reactions. Their interrelations. Arch. Dermatol. 75:547–558, 1957.

A discussion of the two types of eczematous reaction (primary irritant and allergic contact dermatitis), their pathogenesis, interrelations, and differentiation.

53. Fisher AA: Contact Dermatitis. Lea and Febiger, Philadelphia, 1967.

An authoritative review of the problem of contact dermatitis in children and adults.

54. Glaser J: Contact dermatitis. *In* Allergy in Childhood. Charles C Thomas, Springfield, 1956, 157–164.

In a series of 516 allergic infants and children, the incidence of contact dermatitis was 1.55 per cent as compared with an incidence of 12.9 per cent in a series of 200 adults.

55. Epstein WL: Contact-type delayed hypersensitivity in infants and children: induction of rhus sensitivity. Pediatrics 27:51–53, 1961.

The frequency of contact to Rhus allergen (pentadecylcatechol) of 102 infants revealed a relative lack of capacity to react in infants under age one and in young children between one and three years of age.

56. Straus HW: Artificial sensitization of infants to poison ivy. J. Allergy 2:137–144, 1931.

Sensitization to Rhus allergen can be demonstrated within the first month of life.

57. Criep LH: Dermatologic allergy: Immunology, Diagnosis, Management. W.B. Saunders Co., Philadelphia, 1967.

A practical review of basic concepts of immunopathology, diagnosis, and management of cutaneous allergic reactions written for the dermatologist, pediatrician, internist, and allergist.

58. Fisher AA: Contact dermatitis. Poison ivy and related dermatitis. Dermatology 1:43–53, 1978.

An update on Rhus dermatitis and its management.

59. Domonkos AN: Contact dermatitis, drug eruptions, atopic dermatitis and eczema. *In* Andrews' Diseases of the Skin. W.B. Saunders Co., Philadelphia, 1971, 84–139.

An excellent review of the common contact allergens in an update of one of the classic textbooks of dermatology.

60. Fisher AA: Steroid aerosol spray in contact dermatitis. Prophylactic use with particular reference to nickel hypersensitivity. Arch. Dermatol. 89:841–843, 1967.

A combination of dexamethasone and a film formed by isopropyl myristate in Decadron spray affords protection to patients with nickel sensitivity.

61. Leyden JJ, Kligman AM: The case for topical antibiotics. Progress in Dermatology (Dermatology Foundation, Philadelphia) 7:11–14, 1973.

Neomycin appears to be far less a sensitizer than most studies seem to indicate.

62. Parlette HL: Fiberglass dermatitis. Bull. Assoc. Milit. Dermatol. 22:53–55, 1974.

A patchy pruritic dermatitis of the wrists, forearms, and shins of a young man working with fiberglass insulation panels.

63. Champion RH: Autosensitization dermatitis (autoeczematization). *In* Demis DJ, Dobson RL, McGuire J (Eds.): Clinical Dermatology, Vol. 3. (Unit 13:12). Harper and Row, Hagerstown, Maryland, 1977, 1–5.

A thorough review of the problem of autoeczematization and autosensitization dermatitis.

PHOTOSENSITIVITY AND PHOTOREACTIONS

Reactions to the sun's rays have become increasingly common in recent years, owing not only to the ever-expanding number of photosensitizers in our environment, but also to the public's ever-increasing obsession with sunbathing.[1] Sunlight emits a wide spectrum of radiation energy, extending from radio waves through infrared, visible, and ultraviolet (UV) to x-rays. The unit used to specify the wavelength of light is the nanometer (one nanometer is equal to 10 Ångstroms). Visible light is in the range of 400 to 800 nanometers (nm) and is relatively harmless. From 800 to 1800 is the infrared range. It is the ultraviolet (UVL) wavelengths (290 to 400) that cause most cutaneous reactions. Since wavelengths below 220 nm are absorbed by atmospheric gases, including oxygen and nitrogen, and those of less than 290 nm are absorbed by the atmospheric ozone layer, it is the middle ultraviolet (UVB), with wavelengths of 290 to 320 nm, that primarily produces sunburn, suntan, and skin cancer. Long wave ultraviolet light (UVA, 320 to 400 nm) may augment these cutaneous reactions. It is in this range that most drug-induced or chemical-induced photosensitivity reactions occur.[2]

An important factor in sun exposure is the fact that ultraviolet light also reaches the skin through reflection from snow (80 to 85 per cent), sand (17 to 25 per cent), water (5 per cent, but up to 100 per cent when the sun is directly overhead), sidewalks, and turf, and that ultraviolet exposure increases 4 per cent for every 1000 feet elevation above sea level. It must be remembered that on a bright cloudy day with thin cloud cover it is possible to receive 60 to 85 per cent of the amount of ultraviolet radiation that is present on a bright clear day, that hats and umbrellas only provide a moderate degree of protection, and that surfaces with reflectivity greatly increase sunlight exposure.

TANNING AND SUNBURN REACTIONS

A deepening pigmentation due to increased melanization of the skin (referred to as a tan) occurs following ultraviolet exposure. Sunburn is caused by ultraviolet light with wavelengths between 290 to 320 nm. Wavelengths from 290 to 400 nm are mainly responsible for tanning.

Sunburn may be defined as a cutaneous erythema caused by sun exposure at wavelengths between 290 and 320 nm of sufficient degree to cause discomfort. Reactivity may range in severity from a mild asymptomatic erythema to a more intense reaction, with redness accompanied by tenderness, pain, edema, and, and at times, vesiculation and bulla formation.

CLINICAL MANIFESTATIONS. Mild reactions begin approximately 6 to 12 hours after the onset of exposure, reach a peak intensity within about 24 hours, begin to decline gradually over a period of three to five days, and usually result in a tan that reaches its maximum two to three weeks after exposure. Intense reactions begin in a similar manner. Signs and symptoms, however, are more intense and continue to progress, generally reaching their peak on the second day, at which time large blisters may form in the most severely affected areas. After several days the erythema and edema subside and are soon followed by a degree of desquamation relative to the intensity of the clinical reaction. If the sunburned area is extensive, constitutional symptoms may include nausea, malaise, headache, fever, chills, delirium, and in some cases, even prostration.

MANAGEMENT. Treatment for sunburn depends primarily upon the utilization of measures that reduce exposure to strong sunlight. This is especially important for fair-skinned individuals, particularly blue-eyed persons, redheads, blondes, and frecklers who withstand actinic exposure poorly, burn easily, and, over the years, tend to suffer chronic effects of light exposure. Prophylactic measures include timing of outdoor activities to avoid peak ultraviolet exposure between 10:00 A.M. and 2:00 P.M. in the warm seasons of the year. Broad-rimmed hats and long-sleeved clothing help reduce the impact of harmful ultraviolet rays. However, the possibility of reflection must be considered, and it should be recognized that light-textured materials such as T-shirts (especially when wet) only give partial protection.[2]

Sunscreens occupy an important position in the management of ultraviolet exposure. The most common misconception (particularly among teenagers) is the belief that certain preparations can induce or promote a suntan). Sunscreens are topical preparations designed to protect the skin from the effects of ultraviolet light. They act as "screens" that absorb the light at particular wavelengths or as opaque "sunblocking" agents that act as "barriers" and impede the passage of ultraviolet light. Since tanning and sunburn both result from the same ultraviolet waveband, it is difficult to promote one without promoting the other.[2]

It should be noted that many commercially available preparations that claim to promote tanning afford little or no ultraviolet protection. The most effective and cosmetically acceptable sunscreens are those that contain para-aminobenzoic acid (PABA) and its esters, benzophenones, and cinnamates in suitable vehicles that provide penetration of and adherence to the cutaneous surface. Ideally, sunscreens should be applied 30 to 60 minutes before the onset of sun exposure and most should be reapplied after swimming, periods of excessive perspiration, frequent washing, or showering.[3]

Sunscreens may be divided into three types depending upon the wavelengths of sunlight they block. *Short UV sunscreens* screen the sunburn spectrum (290–320 nm). The most effective agents in this group are the formulations of para-aminobenzoic acid (PABA) and its esters (PreSun, PabaFilm, PabaGel, Blockout, Eclipse, Sunbrella, Sundown).

Full-spectrum UV sunscreens screen a wider spectrum that includes both UVB (290–320 nm) and UVA (320–400 nm). These include the benzophenones (Sol-bar) and benzophenone sulfonic acid (Uval). Although the screening effectiveness of these agents is not as great as the short-wavelength ultraviolet sunscreens (PABA and its esters), their advantage is the protection from photosensitivity reactions induced by UVA (320 to 400 nm) wavelengths.

Full-spectrum ultraviolet and visible light sunscreens are opaque formulations that block out all wavelengths between 290 and 700 nm. These include zinc oxide ointment, titanium oxide formulations (A-fil and Maxa-fil), and red petrolatum formulations (RVP, RV Paque, and RV Plus).

When maximum prophylaxis is desired, some physicians recommend the use of a combination of both short ultraviolet and full-spectrum agents. By this technique a sunscreen of the UVB (290–320 nm) sunburn range, such as a para-aminobenzoic acid (PABA) preparations, may be applied and allowed to dry, and then followed by the application of a benzophenone preparation (290–400 nm) such as Sol-bar or Uval.[3] The use of sunscreens has recently been simplified by a classification of sunscreens on the basis of their sun protective factor (SPF) ratings. Thus a sunscreen with a rating of 4 gives limited sunburn protection, 8 gives maximum sunburn protection (allows tanning and limits sunburn), and 15 gives ultraprotection (absorbs burning as well as tanning rays).

Treatment of sunburn consists of cool compresses or cool tub baths in Aveeno Colloidal Oatmeal (Cooper Laboratories), baking soda, or cornstarch; topical corticosteroid formulations; and the use of systemic preparations with analgesic and anti-inflammatory properties, such as aspirin or indomethacin, available as Indocin (Merck Sharp & Dohme). When symptoms are severe, a short couse of systemic corticosteroids (oral prednisone, or its equivalent, in dosages of 20 to 60 mg, with tapering after a period of four to eight days) will abort severe reactions and afford added relief. It should be noted that treatment of sunburn is not listed among the manufacturer's indications for the use of indomethacin, that conditions for its use in childhood have not been established, and that this preparation should not be prescribed for pregnant women, nursing mothers, or children under 14 years of age.

PHOTOSENSITIVITY REACTIONS

Photosensitivity is a broad term used to describe abnormal or adverse reactions to sunlight energy in the skin. Photosensitivity reactions may be phototoxic or photoallergic in nature and endogenous or exogenous in origin. Phototoxic reactions are common and can be likened to a primary irritant reaction. Photoallergy is relatively uncommon and presumably is dependent upon antigen-antibody or cell-mediated hypersensitivity.[4]

Phototoxic reactions refer to a non-immunologic, exaggerated sunburn or sunburn-like reaction characterized by erythema (and, at times, edema), occurring within a few minutes to several hours (usually within a period of two to six hours) after exposure to sunlight and followed by hyperpigmentation and desquamation confined to the exposed areas. This type of sensitivity usually occurs with the first exposure to the photosensitizing substance, when the systemic or percutaneous absorption of the sensitizing substances is in high enough concentration to result in a photo-induced cutaneous reaction.

Histopathologic examination of phototoxic reactions reveals epidermal necrosis, epidermal cell degeneration, and dermal edema, with a mild to moderate infiltrate consisting mostly of polymorphonuclear leukocytes.

Photoallergic reactions are defined as an acquired delayed hypersensitivity dermatitis caused by light energy alone, or by the presence of a photosensitizing substance plus sunlight. Photoallergic reactions are relatively uncommon and develop on initial occurrence after an incubation or refractory period of about nine days. Instead of sunburn-type reactions, photoallergic responses are generally characterized by immediate urticarial or delayed papular or eczematoid lesions that are not followed by hyperpigmentation. After the first sensitization, subsequent photoallergic reactions generally appear within twenty-four hours after even very brief periods of exposure.

Histopathologic features of photoallergic reactions include spongiosis, intra-epidermal vesiculation, infiltration of the epidermis by lymphocytes, and a characteristic, but not necessarily diagnostic, dense perivascular round cell infiltrate.

Immediate Photoallergic Responses (Solar Urticaria)

Solar urticaria is an extremely uncommon type 1 IgE-mediated type of sensitivity characterized by pruritus and erythema. It appears either during or within a few minutes of sunlight exposure and is followed almost immediately by a localized urticarial reaction (without pseudopods) confined to the exposed areas and an irregular flare reaction that extends onto unexposed skin. Although the reaction is generally transient and usually fades within an hour or two, it may, on occasion, last for a much longer period of time.[1]

Solar urticaria usually does not manifest itself until the third or fourth decade of life, and females are affected three times more often than males.[5] It has been reported, however, at as early as three years of age and, at times, may occur during later childhood or adolescence.

Solar urticaria represents a characteristic clinical phenomenon apparently due to or dependent upon a variety of mechanisms.[5] Most patients with this disorder react to ultraviolet light rays shorter than 370 nm. An inborn error of protoporphyrin metabolism (erythropoietic protoporphyria), however, is responsible for some cases, and several categories of reactivity can be differentiated, namely those sensitive to wavelengths in the UVB (290–320 nm), UVA (320–400 nm), and visible light (400–700 nm) ranges. Passive transfer and reverse passive transfer tests have been positive in most case studies in the UV range shorter than 370 nm, thus supporting a proposed allergic nature of the process in this group. The mechanism of response in the other groups, however, remains uncertain.

The diagnosis of solar urticaria is based upon the clinical picture and induction of lesions by natural or artificial light under controlled conditions. The differential diagnosis includes all agents capable of causing urticaria. The relationship to light, and the fact that lesions are confined solely to light-exposed areas, however, is helpful in establishing the true nature of this disorder.

In patients with mild forms of solar urticaria (those in whom the threshold is high) the disorder may be controlled simply by appropriate sunscreens and avoidance of prolonged unprotected sun exposure. Those individuals highly sensitive to sunlight, however, must completely avoid daytime exposure. Antihistamines, antimalarials, adrenocorticosteroids, and psoralens may be beneficial in some select patients, but in the majority of cases these agents appear to be of little or no value. In some individuals it is possible to build up sun tolerance slowly by carefully metered graduated exposures to artificial light. This procedure stimulates pigmentation and possibly depletes the ultraviolet-induced mediators of urticaria responsible for the clinical features seen in association with this disorder.[2]

Delayed Photoallergic Reactions (Polymorphous Light Eruption)

Polymorphous light eruption (PMLE) is a term that was first introduced in 1929 to describe a group of inflammatory dermatoses induced by sunlight. Although the etiology of this disorder remains unknown, it appears to be associated with a phototoxic reaction to ultraviolet rays in the 290 to 480 nm range, with the predominant activity (85 per cent of cases) in the sunburn range (290–320 nm).[6, 7] Although the mechanism or mechanisms of the process have not been established, the clinical patterns, reaction time, histology, and flares of previously involved areas following exposure at distant sites suggest a delayed hypersensitivity response.[1] The fact that this disorder is extremely common in the North American Indians also suggests a possible genetic factor in some individuals with this disorder.[7]

DIAGNOSIS. Despite conflicting results in individual studies, there appears to be no sex predisposition in this disease. Seen in children as well as adults, the disorder usually begins in young and mid-adult life, but may occur at any age from childhood to old age. The clinical eruption consists of a group of pleomorphic or polymorphic lesions that occur one to four days after sunlight exposure on exposed cutaneous areas. The lesions may range from small papules, urticarial, vesicular, or eczematous reactions to large papules, plaques, or patterns resembling erythema multiforme. The areas of the body most commonly involved include the face, the "V" of the neck, and the arms, hands, legs, and feet. Pruritus, although relatively rare, may be severe. Lesions usually involute spontaneously in one to two weeks if no additional exposure to sunlight occurs (Fig. 4–1).

The diagnosis of polymorphous light eruption is suggested by the character of the lesions, their distribution, and their relationship to sun exposure. When the diagnosis remains in doubt, phototesting assists confirmation of the diagnosis and helps differentiate polymorphous light eruption from photocontact reactions and erythropoietic porphyria. This technique consists of exposing uninvolved skin of the forearm to three to five minimal erythema doses (MED) of UVB (rays shorter than 320 nm) every 24 to 72 hours for up to five exposures (this repeated exposure phototest is positive in 70 to 80 per cent of patients with polymorphous light eruption). Some patients with lupus erythematosus (LE), particularly those with systemic LE, acquire sun-induced lesions indistinguishable from those of polymorphous light eruption. Examination for evidence of systemic LE and fluorescent microscopic studies for basement membrane immunofluorescence and antinuclear antibodies, however, serve to differentiate these two disorders.[6]

Microscopic findings in all forms of polymorphous light eruption feature dense perivascular accumulations of round cells in the upper dermis and middermis, with epidermal edema, spongiosis, and vesicle formation in urticarial, eczematous, and papular forms of this disorder. In the vesicular form, subepidermal blisters are present; in the plaque type, histologic lesions are indistinguishable from early lesions of chronic discoid lupus erythematosus.

MANAGEMENT. The treatment of polymorphous light eruption consists of sunscreens, appropriate clothing, and the avoidance of midday sun. If patients severely affected by this disorder anticipate intense or prolonged sun exposure, synthetic antimalarials such as chloroquine, hydroxychloroquine (Plaquenil), and Atabrine are extremely effective. Because of ocular complications associated with these preparations, however, their use should be reserved for severe cases involving short courses of therapy.

Betacarotene, a carotenoid pigment that appears naturally in green and yellow vegetables is available as Solatene (Roche). This preparation absorbs the visible spectrum of light (in the 360 to 600 nm range), with maximum absorption at 450 to 475 nm, and it has been found to be beneficial for patients with this disorder.[8] The usual dose for children under 14 years of age is 30 to 150 mg (one to five capsules) per day, taken with meals. The therapeutic dosage is adjusted for serum carotene levels of 600 to 800 μg per 100 ml of plasma. The only side reactions appear to be a slight yellowish discoloration of the skin, orange-colored stools, and occasional gastrointestinal upset.

Photosensitivity Induced by Exogenous Sources

Exogenous photosensitizers may reach the skin by topical or systemic routes, and their reactions may be phototoxic or photoallergic in nature.

Topical photosensitizers include furocoumarin-containing cosmetic preparations (e.g., Shalomar perfume); fluorescein derivatives, as in indelible lipsticks, and blankophores (optical brighteners) added to detergents.[1, 9, 10]

Coal-tar preparations are time-honored topical therapies for childhood dermatoses. Although these preparations carry a warning regarding possible photosensitivity, documentation of childhood photosensitization from such products is uncommon, and most reports of photosensitivity involve adults contacting coal-tar preparations in industrial settings.

CLINICAL MANIFESTATIONS
Salicylanilide Reactions. Since 1960, halogenated salicylanilides and related antibacterial and antifungal compounds were the most important contact allergenic, photosensitizing agents. They were responsible for the vast majority of reactions reported in the last decade, with an estimated 10,000 cases presumably caused by tetrachlorosalicylanilides in England between 1960

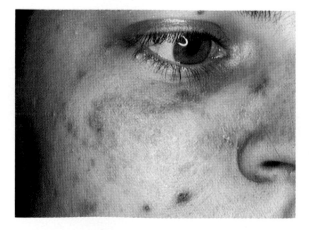

Figure 4–1 Polymorphous light eruption. Erythematous papulovesicular and plaque-like lesions with characteristic distribution on the sun-exposed area of the cheek.

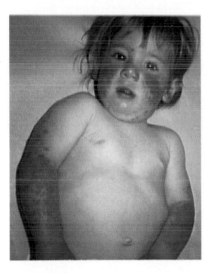

Figure 4–2 Drug-induced photosensitivity. Photoallergic dermatitis on sun-exposed areas of an infant following topical use of hexachlorophene.

and 1962.[4] Although tetrachlorosalicylanilides (TCSA) have been removed from general use, a number of related photosensitizers have been incorporated into soaps and other vehicles to combat infection, reduce body odor, and destroy fungi. These include hexachlorophene, dichlorophene, certain carbanilides, and antifungal agents chemically related to bithionol and tribromosalicylanilide (Figs. 4–2, 4–3).[4, 10, 11] Photosensitivity to salicylanilides probably represents a true delayed hypersensitivity phenomenon, appearing predominantly in 40- to 60-year-old males and relatively uncommonly in childhood.[6, 7]

Sunscreens also, at times, may induce photoallergic-type reactions. One of these, amyl paradimethylaminobenzoate (padimate A), is capable of provoking phototoxic reactions.[12] Photoallergic reactions to blankophores (optical brightening bleaches added to certain detergents) have also been reported by European observers but, fortunately, their use has been largely discontinued in this country.

The hallmark of sunlight-induced photoreaction, whether toxic or allergic, is its characteristic distribution. The exposed areas of the face, neck, upper extremities, and, in women, the anterior aspects of the legs and proximal dorsal areas of the feet are most prominently affected.

Lesions are similar to an exaggerated sunburn reaction. Edema and vesiculation are prominent, and other cutaneous lesions include eczematous, morbilliform, papulovesicular, urticarial, or lichen planus–like reactions. The clinical course is brief, and elimination of the offending drug or sunlight exposure usually results in improvement. In unusual cases, however, the photosensitivity may persist for months after the last known exposure to the offending chemical. Such individuals are known as persistent light reactors.

The action spectrum of topical and systemic photosensitizers is usually in the UVA range (320 to 400 nm). The upper eyelids, subnasal and submental areas, flexures of the wrist, and the antecubital fossae (areas generally not as well exposed to sunlight) tend to be spared. Since UVA passes through plate glass, the eruption may be accentuated on the left side of the face and left arm of drivers who drive automobiles from the left front seat position. Although clothing generally provides protection, reactions can also be produced by penetration of rays through light fabrics worn in summer.

Plant-Induced Photosensitivity (Phytophotodermatitis). Plant-induced photosensitivity (phytophotodermatitis) may at times be responsible for a number of dermatologic reactions. The large majority are phototoxic reactions due to the presence of furocoumarin compounds (psoralens) used in the treatment of psoriasis and vitiligo and found widely in such plants as parsnips, carrots, dill, parsley, figs, limes, and celery (particularly those infected with a fungus that causes pink rot disease). The photo-induced eruption usually begins the day after exposure to the furocoumarin and sunlight, ranges in severity from mild erythema to severe blistering, and eventuates in a characteristic dense inflammatory hyperpigmentation (Fig. 4–4). A bizarre linear streaking configuration of the dermatitis, with subsequent hyperpigmentation, especially on the face, chest, hands, and lower legs of children, is characteristic and highly diagnostic of this disorder (Fig. 4–5).

Berlocque (Berlock) Dermatitis. Several perfumes and colognes contain oil of bergamot, which is extracted from the peel of small oranges that grow in Southern France and Southern Italy.[11] Oil of bergamot contains a furocoumarin (5-methylpsoralen), a potent photosensitizer, and Shalimar perfume, containing 5- and 8-methoxypsoralen, is also a common cause of berlocque dermatitis.

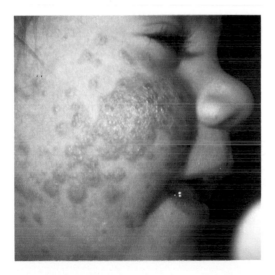

Figure 4–3 Papulovesicular lesions of photoallergic dermatitis due to hexachlorophene.

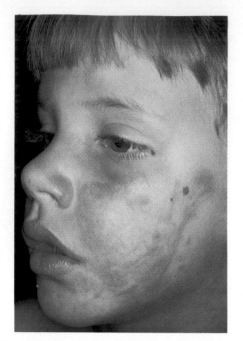

Figure 4–4 Plant-induced photosensitivity (phytophoto-sensitivity). Linear hyperpigmentation on the face of a child following exposure to limes and sunlight.

Hyperpigmentation occurs in bizzare configurations according to areas of application, hence the drop-like or pendant-like configuration and the name berlocque (French) or berlock (German), meaning trinket or pendant. This dermatitis is seen most frequently on the sides of the neck and in the retroauricular areas, the shoulders, breasts, hands, and face of women. When seen in men, the disorder usually occurs on the bearded area and is related to bergamot oil or related substances present in after shave lotions.

Systemic Sources of Photosensitization. Systemic photosensitizers include systemic antibacterial agents (namely demethylchlortetracycline and doxycycline, and only rarely tetracycline, sulfonamides, or nalidixic acid); antifungal preparations (griseofulvin); phenothiazine derivatives, particularly chlorpromazine (Thorazine); sulfonylurea hypoglycemic agents; anovulatory drugs; antihistamines (particularly the phe-

nothiazine congeners); isoniazid, thiazide diuretics; and certain dyes (acridine, methylviolet, and eosin).

DIAGNOSIS. Generally the diagnosis of photoallergic sensitization reactions depends on morphologic and histologic means. Photoallergic testing, however, is particularly valuable in the diagnosis of photoallergic contact dermatitis. By this method duplicate patch tests utilizing suspected photoallergens are applied. One set is uncovered and irradiated with a window glass-filtered ultraviolet light source (one emitting only long wave ultraviolet light rays) 24 hours after application. The following day a comparison is made of the covered and irradiated sites. A positive test reproduces the clinical eczematous lesion at the phototest site.[10]

MANAGEMENT. The management of acute photosensitivity reactions consists of removal (whenever possible) of the offending agent. Protective clothing and full-spectrum sunscreens afford the greatest degree of protection against exposure. Some patients, particularly those with photocontact reactions to halogenated salicylanilides may become persistent light reactors. These patients must avoid even minimal exposure of the sun in order to prevent severe eczematoid reactions. In addition, patients should minimize their exposure to natural sunlight and avoid unnecessary exposure to lamp sources with irradiance in the ultraviolet or visible light spectrum. These include fluorescent bulbs as well as ultraviolet sun lamps.

UNCLASSIFIED PHOTOSENSITIVITY DISORDERS

Juvenile Spring Eruption

Juvenile spring eruption is a disorder of unknown etiology. Perhaps a sunburn reaction of children with light complexions or a form of erythema multiforme, the disorder has been described in England, particularly in boys (sometimes girls) age 5 to 12 in the early spring months on unprotected areas following exposure to sunlight. Most commonly affecting the helix of the ears, occasionally the dorsa of the hands and the trunk, the disorder is characterized by dull-red

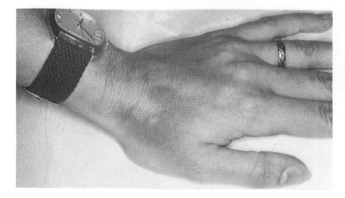

Figure 4–5 Hyperpigmentation on the dorsal aspect of the hands following the use of limes and sunlight exposure.

edematous papules, many of which become vesicular and crusted. The lesions heal within a week, without scarring, unless secondary infection develops. Topical steroids may relieve itching, but sunscreens do not appear to prevent recurrences of this disorder.[13]

Hydroa Aestivale and Hydroa Vacciniforme

Hydroa aestivale (summer prurigo of Hutchinson) and hydroa vacciniforme are rare, possibly related disorders that tend to appear each summer in children on uncovered parts of the body following exposure to sunlight. Males are more often affected than females at a ratio of 2:1. Although the role of heredity has not been clarified, they appear to be transmited as genetic recessive traits and are believed by some authorities to represent variants of polymorphous light eruption. Whereas some believe hydroa vacciniforme to be a more severe form of hydroa aestivale, others use both terms interchangeably and consider distinctions between these disorders to be ambiguous and unnecessary.[14]

To date the mechanism of this disorder has not been clarified. Most current studies suggest a delayed erythema-type reaction to an ultraviolet action spectrum in the UVB (290 to 320 nm) as well as the UVC (254 nm) range. The primary lesion is a pruritic edematous papule, vesicle, or bulla that occurs within hours or days on uncovered surfaces exposed to sunlight. Lesions tend to appear on the face, the "V" of the neck, and extensor surfaces of the extremities and are arranged symmetrically over the nose, cheeks, ears, and dorsal surfaces of the hands. The vesicles or bullae usually develop on an erythematous base and initially are rather tense. These are followed by progressive necrosis that leads to healing with a varioliform scar. Itching and burning as well as mild constitutional symptoms may precede the outbreak of the cutaneous lesions. The vesicles and bullae generally dry up after three or four days with the resultant formation of adherent brown crusts. The course of the disease is usually characterized by recurrent flares after sun exposure and, in most instances, the disorder involutes spontaneously by the late teenage years.

Histopathologic examination of lesions reveals epidermal vesicles, areas of hyperkeratosis with acanthosis, and a perivascular, predominantly lymphocytic and polymorphonuclear infiltrate in the dermis.

Treatment consists of preventive measures such as appropriate sunscreens, proper clothing, and avoidance of the midday sun. Although antimalarial drugs and para-aminobenzoic acids have been used with some therapeutic success, because of potential ophthalmic complications, antimalarial agents must be used with extreme caution, particularly in children. Although not fully studied in children, betacarotene (Solatene), appears to offer relief for individuals with this disorder.[14]

GENETIC DISORDERS ASSOCIATED WITH PHOTOSENSITIVITY

Xeroderma Pigmentosum

Xeroderma pigmentosum is a severe, rare autosomal recessive disease characterized by cutaneous photosensitivity, a decreased ability to repair deoxyribonucleic acid (DNA) damaged by ultraviolet radiation, and a tendency to early development of cutaneous malignancies. The cardinal features of this disorder include sensitivity to light at wavelengths in the UBV spectrum of 290 to 320 nm,[4, 15] premature aging of the skin accompanied by dystrophy, pigmentary changes, and the development of epithelial neoplasms; severe eye involvement; and usually early death from malignancy.

The basic abnormality in xeroderma pigmentosum is attributed to a defect in endonuclease, an enzyme that recognizes ultraviolet light-damaged regions of DNA and excises damaged thymine dimers so that other enzymes (DNA polymerase and polynucleotide ligase) may initiate DNA repair. Recent techniques have led to the discovery of five classes of xeroderma pigmentosum. Although not seen as distinct clinical entities, each of these variants is caused by mutation at a different locus, thus indicating the complexity of the enzyme systems involved in repair of ultraviolet light-damaged DNA.[15, 16]

CLINICAL MANIFESTATIONS. Children with xeroderma pigmentosum develop erythema, freckling, and increased pigmentation after exposure to sunlight. Most cases begin in early childhood. In 75 per cent of cases the first symptoms appear between six months and three years of age and reach the tumor stage (basal cell carcinoma, angiosarcoma, fibrosarcoma, keratoacanthoma, and malignant melanoma) before age 20.

In the acute form the first manifestations appear very early, sometimes shortly after birth or during the first weeks of life, after the first exposure to sun. Initial clinical findings include photophobia, erythema (which sometimes progresses to vesiculation and bulla formation), freckled hyperpigmentation of exposed parts, and subsequent papillomatous or verrucous lesions followed by degenerative and eventual malignant changes. When present at an early age, xeroderma pigmentosum usually presents a relentless course with irreversible skin damage. Although the severity of the disease varies, those individuals with severe forms frequently expire before the age of 10 years, and two thirds of affected children die before the age of 20 (Fig. 4–6).[17]

Many authors have reported the presence of neurologic complications in patients with this disorder. In addition to their cutaneous manifestations, those with the most severe form of xeroderma pigmentosum (termed the *DeSanctis-Cacchione* syndrome) have microcephaly with mental deficiency, premature closure of the sutures, retarded growth and sexual development, choreoathetosis, cerebellar ataxis, shorten-

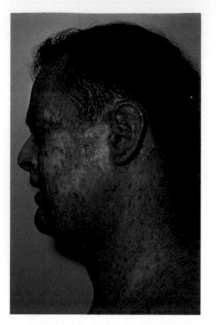

Figure 4–6 Xeroderma pigmentosum. Freckled hyperpigmentation, papillomatous and verrucous lesions on the face and neck (Department of Dermatology, Yale University School of Medicine).

ing of the achilles tendons, and, at times, sensorineural deafness.[15, 18]

Once the possibility of xeroderma pigmentosum is suspected, the clinical features are so distinctive that diagnosis is usually obvious. The characteristic clinical features include erythema, freckling, both hyperpigmentation and depigmentation, an appearance of premature aging, telangiectases, hyperkeratoses, ulcerations, keratoacanthomas, and, after a relatively short period of time, skin cancers. Areas of skin ordinarily protected by clothing remain relatively normal or may eventually show similar features, but to a lesser degree. Conjunctivitis, keratitis, corneal opacities and ulcerations, photophobia, blepharitis, crusting of the eyelids, symblepharon, and ectropion are highly characteristic and said to occur in 60 to 90 per cent of individuals with this disorder.

MANAGEMENT. The treatment of xeroderma pigmentosum consists of genetic counseling, avoidance of ultraviolet light exposure, the use of protective clothing and opaque sunscreen preparations, destruction of individual premalignant and malignant tumors by topical antimetabolite agents such as 5-fluorouracil, early excision of small cutaneous neoplasms, and, at times, resurfacing of severely damaged skin by dermabrasion or with homografts from less severely involved cutaneous surfaces.[19]

Prenatal diagnosis of xeroderma pigmentosum can now be performed. This procedure is simple and reliable and can be used routinely to help establish intrauterine diagnosis of this disorder. Although effective treatment for this defect is not yet available, the information obtained from amniocentesis can be reassuring to the parents if the baby is free of chromosomal aberrations or it can

afford them the chance to decide on termination of pregnancy if abnormalities are found. Although it is usually impossible to detect a heterozygous fetus by amniocentesis, this is of little clinical importance since xeroderma pigmentosum is an autosomal recessive disease and heterozygotes are phenotypically normal.[20, 21]

Hartnup Disease

Hartnup disease (named after the family in whom the disorder was first reported) is a rare autosomal recessive light-sensitive disorder characterized by a pellagra-like cutaneous eruption, neurologic abnormalities, and a specific aminoaciduria (due to a defect in the cellular transport of a group of monoamino-monocarboxylic acids.). The basic defect appears to be a failure in the absorption of tryptophan from the gastrointestinal tract. This results in reduced levels of available tryptophan and, accordingly, nicotinic acid. It has been postulated that a reduction of available tryptophan results in a reduced amount of available nicotinic acid, which, in turn, may be responsible for the pellagra-like photosensitivity. As yet, however, there is no specific proof that the photosensitivity in pellagra and the pellagra-like symptoms are due to a lack of nicotinic acid.

The biochemical defect (aminoaciduria) is a constant feature of Hartnup disease. Clinical manifestations, however, are intermittent, recurrent, and quite variable. The cutaneous eruption usually appears in the spring and summer. It may be present in early childhood, occasionally during early infancy, and, when present, is usually seen in children between three and nine years of age, with symptoms generally becoming milder with increasing age.[18] The cutaneous manifestations consist of a symmetrical distribution of inflammatory macules that tend to coalesce and eventuate in well-marginated red scaly lesions over light-exposed parts of the face, neck, uncovered areas of the arms, and the dorsal aspects of the hands and legs. Cerebellar ataxia is the predominate neurologic feature of Hartnup disease. Seen in over two thirds of those afflicted with this disorder, it seems to occur during periods when the rash is most prominent or following acute episodes of febrile illness.[22]

The diagnosis of Hartnup disease is based upon the clinical picture and demonstration of specific amino acid and indole excretion patterns (not the total aminoacid excretion). Treatment consists of avoidance of sunlight exposure and prolonged oral administration of high doses (40 to 200 mg) of nicotinic acid or nicotinamide. Since nicotinamide does not cause the flushing generally associated with administration of nicotinic acid, the former is generally the drug of choice.

Pellagra

Pellagra is a systemic disturbance caused by a cellular deficiency of niacin due to inadequate intake of nicotinic acid in the diet or to the ingestion of certain antinicotinic substances, such as hydantoin derivatives used in the therapy of epilepsy or the antituberculosis drug isoniazid. This nicotinamide deficiency state may be seen in all ages, but as a result of current nutritional standards and vitamin supplementation, is very rare in infancy and relatively uncommon in children. It is characterized by seasonal recurrences and a classic triad of three D's — dermatitis, diarrhea, and dementia.

The dermatitis may not always be present, but when it appears, it begins as a characteristically asymptomatic or pruritic symmetrical erythematous eruption on areas exposed to sunlight, heat, friction, or pressure. The usual sites of involvement include the face, neck, dorsal surface of the hands, arms, feet, the inguinal region, and, particularly in infants and small children, the diaper area. The eruption begins as well-marginated erythema and superficial scaling on sun-exposed areas resembling sunburn (with or without vesiculation or blister formation) that gradually subsides, leaving a dusky brown-red discoloration. In acute cases the lesions may progress to vesiculation, ulceration, exudation, cracking, and, at times, secondary infection. With chronicity, lesions become more livid, thickened, scaly, and ultimately fissured, atrophic, and deeply pigmented. About the lower neck the eruption may appear as a broad collarette of dermatitis known as *Casal's necklace*. In cases in which the "necklace" is incomplete, the lesions maintain their symmetrical and otherwise characteristic appearance.

Mucous membrane involvement, when present, consists of painful fissures and ulceration. The lips and cheeks are thin and pale, the mouth is dry, the tongue is red and swollen, and aphthous ulcers, fissuring, and angular cheilitis are common.

Neurologic manifestations may appear with or without involvement of the skin and digestive tract. In mild cases they consist of weakness, anorexia, and depression. In more severe cases, delirium, amentia, posterolateral spinal cord degeneration, and pyramidal and peripheral nerve involvement may be noted. The disease tends to be progressive and, if untreated, may eventuate in death within a period of several years.

The recommended daily allowance of niacin is 4 mg for infants and 6 to 12 mg for older children. Treatment of pellagra consists of appropriate dietary management in the form of meat, vegetables, eggs, and milk, supplemented by nicotinic acid or nicotinamide in dosages of 50 to 400 mg of niacin daily. As in the treatment of Hartnup disease, nicotamide is the drug of choice.

Rothmund-Thomson Syndrome (Poikiloderma Congenitale)

Poikiloderma congenitale (Rothmund-Thomson syndrome) is a rare inherited condition transmitted as an autosomal recessive disorder characterized by atrophy, pigmentation, and telangiectasia of the skin in association with juvenile cataracts, shortness of stature, partial or total alopecia, defects of the nails and teeth, and hypogonadism.[23] About 70 per cent of affected individuals are females.

Although the skin may be involved at birth, cutaneous changes generally make their appearance between the third and sixth months of life. Cutaneous features include diffuse erythema and, at times, edema and vesiculation on the cheeks, forehead, chin, ears, buttocks, and extensor surfaces of the arms and legs. As the erythema resolves, the skin begins to show a reticulated pattern of telangiectasia and alterations in pigmentation (both hypopigmentation and hyperpigmentation) with areas of atrophy. Although photosensitivity is a feature of many cases and exposure to sunlight may extend the distribution of the eruption, it probably is not responsible for the poikilodermatous appearance that develops on unexposed as well as light-exposed areas. Cataracts occur in about 40 per cent of reported cases, and defective bone development, which predominantly involves the long bones, occurs in about two thirds of affected individuals.

Bloom's Syndrome

Bloom's syndrome (congenital telangiectatic erythema in dwarfs) is a rare autosomal recessive disorder characterized by a triad of telangiectatic erythema, photosensitivity, and severe intrauterine and postnatal growth retardation.[24] In this disorder, erythema of the cheeks, often resembling lesions of lupus erythematosus, appears, between the second and third week of life, and typically spreads with exposure to sunlight to involve the nose, eyelids, forehead, ears, and lips. Eighty per cent of affected children are males, and 50 per cent are of Jewish descent. Other findings associated with this disorder include café au lait spots, clinodactyly, syndactyly, cryptorchidism, reduced IgM and IgA levels, a high incidence of chromosomal aberrations, and increased predisposition to neoplastic disease, particularly leukemia, during the second and third decades of life.

Cockayne's Syndrome

Cockayne's syndrome (trisomy 10) is a rare, recessively inherited disorder, generally seen in individuals of English lineage, characterized by dwarfism, telangiectatic sun sensitivity, and a 4 to 1 male preponderance. Affected children appear to be normal during infancy and begin to develop signs of the disorder during the second year of life. The cutaneous changes include a facial erythema in a butterfly distribution that develops after exposure to sunlight. Although this light sensitivity eventually disappears, erythema with telangiectasia characteristic of photosensitivity, mottled pigmentation, scarring, and atrophy of these sites remain as prominent features.[1] Loss of subcutaneous fat produces a "bird-like" facies and a tendency toward progressive ataxia, long limbs, and disproportionately large hands and feet, and large protruding ears suggest a "Mickey Mouse"-like appearance. Affected individuals are generally below the tenth percentile for height, and other abnormalities include thickened skull bones, retinal pigmentation, optic atrophy, cataracts, deafness, and mental retardation. There is no effective treatment for this disorder, and most patients die in the second or third decade of life as a result of arteriosclerotic vascular disease.

Kwashiorkor

True pellagrous skin changes can occasionally occur in children with kwashiorkor. In this disorder of infancy and childhood, an inadequate protein intake may result in amino acid (phenylalanine and tyrosine) deficiencies characterized by striking cutaneous and hair changes in association with developmental, mental, and gastrointestinal features, with a high mortality rate in the absence of proper dietary treatment.

The clinical picture generally occurs in children between six months and five years of age and consists of a conspicuous dermatosis that begins as an erythema that blanches on pressure rapidly followed by small dusky purple patches that do not blanch. The eruption has a sharply marginated edge raised above the surrounding skin, much as enamel paint that is lifting up and about to peel off. In contrast to lesions of pellagra, the dermatosis seldom appears on areas exposed to sunlight and tends to spare the feet and dorsal areas of the hands. Photosensitivity, purpura, and excessive bruisability may also be present.

In mild cases the cutaneous eruption is associated with a superficial desquamation; in severe cases there are large areas of erosion. As the disease progresses the entire cutaneous surface develops a reddish or coffee-colored hue, hence the term "red children." Other associated features include circumoral pallor, depigmentation of the hair from its normal black color in African children to a reddish-yellow, gray or straw color. Edema, xerosis, fine branny desquamation, dyschromia with hypopigmentation (perhaps due to phenylalanine deficiency), with cracking along Langer's lines that produces a "mosaic" or "cracked" appearance of the skin, complete the cutaneous picture.

Associated manifestations include mental behavior changes, anorexia, apathy, irritability, growth retardation, edema of the feet and face, a swollen abdomen, hypoproteinemia, and fatty infiltration of the liver. Children afflicted by this disorder are extremely ill and untreated cases carry a mortality rate of 30 per cent or more. Therapy consists of administration of a high protein diet and correction of dehydration and electrolyte imbalance.

THE PORPHYRIAS

The porphyrias comprise a group of genetically determined or acquired disorders of porphyrin, the chemical precursor for hemoglobin synthesis. There are two main categories of porphyric disease in man. Based upon the tissue in which the biochemical lesion is localized, they are classified into erythropoietic or hepatic forms.

Two principal erythropoietic types of porphyria, both inherited, have been described. The first of these, congenital erythropoietic porphyria, is an extremely rare autosomal recessive disorder; the other, congenital erythropoietic protoporphyria, appears to be transmitted as an autosomal dominant trait. The hepatic porphyrias are classified into those that are inherited and those that are acquired.[25] These include acute intermittent porphyria (AIP), acquired hepatic porphyria (porphyria cutanea tarda), and a mixture of the two, congenital cutaneous hepatic porphyria (porphyria variegata).[25] The porphyrins are the only well-established photosensitizers made by the human body. These are substances that produce photodynamic types of phototoxic reactions with a primary action spectrum at about 400 nanometers.[1]

Classification of Porphyrias

1. Erythropoietic
   a. Congenital Erythropoietic Porphyria
   b. Congenital Erythropoietic Protoporphyria
2. Hepatic
   a. Acute Intermittent Porphyria (Autosomal Dominant)
   b. Acquired Hepatic Porphyria (Porphyria Cutanea Tarda)
   c. Porphyria Variegata (A Combination of AIP and PCT)

Erythropoietic Porphyrias

Congenital Erythropoietic Porphyria (Günther's Disease)

Congenital erythropoietic porphyria (Günther's disease) is an extremely rare autosomal recessive disorder characterized by the appearance of red urine during infancy, severe photosensitivity that occurs in the first two or three years of life, splenomegaly, and hemolytic anemia.

Photosensitivity is frequently absent in the neonatal period but generally becomes apparent during the first years of life as exposure to sun increases. Recurrent vesicobullous eruptions on sun-exposed areas of the skin eventually result in multilating ulceration and scarring. Other common clinical features include hypertrichosis manifested as fine blond lanugo hair over the face and extremities, conjunctivitis, keratitis, brown-stained teeth that fluoresce under exposure to Wood's light, hyperpigmentation, hemolytic anemia, and loss of fingernails. The legendary werewolves of the middle ages, with fluorescent teeth and nails, mutilated and deformed ears, nose, and eyelids, and nocturnal habits due to their sensitivity to light, may indeed have been persons afflicted with congenital erythropoietic porphyria.

The biochemical disturbance in this disease appears to be a deficiency of normal enzyme control mechanisms in the formation of hemoglobin at a step prior to the formation of uroporphyrin, resulting in marked overproduction of uroporphyrin I and coproporphyrin I in circulating erythrocytes and bone marrow cells.

The diagnosis of erythropoietic porphyria can be made by the clinical features that appear early in life, fluorescence of the teeth and nails under black light examination, and sharply elevated levels of uroporphyrin I in erythrocytes, plasma, urine, and feces. Splenomegaly, an almost constant feature of this disorder, may remain undetected during the neonatal period only to appear as the child grows older. In the majority of reported cases hemolytic activity is indicated by normochromic anemia, elevated reticulocyte levels, circulating normoblasts, normoblastic hyperplasia of the bone marrow, and increased excretion of fecal urobilinogen. The anemia is thought to be due to hemolysis secondary to an intracorpuscular defect and ineffective erythropoiesis. The color of the urine of patients may vary from faint pink to burgundy or port-wine, depending upon the concentration of uroprophyrin derived from the oxidation of uroporphyrinogen.

The prognosis of erythropoietic porphyria is poor, with few patients surviving into the fourth or fifth decade. Death, when it occurs, is frequently associated with the hemolytic anemia. Treatment includes avoidance of sun exposure and trauma, with resolution of cutaneous manifestations, anemia, and splenomegaly often occurring with protection from light at wavelengths below 510 nm. Splenectomy, although frequently recommended, has had variable success. Window glass and ordinary sunscreen preparations do not protect light waves absorbed by prophyrins. Therefore, appropriate clothing and wide-spectrum sun protectants such as zinc oxide ointment or R V Paque should be used for appropriate topical protection. Oral betacarotene, available as Solatene (Roche), in doses of 30 to 150 mg a day appears to be an effective photoprotective agent for individuals afflicted with this disorder.[8]

Congenital Erythropoietic Protoporphyria (EPP)

Erythropoietic protoporphyria (EPP) is a rare autosomal dominant disorder characterized by mild photosensitivity and slight eczematization and inflammation of exposed skin associated with high concentrations of protoporphyrin in erythrocytes, plasma, and feces. The primary biochemical defect appears to be related to the enzyme ferrochelatase that converts protoporphyrin to heme.

Erythropoietic protoporphyria usually becomes symptomatic between the ages of two and five years. It may present clinically as burning, tingling, or itching of the exposed skin (often manifested by the child's crying when placed in sunshine) following short periods of sunlight exposure. This burning sensation may be followed by pruritic reddened edematous plaques that return to normal within 24 hours, occasionally papulovesicular and petechial eruptions that may persist for longer periods, and chronic changes such as hypopigmentation, hyperpigmentation, and a papular thickening that gives a cobblestone appearance to the skin. In a few patients, hypersplenism with associated hemolytic anemia (which responds favorably to splenectomy) has been reported. It now appears that this disease is quite common and may account for many previously undiagnosed light-sensitive reactions.

Laboratory findings are those of abnormally high protoporphyrin levels in circulating erythrocytes, bone marrow cells, and plasma. Fluorescence of the erythrocytes can be demonstrated by Wood's light or fluorescence microscopy. In contrast to congenital erythropoietic porphyria, fluorescence of teeth and nails is not present, and there is no increase in fecal or urinary uroporphyrins. Of particular interest is the fact that diagnosis has also been facilitated by the recent development of a rapid microfluorometric assay readily available to most well-equipped hospitals.[26]

As in congenital erythropoietic porphyria, window glass does not protect patients with this disorder. The management of erythropoietic protoporphyria, accordingly, is dependent upon limited exposure to sunlight, the use of opaque sunscreens as in congenital erythropoietic porphyria, and the administration of betacarotene (Solatene).

Hepatic Porphyrias

Acute Intermittent Porphyria (AIP)

Acute intermittent porphyria is a rare autosomal dominant disorder characterized by overproduction of porphyrin precursors (aminolevulinic acid and porphobilinogen), episodes of abdominal pain associated with vomiting, constipation, peripheral paresis or paralysis, psychologic manifestations or psychoneuroses provoked by barbiturates, sulfonamides, dapsone, griseofulvin, anticonvulsive agents, sulfonylurea compounds, and estrogens. Although the disease never manifests itself before puberty, the disorder is included here as a matter of completeness. Women seem to have a greater predisposition than men, and photosensitivity is not seen in association with this disorder. Freshly voided urine may be colorless and only darkens on standing and, except for possible laparotomy scars from previous abdominal surgery, cutaneous lesions are absent.

The fundamental problem of diagnosis is the differentiation of acute intermittent porphyria (AIP) from medical or surgical cases of an acute abdomen and from other organic, psychiatric, or neurologic disease. The classic triad of abdominal pain, urine that darkens on standing, and neuropsychiatric symptoms, particularly when associated with multiple laparotomy scars from previous surgery, should raise suspicion of this disorder. Diagnosis can be made by the demonstration of elevated aminolevulinic acid (ALA) and porphobilinogen (PBG) during attacks and by the demonstration of porphobilinogen in the urine by the Watson-Schwartz test.

There is no effective treatment for acute intermittent porphyria. Drugs that are known to precipitate porphyric attacks should be avoided. Bromides have been used with success, propoxyphene (Darvon) is tolerated well, chlorpromazine (Thorazine) is useful for the treatment of acute abdominal pain, and, for severe pain, meperidine (Demerol) is effective.

Acquired Hepatic Porphyria (Porphyria Cutanea Tarda)

Porphyria cutanea tarda (PCT), the most common form of porphyria, appears to be an inborn error of metabolism characterized by the excretion of excessive uroporphyrin and coproporphyrin in both urine and feces. Although most common in adults during the third and fourth decades of life, this disorder has also been seen in children (three cases have been reported in children below 15 years of age, one as young as 2 years of age) and has a high incidence among the Bantus in Africa where home-brewed alcohol or beer with high iron content is ingested.[27]

The exact genetic and enzymatic defect in porphyria cutanea tarda remains unknown. Basically a disease of the liver, it has been shown to be associated with specific enzyme deficiencies (uro- and coprodecarboxylase). The primary cutaneous lesion of porphyria cutanea tarda is a photosensitivity to the uroporphyrin deposited in the skin. Light in the 400 nm range is necessary for production of cutaneous lesions. Skin lesions in this disease consist of vesicles or blisters on light-exposed cutaneous surfaces, especially the dorsal aspect of the hands. Other features include increased fragility of the skin, with erosions and ulcerations as the result of relatively minor trauma, and hypertrichosis and melanosis of the face that appear to be related to sun exposure.

Porphyria cutanea tarda can be precipitated by estrogen therapy, alcoholic cirrhosis, and accidental ingestion of the fungicide hexachlorobenzene (this is not to be confused with the insecticide gamma benzene hexachloride used for the treatment of scabies and pediculosis) responsible for an epidemic of porphyria cutanea tarda in Turkey.[28] Although diabetes mellitus is present in 25 to 50 per cent of patients with porphyria cutanea tarda, the reason for this high association is unknown.

Confirmation of the clinical diagnosis of por-

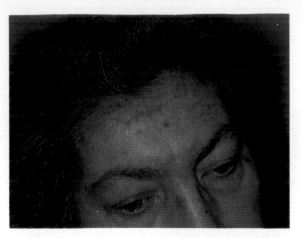

Figure 4–7 Hyperpigmentation, a weather-beaten appearance, and excessive furrowing of the forehead in porphyria variegata.

phyria cutanea tarda can be made by increased levels of uroporphyrin, slightly elevated fecal coproporphyrin and protoporphyrin, and positive fluorescence of the patient's urine with a Wood's light. Treatment consists of phlebotomy, with the number and frequency of phlebotomies dependent upon clinical response, hemoglobin levels, and urinary porphyrin levels. Low-dose chloroquine therapy has also been recommended as an effective form of therapy. The therapeutic effect proposed for chloroquine in this disorder appears to be related to chloroquine destruction of hepatocyte mitochondria and the formation of a water-soluble complex with porphyrin that can be excreted by the kidneys.[29]

Porphyria Variegata

Porphyria variegata (congenital cutaneous hepatic porphyria) is an autosomal dominant disorder that represents a combination of acute intermittent porphyria (AIP) and porphyria cutanea tarda (PCT). This disease, not seen in young children, has its onset after puberty and generally appears in the fourth to fifth decades of life.

Clinical features include sun sensitivity in adult life, with vesicles or blisters on light-exposed surfaces, hyperpigmentation, a weather-beaten or waxy complexion with excessive furrowing of the forehead (cutis rhomboidalis frontalis), scars on the back of the neck and frontal hair margin, milia, and scleroderm-like plaques (Fig. 4–7). The urinary findings overlap those of both acute intermittent porphyria and porphyria cutanea tarda. Treatment consists of avoidance of hepatotoxic agents and sun exposure, repeated phlebotomies, and low-dose chloroquine therapy.

References

1. Epstein JH: Adverse cutaneous reactions to the sun. *In* Malkinson FD, Pearson RW: The Year Book of Dermatology, Year Book Medical Publishers, Chicago, 1971, 5–43.

A thorough analytic presentation of sunlight and its adverse effects.

2. Parrish JA: Photosensitivity and sunburn. *In* Conn HF (Ed.): Current Therapy 1978. W. B. Saunders Co., Philadelphia, 1978, 618–620.

A review of present therapy of cutaneous reactions to sun.

3. Willis I: Photosensitivity. *In* Moschella SL, Pillsbury DM, Hurley HJ Jr (Eds.): Dermatology. W. B. Saunders Co., Philadelphia, 1975, 324–349.

A review of photosensitivity reactions, their prophylaxis, and therapy.

4. Epstein JH: Photoallergy. A review. Arch. Dermatol. 106:741 778, 1972.

A review of photoallergy, its pathogenesis, and its therapy.

5. Sams WM Jr, Epstein JH, Winkelman RK: Solar urticaria, investigation of pathogenetic mechanisms. Arch. Dermatol. 99:390–397, 1969.

A 29 year old man with solar urticaria with an action spectrum between 250 and 330 nanometers.

6. Fisher DA, Epstein JH, Kay D, et al: Polymorphous light eruption and lupus erythematosus: differential diagnosis by fluorescent fluoroscopy. Arch. Dermatol. 101:458–461, 1970.

Polymorphous light eruptions confirmed by phototest techniques.

7. Birt AR, Davis RA: Hereditary polymorphic light eruption of American Indians. Int. J. Dermatol. 14:105, 1975.

An autosomal dominant form of polymorphous light eruption in American Indians (from mid-Canada to South America).

8. Nordlund JJ, Klaus SN, Mathews-Roth MM, et al.: New therapy for polymorphous light eruptions. Arch. Dermatol. 108:710–712, 1973.

Carotenes offer protection for patients with light sensitivity in the 360 to 600 nm range.

9. Freeman RG, Knox JM: The action spectrum of photocontact dermatitis caused by halogenated salicylanilides and related compounds. Arch. Dermatol. 97:130–136, 1968.

Nineteen patients with photocontact dermatitis due to tetrachlorosalicylanilide and related compounds.

10. Epstein JH, Wuepper KD, Maibach HI: Photocontact dermatitis to halogenated salicylanilides and related compounds. Arch. Dermatol. 97:236–244, 1968.

Twenty six patients with photocontact dermatitis associated with halogenated salicylanilides and related compounds.

11. Pathak MA, Epstein JH: Normal and abnormal reactions of man to light. *In* Fitzpatrick TB, Arndt KA, Clark WII Jr, et al.: Dermatology in General Medicine. McGraw-Hill Book Co., New York, 1971, 977–1036.

A comprehensive review of photoreactions and photosensitivity.

12. Kaidbey KH, Kligman AM: Phototoxicity to a sunscreen ingredient. Padimate A. Arch. Dermatol. 114:547–549, 1978.

Amyl paradiamethylaminobenzoic acid (padimate), an ester of para-aminobenzoic acid (PABA) found in popular proprietary sunscreens was found to produce phototoxicity.

13. Ryan TJ: Juvenile spring eruption. *In* Rook A, Wilkinson DS, Ebling FJG (Eds.): Textbook of Dermatology. 2nd ed. Blackwell Scientific Publications, Oxford, 1972, 462.

A papulovesicular eruption seen on the light exposed helix of the ear of children (rarely adults) in England following sun exposure in the early spring months.

14. Bickers DR, Demar LK, DeLeo V, et al.: Hydroa vacciniforme. Arch. Dermatol. 114:1193–1196, 1978.

Two children with hydroa vacciniforme effectively treated with betacarotene (Solatene).

15. Reed WB, Landing B, Sugarman G, et al.: Xeroderma pigmentosum. Clinical and laboratory investigation of its basic defect. JAMA 207:2073–2079, 1969.

On the basis of clinical and laboratory investigation, xeroderma pigmentosum appears to be an autosomal recessive disorder characterized by sunlight sensitivity and multiple cutaneous malignancies.

16. Cleaver JE: DNA damage and repair in light-sensitive human skin disease. J. Invest. Derm. 54:181–195, 1970.

Studies demonstrate the defect in xeroderma pigmentosum to be that of endonuclease, an enzyme that recognizes and initiates repair of an ultraviolet damaged region of DNA.

17. Rook A: Genetics in dermatology. *In* Rook A, Wilkinson DS, Ebling FJG (Eds.): Textbook of Dermatology, 2nd ed. Blackwell Scientific Publications, Oxford, 1972, 91–126.

A review of hereditary and genetic factors and their relationship to cutaneous disease.

18. Reed WB, Sugarman GI, Mathis RA: DeSanctis-Cacchione syndrome. A case report with autopsy findings. Arch. Dermatol. 113:1561–1563, 1977.

The DeSanctis-Cacchione syndrome, a form of xeroderma pigmentosum with neurologic complications.

19. Epstein EH Jr, Burk P, Cohen IK, et al.: Dermatome shaving in the treatment of xeroderma pigmentosum. Arch. Dermatol. 105:589–590, 1972.

Dermabrasion of severely sun-damaged skin in a patient with xeroderma pigmentosum retarded the development of malignant tumors.

20. Ramsay CA, Coltart TM, Blunt C, et al.: Prenatal diagnosis of xeroderma pigmentosum: report of first successful case. J. Invest. Dermatol. 63:392–396, 1974.

Amniotic fluid studies at 16 weeks gestation in a mother with a previous child afflicted with xeroderma pigmentosum revealed a 78 per cent reduction in DNA repair synthesis, thus allowing termination of the pregnancy by prostaglandin and oxytocin infusion.

21. Editorial comment in Malkinson FD, Pearson RS: The Year Book of Dermatology 1975. Year Book Medical Publishers, Inc., Chicago, 1975, 180.

Comments on the article by C. A. Ramsey et al. on the value of early prenatal diagnosis of xeroderma pigmentosum by amniocentesis studies of DNA repair synthesis in amniotic cell culture.

22. Jepson JB: Hartnup disease. *In* Stanbury JB, Wyngaarden JB, Fredrickson DS: The Metabolic Basis of Inherited Disease, 2nd ed. McGraw-Hill Book Co. New York, 1966, 1283–1299.

The metabolic and clinical aspects of Hartnup disease.

23. Silver HK: Rothmund-Thompson syndrome: an oculocutaneous disorder. Am. J. Dis. Child. 111:182–190, 1966.

A review of Rothmund-Thompson syndrome in two brothers.

24. Bloom D: Congenital telangiectatic erythema resembling lupus erythematosus in dwarfs. Am. J. Dis. Child. 88:754–758, 1954.

Three children with facial telangiectatic erythema, photosensitivity, and dwarfism (Bloom's syndrome).

25. Levere RD, Kappas A. The porphyric diseases of man. Hospital Practice 5:61–73, 1970.

A clear and concise analysis of the classification, biochemical derangements, and clinical picture of the porphyrias.

26. Poh-Fitzpatrick MB, Piomelli S, Young P, et al.: Rapid quantitative assay for erythrocyte porphyrins: rapid quantitative microfluorometric assay applicable to diagnosis of erythropoietic protoporphyria. Arch. Dermatol. 110:225–230, 1974.

An accurate, relatively inexpensive quantitative assay for free erythrocyte porphyrins allows rapid diagnosis of erythropoietic protoporphyria (EPP).

27. Kasky A: Porphyria cutanea tarda in a two-year-old girl. Br. J. Dermatol. *90*:213–216, 1974.

A two-year-old girl with small vesicles, crusts, and scars on the face with biochemical findings compatible with a diagnosis of porphyric cutanea tarda.

28. Cam C, Nigogosyan G: Acquired toxic porphyria cutanea tarda due to hexachlorobenzene. JAMA *183*:89–91, 1963.

A report of 348 of an estimated 5000 cases of porphyria cutanea tarda due to accidental consumption of wheat treated with the fungicide hexachlorobenzene ($C_6 Cl_6$).

29. Beeaff D: Dermatologic rounds. Porphyria. Dermatology *1*:15–27 and 56, 1978.

A review of porphyria, its biochemical and cutaneous manifestations.

PAPULOSQUAMOUS AND RELATED DISORDERS

Childhood Psoriasis

Psoriasis is a common inherited disorder characterized by erythematous scaly papules of plaques with a predisposition for the elbows, knees, extensor surfaces of the limbs, the genitalia, and the lumbosacral area. Affecting 1 to 3 per cent of the population, it is uncommon in the Japanese, American Indians, and blacks, particularly those of African origin whose comprise the bulk of the American black population.[1] It usually follows an irregularly chronic course marked by remissions and exacerbations of unpredictable onset and duration.

Despite continuing research and investigation, the etiology of psoriasis remains unknown. Although early studies suggested autosomal dominant transmission with incomplete penetrance, it is apparent that genetic transmission of the psoriatic tendency is more complicated than previously suspected and probably reflects the presence of subpopulations involving different genetic loci. Of interest in this regard are recent studies linking HLA-B13, HLA-B17, HLA-Bw16, and HLA-B37 with psoriasis. Of these, patients with HLA-B17 appear to develop psoriasis at an earlier age than those with HLA-Bw16.[2]

For years it has been stated that psoriasis is uncommon in childhood and rare in those under 3 years of age. Statistical studies, however, reveal that 37 per cent of patients first develop the disease before the age of 20. Twenty-seven per cent of affected individuals develop the disorder before age 15; 10 per cent have the onset of lesions before age 10; 6.5 per cent before age 5; 2 per cent

before age 2; and patients with active lesions present at birth (congenital psoriasis) have been documented (Figs. 5–1 and 5–2).[3-5] In adults the disorder occurs with equal frequency in both sexes. In childhood forms, however, the ratio of females to males is 2:1.[3, 4] Of these, one third have at least one relative with the disorder. In children with at least one affected parent the incidence is said to be three times more common than in those whose parents are unaffected and, although studies of twins may be open to criticism on the basis of selective reporting, up to 72 per cent of identi-

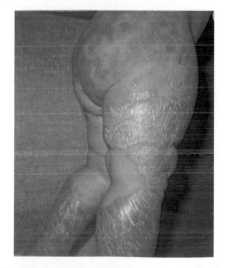

Figure 5–1 Childhood psoriasis in a 10-month-old infant (this patient had the onset of her disorder at 3½ months of age).

83

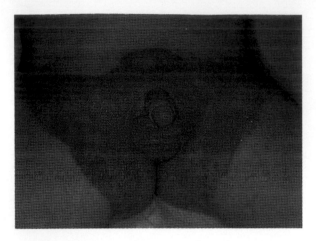

Figure 5–2 Psoriasis in the diaper area of a 3-month-old infant.

cal twins appear to be concordant for this disorder.[6]

The basic cause of psoriasis appears to be related to a marked increase in epidermal cell turnover. Although the factors that initiate this process remain unknown, this increased production and proliferation of psoriatic epidermis appears to be responsible for the scaling and thickening characteristic of psoriatic lesions.[7]

CLINICAL MANIFESTATIONS. Classic lesions of psoriasis consist of round, erythematous, well-marginated patches with a full, rich, red hue covered by a characteristic grayish or silvery-white scale. Lesions almost invariably begin as small, reddish, pinpoint to pinhead-sized papules surmounted by fine scales. These papules coalesce and form patches or plaques that measure from one to several centimeters or more in diameter (Fig. 5–3).

The disorder may present as solitary lesions or countless patches or plaques distributed over wide areas of the body. Although exceptions occur, lesions generally are seen in a bilaterally symmetrical pattern with a distinct predilection for the scalp, elbows, knees, lumbosacral, and anogenital regions. Central portions of the patches may heal and involute so that nummular, annular, gyrate, arcuate, or circinate figures may be produced. Although the classic distribution of psoriasis characteristically occurs on the extensor surfaces (the elbows, knees, and lumbosacral regions), lesions may also be found in a flexural distribution with involvement of the axillae, groin, perineum, central chest, and umbilical region. This variant, termed *psoriasis inversus*, may be seen alone, without involvement of extensor surfaces, in 2.8 to 6.0 per cent of patients, or in association with other regional involvement (in 30 per cent of patients)[8] (Fig. 5–4).

The hallmark of psoriasis is the silvery micaceous (mica-like) scale that is generally attached at the center rather than the periphery of lesions. Removal of this scale results in fine punctate

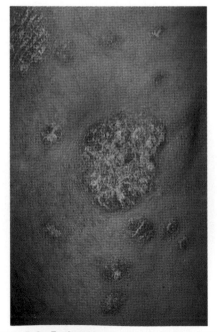

Figure 5–3 Erythematous well-marginated patches of psoriasis with typical micaceous (mica-like) scale.

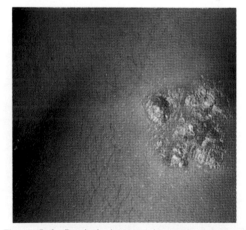

Figure 5–4 Psoriasis inversus in popliteal fossa. Note mica-like scale and fine punctate bleeding points (Auspitz's sign).

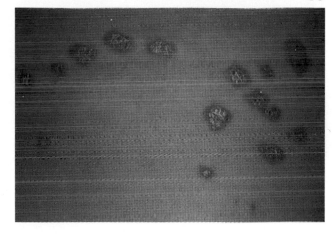

Figure 5–5 Guttate (drop-like) psoriasis.

bleeding points. This phenomenon (termed Auspitz's sign), highly characteristic but not exclusively diagnostic of this disorder, is related to rupture of capillaries high in the papillary dermis of lesions.

The Koebner phenomenon, a special feature seen in psoriasis as well as in certain other skin disorders (verrucae, rhus dermatitis, lichen planus, lichen nitidus, Darier's disease, and pityriasis rubra pilaris), is seen as skin lesions that occur at sites of local injury. While the precise mechanism of the Koebner phenomenon is unknown, it appears to represent a reaction to trauma (an isomorphic response) that follows simple irritation such as a scratch or sunburn, a surgical scar, or a pre-existing disease such as seborrheic or atopic dermatitis. In addition to its clinical value as a diagnostic sign, this phenomenon is frequently seen as a precipitating cause of psoriasis and should be emphasized to all patients afflicted with this disorder.

Guttate Psoriasis. The Koebner phenomenon is particularly significant in childhood psoriasis when drop-like (guttate) lesions appear suddenly over a large part of the body surface (Fig. 5–5). This variant, termed *guttate psoriasis*, may be the first manifestation of the disorder. Generally, but not necessarily, streptococcal in origin, two thirds of patients with guttate psoriasis give a history of an upper respiratory infection one to three weeks before the onset of an acute flare of the disorder.[9] Seen in 14 to 17 per cent of the population, guttate forms of psoriasis generally occur in children and young adults. Lesions are round or oval in configuration, measure from 2 or 3 mm to 1 cm in diameter, and generally occur in a symmetrical distribution over the trunk and proximal aspects of the extremities (occasionally the face, scalp, ears, and distal aspects of the extremities).

Seborrhiasis. The scalp is frequently seen as the initial site of psoriatic involvement. Although psoriatic lesions of the scalp, eyebrows, and ears (the superior and postauricular folds and external auditory meatus) may present as well-demarcated erythematous plaques with thick adherent silvery scales similar in appearance to those on other parts of the body, lesions often tend to be greasy, soft, and salmon-colored, suggesting a diagnosis of seborrhea. In this variant, often termed *seborrhiasis*, lesions may present with features of both seborrhea and psoriasis. Whereas lesions of seborrhea generally remain within the hairline, lesions of psoriasis frequently extend beyond the confines of the hairline onto the forehead, preauricular, postauricular, and nuchal regions (Fig. 5–6). When the true nature of the disorder remains in doubt, appropriate diagnosis may be aided by the fact that lesions particularly resistant to appropriate treatment for seborrhea are more likely to prove to be psoriatic rather than seborrheic in nature.[8]

Pityriasis Amiantacea (Tinea Amiantacea). Another variant of psoriasis of the scalp is known as *pityriasis* or *tinea amiantacea* (asbestos-like). This disorder is unrelated to fungus infection of the scalp and refers to forms of seborrhea or psoriasis of the scalp generally seen in children or adolescents in which crusts are firmly adherent and asbestos-like (Fig. 5–7). When seen as a manifestation of psoriasis, tinea amiantacea frequently is persistent and somewhat resistant to therapy.

Nail Involvement. Although statistics vary, the nails appear to be affected in 25 to 50 per

Figure 5–6 Seborrheic psoriasis (seborrhiasis). Lesions of seborrhea generally remain within the hairline; lesions of psoriasis frequently extend beyond the confines of the hairline.

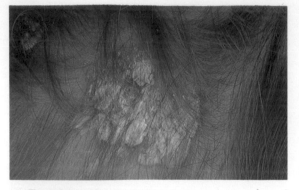

Figure 5-7 Tinea (pityriasis) amiantacea. A severe form of psoriasis of the scalp in which the scales are strongly adherent (asbestos-like).

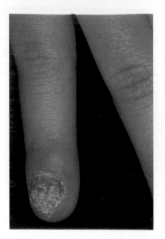

Figure 5-9 Psoriasis of the nail with dystrophy, discoloration, crumbling of the nail plate, and associated secondary candidal infection.

cent of patients with psoriasis.[10] Pitting is probably the best known and most characteristic nail change in psoriasis. Generally seen as small irregularly spaced depressions measuring less than one millimeter in diameter, larger depressions or punched-out areas of the nail plate may also be noted. These pits, formed during the process of keratinization of the nail, probably represent small intermittent lesions in the part of the matrix that forms the superficial layers of the nail plate.[11]

Although psoriatic pitting, when present, is highly characteristic, it must be differentiated from nail pitting seen in alopecia areata and atopic dermatitis. That of atopic dermatitis has a coarse irregular appearance and frequently is associated with nail dystrophy, roughening and discoloration of the nail surface, and a history of recent paronychia or dermatitis of the fingers. Although pitting is said to be an infrequent manifestation of childhood psoriasis, in actuality it is far more common than is realized. This impression is substantiated by a study of 14 infants and small children with psoriasis under age two wherein 79 per cent (11 children) manifested

psoriatic pitting of the nails. Of these, one actually displayed pitting of the nails at the time of birth.[12]

Other psoriatic nail changes include discoloration, subungual hyperkeratosis, crumbling and grooving of the nail plate, and onycholysis (separation of the nail plate from the nail bed) (Figs. 5-8 and 5-9). Onycholysis, also seen in other diseases (onychomycosis, congenital ectodermal defects, hypothyroidism, photoonycholysis due to tetracycline), may be differentiated by a yellow or brown band that separates the white free edge from the normal pink color of the attached portion of the nail. This yellow band, when present, is a particularly valuable clinical feature in the differentiation of psoriasis from onychomycosis (tinea involvement of the nail) and appears to be related to accumulation of large amounts of glycoprotein associated with psoriatic involvement of the hyponychium and nail bed. Subungual keratosis is a common source of secondary bacterial and fungal infection. Bacterial or monilial infections, therefore, are frequently seen in association with psoriasis of the nails (Fig. 5-9).

DIAGNOSIS. The diagnosis of psoriasis can be made on the basis of clinical findings alone or in combination with histologic findings. The histopathologic features of psoriasis include epidermal thickening (acanthosis with elongation of the rete ridges); elongation and edema of the dermal papillae, with thinning of the suprapapillary portions of the epidermis; increased mitoses in the basal layer and lower malpighian layers of the epidermis (in contrast to the presence of mitoses only in a single basal cell layer of normal skin); the presence of immature nucleated cells (parakeratosis) in the stratum corneum, with a diminished or absent stratum granulosum; inflammatory infiltrate (usually lymphocytic or monocytic) in the superficial corium; and focal collection of neutrophils in the stratum corneum or subcorneal layer (Munro microabscesses) (Fig. 5-10).

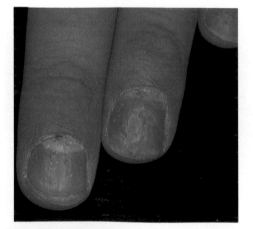

Figure 5-8 Nail psoriasis with pitting, discoloration, subungual keratin, and onycholysis.

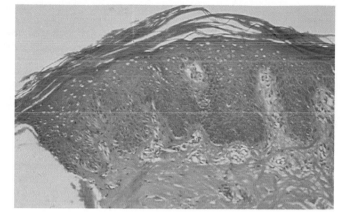

Figure 5-10 Psoriasis. Histologic features include hyperkeratosis, parakeratosis, diminished granular layer, acanthosis, elongation of rete ridges, vascular dilatation, and inflammatory round cell infiltrate.

COURSE. The course of psoriasis in general is prolonged, chronic, and unpredictable. In most patients the disease is not severe and remains confined to localized cutaneous regions. Remissions and exacerbations are the rule in most patients, with a marked tendency to improvement in summer, particularly during long periods of sun exposure. In some patients the disease may undergo spontaneous improvement; in others exacerbations may occur without apparent cause. Although sunlight generally is beneficial, an occasional patient may be photosensitive with resultant exacerbation of lesions in areas exposed to the sun. At times the disorder may remain relatively unchanged for years, but with appropriate therapy satisfactory control of the disease is possible in a majority of patients.

TOPICAL THERAPY. Although studies suggest that childhood psoriasis usually portends a more severe course in adult life,[3] spontaneous remissions lasting for variable time periods occur in 38 per cent of patients, and most patients generally respond well to presently available therapeutic measures.[4, 9] Whatever therapeutic approach is chosen, the patient and his family should receive some degree of instruction as to the pathophysiology and natural course of the disease, with reassurance that most patients, with a little bit of effort, can do much to control the cutaneous aspects of their disorder.

Since psoriasis is a chronic dermatosis characterized by periods of exacerbation, and individual response to therapy frequently varies, it is wise to have a variety of therapeutic modalities available. The nature of the disorder and the lack of a specific cure can be discouraging to the patient, the patient's family, and the physician alike. It is imperative, therefore, that the patient and parents of the patient understand the treatment and the rationale for its use. The approach to medication should be made as simple as possible, since therapy is time-consuming, burdensome, and easily rejected. It is important to let the patient learn day-to-day care and, whenever possible, carry out the routine as independently of parents as possible.[9]

Corticosteroids. Frequently producing dramatic resolution of lesions, corticosteroids are often the mainstay of topical therapy. Although high-potency topical corticosteroids are invaluable in short-term management of severe recalcitrant lesions, most patients with psoriasis respond quite well to moderate or low-potency steroid formulations. Since there is a science to the use of topical corticosteroids, which involves selection of the correct strength corticosteroid in the proper formulation for particular disease processes and specific areas of involvement, an appreciation of the approximate ranking of the potency of these compounds and a review of the pharmacology of these agents is invaluable (see Table 3-1, p. 50).[13]

Formulations of topical corticosteroids are available as creams, ointments, gels, lotions, and sprays. Gel formulations are generally more effective than ointments; corticosteroids in ointment base have greater biological activity than those incorporated into creams or lotions; and creams generally are more effective than lotions. On the scalp, clear solutions (gels, lotions, or sprays) are preferable to ointments and creams; creams or lotions are preferred in the intertriginous areas; and creams or ointments are more convenient and effective on exposed areas. In recent years occlusive dressings utilizing corticosteroid creams under polyethylene film (Saran Wrap) or as flurandrenolide tape (Cordran Tape, Dista) have been utilized to augment the effectiveness of topical therapy. By means of these occlusive dressings the scales soften and the medication can penetrate 10 to 100 times more readily into the skin. Such occlusive dressings are usually used only during sleeping hours (for periods of 6 to 12 hours). Since folliculitis, telangiectases, and atrophic striae may result from prolonged use of corticosteroids under occlusion, care and appropriate precautions should be advised when this form of therapy is recommended.

Prompt resolution of small persistent psoriatic plaques can also be accomplished by intralesional injection of corticosteroid suspension (through a small 30-gauge needle or by dermojet). The steroid most commonly used for intralesional therapy is triamcinolone acetonide (Kenalog) diluted with sterile saline or a local anesthetic (in order to minimize the pain of injection) to concentrations of 2.5 to 10.0 mg per ml. Frequently, only one or two injections may produce satisfactory clearing at the sites of injection. Limitation, however, must be placed on size and number of injections because of associated discomfort and the possibility of steroid atrophy, telangiectasia, or systemic absorption (fortunately, atrophy due to intralesional steroids usually disappears spontaneously, frequently within a period of 6 to 9 months).

Psoriatic nails are extremely distressing to the patient, respond slowly to therapy, and are frequently difficult to treat. This disorder can be treated with triamcinolone acetonide suspension (10 mg per cc) injected into the nail fold just proximal to the diseased matrix by a 30-gauge needle or dermojet (two or three times) at intervals of two to six weeks. Although discomforting to a certain degree, this regimen is beneficial at times and can produce some cosmetic improvement.[14] One per cent 5-fluorouracil (5-FU) in propylene glycol or a combination of benzoyl peroxide gel and a potent topical corticosteroid applied twice daily into the cuticle of chronically involved nails for periods of 4 to 6 months is also reported to be somewhat beneficial. Patients with severe arthropathy or active psoriasis of the nail fold are less likely to respond to 5-FU therapy, and individuals with onycholysis should not be treated with this modality (since an increased tendency to onycholysis occurs in individuals on this form of therapy).[15]

Tar Preparations. Although topical steroids to a great extent have replaced tars in the treatment of many forms of dermatitis, tars still remain a highly effective therapeutic modality, particularly in the management of psoriasis and other chronic dermatoses. The exact mechanism whereby tar exerts its therapeutic effect remains unclear, but it appears to be related to its anti-inflammatory effect and its ability to decrease epidermal proliferation. Cosmetically acceptable tar preparations are now available for baths (Balnetar, Polytar Bath, Zetar Emulsion) and as creams or lotions (Alphosyl by Reed and Carnrick and Tar-Doak Lotion by Doak Pharmacal), and recent formulations of tar in a gel base (Estar gel, Psorigel) are safe, effective, and cosmetically acceptable.

Removal of Scalp Lesions. The scalp frequently presents mechanical difficulties to patients with thick encrustations and scaling. Removal of scales can be facilitated by the use of "P & S" Liquid (Chester A. Baker Laboratories), a specially prepared mixture of phenol and sodium chloride in liquid paraffin, oil, and water. This preparation is highly effective when applied to scalp lesions with a cotton pledget once or twice a day followed 6 to 8 hours later by an appropriate antiseborrheic or tar shampoo. Tar-containing shampoos (such as Ionil-T, Polytar, Pentrax, Sebutone, Vanseb-T, Zetar) are particularly effective and cosmetically acceptable. In stubborn or persistent cases, the use of a corticosteroid lotion or spray formulation (Diprosone, Halog, Kenalog, Valisone) once or twice a day in conjunction with the above regimen is also beneficial. When scaling and crusting are particularly thick and resistant to therapy, incorporation of 3 to 5 per cent salicylic acid to the steroid lotion is helpful.

Sunlight. Most psoriatic patients are benefited by exposure to sunlight and accordingly are frequently better during the summer months. Advantage should be taken of this in planning the summer activities of the psoriatic child. Appropriate sunburn precautions, however, must be utilized since sudden overexposure may result in sufficient epidermal injury to cause exacerbation of the disorder. For those who can arrange exposure to sunlight on a regular basis, this can be an important aspect of therapy, alone or in combination with crude coal tar preparations or their derivatives. Again caution is recommended in an effort to reduce sunburn and photo-sensitization. Although natural sunlight is superior to artificial ultraviolet therapy, ultraviolet treatment, under proper precautions, may be utilized as an adjunct to therapy in an office or at home. Care must be exercised, however, to protect the eyes with moist cotton pledgets or special sungoggles (not sunglasses) and to avoid overexposure resulting in sunburn or exacerbation of the disorder.

The Goeckerman Regimen. Since first introduced over fifty years ago, the Goeckerman regimen has been a highly effective treatment for severe recalcitrant forms of psoriasis.[16] The Goeckerman procedure consists of 5 per cent crude coal tar (Zetar) or one of its derivatives (Estar gel) applied to the entire body at bedtime. In the morning the excess tar is removed with mineral oil and the patient receives ultraviolet light therapy to the entire body (after first testing the patient for the minimal erythema dose to minimize the tendency for sunburn or exacerbation in light-sensitive persons). The amount of ultraviolet is increased gradually (generally by one minute a day) to an erythema or suberythema dose. When properly used, the Goeckerman regimen is safe, highly effective, and within a period of two or three weeks results in clinical remissions for most patients for periods lasting six to eight months. Variations and modifications of this technique include a double Goeckerman (wherein therapy is utilized on a twice-a-day treatment schedule), office or home Goeckerman routines, and modifications of the regimen by use of anthralin instead of tar (as in the Ingram technique). Complications of the Goeckerman regimen include folliculitis, sunburn, or occasional aggravation of the disease (if the patient is sensitive to tar or if therapy is too aggressive).

The Ingram Method. The Ingram method, a standard therapeutic regimen widely used in Great Britain, includes a daily tar bath followed by exposure to a suberythema dose of ultraviolet light and subsequent application of a zinc paste containing anthralin (dioxyanthranol), a derivative of chrysarobin, a traditional modality for persistent psoriatic plaques. In a modification of this regimen, 0.2 per cent anthralin can be incorporated into Lassar's paste with 0.4 per cent salicylic acid (anthralin is unstable in the absence of salicyclic acid and the preparation becomes relatively ineffective). Yellowish-brown to brownish-purple staining of the skin, a side effect of anthralin, generally disappears within a week following discontinuation of this modality or, if desired, may be removed by the use of a salicyclic acid ointment.[17] Although economical and highly effective, it is often difficult to get the patient to use this regimen on a routine outpatient basis.

SYSTEMIC THERAPY. Most drugs given internally for psoriasis have potentially harmful side-effects and should not, in general, be given to children with this disorder. Systemic corticosteroids are double-edged weapons and should not be used in the routine care of psoriasis. They have a role in the management of persistent, otherwise uncontrollable erythroderma, but generally are contraindicated in the treatment of children. Methotrexate, a folic-acid antagonist, although highly effective in the management of severe recalcitrant psoriasis, has serious side effects (ulceration of the mucous membranes of the mouth and throat, gastrointestinal disturbances, lowering of white blood count and platelets, and fibrosis and fatty changes in the liver). Because of its associated side effects, methotrexate should not be used in children.

Photochemotherapy (PUVA) is a form of systemic therapy that combines the use of 8-methoxypsoralen and high intensity long-wave ultraviolet light in the 320 to 400 nm spectrum (UVA). In this outpatient form of therapy, the interaction of a drug (8-methoxypsoralen) and UVA light produces biologic changes of the skin including the conjugation of psoralen with DNA and the inhibition of DNA synthesis.[18] On the basis of encouraging preliminary findings, investigators of leading medical centers have demonstrated excellent therapeutic results in 90 per cent of the patients. Methoxsalen, at a dosage of approximately 0.6 mgm/kg, is given orally two hours before a measured exposure to long-wave (320 to 400 nm [UVA]) ultraviolet light. After the psoriasis has cleared, maintenance therapy is required to prevent recurrence. Although the effectiveness and acceptance of this form of therapy are now well established, this regimen is still considered to be experimental, is not recommended for children, and long-term followup is necessary in order to determine the extent of possible long-term effects such as cataracts, premature actinic damage, or skin cancer.

Psoriatic Arthritis

Arthritis occurs in about 5 to 10 per cent of patients with psoriasis.[19] Although relatively uncommon in adolescents and rarely seen in young children, the onset of this disorder may occur at any age. It appears to affect women more frequently than men and has a peak occurrence in individuals between 30 and 50 years of age.

The course and pathogenesis of psoriatic arthritis are unknown. Instead of the proximal finger and toe joints (which are affected in rheumatoid arthritis) classic psoriatic arthritis involves the distal interphalangeal joints of the hands and feet (Fig. 5–11). In the acute stage the involved joint is red, tender, and swollen. The swelling often includes the juxta-articular tissue, resulting in a blunt "sausage-shaped" appearance of the involved fingers or toes. With long-standing disease, flexure deformities and severe bone destruction may occur with osteoporosis and shortening of the involved distal phalanx. As the lesions progress there is a "whittling" away and tapering of the bones. On radiological examination this resembles a sharpened pencil (the so-called "pencil-in-cup" or "pencil and goblet" deformity) at the metatarsophalangeal and metacarpophalangeal joints. Sacroiliitis and ankylosing spondylitis may also be seen as minor manifestations of psoriatic arthritis.

The psoriatic skin lesions in patients who develop arthritis are identical to those seen in patients who do not manifest joint disease, and there is no relationship between the severity of the cutaneous disease and the development of joint disease. Skin disease usually precedes the development of joint symptoms, often by decades, and nail changes of psoriasis are found more

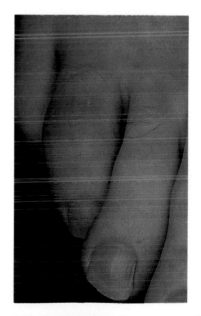

Figure 5–11 Psoriatic arthritis in a teen-ager with inflammatory involvement of the interphalangeal joint.

frequently in patients with psoriasis and arthritis (80 to 90 per cent) than in patients with uncomplicated psoriasis (25 to 50 per cent).

Clinicians generally have little difficulty in the diagnosis of typical cases of psoriatic arthritis. In less typical cases, however, the disorder must be differentiated from rheumatoid arthritis or systemic lupus erythematosus. Compared with rheumatoid arthritis the onset is generally, but not invariably, monoarticular and subacute. It tends to be less painful, and flexural deformity (rather than ulnar deviation) is characteristic of this disease. Psoriatic arthritis is usually associated with nail changes and a severe psoriasis or psoriatic erythroderma. The erythrocyte sedimentation rate is usually elevated but not specific for psoriatic arthritis. There are no subcutaneous nodules, and latex fixation, bentonite flocculation, and sheep cell agglutinations are negative.

Therapy of psoriatic arthritis, similar to that of rheumatoid arthritis, consists primarily of heat, physical therapy, and aspirin. Although folic acid antagonists, particularly methotrexate, have been used with great success in the treatment of severe adult forms of psoriasis and psoriatic arthritis, these preparations, in general, are not recommended for childhood forms of these disorders.

Pustular Psoriasis

There are two conditions to which the term pustular psoriasis has been applied. Localized pustular psoriasis of the palms and soles (pustulosis palmaris et plantaris) is a bilaterally symmetric, chronic pustular eruption that occurs on the palms and soles but is not necessarily associated with evidence of psoriasis on other parts of the body. Generalized pustular psoriasis represents a severe explosive form of psoriasis associated with high fever, severe toxicity, poor prognosis, and frequent relapses.

Localized Pustular Psoriasis. Also termed pustulosis palmaris et plantaris, localized pustular psoriasis is a chronic disorder characterized by deep-seated 2 to 4 mm sterile pustules that develop within areas of erythema and scaling on the palms, soles, or both. Often referred to as *pustular bacterid of Andrews* or *pustular psoriasis of the palms and soles of Barber*, these two terms probably imply clinical variants of the same cutaneous process rather than separate clinical entities.[20] The primary lesion is a subcorneal or intraepidermal pustule or a vesicle that becomes pustular within a period of a few hours. Within a period of several days the pustules resolve and leave a dark yellow or brown scale that is shed, generally within a period of one and a half to two weeks. Stages of quiescence and exacerbation are characteristic. Before the brown crusts of preceding lesions exfoliate, crops of fresh pustules often appear and recurring crops of pustules frequently occur. Accordingly, exfoliating crusted lesions and newly developing pustules may be seen at the same time in the same patient (Fig. 5–12). Although the

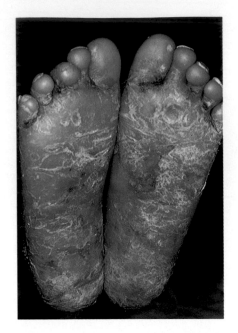

Figure 5–12   Pustular psoriasis of the soles. These lesions generally are raised, horny, quite hard, and covered by a white or grayish-white scale.

etiology of pustulosis of the palms and soles remains unknown, the presence of psoriatic nail changes and lesions in other areas of some affected individuals suggest that this disorder may represent a clinical variant or predisposition to psoriasis vulgaris.

The histologic picture of pustulosis palmaris et plantaris does not resemble that of psoriasis. The chief histologic feature is that of large intraepidermal unilocular pustules containing polymorphonuclear leukocytes (the spongiform pustule of Kogoj) with little if any surrounding spongiosis or inflammation. Although staphylococcal infection may at times occur as a secondary complication, bacterial cultures of these abscesses usually remain sterile throughout the course of the disorder.

The term *acropustulosis* refers to a sterile pustular eruption of the palms and soles of infants and children as well as adults. Lesions may begin on the fingers, toes, or heels, often following trivial injury or local infection. The disorder is characterized by vesicles or small pustules surrounded by psoriasiform or eczematous scaling dermatitis affecting the fingers, toes, palms, and soles. An early vesiculopustular lesion shows hyperkeratosis, sparse parakeratosis, and little or no spongiosis. The epidermis is invaded by lymphocytes and polymorphonuclear leukocytes with surrounding multilocular intraepidermal pustules. Whether this disorder represents a distinct entity or merely a variant of pustulosis of the palms and soles remains open to debate. Although bacterial cultures of pustules are generally sterile, use of antibacterial agents (erythromycin) frequently results in improvement and, at times, in complete remission of this disorder.[20]

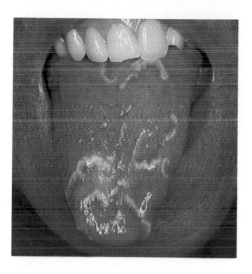

Figure 5–13 Annulus migrans. Psoriasis of the mucous membranes of the tongue in a patient with generalized pustular psoriasis (Zumbusch variety).

Pustulosis of the palms and soles tends to pursue a chronic course characterized by periods of quiescence and exacerbation. Local applications of wet dressings with Burow's solution 1:40 or potassium permanganate 1:5000 frequently help relieve acute flares of the pustular aspect of this disorder. Topical or intralesional corticosteroids often produce temporary subsidence of lesions. Topical tar preparations, although at times helpful in chronic forms of this disorder, are generally not as effective as topical corticosteroids.

Generalized Pustular Psoriasis. Often termed the von Zumbusch variety, generalized pustular psoriasis is a relatively rare, sometimes fatal, severe form of psoriasis characterized by an explosive generalized eruption associated with high fever, leukocytosis, and toxicity. Although the cause is unknown, precipitating factors such as iodides, salicylates, progesterone or penicillin therapy, discontinuation of systemic steroids, acute infection, and emotional upset may be related to the transformation of ordinary psoriasis to the generalized pustular form of this disorder.[18, 19] Generalized pustular psoriasis can occur in infants and children, and a frequent history of antecedent seborrheic dermatitis suggests possible linkage between seborrheic dermatitis and generalized pustular psoriasis in this age group.[21, 22, 23]

Attacks of generalized pustular psoriasis are often preceded by a sensation of burning associated with high fever, leukocytosis, chills, malaise, and polyarthralgia. Previously quiescent psoriatic plaques suddenly develop erythematous halos that soon become studded with superficial pinpoint to two to three millimeter pustules. Sheets of erythema and pustulation spread to involve unaffected skin, with a particular predisposition to the flexures, genital regions, webs of the fingers,

and regions about the fingernails. The nails often become thickened or separated by subungual lakes of pus. Mucous membrane lesions in the mouth and tongue are common (Fig. 5–13). The dermatitis progresses from discrete sterile pustules to shallow subcorneal layers of pus, to dry brownish crusts, and finally to a generalized exfoliative dermatitis. The disease is cyclic in nature and associated with complete clearance of the pustular phase and unexplained exacerbations. Relapses are common and become progressively more severe, often with poor prognosis. Death, when it occurs, is often associated with electrolyte imbalance or associated secondary infection or both.

The histologic picture of generalized pustular psoriasis, as in pustulosis palmaris et plantaris, shows a characteristic spongiform pustule in the upper epidermis (the spongiform pustule of Kogoj). Aside from the presence of spongiform pustules the epidermal changes are very much like those of psoriasis, with parakeratosis and elongation of rete ridges, an infiltrate of lymphocytes and neutrophils in the upper dermis, and neutrophils migrating from the dermis into the epidermis.

Therapy for the acute phase of generalized pustular psoriasis is best managed with soothing, moist compresses and general supportive measures. Although true infection is uncommon, cultures of the skin, blood, and urine should be performed. Occlusive ointments and dressings are contraindicated. Childhood forms of generalized pustular psoriasis appear to carry a better prognosis than adult forms of this disorder and are more likely to resolve spontaneously within a few weeks following bland topical therapy and good general nursing and medical care.[21] As acute stages of this disorder subside, the Goeckerman regimen or topical corticosterids often hasten the involution of stubborn pustules. Systemic corticosteroids appear to be ineffectual and may predispose to severe complications, particularly infection, which at times may prove fatal.[21-23] Although at times advocated for severe generalized pustular psoriasis, the value of methotrexate (in general not recommended for the childhood forms of this disorder) is doubtful and should be reserved only for exceptional cases.

Erythrodermic (Exfoliative) Psoriasis

Erythrodermic or exfoliative psoriasis is a severe generalized disorder that occurs in a small percentage of adults and, on rare occasions, children with psoriasis.[24, 25] Although it may occur spontaneously as an initial manifestation of the disease, it generally occurs in chronic forms of psoriasis following sunburn, excessive ultraviolet exposure, or as a complication of aggressive topical therapy or systemic viral or bacterial disease.

The skin is almost totally involved, with deep erythema, massive exfoliation, and associated abnormalities of temperature and cardiovascular regulation. Erythrodermic psoriasis, therefore, is a serious complication that necessitates hospitalization and skilled management. Although methotrexate has been recommended for adult forms of this disorder, the hazards inherent in the use of folic acid antagonists in early childhood suggest that these agents be employed only in cases where less hazardous measures have been ineffective.[25]

Acropustulosis of Infancy

Acropustulosis of infancy (infantile acropustulosis) is a recently described disease of infancy and childhood that generally appears in black infants between the ages of 2 months and 10 months, and persists, with periods of remission and exacerbation, for a period of about two years[26, 27] (Fig. 5–14). This disorder, seen in infants without family histories of atopy or psoriasis, is characterized by crops of intensely pruritic papulopustular or vesiculopustular lesions that appear for periods of 7 to 10 days, after which time the eruption generally remits for two or three weeks prior to recurrences. Worse in summer than winter, the lesions begin as pinpoint erythematous papules and enlarge into well-circumscribed discrete pustules within 24 hours. Lesions are concentrated on the palms and soles and appear in lesser numbers on the dorsal aspect of the hands, feet, wrists, and ankles, and less occasionally on the face and scalp. New lesions are accompanied by intense pruritus, restlessness, and fretfulness. The eruption is unresponsive to potent topical corticosteroids, the pruritus is relieved only by soporific doses of antihistamine, and the disease resolves spontaneously by the time the patient is two to three years of age.[27]

The differential diagnosis of this disorder includes dyshidrotic eczema, pustular psoriasis, toxic erythema of the newborn, transient neonatal pustular melanosis, scabies, impetigo, and subcorneal pustular dermatosis. The histopathologic features of infantile acropustulosis include large, well-circumscribed intraepidermal pustules filled with polymorphonuclear leukocytes.

Suggested treatment for infantile acropustulosis includes systemic antibiotics such as erythromycin or sulfones. Although this disorder requires further study, Dr. Kahn feels that sulfone (diamino-diphenyl-sulfone, Dapsone), in a dosage of 2 mg/kg/day may be more effective than erythromycin in the management of this disorder.[27]

Reiter's Disease

Reiter's disease is a disorder of unknown etiology characterized by a triad of urethritis, arthritis, and conjunctivitis. In 50 to 80 per cent of patients cutaneous lesions that mimic or closely resemble psoriasis may be seen. Generally recognized as a disorder that primarily affects young males, particularly those between 20 and 40 years of age, it also can affect young children, the youngest reported case being that of a 9-month-old infant. In children the disorder seems to be less severe but otherwise similar to that in adults and, although there are relatively few reports of the disease in this age group, a total of 38 childhood cases have been reported to date.[28-32]

Isolated cases can occur in females, but more than 90 per cent of reported cases have been in males. The syndrome has been associated with an antecedent, apparently infectious dysenteric or urethritic episode, possibly due to *Chlamydia* or *Mycoplasma* (pleuropneumonia-like organisms) that enter the body through inflamed membranes (either intestinal or urethral). Diarrhea is initially seen in 90 per cent of children but only in one-third of adults with this disorder,[29] and recent HL-A typings suggest that heredity may play a significant role in the predisposition of affected individuals to the development of this disorder.[31, 32]

The cutaneous manifestations of Reiter's disease may develop in association with, or indepen-

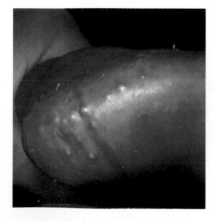

Figure 5–14 Acropustulosis of infancy (infantile acropustulosis). Recurrent pruritic papulopustular lesions on the feet of a 9-month-old black girl.

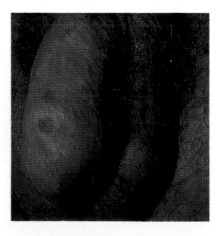

Figure 5–15 Psoriasiform lesions of Reiter's syndrome. When several penile lesions coalesce into a circinate form, it is termed balanitis circinata.

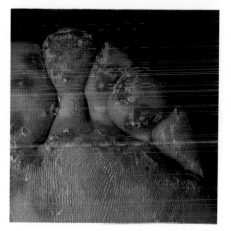

Figure 5-16 Keratoderma blennorrhagicum. Thickened hyperkeratotic psoriasiform lesions on the foot of a patient with Reiter's disease.

dently of, the other features of the disorder. The most characteristic lesions are those that appear over the palms and soles. They begin as pinpoint vesicular or macular lesions that become purulent and eventuate in red scaly psoriasiform lesions (Fig. 5–15). The term *keratoderma blennorrhagicum* refers to the thickened hyperkeratotic, often psoriasiform, yellowish scaly lesions on an erythematous base that have a predilection for the palms and soles (Fig. 5–16).

Oral lesions consist of painless erythema, shallow erosions, and small pustules that may occur on the buccal mucosa, gums, lips, palate, and tongue, and generally resolve spontaneously after a period of several days. Lesions on the tongue, particularly when thickly coated, may simulate a geographic tongue.

The ocular lesions of Reiter's disease are seen in at least 50 per cent of patients. They consist of conjunctivitis, iritis, and, at times, keratitis. Arthritis, the predominant feature of this syndrome, resembles rheumatoid arthritis. It is usually polyarticular and generally involves the sacroiliac joints, knees, ankles, and less frequently, joints of the upper extremities.

Diagnosis of this disorder is aided by the presence of the classic triad, with or without the presence of cutaneous or mucosal lesions. The clinical and histopathologic appearance of cutaneous lesions of Reiter's disease may be identical to or similar to those of psoriasis, but may be differentiated by the presence of ocular, arthritic, and urethral lesions, by HL-A testing, and by a lack of family history of psoriasis.

Treatment consists primarily of bed rest and salicylates for the arthritis; topical corticosteroids for cutaneous lesions; broad-spectrum antibiotics, particularly tetracycline, for the associated urethritis; systemic or intra-articular corticosteroids if symptoms are severe; and, for patients with severe unresponsive disease, immunosuppressive agents (6-mercaptopurine or methotrexate). In view of the excellent prognosis in children, treatment in this age group is symptomatic and consists primarily of bed rest and analgesics.

Pityriasis Rubra Pilaris

Pityriasis rubra pilaris is a chronic skin disorder characterized by small follicular papules, disseminated yellowish-pink scaly plaques surrounding islands of normal skin, and hyperkeratosis of the palms and soles. The papules are an important diagnostic feature of this disorder. They consist of fine, firm, conical papules topped by a central keratotic plug. They are pinpoint in size, arise at the mouth of hair follicles, may or may not be pierced by a central hair, and vary in color from that of normal skin to a yellowish-pink or red.

Available evidence suggests two distinct variants of this disorder — a familial type and an acquired variety. The familial form is inherited as an autosomal disorder that may present at birth or have its onset during infancy or childhood. The acquired type may appear at any age and is generally seen in individuals over 15 years of age.[33] Although the acquired form has no known genetic tendency, many authorities believe that this variant may show mild, easily overlooked features at an early stage and accordingly may merely represent a delayed expression of the inherited form of this disorder.

The cause of pityriasis rubra pilaris is unknown. It appears to represent a disturbance in keratinization in which the precise defect is as yet undetermined. Skin lesions, both clinically and histologically, are suggestive of those seen in phrynoderma (vitamin A deficiency). Vitamin A levels, however, are variable, and the role of vitamin A, if any, remains obscure.[34]

Although little is known about the pathophysiology of this disease, it has been speculated that the involved areas reflect an underlying abnormality in epidermal cell kinetics (decreased transit time and accelerated epidermal proliferation) as significant pathogenetic factors.[35]

CLINICAL MANIFESTATIONS. Pityriasis rubra pilaris, particularly in children, frequently starts gradually with a generalized scaling of the scalp and forehead and a diffuse erythema of the face and ears. In adults the onset is often more acute, and a generalized erythroderma may develop over the course of a few days. The characteristic fine eruption usually appears first on the hands and feet, particularly over the dorsal aspects of the first and second phalanges, the wrists, knees, elbows, sides of the neck, and trunk. On the dorsal aspect of the fingers, the papules remain distinctly follicular and pathognomonic. In other areas, as new lesions occur, they tend to coalesce and form sharply marginated patches (much like plucked chicken skin) and thickened psoriasiform plaques with a coarse texture similar to the surface of a nutmeg grater. The plaques are generally symmetrical and diffuse and contrast sharply with islands of normal skin that occur within the affected areas (Fig. 5–17).

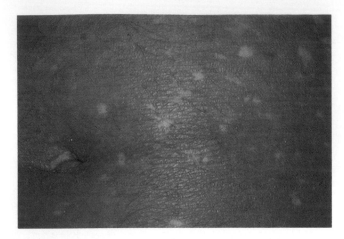

Figure 5–17   Pityriasis rubra pilaris. Islands of normal skin surrounded by areas of erythema.

In adults, at times the eruption can progress to an exfoliative dermatitis with associated systemic symptoms of malaise, chills, fever, and diarrhea. Facial involvement may be seen as a heavy waxy scaling and an associated ectropion of the eyelids. Painful fissures can occur in involved areas of the skin, but pruritus is usually not a prominent feature.

Thickened hyperkeratotic skin frequently develops on the palms and soles. When seen on the soles, this has been referred to as a "keratodermic sandal." The nails are often thickened and opaque, with transverse striations and subungual debris. The characteristic pitting of nails seen in psoriasis, however, is not a feature of this disorder.

The diagnosis of pityriasis rubra pilaris is based primarily upon the acuminate follicular papules with keratotic plugs that appear on the backs of fingers, sides of the neck, and extensor surfaces of the limbs. Salmon-colored scaling plaques, islands of normal skin in the midst of the eruption, and hyperkeratosis of the palms and soles help confirm the clinical impression.

The histologic picture is similar to that of vitamin A deficiency and keratosis pilaris. Although not pathognomonic, it is fairly characteristic and consists of follicular keratosis, diffuse hyperkeratosis, irregular mild acanthosis, and inconstant patchy parakeratosis (particularly near the hair follicles). Liquefactive degeneration of the basal layers of the epidermis with extension along the hair follicles is often present. A mild chronic inflammatory infiltrate in the upper dermis, particularly around hair follicles and superficial vessels, helps complete the histopathologic picture.

The clinical course of pityriasis rubra pilaris is variable. In most cases a protracted clinical course may be anticipated. In 25 to 50 per cent of cases spontaneous clearing may develop after a period of time varying from several months to years. In childhood forms, however, the disorder tends to be persistent and may be characterized by spontaneous remissions and exacerbations.[35, 36]

TREATMENT. Treatment of pityriasis rubra pilaris depends upon suppression of hyperkeratinization; mild forms may require only topical corticosteroids and keratolytic agents. In adults, success has been achieved with large doses of oral vitamin A, varying from 150,000 to 600,000 units a day. In children a lower dose (50,000 units twice a day) has been utilized with complete remission after six and a half weeks of therapy.[37] Adequate therapeutic trial requires treatment for a period of at least three to six weeks. If effective, it can be continued for months before signs of hypervitaminosis A (anorexia, pruritus, dry skin, hair loss, subcutaneous swellings, and painful hyperostoses) occur. After several months of continuous therapy, in an effort to avoid signs of toxicity, oral vitamin A may be discontinued for periods of two to three months or more.

Although discontinuation of therapy often results in relapse, prolonged remissions have been noted. Topical vitamin A acid, of value in certain other hyperkeratinization disorders (ichthyosis vulgaris and lamellar ichthyosis), has been tried but results to date remain inconclusive.[38] Because of their ability to inhibit deoxyribonucleic acid synthesis and cell division, folic acid antagonists (aminopterin and methotrexate) have also been suggested in the therapy of this disorder.[39] Because of potential toxicity associated with these agents, adequate precautions should be taken and antifolic antagonists should be avoided or given with great caution to children, women during the child-bearing period, and patients with renal or hepatic disease.

Mucha-Habermann Disease

Mucha-Habermann disease, also known as acute or guttate parapsoriasis or pityriasis lichenoides et varioliformis, is an acute self-limiting disorder of adults and children characterized by crops of macules, papules, or papulovesicles that tend to develop central necrosis and crusts soon after they arise. Originally described by Mucha of

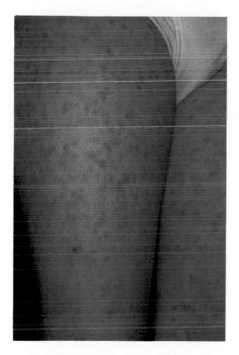

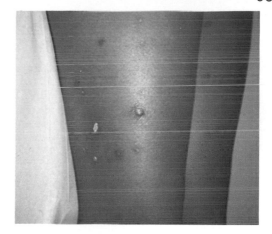

Figure 5-20   Crusted and necrotic varioliform lesions of parapsoriasis lichenoides chronica (Mucha-Habermann disease).

Figure 5-18   Mucha-Habermann disease (guttate parapsoriasis).

Vienna in 1916, and later by Habermann in Germany in 1921, it is frequently referred to by its eponym (Mucha-Habermann disease) because of an unresolved controversy regarding the nosology and etiology of this disorder.[40]

Mucha-Habermann disease appears in two forms and may be see at any age: an acute form (acute guttate parapsoriasis, parapsoriasis varioliformis, pityriasis lichenoides et varioliformis acuta) seen mainly in children and young adults and a chronic form (pityriasis lichenoides chronica, guttate parapsoriasis of Juliusberg) more commonly noted in adolescents and young adults. Acute forms usually begin as an eruption of symmetrical two to three millimeter oval or round reddish-brown macules and papules. The papules occur in successive crops and rapidly evolve into vesicular, necrotic, and sometimes purpuric lesions (Figs. 5-18, 5-19, and 5-20). These develop a fine crust and gradually resolve, with or without a varioliform scar. Occasionally temporary hypopigmentation or hyperpigmentation may result. Although the eruption is usually the first manifestation of the disease, occasionally fever and constitutional symptoms may precede or accompany the cutaneous eruption. Lesions may involve the entire body, but are most pronounced on the trunk, thighs, and upper arms, especially the flexor surfaces. The face, scalp, palms, and soles are frequently spared or may be involved to a lesser degree. The course usually lasts for periods of a few weeks to several months. Although recurrences in a few cases may continue for periods of two or three years, the prognosis is generally good.

Pityriasis lichenoides chronica may begin de novo or may evolve from pityriasis lichenoides acuta. The course of chronic pityriasis lichenoides is variable and may last for periods of six months to several years. It begins with smooth or slightly firm reddish-brown papules that measure several millimeters to a centimeter in diameter. Scales, when present, are adherent, slightly thicker in the center, and can be detached by gentle scraping to reveal a shiny brown surface (a diagnostic feature of this disorder).[41] Over a period of several weeks the individual papules recede, the scale separates spontaneously, and a hyperpigmented or hypopigmented macule results and eventually fades (usually without residual scar).[42] Although sequelae

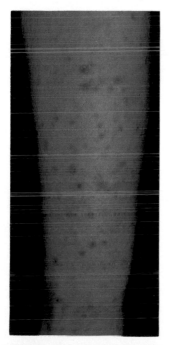

Figure 5-19   Mucha-Habermann disease.

are uncommon, in occasional cases the lesions may progress to form nodules with highly atypical cells, which on histopathologic examination suggest a malignant cutaneous lymphoma. The subsequent clinical course, evolution, and morphology of lesions confirm the benign character of the disorder.[43, 44] Cases that histologically mimic lymphoma have been classified by some authorities as a separate disorder termed "lymphomatoid papulosis";[45] other authors suggest that they merely represent variants of Mucha-Habermann disease.[46] Despite an occasional prolonged and stormy course, Mucha-Habermann disease resolves spontaneously and does not give rise to serious sequelae.[47, 48]

In the early stages Mucha-Habermann disease may be mistaken for chicken-pox, impetigo, pityriasis rosea, allergic vasculitis, or scabies. The duration of the eruption (often in crops), macules and papules interspersed with vesicular, crusted, or hemorrhagic lesions with or without varioliform scarring, and subsequent hypopigmentation or hyperpigmentation help differentiate pityriasis lichenoides from other conditions. When the diagnosis remains in doubt, histopathologic examination of a skin biopsy will often substantiate the proper diagnosis.

The histology of Mucha-Habermann disease varies with the stage, intensity, and extent of the reaction. The prominent feature is a heavy, primarily lymphocytic and histiocytic perivascular infiltrate. Diapedesis of red blood cells occurs in the dermis, and severe intercellular and intracellular edema in the epidermis lead to intraepidermal vesicle formation, necrosis of the epidermis, and finally erosions and eventual crusting.[49]

A number of theories have been proposed concerning the etiology of Mucha-Habermann disease; all to date are unsubstantiated. The clinical and histologic features suggest a vasculitis. Some authors suggest an autoimmune process, a hypersensitivity reaction triggered by various etiologic factors, or an exanthem of viral or rickettsial etiology.[46-50]

Owing to the undetermined etiology and variable nature of this disease, there is to date no well-established form of therapy. Antipruritics, aspirin, and lubricants may be helpful in ame-liorating the symptoms, and topical corticosteroids, tar preparations, and ultraviolet light or sun exposure have been employed with varying success. Tetracycline in high doses (2 gm a day) and erythromycin are reportedly beneficial in some patients,[51] but results are variable and tetracycline should not be administered to children under 12 years of age or to pregnant women during the first trimester. Methotrexate, in dosages of 7.5 to 20 mg weekly by mouth, has resulted in improvement in persistent cases.[52] Relapse, however, usually follows discontinuance of treatment and, again, this form of therapy is not generally recommended, particularly in children or pregnant women.

Pityriasis Rosea

Pityriasis rosea is an acute benign self-limiting disorder that affects males and females equally, with a peak incidence in adolescents and young adults. Although uncommon in children under five years of age, the author has seen it in an 8-month-old and it has been reported in an infant as young as four months of age. Except for a prodrome that may at times consist of headache, malaise, pharyngitis, and lymphadenitis, and occasional reports of mild constitutional symptoms, there is no evidence of systemic involvement, complications, or sequelae. Although the etiology of pityriasis rosea remains unknown, a viral disorder is suggested by the occasional presence of prodromal symptoms, the course of the disease, epidemics with seasonal cluster, reports of similtaneous occurrence in closely associated individuals, and a tendency to life-long immunity in 98 per cent of cases.[53, 54]

The eruption follows a distinctive pattern, and 70 to 80 per cent of cases start with a single isolated lesion, the so-called herald patch (Fig. 5–21). It may occur anywhere on the body, most commonly the trunk, upper arms, neck, and thighs. This characteristic initial lesion is seen as a sharply defined oval area of scaly dermititis (2 to 5 cm in diameter) with a flat, pink or brown center and a red, finely scaled and slightly elevated border. After an interval of 5 to 10 days a secondary generalized eruption appears in crops, characteristically sparing the face (in 85 per cent of individuals), scalp, and distal extremities. These clinically distinctive lesions resemble the herald patch in morphology but are smaller and generally more ovoid in configuration. They may appear as small, pink, finely scaled macules that measure 2 to 10 mm in diameter or as slightly larger dull pink, round or oval patches that measure 0.5 to 3.0 cm in diameter. On the thorax the long axis of individual lesions runs parallel to the lines of skin cleavage in what has been described as a "Christmas-tree" pattern (Fig. 5–22). Typical of these secondary lesions is a fine scaly edge with a characteristic cigarette paper-like "collarette" scale (Fig. 5–23).

Occasionally, particularly in young children, lesions may be predominantly papular, vesicular,

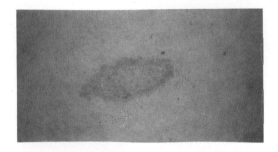

Figure 5–21 Herald patch (pityriasis rosea). Oval lesion with finely scaled elevated border, occasionally misdiagnosed as tinea corporis.

Figure 5–22 Pityriasis rosea. Christmas-tree pattern in lines of cleavage. Note papulovesicular lesions occasionally seen in childhood forms of this disorder.

pustular, urticarial, or even purpuric in nature, particularly during the early stages of the eruption (Fig. 5–22). Less commonly, some patients, particularly children, may show an inverse distribution of lesions on the face, wrists, and extremities, which may or may not spread centrally to include the trunk. This atypical form of pityriasis rosea may be particularly difficult to diagnose if there is no history of a herald patch and if the characteristic morphology of lesions goes unrecognized.

The head and face are frequently affected in children, and the face and neck are occasionally involved in blacks. Involvement of the oral mucous membranes, often overlooked, is unusual but may be seen as red patches that, at times, may appear to be erosive, hemorrhagic, or bullous.[55] In about 25 per cent of cases a moderate itching, particularly in secondary lesions, may be noted. Reports of malaise, headache, adenopathy, low fever, and joint pains have been reported but appear to be rare. Once the secondary cutaneous eruption begins to appear it usually reaches its height within a period of a few days to a week. Healing generally begins after a period of two to four weeks, first in lesions that appeared earliest, and is usually complete by six to twelve weeks. Postinflammatory hypopigmentation (Fig. 5–24) or

hyperpigmentation may frequently be noted, particularly in dark-skinned individuals and may persist for periods of weeks to months after healing is complete.

Diagnosis of pityriasis rosea depends upon recognition of the characteristic appearance and distribution of the oval lesions with their fine peripheral or "collarette" scales. The herald patch may be mistaken for tinea corporis, and the full-blown eruption must be differentiated from lesions of secondary syphilis (a frequent misdiagnosis), drug eruption, Mucha-Habermann disease, seborrheic dermatitis, nummular eczema, and psoriasis (particularly the guttate variety).

The histologic features of pityriasis rosea are not diagnostic and resemble those of a subacute or chronic dermatitis with vascular dilatation, edema, a superficial lymphohistiocytic dermal infiltrate, acanthosis, epidermal spongiosis, mild exocytosis, and, at times, patchy parakeratosis.

Most patients require no treatment beyond reassurance as to the nature and prognosis of the disorder. Pruritus, if present, usually responds to topical antipruritic lotions (calamine lotion, with 0.5 to 1 per cent phenol if desired), antihistamines, colloidal starch or oatmeal baths (Aveeno Colloidal Oatmeal or Aveeno Oilated, Cooper Laboratories), and mild topical corticosteroid formulations. Exposure to ultraviolet light or sunshine

Figure 5–23 Pityriasis rosea. Fine peripheral "collarette" scale.

Figure 5–24 Postinflammatory hypopigmentation following resolution of pityriasis rosea

generally tends to hasten resolution of lesions and, in the summertime, it is not uncommon to see patients with pityriasis rosea under covered areas with little to no evidence of the eruption on sun-exposed regions.

Lichen Planus

Lichen planus is a relatively common dermatosis of unknown etiology that occurs in individuals of all ages. Although 85 per cent of cases occur in adults between 30 and 70 years of age, it has also been recorded in infants, children, and adolescents.[56]

The primary lesion is a small shiny flat-topped polygonal reddish or violaceous papule (Fig. 5–25). Individual papules vary from 2 mm to a centimeter or more in size, may be closely aggregated or widely dispersed, and generally are intensely pruritic.[57] The disorder is usually limited to a few areas, with the flexural surfaces of the wrists, the legs, genitalia, and mucous membranes as the sites of predilection. In chronic forms, the sites of predilection are the flexor surfaces of the wrists, the forearms, and the inner aspects of the knees and thighs.

At times one may detect small grayish puncta or streaks that form a network over the surface of papules. These delicate white lines, termed Wickham's striae, become more visible under magnification with a hand lens or by application of a drop of oil, which renders the horny layers of lesions more transparent. Occasionally lesions may coalesce to form plaques or a linear configuration (the Koebner phenomenon) over sites of minor trauma such as scratch marks (Fig. 5–26).

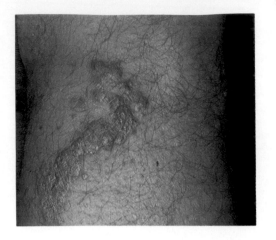

Figure 5–26   Thickened papular lesions of hypertrophic lichen planus with a Koebner phenomenon.

Mucous membrane involvement is seen in 50 to 70 per cent of patients. When present, lesions are usually seen as pinhead-sized white papules forming annular or linear lace-like patterns on the inner aspects of the cheeks (Fig. 5–27). Lesions on the palate, lips, and tongue are less characteristic and, except for their reticulated appearance, may easily be mistaken for areas of leukoplakia.

The etiology of lichen planus is unknown. The principal hypotheses include an infectious (possible viral) origin, a response to stress, and a reaction pattern of genetically predisposed individuals triggered by chemicals or other factors. Of interest, adding partial support to the latter hypothesis, are a group of patients reported to have a congenital deficiency of glucose-6-phosphate dehydrogenase (G-6-PDH) in the epidermis, with resultant attacks of lichen planus precipitated by exposure to certain drugs (lichenoid drug eruptions.[58]

One to 10 per cent of patients with lichen planus demonstrate nail involvement, but lichen planus of the nail without skin lesions is rare.[59] Apparently associated with inflammation of the nail matrix and nail fold, such lesions may involve

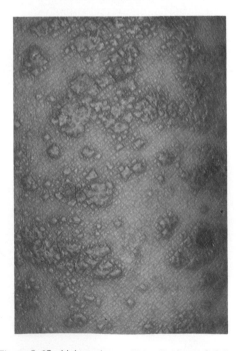

Figure 5–25   Lichen planus. Shiny flat-topped violaceous polygonal papules.

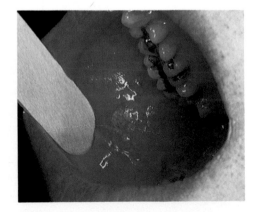

Figure 5–27   White papules of lichen planus in a linear lace-like reticulated pattern on the buccal mucosa.

one, several, or all nails. Occasionally violaceous lines or papules in the nail bed may be seen through the nail plate. Although not pathognomonic of the disorder, nail dystrophy is highly characteristic. It consists of loss of luster, thinning of the nail plate, longitudinal ridging or striation, splitting or nicking of the nail margin, atrophy, overlapping skin folds (pterygia), marked subungual hyperkeratosis, lifting of the distal nail plate, and, at times, complete and permanent loss of the nail.

VARIANTS

Although lichen planus is considered to be papulosquamous in nature, many variations in morphology and configuration may be noted. These variations include vesicular, bullous, actinic, annular, hypertrophic, atrophic, linear, erythematous, and follicular forms.

Vesicular and Bullous Forms. Lesions may appear in part as vesicles or bullae located on top of pre-existing papules (bullous lichen planus). Occasionally bullous lesions may also appear on otherwise normal skin (lichen planus pemphigoid). When other characteristic lesions are not apparent, this variant may be confused with other bullous disorders such as pemphigus vulgaris or dermatitis herpetiformis.

Actinic Lichen Planus. This variant is generally seen in children and young adults of oriental heritage. Often confined to individuals in tropical and subtropical regions, sun-exposed areas are principally involved and pruritus may be mild or absent. Lesions may be pigmented, dyschromic, or granuloma annulare-like, and may be confused with lupus erythematosus. In such cases, individual lesions, course, and histologic features resemble those of true lichen planus. Whether these lesions truly represent lichen planus or not is undetermined.

Annular Lichen Planus. Annular lichen planus, seen in 10 per cent of affected individuals, is a variant that evolves from chronic forms of the disorder and results in a ring-like grouping of lesions. It commonly occurs on the penis and lower trunk, but may occur anywhere. Lesions of granuloma annulare may at times resemble this variant, but few other conditions simulate this disorder.

Hypertrophic (Verrucous) Lichen Planus. Hypertrophic lichen planus is characterized by verrucous plaques covered with fine adherent scales. This variant may involve any region of the body, but most commonly appears on the pretibial areas of the legs and ankles. Lesions may appear as isolated or multiple plaques, or they may be confluent and cover the entire anterior tibial area. Although superficial inspection may suggest a diagnosis of psoriasis, careful examination may reveal small flat-topped polygonal papules that reveal the true nature of the disorder.

Lichen Planus Atrophicus. In this variant lesions tend to be few in number, and atrophy may be the result of resolved annular or hypertrophic lesions.

Linear Lichen Planus. Linear or zosteriform lesions are occasionally seen as an uncommon variant of lichen planus. In this extremely pruritic variant, lesions extend along an extremity or on the trunk, often overlying thrombosed veins and along the course of nerves. Although no explanation for this variant has been satisfactory, it is thought that this form of the disorder may be the result of trauma, or that it may follow dermatomal segments of the skin or distribution of peripheral nerves.

Lichen Planus Erythematosus. Discrete vivid red, soft, non-pruritic lesions of lichen planus that measure 5 to 10 mm in diameter and blanch on pressure may arise on the trunk of affected individuals. Although this variant may at times be associated with mucosal or nail changes and shows typical histologic features of this disorder, the question of whether or not this is a true form of lichen planus is uncertain.

Lichen Planopilaris (Follicular Lichen Planus). This follicular type of lichen planus, also termed folliculitis decalvans of Graham-Little, is seen more frequently in women and generally consists of spinous or acuminate (conical) follicular lesions with typical cutaneous and mucosal lichen planus, follicular lesions and alopecia of the scalp (with or without atrophy), an increased incidence of nail involvement, and erosion of mucous membrane lesions. The end stage of this disorder may be indistinguishable from pseudopelade (a cicatricial form of alopecia of unknown origin) (See Chapter 17).

Lichenoid Drug Eruptions. Many drugs produce an eruption very similar or identical to lichen planus and it is highly probable, at least in some cases, that drugs may precipitate attacks of lichen planus. For years it had been realized that certain drugs (gold and arsenicals) could produce lichenoid eruptions. Not until the Second World War when large numbers of troops taking Atabrine developed drug eruptions was it recognized how closely these disorders resembled typical lichen planus.[57] Recent studies reveal that soldiers who developed such lichenoid drug eruptions were those specifically born with a deficiency of glucose-6-phosphate dehydrogenase (G-6-PDH).[58] Other drugs known to cause lichenoid eruptions include antituberculosis preparations (para-aminosalicylic acid and isoniazid), streptomycin, quinidine, chlorpropamide (Diabinase), the phenothiazines, and paraphenylenediamine salts in color film developers.[60]

When lesions of lichenoid drug eruption closely resemble those of lichen planus, the histologic picture generally also resembles that of lichen planus. Parakeratosis in the stratum corneum and eosinophils in the cellular infiltrate, neither of which are seen in lesions of lichen planus, help differentiate the two disorders.[61]

DIAGNOSIS. Diagnosis of lichen planus is dependent upon the recognition of typical papules of this disorder or one of its variants in location, clinical pattern, or morphology. When the diagnosis is in doubt, histopathologic examination of a cutaneous lesion will generally help to establish the proper diagnosis. The histopathologic picture of lichen planus is that of hyperkeratosis, a thickened granular layer without parakeratosis, destruction of the basal cell layer (liquefactive degeneration), saw-toothing of the rete pegs, and a band-like lymphocytic infiltrate that hugs and invades the lower epidermis.

Although cases of lichen planus occasionally clear in a few weeks, two thirds of affected individuals with acute forms display spontaneous resolution within a period of 8 to 15 months. In most patients the lesions tend to flatten but are often replaced by an area of pigmentation that may persist for periods of months or years. Occasionally the disorder may persist for years, and 10 to 20 per cent of patients suffer one or more recurrences of their disorder.[56]

TREATMENT. There is no specific treatment for lichen planus. Symptomatic relief, however, may be obtained by systemic antihistamines, ataractics such as hydroxyzine (Atarax or Vistaril) in dosages of 10 to 25 mg or more three or four times a day, or sedatives (particularly in individuals in whom stress may be a precipitating factor). Symptomatic relief may also be obtained by colloidal oatmeal (Aveeno Colloidal Oatmeal or Aveeno Oilated) or corn starch baths. Since drug-induced lichen planus may at times present a problem, medications should be discontinued or substituted whenever possible. Local symptomatic treatment with topical corticosteroid preparations is helpful; in lesions that are recalcitrant or hypertrophic, occlusive dressings over topical corticosteroids, Cordran Tape (Dista), or intralesional steroids may be beneficial; and on rare occasions (perhaps one in 20 patients), a short course of systemic steroids may be necessary.

Mucous membrane lesions usually require no therapy. When symptomatic, eroded, or ulcerated, however, topical anesthetics such as Benadryl elixir, Xylocaine viscous, topical corticosteroids (Kenalog in orabase), or intralesional corticosteroids may be beneficial.

Lichen Aureus

Lichen aureus is a rare disorder characterized by slightly elevated, closely packed lichenoid papules with a peculiar rust-like copper or burnt-orange color (not golden as the name suggests) and a thin adherent scale.[62, 63] Since relatively few cases have been recorded to date, little is known of the incidence, pathogenesis, or natural history of the condition. Although most cases recorded to date have been in adults, the disorder has also been seen in children.[7]

The etiology of lichen aureus is unknown. The patches are asymptomatic and usually singular in number or, if multiple, closely grouped. They may be seen on any part of the body and vary in size from one or two centimeters to more in diameter. Lichen aureus is unrelated to lichen planus. Except for a possible association with pigmented purpuric eruptions such as Schamberg's disease or Gougerot-Blum dermatitis, lichen aureus apparently bears no relationship to any other dermatologic or systemic disease.[63]

The histologic picture of lichen aureus is unique. It consists of a normal epidermis, a dense band of lymphocytes and histiocytes separated from the epidermis by a broad band of normal connective tissue, and hemosiderin granules deposited within the histiocytes.

The course of this disorder is generally a protracted one. Lesions occur suddenly and usually remain unchanged for many years. To date, no known effective treatment has been reported.

Lichen Nitidus

Lichen nitidus is a relatively uncommon benign dermatosis that affects individuals of all ages and is most commonly seen in children of preschool and school age. Although the etiology remains unknown, association with lichen planus has been reported and many authorities consider lichen nitidus to be a variant of this disorder.

Individual papules of lichen nitidus are sharply demarcated, pinpoint to pinhead in size,

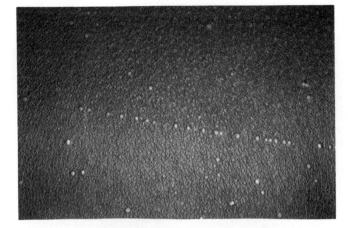

Figure 5–28 Pinhead sized flesh-colored shiny elevated papules of lichen nitidus (note the linear Koebner reaction over a site of trauma).

round or polygonal, and usually flesh-colored (Fig. 5–28). Surfaces of individual lesions are flat, shiny, and slightly elevated, often with a central depression. The eruption is arranged in groups primarily located on the trunk, genitalia, abdomen, and forearms of affected individuals. Linear lesions (Koebner reaction) in lines of trauma are common, and minute grayish flat papules on the buccal mucous membrane have been described. The course is variable. It occasionally clears spontaneously after a period of several weeks but frequently lasts a much longer period of time (occasionally years) with little or no response to treatment.

The histologic features of lichen nitidus are pathognomonic and consist of circumscribed nests of lymphocytes and histiocytes, and occasionally epithelioid and Langerhans giant cells in the uppermost dermis. The overlying epidermis is compressed, occasionally with an area of detachment from the dermis above the center of the lesion, with a characteristic claw-like projection of the rete ridges as though in an attempt to encircle the infiltrate in the manner of a hand clutching a ball.

There is no known effective treatment for lichen nitidus. Antihistaminic preparations, emollients or lubricating lotions with 0.25 per cent menthol and 0.5 per cent phenol for children five and under and 0.5 per cent menthol and 1 per cent phenol for older children, or topical hydrocortisone preparations may help relieve symptoms of pruritus.

Papular Acrodermatitis of Childhood

Papular acrodermatitis of childhood (the Gianotti-Crosti syndrome) is a distinctive, self-limiting dermatosis of childhood characterized by the abrupt onset of non-pruritic lichenoid papules on the face, buttocks, and extremities, generally lasting about 20 days (occasionally longer), with mild constitutional symptoms and acute, usually anicteric, hepatitis (Table 5–1). First recognized in Milan in 1953 and described by Gianotti in 1955 and later by Crosti and Gianotti in 1956, the term "infantile papular acrodermatitis" was designated in 1957.[64, 65]

Since its original description it now appears that this frequently unrecognized disorder is probably worldwide in distribution.[64-67] The disease begins abruptly, and the eruption is often preceded by an upper respiratory infection, generalized lymphadenopathy, hepatomegaly and occasionally splenomegaly, and mild constitutional symptoms. Although adults have also been affected by this disorder, children between 3 months and 15 years of age are usually affected, with a peak incidence between the ages of 1 and 6.[68]

The clinical features of Gianotti-Crosti syndrome are quite distinctive. The eruption consists of a monomorphous, non-pruritic, generally but not necessarily symmetrical, flat-topped 1 to 10 mm flesh-colored, pale pink or coppery red papules that appear in crops and involve the face, buttocks, extremities, palms, soles, and occasionally the upper aspect of the back (Figs. 5–29, 5–30, 5–31, and 3–25).[64-67, 69] Although the trunk is generally spared, a transient eruption may be seen in this region during the initial early phase of the disorder. The rash develops in a few days and lasts for a period of 15 to 20 days or more (occasionally up to eight weeks or more). In infancy the lesions are generally large (5 to 10 mm in diameter); in older children the eruption is often micropapular, one to two mm in diameter. At times the lesions may have a purpuric appearance and, on occasion, a coarse infiltrated tumor-like appearance has been noted. As the rash progresses, lesions frequently tend to become confluent and, particularly on areas subject to trauma, may merge to form plaques of flat-topped lichenoid papules.[61-63]

Constitutional symptoms and systemic manifestations include malaise, low-grade fever, mild generalized lymphadenopathy, hepatomegaly, splenomegaly, and, at times, diarrhea. Hepatitis, when present, begins at the same time or a week or two after the onset of the cutaneous eruption. The rash resolves spontaneously after a variable period of two to eight weeks (usually 15 to 20 days). The lymphadenitis, mainly inguinal and axillary, generally lasts two to three months, and hepatomegaly, when present, generally persists for a three-month period.

Although leukopenia with a relative increase in monocytes (up to 20 per cent) and a mild hypochromic anemia have been reported, laboratory findings generally consist of a normal white blood count and normal erythrocyte sedimentation rate. Abnormal liver function studies with elevation of SGOT, SGPT, LDH, alkaline phosphatase, and bromsulphalein retention without abnormal bilirubin levels have been noted. Liver biopsies done during the dermatitis phase of the disorder reveal a histologic picture indistinguishable from that of acute viral hepatitis.[64]

In 1973 the association with Australian antigen was reported,[64] and in 1976 in Japan an epidemic of the syndrome associated with a very high incidence of hepatitis-B surface antigen (subtype ayw, an uncommon subtype in Japan) was reported.[70] Australian antigen, when present, is generally detectable 10 days or more after the onset of the skin eruption and persists for periods of two months to several years. Evidence of hepatitis manifested by hepatomegaly, elevated serum enzymes, virus-like particles in liver and lymph node specimens, and detection of elevated serum levels of HBS-Ag in some patients makes a viral etiology of this disorder highly probable.

Table 5–1   FEATURES OF GIANOTTI-CROSTI SYNDROME (INFANTILE PAPULAR ACRODERMATITIS)[64, 67, 70]

1. Children 3 months to 15 years (peak between 1 and 6 years).
2. Lichenoid papules (face, buttocks, extremities, palms, soles).
3. Anicteric hepatitis.
4. Lymphadenopathy, hepatosplenomegaly, fever, leukopenia.
5. Hepatitis-B surface antigen in some cases.

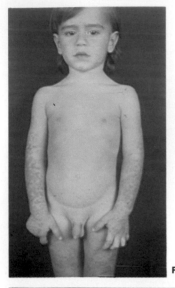

Figures 5–29, 5–30, 5–31 Flat-topped symmetrical lichenoid papules of papular acrodermatitis of childhood (Gianotti-Crosti syndrome) (Courtesy of Professor Ferdinando Gianotti).

Figure 5–29

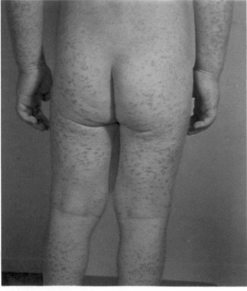

Figure 5–30

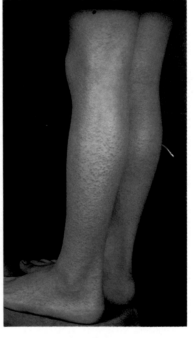

Figure 5–31

Figure 5–32 Microscopic features of Gianotti-Crosti disease. Hyperkeratosis, acanthosis, focal spongiosis, exocytosis, liquefaction and degeneration of basal layer, and lymphomonocytic and histiocytic dermal infiltrate (Courtesy of Professor Ferdinando Gianotti).

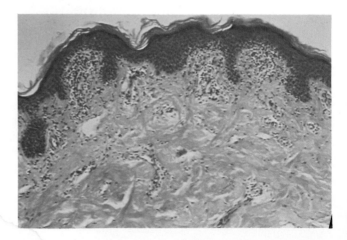

Gianotti has also described a similar disorder that generally affects children of a more limited age group (2 to 6 years) not associated with hepatomegaly or hepatitis virus B surface antigenemia.[71] This disorder, termed "papulovesicular acrolocalized syndrome" consists of small 1 to 5 mm alabaster to rose-pink or purple spherical or hemispherical vesicular papules that are often covered with a hemorrhagic crust. The eruption is symmetrically located on the cheeks, ears, buttocks, and extremities. Pruritus is common, splenomegaly is absent, liver function studies are normal, and hepatitis virus B surface antigenemia (HBS Ag) is absent.[71] Whether this disorder warrants separate classification or not still remains uncertain.

The diagnosis of Gianotti-Crosti syndrome is dependent upon the characteristic clinical findings and histopathologic examination of cutaneous lesions. Microscopic features of the cutaneous eruption include mild acanthosis, hyperkeratosis, focal spongiosis with extensive exocytosis of mononuclear cells, liquefactive degeneration of the basal layer, a dense perivascular lymphomonocytic and histiocytic dermal infiltrate, swelling of the vascular endothelium, and dilatation of dermal capillaries (Fig. 5–32).

Since this syndrome is benign and self-limiting (with a low incidence of familial involvement), treatment with other than symptomatic measures is unnecessary. It should be noted, however, that steroid creams may have an adverse effect on the cutaneous eruption.[66] In view of its apparent association with hepatitis B virus, children with this disorder should be evaluated for possible hepatitis and associated liver involvement.

References

1. Hurley HJ: Papulosquamous eruptions and exfoliative dermatitis. In Moschella SL, Pillsbury DM, Hurley HJ Jr. (Eds.): Dermatology. W. B. Saunders Co., Philadelphia, 1975, 409–458.

   A review of papulosquamous eruptions with emphasis on psoriasis, its pathogenesis, clinical patterns, and management.

2. Krulig L, Farber EM, Grumet FC, et al.: Histocompatibility (HL-A) antigens in psoriasis. Arch. Dermatol. 111:857–860, 1975.

   Studies of 101 psoriatic patients suggest that the HL-A locus (W-17 and W-16) may be a marker for hereditary factors affecting susceptibility to psoriasis.

3. Farber EM, Carlsen RA: Psoriasis in childhood. Calif. Med. 105:415–420, 1966.

   Of 1000 patients with psoriasis 27 per cent developed the disorder at or before age 15. Females were affected in a 2:1 ratio over males in childhood, and patients seemed to be more severely involved in adult life if the disorder had its onset during childhood.

4. Farber EM, Bright RD, Nall ML: Psoriasis. A questionnaire survey of 2144 patients. Arch. Dermatol. 98:248–259, 1968.

   A computerized analysis of 2144 individuals with psoriasis.

5. Lerner MR, Lerner AB: Congenital psoriasis. Arch. Dermatol. 105:598–601, 1972.

   Case histories of three patients with congenital psoriasis,

one of whom developed severe crippling psoriatic arthritis before age 13.

6. Farber EM, Nall MA: Genetics of psoriasis. Twin study. In Farber EM and Cox AJ (Eds.): Psoriasis, Proceedings of the International Symposium. Stanford University Press, Stanford, California, 1971, 7–14.

   A review of the current status of genetic knowledge about psoriasis.

7. Weinstein GD, Frost P: Abnormal cell proliferation in psoriasis. J. Invest. Dermatol. 50:254–259, 1968.

   Studies demonstrate a rapid 37.5 hour germinative cell cycle for psoriatic epidermal cells in contrast to the 19-day cycle of normal epidermal cells.

8. Baker H, Wilkinson DS: Psoriasis. In Rook A, Wilkinson DS, Ebling FJG (Eds.): Textbook of Dermatology, 2nd edition. Blackwell Scientific Publications, Oxford, 1972, 1192–1234.

   A thorough analysis of psoriasis, its pathogenesis, clinical patterns, and therapy.

9. Watson W, Farber EM: Psoriasis in childhood. Pediatr. Clin. North Am. 18:875–895, 1971.

   A review of psoriasis in childhood.

10. Calvert HT, Smith MA, Wells RS: Psoriasis and the nails. Br. J. Dermatol. 75:415–418, 1963.

    Two hundred and sixty patients examined for nail involvement revealed nail changes in 55 per cent of patients. Of these changes, pitting was the most common finding in the fingernails, and yellow discoloration was the most frequent change seen in the toenails.

11. Zaias N: Psoriasis of the nail. A clinicopathologic study. Arch. Dermatol. 99:567–579, 1969.

    The clinical signs of nail psoriasis correlated with psoriatic involvement of the nail components.

12. Farber EM, Jacobs AH: Infantile psoriasis. Am. J. Dis. Child. 131:1266–1269, 1977.

    A report of 14 children under 2 years of age with psoriasis vulgaris.

13. Stoughton RB: A perspective of topical corticosteroid therapy. In Farber EM, Cox AJ (Eds.): Psoriasis: Proceedings of the Second International Symposium, Yorke Medical Books, New York, 1976, 219–226.

    A critical appraisal of topical corticosteroids and their potency.

14. Peachey RDG, Pyre RJ, Harman PRM: Treatment of psoriatic nail dystrophy with intradermal steroid injections. Brit. J. Dermatol. 95:75–78, 1977.

    Thirty-seven patients with psoriatic nail dystrophy showed improvement with intradermal steroid injection (those with onycholysis and more severe types of dystrophy usually show little improvement).

15. Fredriksson T: Topical 5-Fluorouracil in the treatment of psoriatic nails. In Farber EM, Cox AJ (Eds.): Psoriasis: Proceedings of the Second International Symposium, Yorke Medical Books, New York, 1976, 438–439.

    Twenty patients with chronic psoriatic involvement of the nails experienced effective results with topical 5-FU.

16. Perry HO, Soderstrom CW, Schulze RW: The Goeckerman treatment of psoriasis. Arch. Dermatol. 98:178–182, 1968.

    Excellent results to Goeckerman regimen, with remissions varying from 6 to 18 months.

17. Comaish S: Ingram method of treating psoriasis. Arch. Dermatol. 92:56–58, 1965.

    An attempt to introduce this effective therapeutic regimen to American dermatologists.

18. Parrish JA, Fitzpatrick TB, Tannenbaum L, et al.: Photochemistry of psoriasis with methoxsalen and long-wave ultraviolet light. N. Engl. J. Med. 291:1207–1211, 1974.

    An experimental approach (8-methoxy-psoralen and high energy long-wave UVA light) is extremely effective in clearing severe and extensive psoriasis.

19. Cohen GL: Psoriatic arthritis. *In* Progress in Dermatology (Dermatology Foundation, Philadelphia) *10*(2):5–8, 1976.

A careful analysis of psoriatic arthritis with emphasis on its clinical presentation, diagnosis, and therapy.

20. Everall JD, Dowd PM: Pustular psoriasis of the hands and feet. *In* Farber EM, Cox AJ (Eds.): Psoriasis, Proceedings of the Second International Symposium. Yorke Medical Books, New York, 1976, 345–346.

A review of 66 patients with pustular psoriasis supports the view that there is little difference between pustular psoriasis of Barber and pustular bacterid of Andrews.

21. Khan SA, Peterkin GAG, Mitchell PC: Juvenile generalized pustular psoriasis — a report of five cases and a review of the literature. Arch. Dermatol. *105*:67–72, 1972.

A report of five children with generalized pustular psoriasis responding to bland topical therapy.

22. Beylot C, Bioulac P, Julien B, et al.: Generalized pustular psoriasis in infants and children: report of eight cases. Ann. Dermat. et Syph. 100:121–140, 1973.

Of 48 reported cases of pustular psoriasis in children 24 were of the Zumbusch type (with extensive erythema, pustules, scarlatiniform desquamation, and intense malaise).

23. Beylot C, Bioulac P, Grupper C, et al.: Generalized pustular psoriasis in infants and children: Report of 27 cases. *In* Farber EM, Cox AJ (Eds.): Psoriasis, Proceedings of the Second International Symposium. Yorke Medical Books, New York, 1976, 171–179.

A description of 27 cases of generalized pustular psoriasis in children with emphasis on clinical aspects and therapy.

24. Pascher F, Wood WS: Erythrodermic psoriasis in children. Arch. Dermatol. 74:173–176, 1956.

Erythrodermic psoriasis in a 7-year-old girl and a 13-year-old boy.

25. Scott RB, Surana R: Erythrodermic psoriasis in childhood. Am. J. Dis. Child. *116*:218–221, 1968.

Psoriatic erythroderma in a child whose disease began at about 18 months of age and terminated fatally following chicken pox complicated by staphylococcal pyoderma and sepsis while on methotrexate therapy.

26. Kahn G, Rywlin AM: Acropustulosis of infancy. Arch. Dermatol. *115*:831–833, 1979.

Two infants with acropustulosis of infancy, a disorder believed to be distinct from all other disorders of infancy, with pruritic lesions on hands, feet, and face.

27. Jarrett M, Ramsdell W: Infantile acropustulosis. Arch. Dermatol. *115*:834–836, 1979.

Clinical and histologic features in 10 children with infantile acropustulosis.

28. Jacobs A: A case of Reiter's syndrome in childhood. Br. Med. J. 2:155, 1961.

A 9-year-old boy with Reiter's disease manifested by urethritis, conjunctivitis, and arthritis (without cutaneous findings) following a bout of dysentery.

29. Margileth AM: Reiter's syndrome in children: Case report and review of the literature. Clin. Pediatr. *1*:148–151, 1962.

A six-year-old boy with conjunctivitis, urethritis, and arthritis.

30. Moss JS: Reiter's disease in childhood. Br. J. Vener. Dis. 40:166–169, 1964.

Review of 27 cases of Reiter's disease in children, the youngest being 1 year and 9 months of age.

31. Brewerton DA, Caffrey M, Nicholls A, et al.: Reiter's disease. Lancet 2:996–998, 1973.

HL-A antigen found in 25 (76 per cent) of 33 patients with Reiter's disease.

32. Morris R, Metzger AL, Bluestone R, et al.: HL-A: clue to diagnosis and pathogenesis of Reiter's syndrome. N. Engl. J. Med. *290*:554–556, 1974.

Ninety-six per cent of patients with Reiter's syndrome were HL-A W27–positive.

33. Kierland RR, Kulwin MH: Pityriasis rubra pilaris: A clinical study. Arch. Derm. Syph. *61*:925–930, 1950.

Clinical analysis of 58 patients suggests two distinct types of pityriasis rubra pilaris.

34. Leitner ZA, Ford EB: Vitamin A and pityriasis rubra pilaris. Br. J. Dermatol. 59:407–427, 1947.

A comprehensive study of six patients with pityriasis rubra pilaris traced through three generations.

35. Porter D, Shuster S: Epidermal renewal and aminoacids in psoriasis and pityriasis rubra pilaris. Arch. Dermatol. 98:339–343, 1968.

Increased transit times and rapid epidermal turnover in lesions of psoriasis and pityriasis rubra pilaris.

36. Davidson CL, Winkelmann RK, Kierland RR: Pityriasis rubra pilaris. A followup study of 57 patients. Arch. Dermatol. *100*:175–178, 1969.

Fifty per cent of patients with pityriasis rubra pilaris improved after an average period of 2.3 years (with a range of 3 months to 7 years).

37. Huntley CC: Pityriasis rubra pilaris. Am. J. Dis. Child. *122*:22–23, 1971.

Complete remission in a 16-month-old child with pityriasis rubra pilaris after 50,000 units of oral vitamin A twice a day for 6 1/2 weeks.

38. Muller SA, Belcher RW, Esterly NB, et al.: Keratinizing dermatoses — combined data from four centers on short-term topical treatment with tretinoin. Arch. Dermatol. *113*:1052–1054, 1977.

Clinical response to topical vitamin A acid (tretinoin) in patients with ichthyosis vulgaris and lamellar ichthyosis.

39. Brown J, Perry HO: Pityriasis rubra pilaris. Arch. Dermatol. 94:636–638, 1966.

Marked clinical improvement in four patients with pityriasis rubra pilaris treated with folic acid antagonists (aminopterin and methotrexate).

40. Scholtz M: Mucha-Habermann syndrome (parapsoriasis varioliformis) — a critical study with a report of a case. Arch. Derm. Syph. 30:631–644, 1934.

Histopathologic data and clinical picture of Mucha-Habermann syndrome.

41. Harman RRM, Nagington J, Rook A: Virus infections. *In* Rook A, Wilkinson DS, Ebling FJG (Eds.): Textbook of Dermatology. F. A. Davis Co., Philadelphia, 1968, 538–808.

A thorough description of viral disease and certain cutaneous disorders thought to be but not necessarily associated with viral infection.

42. Clayton R, Warin A: Pityriasis lichenoides chronica presenting as hypopigmentation. Br. J. Dermatol. *100*:297–302, 1979.

Widespread hypopigmentation as the conspicuous clinical feature in 7 dark-skinned patients with chronic pityriasis lichenoides.

43. Verallo VM, Haserick JR: Mucha-Habermann's disease simulating lymphocytoma cutis. Arch. Dermatol. 94:295–299, 1966.

Two cases of Mucha-Habermann disease in which the histology suggested a malignant lymphoma.

44. Muller SA, Schulze TC: Mucha-Habermann disease mistaken for reticulum cell sarcoma. Arch. Dermatol. *103*:423–427, 1971.

A case of Mucha-Habermann disease in which reticulum cell sarcoma was diagnosed on the basis of skin biopsies emphasizes the need for clinical re-evaluation when clinical and histopathologic findings are discordant.

45. Macaulay WL: Lymphomatoid papulosis: a continuing self-healing eruption, clinically benign — histologically malignant. Arch. Dermatol. 97:23–30, 1968.

   "Lymphomatoid papulosis." Is this a distinct disorder or merely a manifestation of Mucha-Habermann disease?

46. Marks R, Black MM: The inflammatory reaction in pityriasis lichenoides. Br. J. Dermatol. 87:533–539, 1972.

   Studies suggest that a release of vasoactive substances may play a role in the pathogenesis of pityriasis lichenoides.

47. Ingram JT: Pityriasis lichenoides and parapsoriasis. Br. J. Dermatol. 65:293–299, 1953.

   Pityriasis lichenoides: a self-limiting disease without serious sequelae.

48. Burke DP, Adams RM, Arundell FD: Febrile ulceronecrotic Mucha-Habermann's disease. Arch. Dermatol. 100:200–206, 1969.

   Two cases of acute pityriasis lichenoides with high fever and ulceronecrotic skin lesions.

49. Szymanski FJ: Pityriasis lichenoides et varioliformis acuta —histopathologic evidence that it is an entity distinct from parapsoriasis. Arch. Dermatol. 79:7–16, 1959.

   Clinical and histologic evidence suggest acute pityriasis lichenoides to be a vasculitis distinctly different from chronic pityriasis lichenoides (a low-grade inflammatory process of the epidermis).

50. Clayton T, Haffenden G: An immunofluorescent study of pityriasis lichenoides. Br. J. Dermatol. 99:491–493, 1978.

   Seventy-three per cent of 27 patients with pityriasis lichenoides had IgM and C_3 on direct immunofluorescent studies in superficial dermal vessel walls and along the dermal-epidermal junction, suggesting that immune complexes may play a role in the etiology of this disorder.

51. Shelly WB, Griffith RF: Pityriasis lichenoides et varioliformis acuta: A reported case controlled by high dosage of tetracycline. Arch. Dermatol. 100:596–597, 1969.

   Two grams of tetracycline a day appeared to have a suppressive effect on the course of pityriasis lichenoides.

52. Cornelison RL, Jr, Knox JM, Everett MA: Methotrexate for treatment of Mucha-Habermann disease. Arch. Dermatol. 106:507–514, 1972.

   Improvement of six patients with Mucha-Habermann disease to low dosages of oral methotrexate.

53. Marchall J: Pityriasis rosea. A review of its clinical aspects and a discussion of its relationship to pityriasis lichenoides et varioliformis acuta and parapsoriasis guttata. S. Afr. Med. J. 30:210–217, 1956.

   A review of pityriasis rosea, its epidemiology, clinical appearance, and histopathologic features.

54. Björnberg A, Hellgren L: Pityriasis rosea. A statistical, clinical and laboratory investigation of 826 patients and matched healthy controls. Acta Derm. Venereol. 42 (Suppl. 50):1–68, 1972.

   An in-depth review of pityriasis rosea.

55. Kestal JL, Jr: Oral lesions in pityriasis rosea. JAMA 205:597, 1971.

   Pityriasis rosea in the mouth reveals white lesions, which follow a course similar to that of the cutaneous eruption.

56. Altman J, Perry HO: The variations and course of lichen planus. Arch. Dermatol. 84:179–101, 1961.

   A review of 307 patients with lichen planus.

57. Samman PD: Lichen planus and lichenoid eruptions. In Rook A, Wilkinson DS, Ebling FJG (Eds.): Textbook of Dermatology, Second printing. Blackwell Scientific Publications, Oxford, 1972, 1334–1352.

   A review of the histologic and clinical features of lichen planus, its variants, and other lichenoid disorders.

58. Cotton DWK, Van den Hurk JJMA, Van der Staak WBJM: Lichen planus, an inborn error of metabolism. Br. J. Dermatol. 87:341–346, 1972.

   A group of patients with congenital deficiency of glucose-6-phosphate dehydrogenase with drug-induced attacks of lichen planus.

59. Zaias N: The nail in lichen planus. Arch. Dermatol. 101:264–271, 1970.

   A comprehensive review of nail changes seen in association with lichen planus.

60. de Graciansky P, Boulle S: Skin disease from colour developers. Br. J. Dermatol. 78:297–298, 1966.

   Lichen planus caused by paraphenylenediamine in color film developer.

61. Almeyda J, Levantine A: Lichenoid drug eruptions. Br. J. Dermatol. 85:604–607, 1971.

   A review of drug-induced lichenoid eruptions.

62. Calnan CD: Lichen aureus. Br. J. Dermatol. 72:373, 1960.

   A case report of a 23-year-old patient with lichen aureus.

63. Waisman M, Waisman M: Lichen aureus. Arch. Dermatol. 112:696–697, 1976.

   Aggregated perifollicular gray-brown or rust-colored papules with thin adherent scales on an erythematous background representing hemosiderin.

64. Gianotti F: Papular acrodermatitis of childhood: an Australian antigen disease. Arch. Dis. Child. 48:794–799, 1973.

   A report of 39 children with papular acrodermatitis of childhood all of whom demonstrated the presence of Australian hepatitis antigen.

65. Gianotti F: Papular acrodermatitis of childhood: an Australian antigen disease. Mod. Probl. Paediat. 17:180–189, 1975.

   A review of papular acrodermatitis of childhood presented at the 1st International Symposium on Pediatric Dermatology (Mexico City, 1973).

66. Hjorth N, Kopp H, Osmundsen PE: Gianotti-Crosti syndrome — papular eruption of infancy. Trans. St. John's Hosp. Derm. Soc. 53:46–56, 1967.

   A review of 117 patients with Gianotti-Crosti syndrome.

67. Rubenstein D, Esterly NB, Fretzin D: The Gianotti-Crosti syndrome. Pediatrics 61:433–437, 1978.

   A report of two children (11 and 18 months of age) with the Gianotti-Crosti syndrome and a review of the current status of this disorder.

68. Cloudy AL: Adult papular acrodermatitis. Ann. Derm. Venereol. 104:190–194, 1977.

   A report of three adults with papular acrodermatitis (Gianotti-Crosti syndrome) associated with viral hepatitis.

69. Eiloart M: The Gianotti-Crosti syndrome. Report of forty-four cases. Br. J. Dermatol. 78:488–492, 1966.

   Report of 44 cases plus two others previously reported and a plea for recognition of this often unrecognized distinctive disorder.

70. Ishimaru Y, Ishimaru H, Toda G, et al.: An epidemic of infantile papular acrodermatitis (Gianotti's disease) in Japan associated with hepatitis-B surface antigen subtype ayw. Lancet 1:707–709, 1976.

   Ninety-three per cent of patients with infantile papular acrodermatitis of childhood with hepatitis B surface antigen subtype ayw suggest this disorder to be a manifestation of hepatitis B virus infection in children under age 3.

71. Gianotti F: Infantile papular acrodermatitis: acrodermatitis papulosa and infantile papulovesicular acrolocalized syndrome. Hautarzt 27:467–472, 1976.

   A review of infantile papular acrodermatitis and "acrolocalized infantile papulovesicular syndrome."

6

DISORDERS OF THE SEBACEOUS AND SWEAT GLANDS

DISORDERS OF THE SEBACEOUS GLANDS

Acne Vulgaris

Although th basic cause of acne vulgaris remains unknown, considerable data concerning its pathogenesis accumulated in recent years allows a rational and therapeutically successful approach to the management of this disorder. Acne therefore should never be dismissed as being of no consequence, with mere reassurance that the patient will outgrow it, for the psychological scars and trauma are often deeper and more disastrous than the blemishes displayed on the cutaneous surface alone. To date there is no single treatment for acne. The choice of therapy must be individualized for each patient, with appropriate modifications as the activity of the disease fluctuates. The success of therapy depends upon the cooperation of the patient and the interest, enthusiasm, and careful selection of medications on the part of the physician (Fig. 6–1).

Acne vulgaris, a disorder of the pilosebaceous apparatus, is the most common skin disorder of the second and third decades of life and for years has been a perplexing enigma to patients and physicians alike. Recent scientific advances have finally dispelled much of its mystique and mythology,

allowing a rational and highly successful approach to the therapy of this disorder. Its name is attributed to the Greek and Latin words "akmē" and "acme," respectively, no doubt owing to the fact that this condition is most prominent during adolescence, the so-called peak of life. The word vulgaris is derived from the Latin adjective meaning ordinary or common and denotes an average form of acne rather than a disorder with a coarse or derogatory connotation.

INCIDENCE. The tendency to develop acne is often familial and is thought to be inherited as an autosomal dominant trait. However, because of the high prevalence of this disorder, its exact genetic pattern remains undetermined. Actually we know very little about the genetics and epidemiology of acne. Hereditary influences can easily be appreciated by taking histories and looking for scars among first-order relatives; yet, except for Nierman's study showing 98 per cent concordance for the presence of acne in identical twins, controlled data are lacking.[1] Acne therefore probably represents a polygenic disorder in which the clinical expression represents the sum of the action of many genes.[2]

Adolescence is the period of life between childhood and adulthood. It begins with puberty, which may appear at any time between 9 and 17

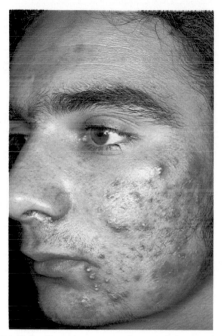

Figure 6–1 Comedones, papules, pustules, cysts, and nodules on the face of a 20-year-old male with acne vulgaris.

years of age. The physiologic mechanism that triggers the changes associated with the onset of puberty is unknown, but it appears to involve the release of gonadotropic hormone from the anterior pituitary, which in turn stimulates ovarian secretion of estrogen and the production of androgen by the testicles, ovaries, and adrenal cortex. These steroid hormones are responsible for the production of the secondary sex characteristics as well as the cutaneous disorders associated with adolescence.

Although acne may be present at birth, as the result of hormonal stimulation of sebaceous glands that have not yet involuted to their childhood state of immaturity (neonatal acne), it is frequently not until puberty that acne becomes a common problem. It may develop as early as the fifth to eighth year of life, and in girls may precede menarche by more than a year. In girls its peak is reached between the ages of 14 and 17; in boys the greatest severity is noted between 16 and 19 years of age.[3] It is seen slightly more often in males than in females, the disparity between the sexes becoming more apparent as the severity of the disorder increases. Depending on one's definition of acne, approximately 85 per cent of high school students between 15 and 18 years of age have some degree of this disorder.[4, 5] Mild forms, however, appear to be so prevalent that if one considers an occasional comedo and papule as acne, the disorder might be regarded as a physiologic phenomenon with estimates of its presence reaching almost 100 per cent of individuals.[6] In 80 per cent of patients, the incidence and severity of acne appears to decline at about 22 to 23 years of age; in 10 per cent of

patients active lesions may occur even into the thirties or forties.[3, 4]

ETIOLOGY. An understanding of the physiological basis of acne can simplify one's therapeutic approach and can produce results far better than heretofore have been attainable. Acne usually begins one or two years prior to the onset of puberty as a result of androgenic stimulation of the sebaceous glands and is attributable to an abnormal keratinization process that results in obstruction of the pilosebaceous unit. Sebaceous glands are present in all human skin except the palms, soles, dorsa of the feet, and perhaps the lower lip. The highest concentrations are noted on the face, chest and back, with a total of 15,000 to 20,000 glands on the face alone. Each gland is composed of several lobules that lead into a common excretory duct. These glands, holocrine in nature, are devoid of motor innervation and depend solely upon androgenic stimulation.

Recent studies have demonstrated that the increasing flux of circulating testosterone is taken up by the sebaceous gland and converted to dihydrotestosterone by the enzyme 5-alpha-reductase. Current research suggests that dihydrotestosterone is the tissue androgen that causes hypertrophy of the sebaceous gland and an increased production of sebum associated with this disorder. Acne patients appear to convert testosterone to dihydrotestosterone more readily than unaffected individuals. In males the testicles are the major source of androgen for sebaceous gland development. In females androgens, in normal amounts, are derived from the ovary and adrenal gland. The androgenic stimulation of sebaceous glands does not imply a hormonal imbalance, merely a normal physiologic phenomenon that sets the stage for the subsequent changes seen in acne. In females the endogenous androgen secretion is approximately two thirds that of males, with acne accordingly less common and less severe in women than it is in men.[7]

In addition to excessive sebum production, patients with acne have one other major abnormality of the sebaceous follicle, namely a change in the process of keratinization. Acne thus develops in the sebaceous follicles and is initiated by an altered keratinization process of the follicular canal that results in obstruction of the pilosebaceous unit. The cause of this abnormality of keratinization is unknown, although patients with a predisposition to acne appear to have a tendency for irritation to the follicular wall by free fatty acids.[8] When the normal flow of sebum onto the skin surface is obstructed by this follicular hyperkeratosis, comedones are formed, thus initiating the process of acne (Fig. 6–2).

In terms of pathogenesis, two types of comedones are formed—open comedones (blackheads) and closed comedones (whiteheads) (Figs. 6–3 and 6–4).[9] The open comedo is composed of an epithelium-lined sac filled with keratin and lipid, with a widely dilated orifice. For years there has been much speculation regarding the genesis of

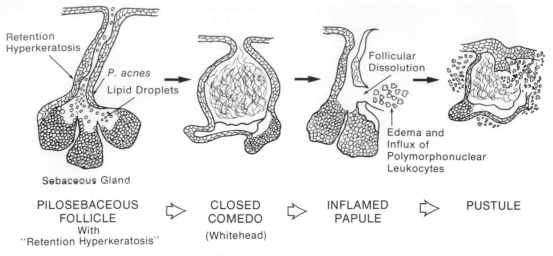

Retention Hyperkeratosis

P. acnes

Lipid Droplets

Sebaceous Gland

Follicular Dissolution

Edema and Influx of Polymorphonuclear Leukocytes

PILOSEBACEOUS FOLLICLE
With "Retention Hyperkeratosis"

CLOSED COMEDO
(Whitehead)

INFLAMED PAPULE

PUSTULE

Figure 6–2   The pathogenesis of acne. (Adapted from Hurwitz S: Am. J. Dis. Child. *133*:536–544, 1979.)

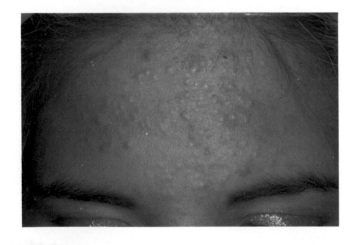

Figure 6–3   Closed comedones (whiteheads) and papules on the forehead of a patient with acne vulgaris.

Figure 6–4   Multiple open comedones (blackheads) on the forehead of a 14-year-old male with acne vulgaris.

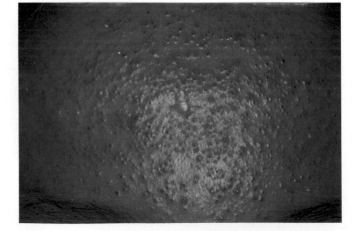

the blackened tip of the open comedo. Contrary to popular misconception, the color is not caused by exogenous dirt or lack of hygiene. Although various theories suggest compaction and oxidation of the keratinous material at the follicular orifice as the cause of the brown to black discoloration, recent histochemical and histologic studies suggest that melanin also plays a role in the etiology of open comedones.[10, 11] Blackheads, though unsightly, are easily managed and rarely create problems in acne. The contents of the open comedones easily escape to the skin surface; follicular disruption and inflammation, therefore, rarely occur, except when the comedones are traumatized by the patient.

Conversely, it is the whitehead, or closed comedo, that is responsible for the problems seen in acne. These lesions are seen as small, skin-colored, slightly elevated papules just beneath the skin surface (their visualization may be enhanced by a slight stretching of the overlying skin) (Fig. 6–3). The closed comedo has a microscopic opening that keeps its contents from escaping. It continues to form keratin and some sebum, and when the follicular wall ruptures, it acts as a veritable time bomb and expels sebum into the surrounding dermis, thus initiating the inflammatory process.[9] The clinical appearance of the resulting inflammatory lesion is dependent not only on the size of the comedo in which the rupture occurs but also on the location of the inflammatory reaction in the dermis. Thus, if the inflammatory nidus is close to the surface, the lesion will usually be a pustule; deeper inflammation results in a larger papule or nodule.[12]

Some authors feel that stressful events such as emotional tension, lack of sleep, and menses in the female patient result in increased sebum formation that tips the balance and creates a breach in the follicular epithelium. This break permits leakage of the irritating follicular contents, thus initiating the inflammatory reaction within the dermis. The explanation for the worsening of acne vulgaris after stressful situations is unclear, but it appears to be related to an increased adrenocortical response by way of the pituitary-adrenal pathway.[12]

Sebum is made up of a mixture of triglycerides, wax esters, squalene, and sterol esters. Currently, free fatty acids, particularly those with short chains (C_8 to C_{14}), are believed to play an important role in comedogenesis and the formation of inflammatory lesions.[13] Free fatty acids, however, are not found in the lipids normally present within the sebaceous canal. Their release appears to be the result of hydrolysis of triglycerides within the pilosebaceous follicles (to diglycerides, monoglycerides, and finally glycerol) by lipases, with release of physiologically active molecules of free fatty acids at each step of the process. An ordinarily harmless bacteria, the anaerobic *Propionibacterium acnes* (formerly termed *Corynebacterium acnes*), appears to be the major source of lipolytic enzymes within the pilosebaceous follicle.[13-19]

CLINICAL MANIFESTATIONS.   Acne usually presents as a variety of lesions in which the comedo is pathognomonic. In its mildest form it is limited to open comedones (blackheads) and closed comedones (whiteheads) (Figs. 6–3 and 6–4). As the disorder increases in severity, patients may develop papules, pustules, nodules, or cysts (Figs. 6–1, 6–4 and 6–5). The term cyst is actually a misnomer; in this case it denotes a large nodular lesion that has undergone suppuration, thus resembling an inflamed cyst.

The primary sites of acne are the face, chest, back, and shoulders (Fig. 6–6). There is often a seasonal variation, acne being least active in summer and most severe in winter. As acne lesions resolve they are frequently followed by temporary postinflammatory redness and hyperpigmentation. Although patients commonly regard these as active lesions and potential scars, this discoloration gradually subsides once the condition is controlled. In the more severe pustular and cystic forms of acne, sheaths of epithelium from remaining follicular walls tend to encapsulate the inflammatory areas with subsequent fibrous contraction and eventual cicatricial formation. The scars usually present as sharply punched out pits or as hypertrophic and keloid scars (Figs. 6–7 and 6–8). The severity of the scarring depends upon the depth and intensity of the inflammation and the patient's susceptibility to cicatrization.

TREATMENT.   For years the treatment of acne was hindered by mythical concepts of etiology, a lack of concern for the physical and psychological trauma of those affected with severe forms of this disorder, and the perpetuation of ineffec-

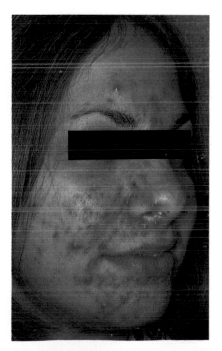

Figure 6–5   Papules, pustules, cysts, and nodules in a 16-year-old girl with acne vulgaris.

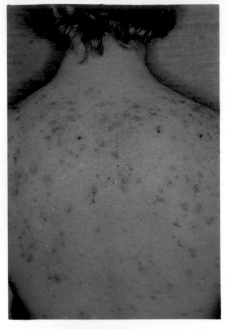

Figure 6–6 Severe acne vulgaris with scarring on the back.

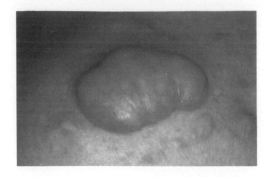

Figure 6–8 Keloidal acne scarring on the shoulder of a 16-year-old male with acne vulgaris.

tive therapeutic regimens based upon misconception and misinformation. No concerned physician should fail to recognize the deep emotional trauma suffered by patients with acne, nor should he ignore the tremendous benefits, both physical and emotional, that today's effective therapeutics can evoke. It is indeed a grievous injustice for either

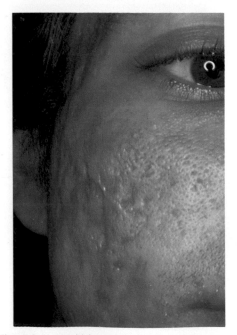

Figure 6–7 Keloidal and atrophic "ice-pick" scars on the cheek of a young man with acne vulgaris.

parent or physician to regard acne as evanescent or untreatable, for the psychological scars that accompany this disorder can frequently be far more devastating and destructive than the visible cutaneous aberrations caused by the disease itself.

As yet there is no single treatment for acne vulgaris. Therapy must be individualized with appropriate variations and modifications as the degree or severity of the disorder fluctuates. Success of acne therapy depends upon (1) prevention of follicular hyperkeratosis, (2) reduction of *Propionibacterium acnes* and free fatty acids, and (3) elimination of comedones and the papules, pustules, cysts, and nodules that result from them. Today this goal can be achieved by proper selection of available medications, coupled with the cooperation of the patient, and the knowledge, continued interest, and enthusiasm of the physician and his staff, usually within 6 to 12 weeks of treatment. Once this has been accomplished, therapy must be continued faithfully for as long as the tendency toward acne persists. Unfortunately, as with so many long-term programs, patients occasionally develop a false sense of security and tend to modify their therapy, often with regrettable effects. In order to achieve the best long-term results, patients should be forewarned of this possibility and encouraged to continue treatment as long as their tendency to acne persists.[20]

Diet. Recent controlled studies refute the value of dietary restrictions imposed upon acne patients. For years the elimination of various foods such as chocolate and cola drinks, sweets, milk, ice cream, fatty foods, shellfish, and iodides dominated many of the futile approaches to acne control. The misconception that iodine is injurious to patients with acne originated with the concept that iodides administered orally as medication occasionally initiate a papulo-pustular acneform eruption (iodism). A large-scale epidemiological investigation of over 1000 North Carolina high school students revealed that dietary iodine exerts no influence on either the prevalence or the severity of acne.[21] The concept that chocolate exerts an adverse effect on acne has also been challenged. In a carefully controlled double-blind study, it was found that this too failed to affect either the course of acne vulgaris or the composition of sebum.[22] For those patients who attest to flares following certain foods, it is judicious to eliminate the suspicious agents until their true influence can be appropriately and individually assessed.

Topical Therapy. Appropriate topical therapy is essential to the successful management of acne. With presently available pharmacological agents, frequently topical drugs are the only modalities necessary for therapy of even some of the most severe forms of acne vulgaris. For years various drying and exfoliating agents (abrasive soaps, astringents, ultraviolet light, sulfur, resorcinol (resorcin), and salicylic acid), alone or in various combinations, were the focus of acne therapy. Whereas such preparations may indeed cause drying and peeling, remove oils from the surface of the skin, and suppress individual lesions to a limited degree, they fail in the effective prevention of new lesions and actually impede the proper utilization of the effective topical agents currently available for the treatment of acne vulgaris.

Propionibacterium acnes organisms are the source of lipases responsible for the breakdown of sebum into irritating free fatty acids. These anaerobic diphtheroids live beneath the skin surface, within the pilosebaceous follicle, where they are inaccessible to most previously available topical antibacterial agents. Therefore, contrary to many advertising claims, soaps containing hexachlorophene and other antibacterial agents are also probably ineffective in the therapy of acne vulgaris.

Of the available topical agents, those that have had the greatest popularity include sulfur, resorcin, salicylic acid, benzoyl peroxide, and vitamin A acid (tretinoin). Sulfur and resorcinol have been used in varying concentrations of from 1 to 5 per cent and 1 to 10 per cent respectively. Their efficacy is limited and seems to be related to their capacity to produce erythema and desquamation. They tend to help dry and peel existing comedones, papules, and pustules, but fail in attempts to limit the formation of closed comedones (whiteheads) and the lesions that result from them.

Benzoyl peroxide and vitamin A acid (tretinoin), though potential irritants, appear to be the most effective topical agents. Based on our current understanding of the pathogenesis of acne, these two agents offer a highly effective therapeutic approach that can be tailored to each patient. Although success in the management of acne vulgaris can be achieved by the use of topical tretinoin or benzoyl peroxide alone, it appears that under proper management the therapeutic effect can be increased substantially by the use of the two agents in combination.[23, 24]

Salicylic Acid. Salicylic acid is categorized as a "keratolytic" agent and has been used in a wide variety of cutaneous disorders. The concentration of salicylic acid in most proprietary acne preparations, however, is often too low, or it is formulated with other agents that may handicap its activity.[6] When used in the treatment of acne, it may be used in concentrations of 5 per cent to 10 per cent salicylic acid in equal parts of 85 per cent ethanol and propylene glycol, or as 5 per cent salicylic acid in a hydroalcoholic gel containing 40 per cent alcohol, available as Saligel (Stiefel). Although somewhat less effective than tretinoin or benzoyl peroxide, salicylic acid formulations may be used for patients with mild comedonal acne, for those who have difficulty with or do not like to use the more potent formulations of tretinoin, or as an alternate to tretinoin in combination with benzoyl peroxide.[25]

Benzoyl Peroxide. In 1934, topical benzoyl peroxide was first introduced in the therapy of acne vulgaris. Unfortunately, a lack of appreciation of the role of the vehicle in delivery of medication to the skin prevented consistently effective results and more widespread use of this modality. During the 1960's this chemotherapeutic agent was introduced, initially in lotion form, and more recently in a series of more potent gel formulations. With these newer vehicles, the benzoyl peroxide appears to penetrate the pilosebaceous follicle more effectively. Benzoyl peroxide $(C_{14}H_{10}O_4)$ is currently available in lotion form (Benoxyl, Loroxide, Oxy-5, Persadox, Vanoxide) or in the more potent gel formulation (Benzac, Benzagel, Desquam-X, Panoxyl, Persa-Gel, Xerac-BP, or Zeroxin gel), both of which are available in 5 per cent and 10 per cent concentrations. Although the precise and complete mechanism of action of benzoyl peroxide is not fully understood, these preparations offer more than a form of epidermal irritation. They cause a fine desquamation ("keratolysis"), help reduce the level of free fatty acids, appear to be bactericidal for *P. acnes,* inhibit triglyceride hydrolysis, and decrease inflammation of acne lesions. Whether the therapeutic effect is based upon benzoyl peroxide's exfoliative or possible antibacterial effect, or a combination of these two, remains open to conjecture.

Benzoyl peroxide is potentially irritating and drying, particularly when used excessively or in association with abrasive soaps or astringents or both. Therapy must be individualized and initiated gradually, particularly in fair-skinned or atopic individuals. A relatively low incidence of irritant or allergic contact dermatitis (up to 1 to 2.5 per cent) suggests a certain degree of caution in its use in the treatment of acne.[26] A test for possible allergic contact dermatitis, perhaps by an open patch test on the volar aspect of the patient's wrist, prior to the initiation of therapy, therefore, appears to be a sensible precautionary measure.

Following an initial test application, benzoyl peroxide should be applied as a thin film, initially every day or every other day, and rubbed in gently, gradually increasing the frequency and strength of the preparations as tolerance is developed (generally within a period of two or three weeks).[25] The 10 per cent gel is potentially more drying and irritating. Therefore it is often a good

Table 6-1 ACTION OF BENZOYL PEROXIDE

1. Irritant and keratolytic
2. Suppresses *P. acnes*
   a. Inhibits triglyceride hydrolysis
   b. Lowers free fatty acids
   c. Decreases inflammation in acne lesions

idea to start with the lower strength formulation and work up to higher concentrations as tolerance to the medication develops. If irritation or excessive dryness develops, the preparation may be discontinued for a period of several days. Lubricants may then be used for a period of one to several days until the irritation resolves. Once the irritation or dryness disappears, therapy can be resumed gently and cautiously as a degree of tolerance is established. Although clinical dryness and exfoliation were thought to be helpful and resulted in a more effective therapeutic response, our studies show that when benzoyl peroxide is applied properly in a thin film (with a certain degree of care and caution) most patients will achieve success without the unpleasant side effects of dryness, redness, or irritation. Most problems with benzoyl peroxide, accordingly, appear to be related to overzealous or improper application of the prescribed formulations (Table 6–1 and Fig. 6–9).[25]

Vitamin A Acid (Retinoic Acid, Tretinoin). For years, vitamin A has been administered orally to patients with acne vulgaris in the hope of reducing hyperkeratosis of the sebaceous follicle. Unfortunately, therapeutic effect requires dosage in the toxic range of 400,000 to 700,000 units a

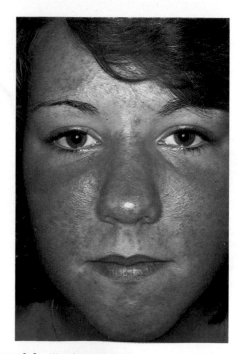

Figure 6–9 Allergic contact dermatitis due to the use of benzoyl peroxide in the treatment of acne vulgaris.

day.[27] In an effort to find a way of delivering a substantial dose of this drug to the target area without exacting the penalty of systemic toxicity, the use of tretinoin (topical vitamin A acid) in the therapy of acne vulgaris was proposed in 1969.[28]

Available as Retin-A, in liquid (0.05 per cent), as Retin-A cream (0.05 to 0.1 per cent), and Retin-A gel (0.01 or 0.025 per cent), tretinoin seems to have several beneficial effects on the skin of patients with acne vulgaris. Included among these benefits are an increased cell turnover within the pilosebaceous ducts and a decreased cohesiveness of epidermal cells. This stimulates dehiscence of horny cells, which results in a thinning of the horny layer, an increased cell turnover, a decreased comedo formation, a sloughing and expulsion of existent comedones from their sebaceous follicles, a reduction of inflammatory lesions arising from comedones, and transepidermal penetration of benzoyl peroxide and topical antibiotics (Table 6–2).[28, 29, 30]

It is unfortunate that vitamin A acid (tretinoin), perhaps the single most effective topical remedy for acne, is potentially irritating and improperly utilized by so many physicians.[30, 31] Because of its known capacity to cause severe irritation and peeling, topical vitamin A acid therapy should be initiated conservatively, on an alternate-day or occasionally on an every-third-day regimen, preferably with the less irritating gel or cream formulation. If tolerated, the patient may then gradually use the more potent cream, gel, or liquid preparations. Patients should be instructed to wash with a mild soap, no more than two or three times a day, and to wait at least 30 minutes after washing (to ensure that the skin is completely dry) before the application of tretinoin. If prolonged sun exposure is anticipated, patients must be cautioned to use a sun-protective lotion (see Chapter 4).

Vitamin A Acid and Benzoyl Peroxide. The art of medicine is predicated on the physician's ability to balance side effects against the potential benefits of various pharmacological agents. Although success in the management of acne vulgaris can be achieved by the use of vitamin A acid or benzoyl peroxide alone, the therapeutic effect is substantially increased by the use of the two agents in combination. When the two agents are used in combination (one in the morning and one at night), there appears to be less irritation than when tretinoin is used alone, the use of systemic antibiotics can be decreased and often eliminated, and dramatic therapeutic success can be achieved in a relatively short period of time in a high

Table 6–2 ACTION OF VITAMIN A ACID (TRETINOIN)

1. Thins epidermis
   a. Increased cell turnover
   b. Decreased cohesiveness of epidermal cells
2. Reverses comedo formation
   a. Increased cell turnover in pilosebaceous ducts
   b. Sloughing and expulsion of existing comedones
3. Increases transepidermal penetration

percentage of patients, even those with severe pustulocystic forms of this disorder.[23, 24]

In 1972 the combination of tretinoin and benzoyl peroxide (although not recommended in the package insert) was suggested for the topical therapy of acne vulgaris.[23] In addition to its keratolytic effect, it was proposed that benzoyl peroxide could suppress *P. acnes*, inhibit triglyceride hydrolysis, and lower free fatty acid levels in sebum; tretinoin would simultaneously thin the epidermis, lessen follicular hyperkeratosis, and enhance penetration of benzoyl peroxide. It was theorized that this combination of two potent topical medications could produce an additive, possibly synergistic, effect and could result in a more effective therapeutic approach to the management of acne vulgaris.

In an attempt to test this hypothesis, during the five year period between 1972 and 1977 I treated 1207 patients having varying degrees of acne vulgaris with topical tretinoin (vitamin A acid) in combination with benzoyl peroxide.[24] Of these, 847 (70.2 per cent) had moderate to severe cases of acne vulgaris, many of them unresponsive to previous conventional therapeutic regimens (Table 6–3); 512 (42.4 per cent) were treated simultaneously with antibiotics; and 695 (57.6 per cent) received no antibiotics. The steps taken in the regimen I used follow.

Step 1. Most patients were seen initially at four-week intervals and then less frequently as their acne responded to therapy. Education of the patient prior to the initiation of therapy was essential. A careful history was taken, the nature of the disease was explained, potential pitfalls were discussed, and treatment was outlined in detail.

Step 2. Tretinoin (Retinoic acid) was used in the form of Retin-A swabs (0.05 per cent), Retin-A Gel (0.025 per cent), or Retin-A cream (0.05 or 0.1 per cent) depending upon the complexion of the patient and his tolerance to the medication. For persons with potentially irritable skin (light-complexioned blonds and redheads, particularly women), tretinoin cream was prescribed initially (0.05 per cent cream was initiated conservatively on an alternate-day or occasionally on an every-third-day regimen). For those with a more ruddy complexion, tretinoin cream in a 0.1 per cent concentration or tretinoin gel in a 0.025 per cent concentration was employed. As a satisfactory tolerance to the milder cream formulation was demonstrated (generally within the first 7 to 14 days of treatment) the frequency of administration was increased to daily application with gradual introduction to the higher concentration cream, gel, or liquid formulations.

To minimize possible adverse cutaneous reactions, all recommended precautions for tretinoin were carefully emphasized and strictly implemented. Patients were instructed to wash with a mild soap (Dove, Aveenobar, Neutragena, or Purpose)[32] no more than two or three times a day, and to wait at least 30 minutes after washing (to insure that the skin was completely dry) before the application of tretinoin. They were also advised to avoid all local medications. Only oil-free noncomedogenic cosmetics were allowed, and excessive sun exposure was limited. If prolonged sun exposure was anticipated, patients were cautioned to use a sun-protective preparation.[32a]

Step 3. Benzoyl peroxide was used as benzoyl peroxide gel in a 10 per cent concentration, but not before testing for possible allergy by open patch tests on the volar aspect of the wrist. Since it has been suggested that benzoyl peroxide might oxidize tretinoin if the two preparations were applied simultaneously, all patients were instructed to apply the two medications separately (one in the morning and the other at night).[23]

Step 4. Oral antibiotics were prescribed for only those patients with severe pustular or cystic forms of acne vulgaris. Once the inflammatory aspect improved, the antibiotic dose was reduced and whenever possible was completely discontinued.

Step 5. To assure a minimum of complications, patients were instructed to maintain close telephone communication (including collect or personal calls for those calling from long distances), particularly during the first weeks of treatment. At each office visit therapy was reviewed, comedones were extracted, liquid nitrogen was applied to individual lesions, and large pustulocystic lesions were treated by intralesional steroid injection. If irritation occurred, patients were instructed to discontinue treatment for a few days, a moisturizer was used for a day or two, and then treatment was reinstituted, slowly and cautiously as tolerated. Careful re-evaluation at each visit revealed the fact that most side effects, when present, were associated with excessive or inappropriate application of the preparations, or failure to follow the precautions carefully outlined at the onset of therapy.

Results. Although success in the management of acne vulgaris can often be achieved by the use of topical tretinoin or benzoyl peroxide alone, the therapeutic effect appears to be substantially increased by the use of the two agents in combination.[24] Of 1207 patients treated by this combination, 89.1 per cent demonstrated good to excellent results within a period of six to twelve weeks; 61.1 per cent had excellent results (90 to 98 per cent clearing of lesions); 28.0 per cent had good results (80 to 90 per cent clearing); 6.6 per cent demonstrated fair results (60 to 80 per cent clearing); and 4.3 per cent had poor results or were lost to follow-up. In the latter category, 0.4 per cent had poor results (less than 60 per cent clearing) and 3.9

Table 6-3 SEVERITY OF ACNE ACCORDING TO SEX[24]

	Mild	Moderate	Severe	Total
MALES	105	336	86	527 (43.7%)
FEMALES	255	367	58	680 (56.3%)
	360	703	144	1207

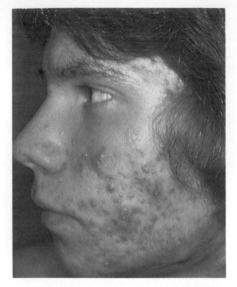

Figure 6–10 Sixteen-year-old boy with grade III–IV acne (large papules, pustules, and cystic lesions) before treatment with vitamin A acid and benzoyl peroxide.

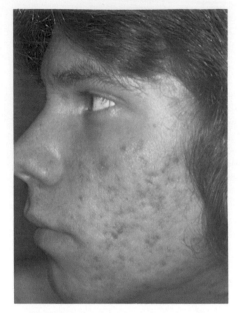

Figure 6–12 After 9 weeks of treatment.

per cent were lost to follow-up (Figs. 6–10, 6–11, 6–12, 6–13, and Table 6–4).

Systemic antibiotics are often required for the effective treatment of inflammatory lesions of acne vulgaris. In this study, 58 per cent of the patients were controlled solely by the combined usage of topical tretinoin and benzoyl peroxide (of the last 300 patients, as sophistication and experience with the combination were achieved, only 15 per cent required systemic antibiotics).

In this series, 3.8 per cent of patients were found to be sensitive to or irritated by the benzoyl peroxide gel. These patients were treated with a combination of vitamin A acid and topical erythromycin (2.0 to 2.7 per cent) in an ethanol-propylene glycol solution. In addition to the use of benzoyl peroxide as a 10 per cent gel, studies were begun on the use of 20 per cent benzoyl peroxide gel, with or without 10 per cent sulfur, as 20 per cent Zeroxin gel (Syosset Laboratories). It was found that 20 per cent benzoyl peroxide could be utilized in almost all patients (a small amount rubbed

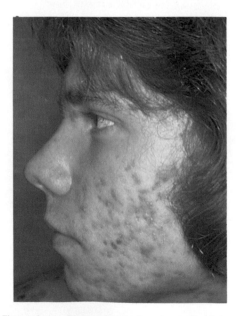

Figure 6–11 Same patient after six weeks of treatment with vitamin A acid gel (0.025%) in the morning and benzoyl peroxide gel (10%) in the evening.

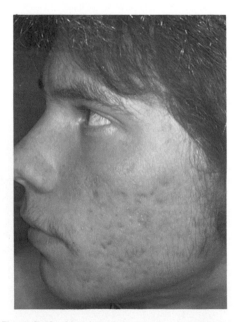

Figure 6–13 After 14 weeks of treatment. Patient received systemic tetracycline (500 mg 2 times a day initially, with gradual reduction and eventual discontinuation).

Table 6–4 RESULTS OF 5-YEAR STUDY OF COMBINED TRETINOIN AND BENZOYL PEROXIDE THERAPY

Extent of Clearing	Number	Per Cent
Excellent (90–98%)	737	61.1
Good (80–90%)	338	28.0
Fair (60–80%)	80	6.6
Poor (less than 60%)	5	0.4
Lost to follow-up	47	3.9
Total	1207	100.0

into the individual lesions) after the application of the usual 10 per cent benzoyl peroxide gel, with good clinical results. A few hardy patients even found that with care they could substitute 20 per cent benzoyl peroxide gel (instead of the 10 per cent formulation) in combination with tretinoin with even better results and relatively little irritation.

Antibiotics

Systemic Antibiotics. Systemic antibiotic therapy suppresses *P. acnes* and inhibits bacterial lipases, causing a reduction in the concentration of free fatty acids (the primary irritant of sebum). For years, broad-spectrum antibiotics have been invaluable in the treatment of inflammatory pustules, nodules, and cystic lesions. Today, however, the use of systemic antibiotics can be decreased and often eliminated as experience and sophistication in the use of effective topical agents are developed.[24] Since little or no improvement can be expected with non-inflammatory lesions, antibiotics are unnecessary in patients in whom these lesions appear as the sole manifestation of their acne problem.

When antibiotics are considered necessary, tetracycline, the antibiotic most frequently prescribed, is effective, inexpensive, and relatively free of side effects.[33, 34] Erythromycin, clindamycin, and minocycline are also beneficial when inflammatory and pustular lesions fail to respond to oral tetracycline. Of these three, erythromycin is the least expensive and has the fewest complications.

Long-term systemic use of clindamycin is not recommended owing to the possibility of induced pseudomembranous ulcerative colitis. This complication to clindamycin appears to be due to a toxin that is liberated by *Clostridium difficile*, which is able to grow in large numbers in the intestinal tract of some patients who receive clindamycin or other antibiotics.[35] In such individuals it has been found that the problem responds rapidly to the oral or intravenous administration of vancomycin hydrochloride.

Minocycline appears to have merit in those patients unresponsive to tetracycline or erythromycin therapy. Caution must be exercised, however, since this tetracycline derivative appears to have an affinity for the central nervous system, with a resulting high incidence of headaches and dizziness. This problem can frequently be eliminated by administration of the minocycline in small dosages immediately after mealtime.

The use of sulfone (diaminodiphenylsulfone) has been suggested for the management of very severe, resistant, nodulocystic, and conglobate acne. This preparation should be used with extreme caution, with full awareness of the risk of hemolytic anemia, cyanosis, and methemoglobinemia. Penicillin and its derivatives appear to be ineffective in the treatment of acne. Sulfa drugs have been used, but their clinical results are not as favorable as those of the broad-spectrum antibiotics.

Tetracycline therapy generally begins with a dosage of 500 to 1000 mg a day. This is gradually decreased to the lowest optimal level, usually to a dosage of 250 mg per day or every other day, until clinical improvement allows its discontinuation. The capacity for tetracycline to bind to certain types of cells and to intracellular organelles is well documented; however, it takes several weeks to develop an effective level of tetracycline in the skin.[36] Antibiotic treatment, therefore, should be used for a minimum of three to four weeks before results are appreciable. Tetracyclines are incompletely absorbed from the gastrointestinal tract and may be impaired by food, iron supplements, milk, aluminum hydroxide gel, and calcium-magnesium salts. To assure optimal absorption, patients should be instructed to take this medication on an empty stomach, preferably one hour before or two hours after mealtime.

Low dosage tetracycline therapy may be continued for many months with relatively few side effects.[33] The most frequent complication of antibiotic therapy in female patients is vaginal moniliasis. This complication, less frequently seen in young adolescents, is proportionally more common in women who take oral contraceptives concomitantly with their systemic antibiotics. Patients taking tetracycline occasionally manifest gastrointestinal irritation (epigastric distress, anorexia, nausea, or vomiting) after ingestion of tetracycline or its derivatives, and on occasion esophageal ulcerations have been associated with its use.[37] Enteric symptoms (cramps and diarrhea) are believed to result from alteration of normal intestinal flora, with overgrowth of yeasts and resistant bacteria. Complications based upon antigen-antibody mechanisms (urticaria, angioneurotic edema, erythema multiforme, and fixed eruptions), although reported, are relatively rare.

The incidence of photoreactivity to oral tetracycline is unknown, but appears to be extremely low, except for demethylchlorotetracycline hydrochloride (demethylchlorotetracycline, Declomycin) in which photosensitivity appears to develop in about 20 per cent of cases. Recent reports also describe brown discoloration and onycholysis as well as an unusual porphyria-like photosensitivity with bullae on the hands of patients on tetracycline therapy (Fig. 6–14).[38, 39, 40] Occasionally, patients on long-term tetracycline therapy may develop a gram-negative folliculitis due to *Escherichia coli*, *Klebsiella*, or *Proteus* overgrowth.[41, 42] This complication is manifested by a

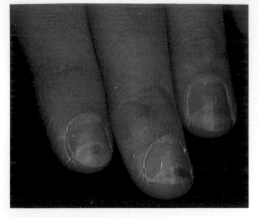

Figure 6–14 Photo-onycholysis as a complication of oral tetracycline hydrochloride therapy for acne vulgaris.

pustular folliculitis along the ala nasi or by deep nodulocystic lesions of the face.

The possibility that tetracycline will stain the teeth precludes its use for children under 12 years of age and for women after the first trimester of pregnancy. The deposition of the drug in the teeth is thought to be the result of its chelating properties, with the formation of a tetracycline-calcium orthophosphate complex. In time, exposure to light results in slow oxidation with a change in color of affected teeth from yellow to a cosmetically objectionable grayish-brown or gray (Fig. 6–15). The ingestion of outdated tetracycline may cause severe toxicity. It is particularly dangerous in patients who use "leftover" medication and who start and stop therapy on their own without proper medical guidance.

Although many questions have been raised concerning the safety of long-term use of tetracycline or erythromycin in acne, in general these drugs appear to be relatively safe, with no evidence of significant deleterious effect. Nevertheless, complete baseline blood counts and screening studies for hepatic and renal functions every 6 to 12 months appears to be a good precautionary measure when long-term use is contemplated.

Topical Antibiotics. It is desirable to avoid oral or systemic therapy in the treatment of skin

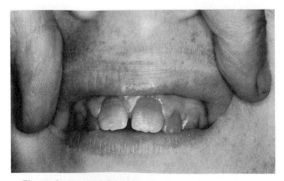

Figure 6–15 Staining of teeth due to the oral administration of tetracycline hydrochloride during early childhood.

diseases if an equally potent topical agent can be used. Recent investigations have shown that topical tetracycline, topical erythromycin, and topical clindamycin, when used in appropriate vehicles, can inhibit the growth of *Propionibacterium acnes* and produce a decrease in comedones, papules, and pustules in acne patients. Although studies are incomplete and these products are just becoming available commercially, it appears that topical antibiotics may to a great degree replace oral antibiotic therapy in the near future.[43, 44, 45]

In 1974 it was shown that a 2 per cent erythromycin solution applied three or four times a day could produce clinical improvement in patients with acne.[43] Subsequent studies have confirmed a somewhat similar clinical response to the use of topical tetracycline and clindamycin.[44, 45] Recent studies further suggest that topical antibiotics appear to be more effective in patients with predominantly papular or nodular acne (particularly those in their 20's and 30's), and that the presently available topical antibiotics are not as effective as benzoyl peroxide in the treatment of acne vulgaris.[46]

Topical antibiotics are used widely today for the treatment of acne; of these only one is currently approved by the Food and Drug Administration. This preparation, topical tetracycline hydrochloride (Topicycline, Procter and Gamble), contains 2.2 mg of tetracycline per ml, 4-epitetracycline hydrochloride, and sodium bisulfite in a base of 40 per cent ethanol, *n*-decyl methyl sulfoxide (DMSO) and sucrose esters. Topical tetracycline, however, may stain or sting and will induce fluorescence under black light, which is used in certain discotheques and night clubs. I therefore prefer to use topical erythromycin or clindamycin, particularly in those relatively few patients who are allergic or sensitive to benzoyl peroxide formulations, as a supplement to the topical use of tretinoin or benzoyl peroxide (alone or in combination), or in an effort to limit or avoid long-term use of systemic antibiotics.

Although to date studies remain inconclusive, it appears, at least by clinical impression, that topical clindamycin has a slight advantage over topical tetracycline and topical erythromycin formulations.[47] When clindamycin was first introduced as a topical agent for the management of acne vulgaris, the question was raised as to whether or not pseudomembranous colitis might occur in individuals who were so treated. It now appears that pseudomembranous colitis is not a major problem with topical clindamycin; to date I have used topical clindamycin in over 500 patients for the management of acne vulgaris and have had no reports of diarrhea from such use.

A great variety of vehicles are currently used for the formulation of topical antibiotic agents. The stability of many of these various topical antibiotic formulations, however, is not clearly defined. A popular topical clindamycin preparation that maintains 90 per cent of its activity for a year at room temperature may be prepared by dissolving four clindamycin hydrochloride capsules (Cleocin) (150 mg each), equaling 600 mg, in 48 ml of 70 per cent isopropyl alcohol, 6 ml of water, and 6 ml of propylene glycol. Other acceptable formulations of erythromycin or clindamycin may be prepared by dissolving erythromycin base Filmtabs (Abbott) or the contents of clindamycin hydrochloride (Cleocin) capsules in Neutrogena Vehicle/N (Neutrogena Dermatologics). In this vehicle erythromycin appears to maintain potency for a period of two or three months at room temperature, or for a period of four to six months under refrigeration.

I also use 2.7 per cent solutions of erythromycin in E-Solve lotion (Syosset Laboratories)[48] or a 1 to 2 per cent solution of clindamycin that is made by dissolving two to four 150 mg clindamycin hydrochloride capsules in 28 ml of C-Solve lotion (Syosset Laboratories). If kept under refrigeration, topical erythromycin in E-Solve lotion maintains stability for one year and topical clindamycin (Cleocin) in C-Solve lotion maintains its stability for one year at room temperature. Better clinical results may yet be achieved as newer forms of topical antibiotics are introduced and as experience and sophistication in the use of these agents is developed.

Estrogens. Although acne is not listed among the manufacturers' indications for use of anovulatory drugs, these preparations have been useful in the treatment of women over 16 years of age with severe, recalcitrant, pustulocystic acne. These agents produce good results, but not without a certain element of potential risk. Anovulatory drugs suppress the androgenic stimulation of sebum production, and when adequate amounts of estrogen are used, are beneficial in 50 to 70 per cent of patients.

It is important to weigh the risks and benefits when the use of estrogens is contemplated in the treatment of acne. Side effects to be considered include nausea, weight gain, monilial vaginitis, chloasma, hypertension, and thromboembolic phenomena. I prefer to restrict the use of estrogens to those few females, over 16 years of age, with severe recalcitrant pustulocystic acne, or to those who elect a course of anovulatory drugs for reasons other than their acne. Estrogens should never be prescribed in males, since the dose required for sebum suppression will produce feminizing side effects, nor should they be administered to patients under the age of 16 when possible bone growth inhibition is a consideration.

If estrogen is used, it should contain a minimum of 80 to 100 micrograms of ethinyl estradiol or its 3-methyl ether derivative (mestranol). This amount is present in Enovid-E, Ovulen, Ortho-Novum 2 mg, Norinyl, and Oracon; it is not present in Ovral, Demulen, or Enovid. Although sebum production occasionally decreases during the first or second cycle of drug administration, it usually takes three or four cycles (12 to 16 weeks) for a maximum effect to be achieved. In two thirds of patients a temporary acne flare may occur during the first two cycles of therapy. Patients should be forewarned of this possibility and reassured that this effect is only temporary.[49]

Oral Retinoids.   Two new oral retinoids (13-cis-retinoic acid and an aromatic retinoid ethyl ester) have shown promise in the management of acne vulgaris, lamellar ichthyosis, psoriasis, pityriasis rubra pilaris, keratosis follicularis (Darier's disease), and some cases of epidermolytic hyperkeratosis. The 13-cis-retinoic acid is being used experimentally in the United States, and the aromatic ester of retinoic acid is being used primarily in Europe.

Peck and his associates at the National Institutes of Health found that oral administration of 80 to 240 mg/day (average, 140 mg/day) of 13-cis-retinoic acid cleared the skin in 12 of 14 patients with cystic acne vulgaris.[50] Studies of skin surface lipid show that the composition of the lipid film is greatly altered, that the cholesterol content is increased, and that the percentage of squalene and wax esters is decreased with the administration of oral retinoids.[51] This appears to be due to marked inhibition of the synthesis of sebum, a secretory product of the sebaceous gland, at the level of DNA transmission. Side effects, especially cheilitis and facial dermatitis, xerosis, conjunctivitis, rhinitis sicca, epistaxis, skin fragility, pruritus, fingertip peeling, headache, appetite changes, inflamed urethral meatus, hair changes, arthralgia, and paronychia have been noted, but none of these has been serious enough to require discontinuation of therapy. Increase in the erythrocyte sedimentation rate (ESR) and a slight temporary elevation of serum glutamic pyruvic transaminase (SGPT), serum glutamic oxalicacetic transaminase (SGOT), and alkaline phosphatase levels have also been observed occasionally, but the changes have been reversible and are not considered to be major problems. At this time the use of oral retinoids is experimental; all patients undergoing treatment are on investigational protocols, and the availability of oral retinoids currently appears to be two or three years away.[50, 51]

Oral Zinc Therapy.   In 1977 it was suggested that oral zinc in a dosage of 0.2 gm (200 mg) daily might be effective for the treatment of patients with moderate to severe forms of acne vulgaris. In a double-blind study of 64 patients a substantial reduction of papules, pustules, and infiltrates was noted by the end of four weeks of therapy.[52] Another study suggests that zinc may have a beneficial effect on pustules, but not on comedones, papules, infiltrates, or cysts. However, the effect of placebo in acne varies between 19 and 56 per cent improvement according to the literature, so the 37 per cent improvement in pustules attributed to zinc in this study may prove to be a placebo effect.[53]

A subsequent double-blind study of 22 patients with acne who received 411 mg of zinc sulfate monohydrate or a lactose placebo daily showed no statistical difference in lesion counts (papules, pustules, open comedones, and closed comedones) between the 12 zinc-treated and the 10 lactose placebo-treated patients despite evidence of zinc absorption in serum and urinalyses of the treated patients.[54] Furthermore, it should be noted that as little as one 220 mg capsule of zinc sulfate a day has caused high plasma zinc levels with nausea and vomiting and that anemia secondary to a bleeding gastric erosion has been reported in a 15-year-old girl following the use of 220 mg of oral zinc sulfate twice a day for one week for the treatment of acne vulgaris.[55, 56] The divergence of results among various clinical studies may reflect the difficulties inherent in the characteristics of patient populations, or, perhaps, differences in design study. Hopefully, further studies eventually will determine what role, if any, zinc has in the pathogenesis or management of this disorder.

Acne Surgery. Acne surgery, the mechanical removal of comedones, pustules, and cysts, though time consuming, is extremely important for the rapid involution of individual acne lesions. This procedure is helpful only when properly done. The removal of open comedones does not materially influence the course of acne. However, it is desirable that they be removed for cosmetic purposes. Closed comedones should be removed to prevent rupture and spilling of their inflammatory contents into the surrounding dermis. For stubborn lesions, the procedure may be assisted by nicking the surface of the lesion with a sharp needle and expressing the contents with a comedo extractor. When improperly performed, inaccurate placement of the comedo extractor or overzealous manipulation may cause damage and irritation to the overlying skin, or rupture of the comedo wall with escape of sebum and further formation of inflammatory lesions.

Intralesional Acne Therapy. When cystic lesions are drained, a slightly larger incision is occasionally necessary. Whenever possible a small gauge sterile needle is preferred over a scalpel blade in an effort to minimize potential scarring. Intralesional corticosteroid injection usually results in rapid involution of nodular and cystic lesions. The injection of 0.1 to 0.3 ml of triamcinolone acetonide (in a concentration of 2.5 to 10.0 mg per ml) is recommended. With proper use of intralesional corticosteroid injection, incision and drainage of lesions is rarely required, and scars can frequently be avoided. Extreme caution should be exercised, since atrophy of the skin may occur when the injection is high in the dermis, particularly when the amount of concentration of steroid is excessive (Fig. 6–16). This atrophy fortunately generally disappears spontaneously within six months to one year.

Phototherapy. The value of artificial ultraviolet light is debatable. Its major effect is to give the patient a feeling of well-being, mild erythema, desquamation, and a resultant tan, which helps to conceal acne lesions. The risk of over-exposure and conjunctival inflammation from failure to shield the eyes suggests caution and a limitation on the use of ultraviolet light as a method of home

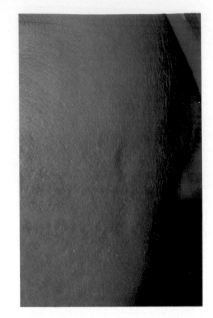

Figure 6–16   Temporary dermal atrophy on the cheek following intralesional corticosteroid injection in the treatment of pustulocystic acne vulgaris.

therapy. Of particular note are recent studies suggesting that long-term ultraviolet light may result in increased sebum production and acceleration of follicular hyperkeratosis, thus leading to comedo formation.[57] It appears, therefore, that the adverse effects of ultraviolet light may outweigh its benefit as a possible adjunct to acne therapy.

X-ray. Once widely employed in the treatment of acne, the use of x-ray has generally been abandoned as more effective forms of therapy have developed. Superficial x-ray treatment has been shown to reduce the size of sebaceous glands; however, acne often recurs when the glands regenerate after three to four months.

Cryotherapy. Cryotherapy appears to be helpful in the hands of some dermatologists. Erythema and desquamation may be produced by a carbon dioxide "slush," made of powdered dry ice and acetone. A piece of gauze held in a clamp is used to apply the slush by lightly brushing the skin. Involution of isolated persistent acne lesions may also be accelerated by local application of solid carbon dioxide dipped in acetone or by liquid nitrogen on a simple cotton applicator applied carefully to individual lesions. This technique effectively hastens involution of small pustular lesions; more vigorous liquid nitrogen application (15 to 30 seconds or more) appears to help resolution of cystic lesions and keloidal scars, particularly those measuring 1.0 to 1.5 cm in diameter or less.

Scar Removal. Acne scars may improve spontaneously to a surprising degree over a period of two to three years, but often the patient's final appearance is less than desirable. Topical chemotherapy with 20 to 30 per cent trichloroacetic acid appears to help some patients with persistent pitting.

Dermabrasion, popular in the past, still offers hope for improvement in those with residual scarring and persistent nodular lesions. It is important to note that following dermabrasion a small percentage of individuals who pigment easily occasionally develop hyperpigmentation, which may be more unattractive than the original scars. Other possible complications of dermabrasion include infection, further scarring, occasional hypopigmentation, or an inability to tan properly over treated areas.

Medical grade liquid silicone (dimethyl polysiloxane) has been found to be of value in the reconstruction of deep pits and atrophic scars. It is currently available only as an investigational drug, and the number of physicians now authorized to use it is strictly limited.[58] Some controversy still exists, but this liquid silicone, or maybe bovine collagen, may prove to be safe and effective for the correction of atrophic acne scars. Dermabrasion, collagen, and liquid silicone should be used only in selected cases, by a dermatologist or plastic surgeon familiar with the techniques and potential consequences.

MISCELLANEOUS ACNE DISORDERS

Neonatal Acne

Occasionally infants develop an eruption that resembles acne vulgaris as seen in adolescents. Although the etiology of neonatal acne (acne neonatorum) is not clearly defined, it appears to develop as a result of hormonal stimulation of sebaceous glands that have not yet involuted to their childhood state of immaturity. Although testosterone synthesis occurs in the fetal testis and adrenal gland between the 9th and 15th weeks of intrauterine life, steroid synthesis in the fetal ovary is relatively limited. This disparity may explain the apparent higher incidence of acne neonatorum in male infants.[59, 60]

Lesions of acne neonatorum may be present at birth or may appear in early infancy. Lesions characteristically present as erythematous papules or pustules, and rarely as comedones, usually confined to the cheeks, occasionally the chin and forehead. In contrast to adolescent acne, the chest and back are not affected.

Infantile Acne

The term acne neonatorum has also been applied to a more serious type of acne that generally does not make its appearance until the infant is three or four months of age, or sometimes older (Fig. 6–17). This disorder deserves a separate designation (infantile acne). Lesions may be fairly numerous, and comedones (mainly on the cheeks) often predominate. Individual lesions may be quite inflammatory, papules and pustules are common, and at times, nodules (occasionally healing with scar formation) may be apparent.[6]

The course of infantile acne varies consider-

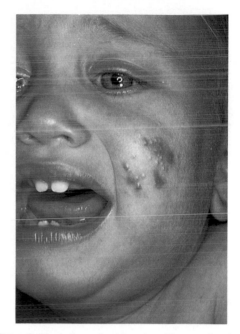

Figure 6–17 A 3-month-old male with comedonal and papular acne on the cheek (infantile acne).

ably. The lesions may be limited to a few comedones that clear after a few weeks. Most cases disappear within the first two or three years of life; others reportedly have persisted for up to 11 years. Cases with early onset and strong family history are generally the most persistent and subject to severe resurgence at puberty. Infants with acne neonatorum or infantile acne generally have no evidence of sexual precocity; those with persistent involvement, however, should be investigated for evidence of precocity or abnormal virilization. If endocrine abnormality is suspected, 17-ketosteroid excretion should be evaluated. During the first few weeks of life this normally may be elevated. A level of 0.5 mg in a 24-hour urine after two weeks of age, however, should be considered excessive, suggesting further investigation for gonadal or adrenal cortex hyperfunction.

Acne neonatorum must be differentiated from milia of the newborn, a disorder manifested by multiple 1 to 2 mm white or yellowish-white follicular papules (Fig. 6–18). Milia of the newborn usually occurs on the face, particularly the nose, cheeks, chin, and forehead, as a normal phenomenon in up to 40 per cent of full-term infants and children during the first few years of life.

In mild cases of acne neonatorum, therapy is generally unnecessary; daily cleansing with soap and water may be all that is required. Exogenous oil such as baby oils and lotions may aggravate this disorder and should be avoided. Occasionally mild keratolytic agents containing 3 to 5 per cent sulfur, salicyclic acid, or resorcin may be helpful. In the more severe cases of infantile acne, benzoyl peroxide lotions in a 5 per cent concentration may

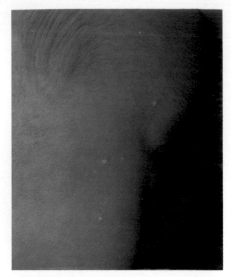

Figure 6–18   Milia neonatorum. One to 2 millimeter white follicular papules over the cheeks and forehead (a common phenomenon seen in up to 40 per cent of full-term infants).

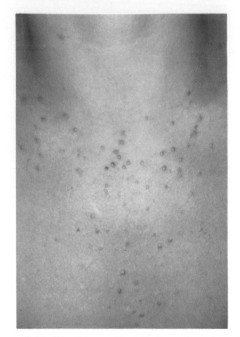

Figure 6–19   Steroid acne. Smooth dome-shaped papules on the upper chest following administration of systemic corticosteroids.

be utilized. Although topical vitamin A acid can be used for severe cases of neonatal acne, this preparation is potentially irritating, and most parents of children with this disorder prefer to use milder therapeutic agents. Management, therefore, should be determined by the degree of peeling or irritation and individual tolerance to available preparations.

Drug Acne

Steroid acne, although not commonly seen in small children, occasionally occurs in older children and adults following the administration of ACTH and corticosteroids. Identical lesions can also be produced by application of potent topical steroid formulations.[61] The lesions represent a folliculitis rather than a stimulation of the sebaceous glands. Lesions consist of dull red, smooth, dome-shaped papules or small pustules and are seen primarily on the upper trunk, arms, and neck. The face may be involved, but to a lesser degree (Fig. 6–19).

Iodides and bromides, particularly after long periods of administration, may induce an inflammatory acneform eruption, chiefly follicular pustules in the typical acne areas (face and upper trunk), as well as elsewhere. Usually it is caused by the iodine content of therapeutic agents rather than the use of iodized salt. Antituberculous drugs such as isoniazid may also cause an acneform eruption, starting with the face and spreading to the trunk and even beyond, without pustule or comedo formation. It consists primarily of reddish-brown papules somewhat resembling those of steroid acne. Anticonvulsive drugs (Dilantin and Tridione) and antidepressants (lithium-containing compounds) after a month or so of therapy are also

known to exacerbate acne in susceptible persons (Fig. 6–20).

ACNE OF EXTERNAL ORIGIN

Pomade Acne

A variety of external agents can induce acne-like eruptions upon repeated exposure to the skin

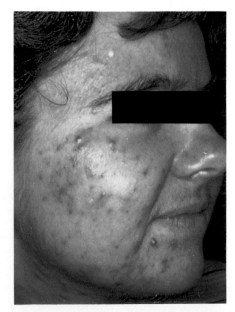

Figure 6–20   Exaggeration of acne in a 20-year-old woman on anticonvulsant drug therapy.

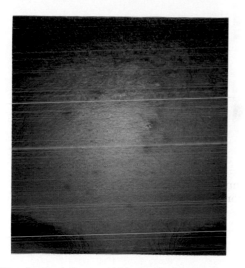

Figure 6–21 A 5-year-old black girl with multiple comedones and papules on the forehead due to the use of grooming substances on the hair and scalp ("pomade acne").

of susceptible individuals. These include greasy or oily suntan preparations, heavy makeup bases, and grooming agents. An acneform eruption induced by various grooming substances used on the scalp has been termed "pomade acne."[62] This disorder, seen chiefly on the forehead and temples in blacks, consists of closely set, rather uniform, closed comedones. The cheek and chin may also be involved if the pomade is rubbed over the entire face. In more advanced cases, papular or papulopustular lesions may be noted (Fig. 6–21). They improve with discontinuation of the offending comedogenic preparation and the use of appropriate topical keratolytic agents.

Occupational Acne

Acnegenic agents such as relatively unrefined oils, greases and waxes derived from petroleum, and animal and vegetable oils can produce eruptions in workers in gas stations, garages, and restaurants, particularly those specializing in hamburgers and french fries. The eruption appears at the sites of contact, particularly the face, back, upper extremities, and neck.

"Acne Cosmetica"

Acne cosmetica is a variant of acne occurring in women, usually over 20, as a result of the frequent use of cosmetics, particularly those containing lanolin, petrolatum, certain vegetable oils, butyl stearate, isopropyl myristate, sodium lauryl sulfate, lauryl alcohol, and oleic acid.[63, 64] Lesions are predominantly small, scattered closed comedones on the face and should be differentiated from acne vulgaris that may persist into adult life. Though common in women who never had acne vulgaris, women with a history of adolescent acne seem to be the most susceptible. A prominent

feature is a coarse facial appearance associated with dark prominent follicles, often more distressing to the patient than the actual acne-like lesions seen in this disorder. The most extensive eruptions are seen in women who attempt to mask the lesions under a heavy coating of cosmetics.

Acné excoriée des jeunes filles

Acné excoriée des jeunes filles is a form of acne most frequently seen in adolescent girls. Often associated with various degrees of emotional stress, it occasionally may be seen in boys, but to a lesser degree. Excoriating or squeezing of acne lesions may vary from mild irritation to severe scarring and occasional gross mutilation (Fig. 6–22). In the mild forms a simple explanation and local therapy may be all that is required to control the situation. In severe forms intensive psychiatric therapy may be required to control the underlying psychiatric basis of this disorder.

Pyoderma Faciale

Pyoderma faciale is a relatively uncommon form of acne usually seen in women in their early twenties. It is characterized by a sudden fulminating onset of pyoderma localized to the face with superficial or deep abscesses intercommunicating with one another through channels or sinus tracts.[65] The condition is marked by a reddish cyanotic color of the involved areas with sharply demarcated borders, an absence of comedones, and strict localization to the face. Keloidal scars are often seen as a prominent feature of this disorder.

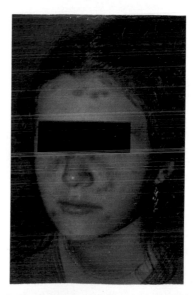

Figure 6–22 A 16-year-old girl with excoriated acne vulgaris (acné excoriée des jeunes filles).

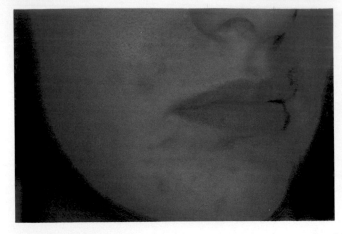

Figure 6–23 A 17-year-old girl with perioral dermatitis—discrete erythematous papules, papulovesicles, and pustules on the chin, upper lip, and the lower aspect of the cheeks, with sparing of the vermilion border of the lips.

Acne Conglobata

Acne conglobata is another suppurative form of acne vulgaris that is usually chronic and seen in men from 18 to 30 years of age. It is characterized by cysts, abscesses and burrowing sinus tracts. Healing often results in cosmetically disfiguring keloidal scars.

Perioral Dermatitis

A relatively common distinctive skin eruption resembling acne occurs primarily in young women. It was originally described by Frumess and Lewis in 1957 under the title of "light-sensitive seborrheid."[66]

The eruption consists of discrete, 1 to 3 mm erythematous papules, papulovesicles, and papulopustules. The eruption is symmetrical and affects the chin and nasolabial folds, sparing a clear zone around the vermillon border (Fig. 6–23). As the papules resolve they are often replaced by a diffuse redness or erythematous scale; itching is rare and never severe, but a sensation of burning is frequently noted. Histologic features include non-specific inflammation and parakeratotic scaling around the follicular opening.

The etiology of this disorder is uncertain, but the eruption is distinctive owing to its peculiar localization and sex and age distribution. Marks and others suggest an external irritant, possibly cosmetics or topical steroids, as provoking or perpetuating stimuli of this disorder.[67, 68] Its clinical resemblance to acne, the fact that potent topical steroids can induce or aggravate the disorder, and its response to tetracycline therapy and mild topical keratolytic agents suggest that it is a distinctive acne variant.

DISORDERS OF THE APOCRINE GLANDS

Fox-Fordyce Disease

Fox-Fordyce disease (apocrine miliaria) is a chronic itching papular eruption of apocrine gland-bearing areas, principally the axillae, the mammary areolae, and the pubic and perineal regions. Seen primarily in young women, this disorder is of unknown etiology but appears to be a form of apocrine sweat retention associated with obstruction and rupture of the intraepidermal portions of the affected apocrine glands. The disease is more common in women, with an estimated ratio of affected females to males of 9 or 10 to 1. It has its onset between 13 and 35 years of age, and is not seen before puberty owing to prepuberal quiescence of the apocrine glands.

Lesions of Fox-Fordyce disease are small, usually smooth and rounded papules that are principally follicular in location (Fig. 6–24). Itching, often paroxysmal and aggravated by emotional stress, is a prominent symptom of this disorder. The histologic picture is characterized by obstruction of the apocrine duct at its entrance into the follicular wall and an inflammatory infiltrate that surrounds the upper third of the hair follicles in involved areas.

The management of this disorder is still less

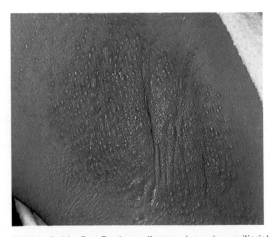

Figure 6–24 Fox-Fordyce disease (apocrine miliaria). Small round follicular papules in the axilla of an adolescent girl.

than satisfactory. Topical corticosteroids have limited value. Intralesional steroids are helpful and can produce a temporary remission for periods of six to eight months. Surgical excision of the affected areas with plastic repair, although effective, is rarely justified. Estrogen therapy (Premarin in a 1.25 mg dose daily), although not universally successful, appears to be beneficial in some women with this disorder.

Hidradenitis Suppurativa

Hidradenitis suppurativa is a chronic suppurative and cicatricial disease of the apocrine sweat glands in the axillary, inguinal, and anogenital regions. The disease affects blacks and females more often than whites or males, usually develops after puberty, and appears to be related to keratinous plugging of the apocrine duct, associated bacterial infection, and rupture of the involved area with extension of the infection to adjacent areas.

The earliest clinical sign of hidradenitis suppurativa is a painful, inflammatory abscess-like swelling, usually 0.5 to 1.5 cm in diameter, in the affected apocrine areas. Within a period of hours to days the abscess frequently grows in size and, if untreated, will often perforate the overlying skin. There is then a seropurulent drainage. The abscess heals by deep fibrosis, resulting in intercommunicating sinus tracts and band or bridge-like hypertrophic scars (Fig. 6–25).

Bacteriologic study of early lesions usually reveals coagulase-positive staphylococci or streptococci, probably representing secondary infection and not the cause of hidradenitis. Occasionally *E. coli*, *B. proteus*, or *P. aeruginosa* contaminates the flora.

In the early stages of hidradenitis suppurativa, sections of the skin show keratinous obstruction of the apocrine duct and often of the associated hair follicle orifice, ductal and tubal dilation,

and associated inflammatory changes. As the process becomes more chronic, there is fibrosis and scarring, with destruction of the apocrine gland, eccrine gland, and pilosebaceous apparatus. In the healing stage, one sees deep tortuous invaginations of the epidermis filled with keratin and representing the sinus tracts.

Optimal therapy of hidradenitis suppurativa depends upon early and accurate diagnosis, prolonged antibacterial therapy, intralesional steroids, incision and drainage of abscesses, and, in recalcitrant cases, total excision of the affected region. Early in the disease, broad-spectrum antibiotics and elimination of the local factors might reverse the process, but in the chronic phase surgery remains the only curative mode of therapy. Repeated incision and drainage of abscesses and incomplete excision of infected tracts, however, are often harmful since they permit extension of the infection and an increase in fibrosis and tract formation. Advanced cases, therefore, have a more pessimistic outlook. In such cases both recurrence and complication rates are lowest after total excision of the hair bearing area, followed by coverage with a split thickness skin graft.[69, 70]

DISORDERS OF THE ECCRINE GLANDS

The eccrine sweat glands are distributed over the entire skin surface and are found in greatest abundance on the palms and soles and in the axillae. They represent the principal means of maintaining homeostatic balance by evaporation of water. Their secretion depends upon their sympathetic nerve supply which is controlled by stimuli of three types: thermal, mental, and gustatory. By these mechanisms, the quantity and quality of sweat may be varied.

Hyperhidrosis

Hyperhidrosis is a disorder characterized by an excessive production of perspiration in response to heat or emotional stimuli. Topical and systemic therapy can be temporarily suppressive but are basically unsatisfactory. Treatment with systemic anticholinergic agents (atropine, 0.01 mg per kg every 4 to 6 hours, or Pro-Banthine, 1.5 mg per kg per 24 hours), effective to variable degrees, is limited by side effects such as mucous membrane dryness, blurred vision, and mydriasis. Sedative or tranquilizing drugs appear to be beneficial for axillary or palmar hyperhidrosis, as are aluminum salts applied locally (10 to 25 per cent aluminum chloride in distilled water). Drysol (Person and Covey), a solution of 20 per cent aluminum chloride in alcohol, is cosmetically acceptable and beneficial for most patients with this disorder.

In palmar hyperhidrosis, local astringents of value are those that inhibit the production of perspiration (Burow's soaks 1:40 or potassium permanganate 1:4000). Dusting powders, such as ZeaSorb, may be helpful. Plantar hyperhidrosis

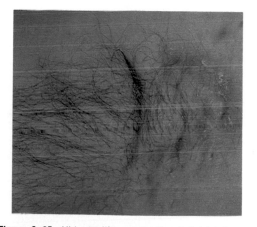

Figure 6–25 Hidradenitis suppurativa. Painful inflammatory abscess-like swellings with deep fibrosis, intercommunicating sinus tracts, and hypertrophic scars in the axilla.

may be suppressed with a solution of 10 per cent glutaraldehyde buffered with sodium bicarbonate to a pH of 7.5 (1.65 gm of $NaHCO_3$ per ml) applied topically daily or every other day. This solution causes staining and therefore is not a useful modality for treatment of the palms.

Dyshidrosis

Dyshidrosis (pompholyx) is a term applied to a condition of recurring vesiculation of the palms and soles in which hyperhidrosis and retention of sweat precedes the eruption. Although this condition may not be a disorder of the sweat glands per se, hyperhidrosis is an important accessory factor; treatment directed toward the hyperhidrosis may prove beneficial. Topical steroid formulations and efforts to minimize excessive perspiration are helpful in controlling this disorder.

Anhidrosis

Anhidrosis is an abnormal absence of perspiration from the surface of the skin in the presence of appropriate stimuli, often resulting in hyperthermia. This condition may be caused by a deficiency or abnormality of the sweat glands (as in anhidrotic ectodermal dysplasia) or of the nervous pathways from the peripheral or central nervous system leading to the sweat glands (as in syringomyelia, leprosy, anticholinergic drug therapy, or sympathectomy). Cool baths, air conditioning, light clothing, and reduction of the causes of normal perspiration help to relieve symptoms.

Bromhidrosis

Bromhidrosis is an embarrassing malodorous condition in which an excessive, usually offensive, odor emanates from the skin. It may be of two types: apocrine (resulting from bacterial degradation of apocrine sweat) and eccrine (from the microbiological degradation of stratum corneum softened by excessive eccrine sweat).

The human skin is populated with two distinct types of sweat glands, the eccrine and apocrine glands. Apocrine glands are found in only a few areas: in the axillae, perianal region, and the areolae of the breasts. They are poorly developed in childhood but, triggered by androgen production, begin to enlarge with the approach of puberty. Apocrine secretion is sterile and odorless when it initially appears on the cutaneous surface.[71] The term apocrine bromhidrosis refers to an exaggeration of the axillary odor normally noted by all postpubertal individuals. Short-chain fatty acids, products of bacterial degradation of this secretion by gram-positive organisms (coagulase-negative staphylococci and diphtheroids) are responsible for the malodor associated with this disorder.[71, 72] Eccrine bromhidrosis refers to the excessive odor produced by bacterial action on the stratum corneum when it becomes macerated by eccrine sweat. This disorder occurs on the plantar surfaces of the feet and intertriginous areas, particularly the inguinal region.

Bromhidrosis is best managed by regular thorough cleansing, preferably with an antibacterial soap, the use of commercial deodorants, the application of topical antibiotics and dusting powder to the affected areas, and frequent changes of clothing. Topical application of aluminum salts (10 to 25 per cent aluminum chloride in alcohol or distilled water) may help relieve the hyperhidrosis often associated with this disorder. Oral anticholinergic drugs (Pro-Banthine, 1.5 mg per kg per day) may help axillary eccrine hyperhidrosis, but there is little evidence of their effect upon apocrine gland secretion.

Plantar bromhidrosis is managed by careful and scrupulous hygiene, preferably with germicidal soaps, the use of dusting powders (ZeaSorb) to absorb excessive perspiration, topical aluminum chloride preparations (Drysol) to limit hyperhidrosis, and the avoidance of shoes and sneakers whenever possible. Disagreeable odors may be reduced by soaks with Burow's solution (1:40) or potassium permanganate (1:4000).

Miliaria

Miliara, a common dermatosis caused by sweat retention, is characterized by a vesicular eruption secondary to prolonged exposure to perspiration, with subsequent maceration and obstruction of the eccrine ducts. The pathophysiologic events that lead to this disorder are keratinous plugging of eccrine ducts followed by disruption of the duct and escape of the eccrine sweat into the skin below the level of obstruction. Recent studies suggest that increased perspiration causes hydration of the horny layer with an increase in the aerobic bacterial flora.[73] Subsequent release of a "toxin" secreted by these aerobic cocci injures luminal cells and precipitates a cast within the lumen. Cell membranes subsequently become more permeable and allow extravasation of sweat through the damaged sweat ducts, resulting in the clinical picture of miliaria rubra. Thereafter, as reparative processes come into play, the occluding mass moves upwards, finally occupying the coils of ducts within the horny layer. These observations explain the sequence of miliaria crystallina, rubra, and profunda.

Thus we see three forms of this disorder: miliaria crystallina (sudamina), miliaria rubra (prickly heat), and miliaria profunda (a more severe form of miliaria rubra commonly seen in the tropics). Although frequently seen in children, adolescents, and adults, the incidence of miliaria is greatest in the first few weeks of life owing to a relative immaturity of the eccrine ducts that favors poral closure and sweat retention.

In infants miliaria is seen as crops of crystal-clear pinpoint superficial vesicles without an inflammatory areola as miliaria crystallina (sudamina) or as miliaria rubra ("prickly heat"), which is characterized by small discrete erythematous, often pruritic papules, vesicles, or papulovesicles (see Fig. 2–3).

Miliaria Crystallina. Characterized by clear, thin-walled vesicles, 1 to 2 mm in diameter, miliaria crystallina develops in crops on otherwise normal-appearing skin. The vesicles are asymptomatic and occur most frequently in intertriginous areas, particularly in the neck and axillae, or on parts of the trunk covered by clothing.

Lesions of miliaria crystallina are highly characteristic and easily differentiated from other vesicular diseases. When the diagnosis is in doubt, rupture of vesicles with a fine needle results in release of the clear, entrapped sweat. In miliaria crystallina the obstruction is quite superficial; histopathologic examination of lesions reveals vesicles either within or directly beneath the stratum corneum. On serial sectioning the vesicles can be seen to be in direct communication with ruptured sweat ducts.

Miliaria Rubra "Prickly heat" is the most frequently seen and most important clinical form of miliaria (see Fig. 2–3). Lesions have a predilection for the covered parts of the skin, especially where there is friction from clothing, particularly the forehead, upper trunk, volar aspects of the arms, and body folds. They are characterized by pruritic, discrete, but closely aggregated, small papules, vesicles, or papulovesicles surrounded by erythema. The fact that lesions of miliaria rubra are always extrafollicular helps in the differentiation of this disorder from the papules or pustules of folliculitis. Miliaria rubra, therefore, can be differentiated by close inspection, especially under slight magnification with a hand lens, by typical papules or vesicles surrounded by an erythematous areola, without penetrating hairs, which characterize the eruption seen in lesions of folliculitis. Histologic examination of lesions of miliaria rubra reveals varying degrees of spongiosis and vesicle formation within the epidermal sweat duct and adjacent epidermis, with or without a hyperkeratotic or parakeratotic plug above the area of spongiosis.

Miliaria pustulosa is a variant of miliaria rubra consisting of distinct superficial pustules not associated with hair follicles. Lesions tend to occur in areas of skin that have had previous inflammation and frequently appear coexistent with lesions of miliaria rubra.

Miliaria Profunda. A more pronounced form of miliaria, miliaria profunda is uncommon except in the tropics. This disorder nearly always follows repeated attacks of miliaria rubra and is characterized by firm whitish 1 to 3 mm papules. Lesions are most prominent on the trunk, but may also be seen on the extremities. The deep location of the sweat retention in miliaria profunda results in papular rather than vesicular lesions. Erythema and pruritus are not seen in association with this disorder. Although miliaria profunda may at times resemble cutis anserina ("goose flesh"), the nonfollicular location of lesions of miliaria profunda

helps in the differentiation of these two disorders. Histologic examination of lesions of miliaria profunda demonstrates rupture of the sweat duct in the upper dermis, with or without surrounding edema and inflammatory infiltrate.

The key to the management of miliaria is avoidance of excessive heat and humidity. In infants generally all that is required is reassurance and advice on proper clothing and temperature regulation. Cool baths, light clothing, and air conditioning are invaluable. Calamine lotion, with or without 0.25 per cent menthol and 0.5 per cent phenol, is effective but has a tendency to cause excessive dryness, when this occurs, emollient creams such as Eucerin may be helpful. Resorcinol, 3 per cent in alcohol or Cetaphil lotion, is therapeutically beneficial in this disorder.

Granulosis Rubra Nasi

Granulosis rubra nasi is a rare chronic disease that occurs on the nose (occasionally the cheeks and chin) of prepuberal children, with the highest reported incidence between the ages of 7 and 15 years of age. It is characterized by diffuse redness, persistent hyperhidrosis, and discrete pinpoint to pinhead-sized red or brownish-red macules and soft papules on an erythematous base. Vesicles and small cystic lesions have also been seen in some patients with this disorder.[74]

The etiology of granulosis rubra nasi is unknown, but it appears to represent an inherited disorder. The role of the sweat glands and cutaneous vasculature is obscure, although occasionally this disease is associated with hyperhidrosis of the palms and soles.

Histologic examination of a cutaneous biopsy is characterized by dilatation of the dermal blood vessels and lymphatic channels with an inflammatory infiltrate about the sweat ducts, sometimes associated with occlusion and dilatation and cyst formation.

No effective local or systemic therapy is available for this disorder, although simple drying lotions, tinted to help obscure the erythema, may provide symptomatic and cosmetic relief. Although granulosis rubra nasi may sometimes persist into later years, reassurance that the disorder usually disappears at puberty is helpful.

References

1. Nierman H: Bericht über 230 Zwillinge mit Hautkrankheiten. Z. Menschl. Vererb. Konstitutional. 34:483–487, 1958.

   A study of 230 twins reveals 98 per cent concordance of acne in identical twins.

2. Kligman AM: An overview of acne. Journal Invest. Dermatol. 62:268–287, 1979.

   A critical appraisal of acne vulgaris with emphasis on its anatomy and pathophysiology.

3. Strauss JS: Diseases of the sebaceous glands. In Fitzpatrick TB et al.: Dermatology in General Medicine. McGraw-Hill Book Company, New York, 1971, 353–375.

A comprehensive review of acne vulgaris, its pathogenesis, and treatment.

4. Ebling, FJG, Rook A: The sebaceous gland — Acne vulgaris. *In* Rook A, Wilkinson DS, Ebling FJG: Textbook of Dermatology, 2nd edition. Blackwell Scientific Publications, Oxford, 1972, 1545–1558.

   A review of incidence, etiology, pathogenesis, clinical features, and therapeutic approaches to acne vulgaris.

5. Emerson GW, Strauss JS: Acne and acne care — A trend survey. Arch. Dermatol. *105*:407–411, 1972.

   A statistical survey and analysis of acne, its incidence, and severity in 1023 high school students.

6. Plewig G, Kligman AM: Acne: Morphogenesis and Treatment. Springer-Verlag, New York, Heidelberg, Berlin, 1975.

   A richly illustrated treatise on acne depicting gross and microscopic features and therapeutic strategies to aid in the management of this disorder.

7. Strauss JS, Kligman AM, Pochi P: The effect of androgens and estrogens on human sebaceous glands. J. Invest. Dermatol. *39*:139–155, 1962.

   Studies on the effect of estrogens and androgens on human sebaceous glands.

8. Van Scott EJ, McCardle RC: Keratinization of the duct of the sebaceous gland and growth cycle of the hair follicle in the histogenesis of acne in the human skin. J. Invest. Dermatol. 27:405–429, 1956.

   Hyperkeratinization of the execretory duct of the sebaceous gland is shown to be the earliest histologic change in acne.

9. Strauss JS, Kligman AM: The pathologic dynamics of acne vulgaris. Arch. Dermatol. 82:729–790, 1960.

   A classic study in the pathogenesis of acne vulgaris.

10. Blair C, Lewis CA: The pigment of comedones. Br. J. Dermatol. 82:572–583, 1970.

    Histochemical techniques confirm the presence of melanin granules within the horny compacted cells of the tips of blackheads.

11. Kaidbey, KH, Kligman AM: Pigmentation in comedones. Arch. Dermatol. *109*:60–62, 1974.

    Melanocytes as the source of color in blackheads (open comedones.)

12. Pochi PE: in Demis DJ, Dobson RL, McGuire J: Acne Vulgaris. *In* Clinical Dermatology, Unit 10-2. Harper and Row, Hagerstown, Maryland, 1977.

    An up-to-date concise review of acne, its pathogenesis, and therapy.

13. Kellum, RE: Acne vulgaris. Studies in pathogenesis: Relative irritancy of free fatty acids from C_2 to C_{16}. Arch. Dermatol. 97:722–726, 1968.

    Repeated applications of free fatty acids to human skin under occlusive patch tests revealed a greater irritancy and penetration by the C_8 to C_{14} range of fatty acids.

14. Kligman AM, Katz AG: Pathogenesis of acne vulgaris. Comedogenic properties of human sebum in external ear canal of the rabbit. Arch. Dermatol. 98:53–66, 1968.

    Sebum contains substances that fuel the process of acne.

15. Kligman AM, Wheatley VR, Miles OH: Comedogenicity of human sebum. Arch. Dermatol. *102*:267–275, 1970.

    The components in human sebum that mediate the formation of comedones.

16. Kellum RE, Strangfeld K, Ray LF: Acne vulgaris. Studies in pathogenesis: triglyceride hydrolysis by *Corynebacterium acnes* in vitro. Arch. Dermatol. *101*:41–47, 1970.

    Distinctive strains of *Corynebacterium acnes* appear to inhabit the sebaceous follicles of the acne patient—strains with particular abilities to hydrolyze certain triglycerides to free fatty acids.

17. Marples RR, Kligman AM, Lautis LR, et al.: The role of aerobic microflora in the genesis of fatty acids in human surface lipids. J. Invest. Dermatol. 55:173–178, 1970.

    After eliminating each of the lipase-producing groups of organisms by selective antibiotics, *Corynebacterium acnes* was shown to be mainly responsible for lipolysis of triglycerides.

18. Shalita AR: Genesis of free fatty acids. J. Invest. Dermatol. 62:332–335, 1974.

    Experimental evidence supports the hypothesis that the free fatty acids of skin surface lipids are derived from sebum triglycerides through the activity of microbial lipases.

19. Strauss JS, Pochi, PE, Downing DT: The role of skin lipids in acne. Cutis *17*:485–487, 1976.

    The generation of free fatty acids by intrafollicular hydrolysis of sebum triglycerides appears to be of considerable importance in the pathogenesis of acne.

20. Hurwitz S: Diseases of the sebaceous glands — Acne. *In* Gellis S, Kagan BM: Current Pediatric Therapy, 8. W. B. Saunders Co., Philadelphia, 1978, 506–508.

    A therapeutic approach to acne based upon present knowledge of pathogenesis and therapy.

21. Hitch JM, Greenburg BG: Adolescent acne and dietary iodine. Arch. Dermatol. *89*:898–911, 1961.

    Although iodine in medications can cause an acneform eruption, dietary iodine appears to have little effect on the prevalence or severity of acne.

22. Fulton JE, Plewig G, Kligman AM: The effect of chocolate on acne vulgaris. JAMA *210*:2071–2074, 1969.

    Ingestion of large amounts of chocolate influences neither the production nor composition of sebum, nor does it affect the course of acne vulgaris.

23. Fulton JE, Jr, Farzad-Bakeshandeh A, Bradley S: Studies on the mechanism of the action of topical benzoyl peroxide and vitamin A acid in acne vulgaris. J. Cutan. Pathol. *1*:191–200, 1974.

    Although systemic tetracycline remains the most frequent treatment for acne vulgaris, this report indicates that topical therapy can clear the majority of cases within the initial three months of therapy.

24. Hurwitz S: The combined effect of vitamin A acid and benzoyl peroxide in the treatment of acne. Cutis *17*:585–590, 1976.

    The combination of vitamin A acid and benzoyl peroxide, when used properly, offers a well-tolerated, extremely effective therapeutic approach to the topical management of acne vulgaris.

25. Hurwitz S: Acne vulgaris. Current concepts of pathogenesis and treatment. Am. J. Dis. Child. *133*:536–544, 1979.

    An overview of acne vulgaris and current concepts of pathogenesis and management.

26. Eaglstein, WH: Allergic contact dermatitis to benzoyl peroxide — report of cases. Arch. Dermatol. 97:527–528, 1968.

    Allergic contact dermatitis to topical benzoyl peroxide preparations suggests a certain degree of caution in their use.

27. Lynch FW, Cook, CD: Acne vulgaris treated with vitamin A. Arch. Dermatol. 55:355–357, 1947.

    Oral vitamin A, even when given in dosages of 100,000 units a day, was not effective in the treatment of a group of university students with acne.

28. Kligman AM, Fulton JE, Jr, Plewig G: Topical vitamin A acid in acne vulgaris. Arch. Dermatol. 99:469–476, 1969.

    Topical vitamin A acid, when used properly, can be most beneficial for the treatment of patients with extensive comedo-papular acne.

29. Strauss JG, Pochi PE, Downing DT: Acne: perspectives. J. Invest. Dermatol. 62:321–325, 1974.

    A review of the pathogenesis of acne and exploration of future aspects of therapy.

30. Hurwitz S: Acne vulgaris. Pediatr. Ann. 5:772–781,1976.

    A clinical approach to acne, its pathogenesis, and treatment.

31. Kligman AM, Mills OH, Jr, Leyden JJ, et al.: Letters to the Editor: postscript to vitamin A acid therapy for acne vulgaris. Arch. Dermatol. 107:296, 1973.

    Appropriate precautionary instructions to patients can relieve the irritation formerly associated with vitamin A acid therapy.

32. Frosch PJ, Kligman AM: The soap chamber test. A new method for assessing the irritancy of soaps. J. Am. Acad. Dermatol. 1:35–41, 1979.

    Studies of irritancy (scaling, redness, and fissuring) of eighteen well-known toilet soaps contrast with a number of previous studies that failed to show differences among soaps or concluded that soaps are innocuous.

32a. Kligman LH, Akin FJ, Kligman AM: Sunscreens prevent ultraviolet photocarcinogenesis. J. Am. Acad. Dermatol. 3:30–35, 1980.

    Sunscreens tested on hairless albino mice appear to prevent tumor formation over a 30-week period.

33. Committee on Drugs: The treatment of acne with antibiotics. Pediatrics 48:663–665, 1971.

    Tetracycline is beneficial in inflammatory or pustular acne with little evidence of toxicity, even with occasional long-term therapy.

34. Clendenning WE: Complications of tetracycline therapy. Arch. Dermatol. 91:628–632, 1965.

    A review of complications associated with the systemic use of tetracycline.

35. George RH, Symonds JB, Dimock T, et al.: Identification of Clostridium difficile as a cause of pseudomembranous colitis. Br. Med. J. 1:695, 1978.

    High titers of Clostridium difficile toxin in 8 patients with pseudomembranous colitis identify Cl. difficile as a cause of this disorder.

36. Freinkel RK, Strauss JS, Yip SY, et al.: The effect of tetracycline on the composition of sebum in acne vulgaris. N. Engl. J. Med. 273:850–854, 1965.

    The therapeutic efficacy of antibiotics in acne vulgaris may be attributable, at least in part, to suppression of lipolytic activity within the sebaceous follicle.

37. Crowson TD, Head LH, Ferrante WA: Esophageal ulcers associated with tetracycline therapy JAMA 235:2747–2748, 1976.

    Three patients with esophageal ulceration presumably associated with the ingestion of tetracycline or its derivative doxycycline (Vibramycin).

38. Frank SB, Cohen HJ, Minkin W: Photo-onycholysis due to tetracycline hydrochloride and doxycycline. Arch. Dermatol. 103:520–521, 1971.

    Three patients on tetracycline and doxycycline developed photosensitivity and onycholysis.

39. Kestel JL, Jr: Tetracycline-induced onycholysis unassociated with photosensitivity. Arch. Dermatol. 106:766, 1972.

    Two patients with sun exposure while on tetracycline developed discoloration and separation of the nails.

40. Epstein, JH, Tuffanelli DL, Seibert, JS, et al.: Porphyria-like cutaneous changes induced by tetracycline. Arch. Dermatol. 112:661–666, 1976.

    Blisters similar to those seen in porphyria can develop as a complication of tetracycline therapy.

41. Fulton JE, Jr, McGinley K, Leyden J, et al.: Gram negative folliculitis in acne vulgaris. Arch. Dermatol. 98:349–353, 1968.

    A previously unrecognized complication of tetracycline therapy in acne.

42. Leyden J, Marples RR, Mills OH, et al.: Gram-negative folliculitis. A complication of antibiotic therapy in acne vulgaris. Br. J. Dermatol. 88:533–538, 1973.

    Fifty cases of gram-negative folliculitis in a series of 1200 patients with acne vulgaris.

43. Fulton JE, Jr, Pablo G. Topical antibacterial therapy for acne. Arch. Dermatol. 110:83–86, 1974.

    Two per cent erythromycin base applied three or four times daily in ten patients produced a decrease in papules and pustules in two weeks and a reduction of comedones after two months.

44. Resh W, Stoughton RB: Topical antibiotics in acne vulgaris. Clinical response and suppression of C. acnes in open comedones. Arch. Dermatol. 112:182–184, 1976.

    Studies with topical preparations of erythromycin, tetracycline, and clindamycin demonstrate that topically applied antibiotics can depress P. acnes in comedones and improve the course of the disease.

45. Frank SB: Topical treatment of acne with a tetracycline preparation: Results of a multi-group study. Cutis 17:539–545, 1976.

    A study of 300 patients treated with a tetracycline topical solution.

46. Fulton JE, Jr, Bradley S: The choice of vitamin A acid, erythromycin, or benzoyl peroxide for the topical treatment of acne. Cutis 17:560–564, 1976.

    Retinoic acid, benzoyl peroxide, and topical erythromycin (their advantages and disadvantages) in the treatment of acne.

47. Stoughton RB: Topical antibiotics for acne vulgaris. Current usage. Arch. Dermatol. 115:486–489, 1979.

    A review of the current status of topical antibiotics in the treatment of acne.

48. Fisher AA: Erythromycin "Free Base" — A non-sensitizing topical antibiotic for infected dermatoses and acne vulgaris. Cutis 20:17–35, 1977.

    Erythromycin base in a non-sensitizing lotion — a cosmetically acceptable preparation for the treatment of papulopustular acne.

49. Strauss JS, Pochi PE: Effect of cyclic progestin-estrogen therapy on sebum and acne in women. JAMA 190:815–819, 1964.

    Drugs containing estrogen in the management of recalcitrant pustulocystic acne in women.

50. Peck GL, Yoder FW: Treatment of lamellar ichthyosis and other keratinizing dermatoses with an oral synthetic retinoid. Lancet 2:1172–1174, 1976.

    Short-term treatment with 13-cis-retinoic acid produced excellent results in five patients with lamellar ichthyosis, in two of three patients with Darier's disease, and in one patient with pityriasis rubra pilaris.

51. Peck GL, Olsen TG, Yoder FW, et al.: Prolonged remissions of cystic and conglobate acne with 13-cis-retinoic acid. N. Engl. J. Med. 300:329–333, 1979.

    Complete resolution of severe, chronic, treatment-resistant cystic and conglobate acne in 13 of 14 patients treated with oral 13-cis-retinoic acid and the apparent persistence of this beneficial effect for periods lasting for as long as twenty months after discontinuation of therapy.

52. Michaelsson G, Juhlin L, Vahlquist A: Effect of oral zinc and vitamin A in acne. Arch. Dermatol. 113:31–36, 1977.

    In a study of 64 patients with acne, the number of acne lesions was significantly decreased in the zinc-treated group.

Although data appear to support the efficacy of zinc therapy in acne, further double-blind studies are required to substantiate this finding.

53. Weimar VM, Puhl SC, Smith WH, et al.: Zinc sulfate in acne vulgaris. Arch. Dermatol. *114*:1776–1778, 1978.

In a study of 40 patients, oral zinc appeared to have a somewhat beneficial effect on pustules but not on comedones, papules, infiltrates, or cysts.

54. Orris L, Shalita AR, Sibulkin D, et al.: Oral zinc therapy of acne. Arch. Dermatol. *114*:1018–1020, 1978.

In a double-blind controlled study on 22 male subjects that lasted eight weeks there was no statistically significant difference in lesion counts in the zinc-treated and lactose placebo-treated patients.

55. Glover SC, White MI: Zinc again. Br. Med. J. *2*:640–641, 1977.

A warning of potential side effects due to oral zinc sulphate and unphysiological zinc level concentrations in human plasma.

56. Moore R: Bleeding gastric erosion after oral zinc sulphate. Br. Med. J. *1*:754, 1978.

Epigastric discomfort and gastrointestinal bleeding in a 15-year-old English girl developed within one week after the initiation of 220 mg of oral zinc sulphate twice a day for the treatment of acne.

57. Mills OH, Porte M, Kligman AM: Enhancement of comedogenic substances by ultraviolet radiation. Br. J. Dermatol. *98*:145–150, 1978.

Solar-simulating irradiation enhancement of the degree of follicular hyperkeratosis suggests that the adverse effects of sunbathing and ultraviolet light outweigh their benefit in the treatment of acne.

58. Rees TD: The current status of silicone fluid in plastic and reconstructive surgery. J Dermatol. Surg. *2*:34–38, 1976.

Medical-grade liquid silicone (dimethyl polysiloxone) appears to be of value in the correction and reconstruction of deep pits and atrophic scars of acne.

59. Giknis FL, Hall WK, Tolman MM: Acne neonatorum. Arch. Dermatol. *66*:717–721, 1952.

A case of acne neonatorum with onset at 7 weeks, with a review of 17 patients with this disorder.

60. Pochi PE, Strauss JS: Endocrinologic control of the development and activity of the human sebaceous gland. J. Invest. Dermatol. *62*:191–201, 1974.

The fetal endocrine system and sebaceous gland development in acne neonatorum.

61. Plewig, G, Kligman AM: Induction of acne by topical steroids. Arch. Dermatol. Forsch. *247*:29–52, 1973.

Potent topical steroids can produce "steroid acne."

62. Plewig G, Fulton JE, Kligman AM: Pomade acne. Arch. Dermatol. *101*:580–584, 1970.

The physician should be alert to this disorder, which is seen particularly on the forehead in Negroes using greasy hair grooming formulations.

63. Kligman AM, Mills OH: "Acne cosmetica." Arch. Dermatol. *106*:843–850, 1972.

Low-grade acneform eruptions can be attributed to cosmetics.

64. Fulton JE, Jr, Bradley S, Agundez A et al.: Non-comedogenic cosmetics. Cutis *17*:344–351, 1976.

A scale of comedogenicity of some of the popular cosmetic formulations.

65. O'Leary PA, Kierland RR: Pyoderma faciale. Arch. Dermatol. *41*:451–462, 1940.

A fulminating form of facial acne characterized by superficial and deep abscesses.

66. Frumess, GM, Lewis, HM: Light-sensitive seborrheid. Arch. Dermatol. *75*:245–248, 1957.

This unique perioral eruption was initially thought to be a light-sensitive disorder.

67. Hjorth N, Osmundsen P, Rook AJ, et al.: Perioral dermatitis. Br. J. Dermatol. *80*:307–313, 1968.

Perioral dermatitis is characterized by an erythematous eruption of the chin and upper lip with sparing of the perivermilion border.

68. Marks R, Black MM: Perioral dermatitis. A histologic study of 26 cases. Br. J. Dermatol. *84*:242–247, 1971.

Histologic findings suggest external irritants as provocative or perpetuating stimuli to perioral dermatitis.

69. Knaysi GI, Cosman B, Crikelair GF: Hidradenitis suppurativa. JAMA *203*:73–76, 1968.

In 45 patients (with 83 surgical procedures for hidradenitis suppurativa) the lowest recurrence and complication rates were obtained following total excision of the hair-bearing areas with split thickness skin graft coverage.

70. Dvorak VC, Root RK, MacGregor RR: Host-defense mechanisms in hidradenitis suppurativa. Arch. Dermatol. *113*:450–453, 1977.

Hidradenitis suppurativa is related to local obstruction of apocrine glands, not to a generalized defect of host defense mechanism.

71. Shelley WB, Hurley HJ, Nichols AC: Axillary odor: Role of bacteria apocrine sweat, and deodorants. Arch. Derm. Syph. *68*:430–446, 1953.

Axillary micro-organisms are responsible for axillary odor.

72. Shehadeh, NH, Kligman, AM: Bacteria responsible for axillary odor, II. J. Invest. Dermatol. *41*:3, 1963.

Gram-positive organisms, coagulase-negative staphylococci, and diphtheroids generate axillary odor.

73. Hölzle E, Kligman AM: The pathogenesis of miliaria rubra. Role of the resident microflora. Br. J. Dermatol. *117*:99–137, 1978.

Studies demonstrate that the degree of sweat suppression and miliaria after a thermal stimulus was directly proportional to the increase in density of resident aerobic bacteria, notably cocci.

Aram H, Mohagheghi AP: Granulosis rubra nasi. Cutis *10*:463–464, 1972.

A case of granulosis rubra nasi of four years' duration in a 12-year-old girl.

7

HEREDITARY SKIN DISORDERS — THE GENODERMATOSES

The genodermatoses represent a group of cutaneous disorders dependent upon genetic as opposed to environmental causes. This chapter discusses the significant hereditary dermatoses — ichthyoses, ectodermal dysplasias, disorders of collagen and elastic tissue, and errors of metabolism with dermatologic consequences, with emphasis on aids to clinical recognition, recent concepts of pathophysiology, and advances in therapeutics.

ICHTHYOSIS

Ichthyosis refers to hereditary cutaneous conditions characterized by dryness and scaling. Until recently, ichthyosis classification relied upon primarily descriptive and confusing clinical and histologic criteria, which offered little understanding of etiology or pathogenesis. The introduction of reliable measurements of cellular kinetics has provided clearer understanding and organization of the ichthyosiform dermatoses.[1, 2] The combination of cellular kinetics and clinical, histologic, and genetic criteria allows these disorders to be divided into four major classes:

1. Ichthyosis vulgaris (autosomal dominant)
2. Sex-linked ichthyosis (X-linked recessive)
3. Lamellar ichthyosis (autosomal recessive)
4. Epidermolytic hyperkeratosis (autosomal dominant)

In the past, lamellar ichthyosis and epidermolytic hyperkeratosis have been designated as the non-bullous and bullous congenital ichthyosiform erythrodermas respectively. To emphasize that these are two distinct, unrelated forms of ichthyosis, Frost and Van Scott suggest, on the basis of clinical and histologic findings, that the non-bullous form be called "lamellar ichthyosis" and the bullous form, "epidermolytic hyperkeratosis." These designations have found wide acceptance and will be utilized in subsequent references.

Pathogenesis of the ichthyoses appear to involve:

1. an increased rate of arrival of cells at the skin surface (this has been determined by epidermal mitotic activity and cellular transit time)

2. a decrease in the rate of cell removal (increased adhesiveness of the stratum corneum)

3. an abnormal transepidermal water loss[3]

All four major types of ichthyosis demonstrate abnormalities of the third mechanism, an increased transepidermal water loss with resultant loss of suppleness and moisture content of the integument. Excessive scaling seen in ichthyosis vulgaris and X-linked ichthyosis is probably related to the second mechanism (increased adhesiveness of the cells of the stratum corneum with normal cellular transit rates). In lamellar ichthyosis and epidermolytic hyperkeratosis the thickening of the stratum corneum appears to be related to cellular kinetics (a decreased transit time of the epidermal cells from basal layer to stratum corneum).

Ichthyosis Vulgaris

Ichthyosis vulgaris, transmitted as an autosomal dominant trait, is the mildest, most common form of ichthyosis (Table 7–1). Because it is often overlooked or undiagnosed, its incidence can only be estimated as 1 in 250 to 1000 persons.

This disorder, not present at birth, is first noted in childhood, usually after the first three months of life. It is often milder and more localized than other types of ichthyosis. Scales are most prominent on the extensor surfaces of the extremities particularly in cold and dry weather (Figs. 7–1, 7–2, 7–3). Scales on the pretibial and lateral aspects of the lower leg are large and plate-like, resembling fish scales; the flexural areas are characteristically spared. In other areas small, white, bran-like scales may be seen. Scaling of the forehead and cheeks, commonly involved during

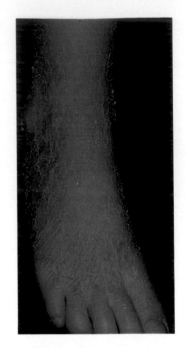

Figure 7–1 Large plate-like scales on the ankle and dorsal aspect of foot in a patient with ichthyosis vulgaris.

childhood, generally diminishes and clears with age.

Keratosis pilaris (Fig. 3–5), frequently associated with ichthyosis vulgaris, is most predominantly seen over the arms, buttocks, and thighs. The palms and soles may show a moderate degree of chapping with accentuation of palmar markings (Fig. 3–6), and a discrete hyperkeratosis may be seen on the elbows, knees, and ankles. Patients with ichthyosis often reveal an atopic background with a tendency toward eczema, asthma, or hay fever.

Skin biopsy is helpful for differentiating this disorder from other forms of ichthyosis. A moderate thickening of the stratum corneum is charac-

Table 7–1 ICHTHYOSIS VULGARIS

a. Incidence approximately 1:300 (250–1,000)
b. Develops after 3 months
c. Large lamellar scales
   1. face, back, extensors
   2. spares flexures
d. Favorable course (improves with age)
e. Mx: hyperkeratosis of stratum corneum with decrease in granular layer

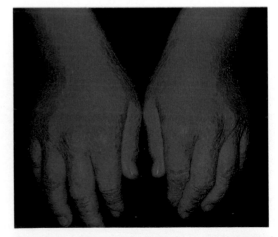

Figure 7–2 Ichthyosis vulgaris on the extensor aspect of hands and fingers.

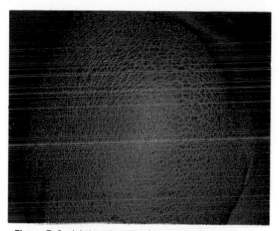

Figure 7–3 Ichthyosis vulgaris—typical large adherent scales on the shoulder.

Table 7–2 X-LINKED ICHTHYOSIS

a. Affects males
b. First 3 months (collodion membrane)
c. Ichthyosis nigricans
   1. large yellow to black scales
   2. all body surfaces (except palms and soles)
   3. central face, neck, and flexures
d. Corneal opacities (males, and female carriers)
e. Same or worse with age
f. Mx: Hyperkeratosis with increased granular layer

teristically present; the granular layer is usually reduced or absent in contrast to the normal stratum granulosum of other ichthyoses.

Sex-linked Ichthyosis

This disease, transmitted as an X-linked recessive trait, is seen primarily in males. Although an affected homozygous female has been described, female carriers generally do not develop the full clinical picture but may manifest partial abnormalities. This phenomenon appears to be explained by the Lyon principle (formerly the Lyon hypothesis). In this hypothesis one X chromosome in each cell of a normal XX female carrier of an X-linked recessive trait shows a reduced level of the gene product and is not fully expressed. Accordingly the phenotypes of such heterozygous females may present only mild manifestations of the X-linked disorder.[1]

The prevalence of this dermatosis is unknown; Wells and Kerr's study in England, however, estimated the incidence at approximately one in 6000 males.[5] Although the exact biochemical basis of X-linked ichthyosis is not fully understood, recent studies suggest that steroid sulfatase deficiency is associated with at least some cases of this condition.[6] Steroid sulfatase activity determination will permit the identification of maternal carriers and, in cultured amniotic cells, provides prenatal diagnosis of this disorder.

Sex-linked ichthyosis begins early in infancy, usually within the first three months of life; occasionally as late as one year. Some infants have a collodion-like membrane at birth (Fig. 7–4). This form of ichthyosis generally involves the entire body with accentuation on the abdomen, back, front of the legs, and feet, with sparing of the palms and soles, central face, and flexural areas. Scales are large in size, yellowish-brown to black in color, giving the patient an unwashed appearance (this gave rise to the name "ichthyosis nigricans"). Patients may shed or moult their scales episodically, particularly in the spring and fall months (Table 7–2).

Deep corneal opacities may be found in almost all affected males and, with less consistency, in female carriers of this disorder. The opacities are discrete, diffusely located near Descemet's membrane or deep in the corneal stroma, and on slit lamp examination the corneal opacities appear as gray-white filaments, commas, dots, or coronas in the deep stroma and do not affect vision.[7] Slit lamp examination of the eyes, therefore, is useful for identification of individuals with this dermatosis.

Skin biopsy is of value for differentiation of sex-linked ichthyosis from the dominant form of ichthyosis vulgaris. In the sex-linked disorder, there is a moderately increased stratum corneum, granular layer, and stratum malpighium. In the autosomal dominant form the granular layer is reduced or absent.

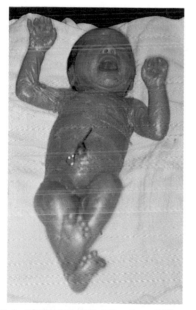

Figure 7–4 "Collodion baby." Parchment-like membrane with beginning cracking and desquamation (Department of Dermatology, Yale University School of Medicine).

Lamellar Ichthyosis

Lamellar ichthyosis (non-bullous congenital ichthyosiform erythroderma) is a rare autosomal

Table 7–3 LAMELLAR ICHTHYOSIS (Non-Bullous CIE)

a. Rare (1:300,000)
b. At birth or soon after
   (collodion baby, ectropion in one third)
c. Large lamellar scales
   1. grayish-brown
   2. adherent in center
   3. face, trunk (flexures, palms and soles)
d. Same or worse with age
e. Mx: marked hyperkeratosis, prominent granular cell
   layer

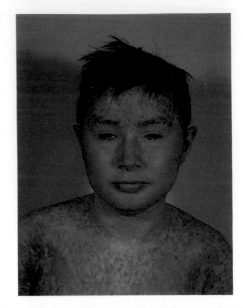

Figure 7–6 Lamellar ichthyosis. Prominent quadrangular scales on the forehead and chest. Note contrasting shiny cheeks. (Mirrer E, McGuire JS: Lamellar ichthyosis — response to retinoic acid (tretinoin). A case report. Arch Dermatol. 102: 584, 1972).

recessive disorder characterized by a collodion membrane that may envelop the infant at birth (hence the term "collodion baby").[8] (See Table 7–3 and Fig. 7–4.) In this disorder a collodion or parchment-like membrane is usually present at birth; on occasion, however, skin findings are not evident until approximately three months of age. The cutaneous covering dries out and is gradually shed in large sheet-like layers, leaving a residual redness and hyperkeratosis. As the infant grows the scaling becomes less prominent, slowly clearing in some cases. In others it develops into a severe skin disorder characterized by lamellar or plate-like scales covering the entire body.

Lamellar scales are large, quadrangular, yellow to brown-black in color, often thick and centrally adherent with raised edges resembling armor plates (hence the term lamellar ichthyosis) (Fig. 7–5). Scales are most prominent over the face, trunk, and extremities, with a predilection for the flexor areas. Cheeks are often red, taut, and shiny; more scales appear on the forehead than on the lower portion of the face. The scalp is often scaly with partial hair loss. Ectropion is common, but the eye itself remains unaffected (Fig. 7–6).[9]

The palms and soles are almost always affected in lamellar ichthyosis; severity varies from increased palmar markings to a thick keratoderma with fissuring. Involvement of the nails is variable. They may be stippled, pitted, ridged, or thickened, often with a collection of subungual keratin.

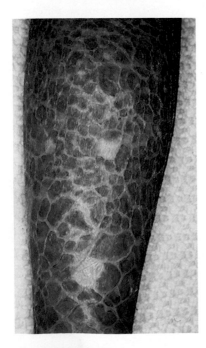

Figure 7–5 Large, thick, centrally adherent quadrangular scales with raised edges (resembling armor plates) on the legs of a patient with lamellar ichthyosis.

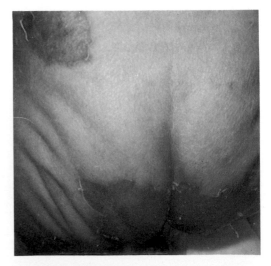

Figure 7–7 Epidermolytic hyperkeratosis (bullous congenital ichthyosiform erythroderma). The presence of bullae (present here in a 2-day-old infant) helps differentiate this disorder from other types of ichthyosis.

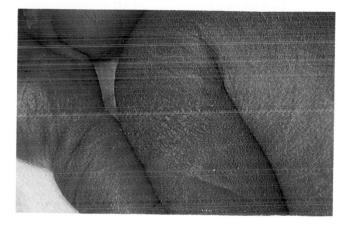

Figure 7–8 Epidermolytic hyperkeratosis Thick verruciform scales in the same patient at 6 months of ago.

Histology of lamellar ichthyosis is similar to that of the sex-linked form of ichthyosis. The epidermis shows marked hyperkeratosis with occasional patchy parakeratosis, increased thickness of the granular layer, acanthosis, and variable papillomatosis. Studies of epidermal kinetics suggest that an increased mitotic activity and an associated rapid epidermal transit time are responsible for the skin changes seen in this disorder.

Epidermolytic Hyperkeratosis

Epidermolytic hyperkeratosis (bullous congenital ichthyosiform erythroderma) is a distinctive, dominantly inherited form of ichthyosis characterized by verruciform scales particularly prominent in the flexural area. Bullae generally appear within the first week of life (often within a few hours after delivery) (Fig. 7–7); hyperkeratosis often appears from the third month on (Fig. 7–8).[10] The presence of bullae is highly characteristic of this disorder. The blisters occur in crops and vary in size from 0.5 cm to several centimeters in diameter. They are superficial, tender, and frequently painful, and when ruptured, discharge clear fluid and leave raw denuded areas. Secondary infection with beta hemolytic streptococcus or *Staphylococcus aureus* is commonly seen in association with this disorder (Table 7–4).

Thick grayish-brown scales cover most of the skin surface; the flexural creases and intertriginous areas show marked involvement, often with furrowed hyperkeratosis (Fig. 7–9). Palms and soles are frequently affected and may show varying degrees of scaling (Fig. 7–10).[9] This hyperkeratosis is often generalized, with a thick covering of prominent verruciform scales over the hands, feet, wrists, and ankles (Figs. 7–11 and 7–12). A disagreeable body odor is frequently

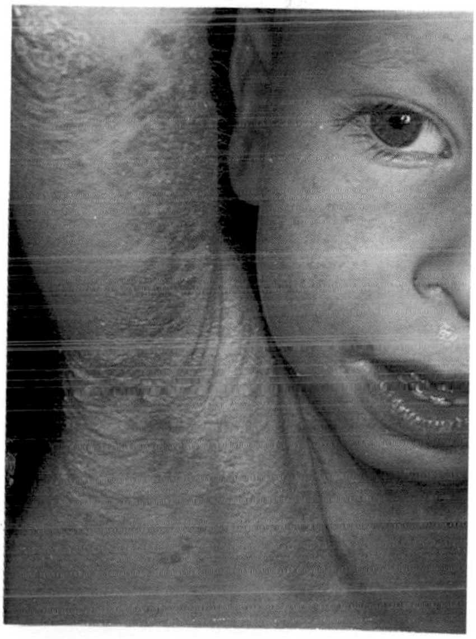

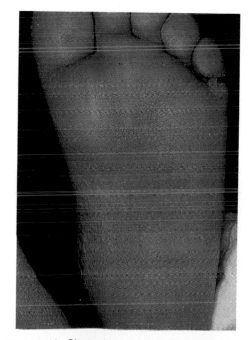

Figure 7–9 Epidermolytic hyperkeratosis. Thick grayish-brown scales in flexural creases.

Figure 7–10 Plantar hyperkeratosis in a patient with epidermolytic hyperkeratosis.

Table 7–4 EPIDERMOLYTIC HYPERKERATOSIS
(Bullous CIE)

a. Generally at birth, with bullae in first week
b. Secondary infection common
c. Hyperkeratosis after third month
   1. flexures (furrowed hyperkeratosis)
   2. elbows, knees, wrists, ankles
   3. palms and soles
d. Same or worse with age
e. Mx: marked hyperkeratosis, thickened granular layer,
   vacuolization of epidermal cells

associated with severe forms of this disorder. Histologically, linear epidermal nevi and their systematized variant, nevus unius lateris, appear to be closely related to localized variants of this disorder. When this involvement is bilateral, it is termed ichthyosis hystrix.

As in lamellar ichthyosis, the epidermal turnover has been described as six times that of normal epidermal tissue.[2] Skin biopsies show distinctive histologic changes. An extreme degree of hyperkeratosis is associated with vacuolization (due to intracellular edema) of epidermal cells in the upper and midportions of the stratum malpighium.[11] Vacuolization or ballooning of the squamous cells is responsible for their dehiscence, and since this often results in formation of microvesicles and bullae, epidermolytic hyperkeratosis has been classified as "bullous congenital ichthyosiform erythroderma."

Harlequin Fetus

The term harlequin fetus refers to a severe and dramatic form of congenital ichthyosis. Whereas mild and moderately severe forms of ichthyosis are relatively common disorders, this represents a rare condition with less than 100 cases described in the world's literature. Because of the rarity of this condition and the short life span of affected individuals (6 weeks or less), the place of this disorder in the spectrum of ichthyoses remains controversial. The presence of familial cases and consanguinity among the parents of some of the patients suggest that the disorder is inherited as an autosomal recessive trait. Although the nature of the abnormality is not clear, x-ray

diffraction analysis of the stratum corneum in one case revealed the presence of an unusual fibrous protein, suggesting a defect in epidermal keratin. On the basis of x-ray diffraction studies, keratins have been found to exist in two forms, alpha and beta. In this disorder cross–beta-fibrous protein (rather than the usual alpha-fibrous protein of normal keratin) appears as a major component of the stratum corneum,[12] and a defect in epidermal lipid metabolism has been postulated as the biochemical abnormality in the skin.[13]

The disorder is manifested by a gross appearance and severe hyperkeratosis characterized by deep reddish-brown or purple fissures that divide the thickened gray or yellow-colored skin into polygonal, triangular, or diamond-shaped plaques that simulate the traditional costume of a harlequin. The skin is dry and hard and has been likened to that of a baked apple, the bark of a tree, morocco leather, and tortoise, elephant, and crocodile skin. Rigidity of the skin about the eyes results in marked ectropion, everted O-shaped lips with a gaping fish-mouth deformity, and a distorted, flattened, and undeveloped appearance to the nose and ear, all of which add to the grotesque clown-like appearance of the infant.

The nails of the harlequin fetus may be hypoplastic or absent. Rigidity of the skin restricts respiratory movements, sucking, and swallowing. Extreme inelasticity of the skin is associated with flexion deformity of all joints of the limbs. The hands and feet are ischemic, hard, and waxy in appearance, often with poorly developed digits and an associated rigid and claw-like appearance.

Histopathologic examination of the skin of affected infants is characterized by perforation of the epidermis by distorted and fragmented hair shafts, extreme hyperkeratosis, a grossly deficient or absent granular layer, and plugging of eccrine sweat ducts and sebaceous follicles by hyperkeratotic debris.

Therapy is ineffective and most infants born with this disorder are stillborn or expire within the neonatal period (usually during the first few hours or days following delivery). The longest survival reported to date has been six weeks. Death is frequently a result of pneumonia associated with

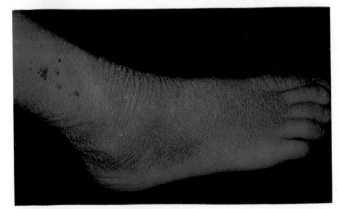

Figure 7–11 Epidermolytic hyperkeratosis. Verruciform scales on the dorsal aspect of the foot.

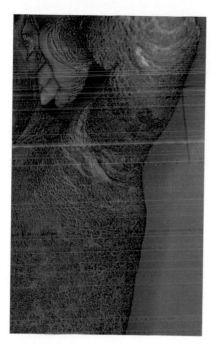

Figure 7–12 Thick grayish-brown verruciform scales (epidermolytic hyperkeratosis).

Figure 7–13 Peripheral double-edged polycyclic scaly lesions of ichythyosis linearis circumflexa. This patient also had trichorrhexis invaginata (this combination has been termed Netherton's disease).

hypoventilation due to thoracic rigidity or sepsis as a result of cutaneous infection.[14]

UNCLASSIFIED ICHTHYOSIS

In addition to the major types of ichthyosis, there are numerous syndromes in which ichthyosis is a constant or variable feature but where clinical and histologic description does not permit appropriate classification.

Erythrokeratodermia Variabilis

Erythrokeratodermia variabilis is an uncommon, dominantly inherited ichthyosis characterized by two distinct types of lesions: (1) symmetrically distributed, sharply marginated areas of erythema that undergo changes in size, shape, and distribution during a period of days and (2) plaques with thick, yellow-brown scales that occur in most of the erythematous areas. Lesions may be found on the face, trunk, or extremities and have a chronic course with variable remissions and exacerbations. Although lesions are usually noted at birth or shortly thereafter during the first year of life, in a few individuals the onset has been noted during late childhood or early adulthood.[15]

Ichthyosis Linearis Circumflexa

Ichthyosis linearis circumflexa is an autosomal recessive disorder characterized by migratory, polycyclic scaly lesions with a peripheral double-edged scale (Fig. 7–13). Partial remissions have been noted, but there is little tendency to sponta-

neous resolution. In a survey of 15 patients with ichthyosis and structural defects of the hair shaft it appears that ichthyosis linearis circumflexa is frequently seen in association with Netherton's syndrome, but all patients with ichthyosis linearis circumflexa do not have hair shaft abnormalities.[16]

Netherton's Syndrome

Netherton's syndrome is a rare condition described as a combination of ichthyosis, atopy, and hair shaft deformities (usually trichorrhexis invaginata, occasionally trichorrhexis nodosa or pili torti). Although the number of reported cases is too small for a thorough genetic analysis, the syndrome is thought to be determined by an autosomal recessive gene of variable expressivity. The ichthyotic changes have usually been described as ichthyosis linearis circumflexa; however, it has been noted that individuals may also manifest lamellar ichthyosis or ichthyosis vulgaris in combination with their hair shaft abnormality.[16]

Refsum's Disease

Refsum's disease is a rare autosomal recessive disorder with ichthyosis, retinitis pigmentosa, and chronic polyneuritis with deafness, progressive flaccid paralysis, and ataxia. Other ocular findings include night-blindness, concentric constriction of the visual fields, nystagmus, cataracts, and rarely photophobia. Mild scaling of the skin is variable, and a generalized branny desquamation of dirty-brown scale appears to be the most characteristic cutaneous change in individuals with this disorder.

A block in the degradation pathway of phytanic acid appears to be the significant metabolic defect.[17] The diagnosis is based on the demonstration of increased levels of phytanic acid in the patient's serum, tissue, or urine. Therapy consists of a chlorophyll-free diet and avoidance of phytanic acid–containing foods.

Rud's Syndrome

Rud's syndrome is a rare recessive disorder characterized by ichthyosis, mental deficiency, epilepsy, dwarfism, and sexual infantilism. The cutaneous findings vary from a mild, generalized, branny desquamation to a severe ichthyosis resembling "snakeskin" with predilection for the extensor surfaces of the extremities.[18]

Frequent and recurring seizures prove to be a difficult management problem, and patients usually require institutional care because of severe mental retardation. Other associated anomalies include arachnodactyly, structural defects of the hands and feet, hypoplastic or absent teeth, alopecia, nerve defects, and various ophthalmologic defects, namely strabismus, retinitis pigmentosa, cataracts, ptosis, blepharospasm, and nystagmus.

Sjögren-Larsson Syndrome

Sjögren-Larsson syndrome is a rare autosomal recessive disorder that combines generalized ichthyosis, spastic paralysis, mental retardation, and, at times, retinitis pigmentosa and epilepsy. Ichthyosis is present at birth and is characterized by a generalized fine scaling with accentuation in the flexures, a varying degree of erythroderma, and hyperkeratosis of the palms and soles.[19] As in Rud's syndrome, the cutaneous findings are relatively insignificant in comparison to the neurologic defects. The histologic features are consistent with those observed in patients with lamellar ichthyosis (hyperkeratosis, acanthosis and papillomatosis of the epidermis, and a normal to slightly increased granular layer).

Conradi's Disease

Conradi's disease is a rare congenital disorder of variable expression also termed chondrodysplasia punctata and chondrodysplasia congenita punctata. In about one-fourth of affected subjects this multisystem defect syndrome is characterized by ichthyosis of the skin similar to that of the collodion baby at birth, followed by hyperkeratotic yellow-white adherent scales arrounged in whorl and swirl patterns on the trunk and limbs, rough and erythematous intervening skin, and hyperkeratosis of the palms and soles. The erythema and ichthyosiform dermatosis generally disap-

pear by three to six months only to be followed, in some cases, by blotchy pigmentation in the pattern of incontinentia pigmenti, follicular atrophoderma, and patchy cicatricial alopecia. Follicular atrophoderma is a late manifestation and seems to occur at sites previously affected with hyperkeratosis, and the hyperpigmented changes seen in some patients may represent postinflammatory changes rather than true incontinentia pigmentation.[20, 21, 22] Associated skeletal changes include shortening of the femur and humerus, dwarfism, and flexion contraction of large joints, due not only to shortening of the bone but also to replacement of muscle by fibrous tissue. Bilateral cataracts with or without optic atrophy, nasal bone dysplasia with saddle nose deformity, and a high arched palate constitute other features of this disorder.

Two major types of chondrodysplasia punctata with different prognoses, radiologic changes, and modes of inheritance have been distinguished. These have been described as type 1, the Conradi-Hunerman syndrome, and type 2, rhizomelic dwarfism. Type 1 has been associated with advanced paternal age and appears to follow an autosomal dominant inheritance. The type 2 form seems to be inherited as an autosomal recessive trait.

Type 1 patients have been further subdivided into three subgroups: (a) infants of low birth weight and small stature with mild to severe skeletal effects who die early in infancy; (b) moderately affected infants, predominantly girls, often with cataracts and skin manifestations who have a relatively good prognosis; and (c) children with mild symmetrical epiphyseal changes and no cutaneous manifestations or cataracts who have an excellent prognosis.

Type 2, the rhizomelic form, is associated with psychomotor retardation and spasticity. Most infants with this form of the disorder die within the first year of life from cardiovascular, gastrointestinal, or respiratory involvement. Stippling of the epiphyses occurs in both types of chondrodysplasia punctata (detectable in radiologic examination of the fetus and persisting until 3 to 4 years of age), and cataracts occur in 17 per cent of patients with Type 1 disorder and in 92 per cent of those with the rhizomelic form.[22]

TREATMENT

The management of all types of dry skin consists of retardation of water loss, rehydration and softening of the stratum corneum, and alleviation of scaliness and associated pruritus (Table 7–5). Ichthyosis vulgaris and X-linked ichthyosis can be managed quite well by topical application of emollients and the use of keratolytic agents to facilitate removal of scales from the skin surface. Limited baths with a mild soap and hydration of dry skin by frequent use of lubricating creams or lotions over moisture is helpful. Urea, in concentrations of 10 to 20 per cent (in a cream, lotion, or ointment base), has a softening and

Table 7–5   TREATMENT OF ICHTHYOSIS

1. Lubricants
   a. 10–20% urea
   b. 40–60% propylene glycol
   c. alpha hydroxy acids (5% lactic acid)
   d. Saran wrap
2. Keratolytics
   a. 3–6% salicylic acid
   b. Keralyt Gel
      (6% salicylic acid in propylene glycol)
3. Vitamin A acid (tretinoin)
4. Antimetabolites? (lamellar ichthyosis, epidermolytic hyperkeratosis)

moisturizing effect on the stratum corneum and is helpful in the control of dry skin and pruritus. Propylene glycol (40 to 60 per cent in water), applied overnight under plastic occlusion, hydrates the skin and causes desquamation of scales.

Salicylic acid is an effective keratolytic agent and at concentrations between 3 and 6 per cent promotes shedding of scales and softening of the stratum corneum. When it is used to cover large surface areas for prolonged periods, however, care should be taken to ensure that salicylate toxicity does not occur. A keratolytic gel containing salicylic acid and propylene glycol, available as Keralyt gel (Westwood Pharmaceuticals), a proprietary preparation containing 6 per cent salicylic acid in propylene glycol, is frequently helpful following hydration of the involved area. This preparation, when used either alone or under occlusive poly-

ethylene wrapping, has been most successful in patients with ichthyosis vulgaris and X-linked ichthyosis.[23] Studies also suggest that alpha hydroxy preparations such as lactic or pyruvic acid may be beneficial in the treatment of ichthyosiform dermatoses. Lactic acid is available as a proprietary preparation (Lacticare lotion, Steifel) or may be added to lubricating lotions or emollient creams. While 5 to 10 per cent concentrations have been used, 2 to 5 per cent concentrations appear to be less irritating, more readily tolerated, and better for use on large areas of the body.[24]

The treatment of lamellar ichthyosis by frequent lubrication or the addition of urea, salicylic acid, or lactic acid to lubricating creams or lotions, although encouraging, is not as effective as in the treatment of ichthyosis vulgaris and X-linked ichthyosis. Oral vitamin A has been used in the treatment of lamellar ichthyosis but appears to be ineffective except in large doses. The hazards of toxicity, therefore, preclude its use in infants and small children with this disorder. Topical vitamin A acid, although potentially irritating, is beneficial in the treatment of lamellar ichthyosis (Fig. 7–14).[9, 25] This preparation should be used cautiously on a daily or alternate-day routine.

The oral retinoid 13-*cis*-retinoic acid has been used experimentally, and in dosages of 1 mg/kg daily for one or more courses of 16 weeks appears to be beneficial in the management of several keratinizing dermatoses. Although not yet available, this preparation has been effective for most patients with lamellar ichthyosis, for some patients with Darier's disease and pityriasis rubra pilaris, and for some individuals with epidermolytic hyperkeratosis.[26] The therapy of epidermolytic hyperkeratosis is similar to that of lamellar ichthyosis, with the exception that antibiotics are frequently required to control the secondary infection of bullous lesions.

CONGENITAL ECTODERMAL DEFECTS

Ectodermal dysplasia is a descriptive term for an inherited group of defects involving the skin and its appendageal structures. These defects include hidrotic ectodermal dysplasia, anhidrotic ectodermal dysplasia, and congenital aplasia cutis. Although these defects share involvement of similar structures (the integument and its appendages) they are distinct nosological entities, with individual histologic and clinical manifestations. Genetically they are not related to one another.

Hidrotic Ectodermal Dysplasia

The hidrotic type of ectodermal dysplasia is an autosomal dominant disorder of keratinization characterized by dystrophy of the nails, hyperkeratosis of the palms and soles, and defects of the hair. Most cases have been reported in French-Canadian families. Unlike anhidrotic ectodermal dysplasia, which is an X-linked recessive disorder and more common in males, hidrotic ectodermal

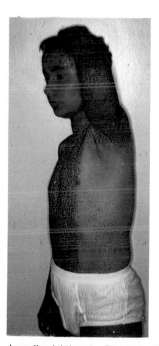

Figure 7–14   Lamellar ichthyosis. The patient's left side was treated with topical tretinoin (vitamin A acid). (Mirrer F, McGuire JS: Lamellar ichthyosis—response to retinoic acid (tretinoin) A case report. Arch. Dermatol. 102:548, 1972).

dysplasia is of equal sex incidence, shows no abnormality of sweating, and although dental caries may be present, includes normal teeth and facies.

There is some evidence that hidrotic ectodermal dysplasia is caused by a defect in keratinization due to a molecular abnormality of keratin.[27] In 30 per cent of individuals with this disorder, however, there may be no obvious defect other than dystrophy of the nails. Although nail dystrophy is the primary feature of this syndrome, various nail changes may occur, none of which is characteristic. Nails grow slowly and may appear thickened or thinned, striated, discolored, brittle, or hypoplastic. Paronychial infections are common and may result in partial to complete destruction of the nail matrix.

Body hair may be sparse; eyebrows and eyelashes may be thinned or absent. Scalp hair, generally normal during infancy and childhood, may become thin, fragile, or sparse to absent following puberty. Keratoderma (hyperkeratosis) of the palms and soles is common and occasionally extends to involve the sides and dorsa of affected hands and feet. Extreme hyperkeratosis of the palms and soles may be controlled to a degree by topical keratolytic agents (3 to 6 per cent salicylic acid or 10 per cent urea in an emollient cream).

Anhidrotic Ectodermal Dysplasia

Anhidrotic ectodermal dysplasia is thought to be a sex-linked recessive disorder in which more than 90 per cent of affected patients have been males. It is characterized by partial to complete absence of eccrine sweat glands, hair and dental abnormalities, and associated congenital defects.

Clinical findings in this condition are absent or reduced sweating, hypotrichosis, and defective dentition. Abnormal absence of perspiration from the surface of the skin in the presence of an appropriate stimulus often results in hyperthermia. Patients may appear normal at birth but soon develop intermittent fevers during hot weather or following exercise or meals.

Affected individuals often appear more like each other than like their own siblings; classic features may be present by the age of one year. Most have a distinctive pathognomonic facies — a square forehead with frontal bossing, saddle nose, wide cheekbones with depressed cheeks, thick everted lips, and prominent chin. Ears may be small, satyr-like (pointed), low-lying, and anteriorly placed.[28]

Skin is soft, thin, white, and shiny, often feminine-like in quality, with easily seen cutaneous vasculature. Alopecia is often the first feature to attract attention but is seldom complete. Nails are defective in 50 per cent of cases and may be thin, brittle, or ridged. Gross deformities are uncommon.

Dentition is generally delayed and dental anomalies varying from complete to partial absence of teeth may be noted. Incisors and canines are often discolored, peg-shaped or conical, and

pointed with inward curving. Occlusion is poor and caries are commonly seen. General physical development is often stunted. Mental development is retarded in 30 to 50 per cent of cases, and life expectancy is normal or slightly reduced.

Therapy is difficult and should be directed toward temperature regulation, restriction of excessive physical exertion, choice of suitable occupation, and avoidance of warm climates. Cool baths, air conditioning, light clothing, and the reduction of the causes of normal perspiration are beneficial. Regular dental supervision may help preserve teeth and reduce cosmetic disfigurement.

Aplasia Cutis Congenita

This disorder presents a localized congenital absence of the epidermis, dermis, and at times the subcutaneous tissue. The inheritance of this disorder is uncertain. A number of familial cases, however, suggest an autosomal mode of inheritance[29, 30] (see Chapter 2).

Sixty per cent of lesions appear on the vertex of the scalp as sharply marginated erosions (1–2 cm in diameter). Skin defects may be solitary or multiple in number; they are frequently round or oval but may be elongated, triangular, or stellate in configuration (see Fig. 2–11). Occasionally they occur on the trunk or limbs and often are located symmetrically over the patellae.

At birth the surface of the lesion may be covered by a smooth membrane, which may be ulcerated or crusted. As healing occurs the raw area is replaced by a smooth, gray, parchment-like atrophic scar tissue devoid of appendageal structures (hair, eccrine, and sebaceous glands).

Following delivery, scalp lesions may be misdiagnosed and considered to be the result of birth trauma or forceps injury. The sharply punched-out configuration and characteristic location of lesions are diagnostic and should lead to the recognition of this disorder.

Treatment during the newborn period consists of control of secondary infection. As the child matures, most scars become inconspicuous and require no correction. Obvious scars may be treated by multiple punch-graft hair transplants or surgical excision with plastic repair.

CONGENITAL DERMAL DEFECTS

Hereditary disorders of the dermal tissue generally involve one element of the connective tissue. Three types of fiber form the connective tissue of the dermis — collagen, reticulum, and elastin. The mucopolysaccharides are a major component of the ground substance between these fibers. Discussion in this section will include the disorders of collagen, the largest constituent of the connective tissue (Ehlers-Danlos syndrome), and the disorders of elastin (cutis laxa and pseudoxanthoma elasticum). The mucopolysaccharidoses will be reviewed in another section.

DISORDERS OF COLLAGEN

Ehlers-Danlos Syndrome

Ehlers-Danlos syndrome is a disorder of collagen characterized by increased cutaneous elasticity (Fig. 7–15), hyperextensibility of the joints (Fig. 7–16), and fragility of the skin, with formation of pseudotumors and large gaping scars (Fig. 7–17). There are at least seven variants of the syndrome. Types 1, 2, and 3 are characterized by autosomal dominant inheritance, type 4 is autosomal recessive; type 5 is X-linked recessive; and types 6 and 7 are autosomal recessive.[31, 32] The collagenous defect appears to be the manner in which collagen bundles are joined to one another (a defective wickerwork arrangement), which results in increased mobility and rubber-like stretchability of the skin and joints.[32, 33, 34]

To date specific defects have been noted in the most common autosomally dominant Ehlers-Danlos syndrome (EDS) types 1, 2, and 3. Type 4 Ehlers-Danlos syndrome (the Sack type) is characterized by an absence of type III collagen; the defect in type 5 EDS is a deficiency of lysyl oxidase; and deficiencies of lysyl hydroxylase and p-collagen peptidase respectively are seen as features of type 6 and type 7 Ehlers-Danlos syndrome.[35, 36]

In general, infants with Ehlers-Danlos syndrome are prone to premature birth because of early rupture of membranes (the placenta is determined entirely by the fetal genotype and therefore its membranes have the same fragility as other structures in this disorder). The skin of affected individuals is velvety and soft in texture, and on palpation has a peculiar, doughy consistency. It is hyperelastic, yet not lax except in late stages. After being stretched it returns to its normal position as soon as released (Fig. 7–15).

In addition to this abnormal elasticity the skin is extremely fragile, and minor trauma may produce gaping "fish-mouth" wounds. It has poor tensile strength and cannot hold sutures properly. This leads to frequent dehiscence, poor healing, and the formation of wide, papyraceous, wrinkled

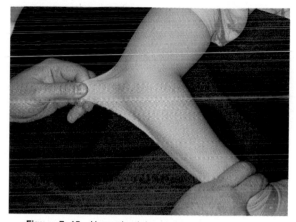

Figure 7–15 Hyperelasticity of skin overlying the elbow (Ehlers-Danlos syndrome) (Braverman IM: Skin Signs of Systemic Disease. W. B. Saunders Co., Philadelphia, 1970).

hernia-like scars, particularly over areas of trauma (such as the forehead, elbows, and knees). Blood vessels are fragile, resulting in hematomas. The resolution of hematomas is accompanied by fibrosis, which produces soft subcutaneous pseudotumors (Fig. 7–17). Except for areas of skin that have been altered by trauma, histopathologic examination of the skin of individuals with Ehlers-Danlos disease reveals no obvious alteration in either elastic or collagen fiber.

Hyperextensible joints may result in "double-jointed" fingers or frequent subluxation of larger joints (Fig. 7–16). This may occur spontaneously or follow slight trauma. Muscle tone is often poor, and inguinal and diaphragmatic hernias are common. Anomalies of the heart and dissecting aortic aneurysms have been described, and although life expectancy is generally normal, premature deaths have occurred from gastrointestinal bleeding, rare

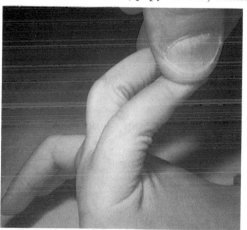

Figure 7–16 Hyperextensibility of the fingers in Ehlers-Danlos syndrome.

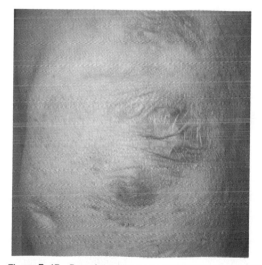

Figure 7–17 Pseudotumors and papyraceous scars on the knee in Ehlers-Danlos syndrome.

bowel perforation, and rupture of cardiovascular defects.[37]

It has been noted that type 1 Ehlers-Danlos patients are characterized by loose hyperextensible skin, hypermobile joints, pseudotumors, and paper-thin scars; type 2 is characterized by loose skin, hypermobile joints, and bleeding problems; type 3 by lax joints and variable bruising; and patients with type 4 EDS have thin skin, fragile and inextensible connective tissues with a tendency to keloid and contracture formation, a characteristic pinched facies, acrogeria (premature aging of the skin of the hands and feet), ecchymoses, and a tendency toward ruptures of large arteries of the bowel. Patients with Ehlers-Danlos syndrome type 6 tend to have scoliosis and are prone to retinal detachments, and type 7 patients have lax joints, a characteristic facies, and, in some individuals, a tendency to short stature.[36, 38]

Management of patients with Ehlers-Danlos syndrome is mainly supportive in nature and should include genetic counseling. The possibility of premature birth should be discussed and cutaneous, skeletal, and ocular difficulties (possible retinal detachment and abnormalities of the lens) should be emphasized. Surgical procedures present problems because tissues are friable and difficult to suture. Edges of gaping wounds should be kept approximated with appropriate sutures and adhesive closure to facilitate healing. Precautions must be taken to minimize trauma to the skin and joints. Pressure bandages over hematomas may help prevent pseudotumor formation.

DISORDERS OF ELASTIN

Cutis Laxa

Cutis laxa (generalized elastolysis) is an extremely rare disorder of the elastic tissue characterized by inelastic, loose, and pendulous skin, which results in an aged, bloodhound-like appearance. To date there appear to be three known genetic forms — a severe autosomal recessive form; a less commonly observed, relatively benign autosomal dominant form, with a tendency to spontaneous improvement; and a rare X-linked form in which there is a deficiency of lysyl oxidase (the collagen and elastin crosslinking enzyme).[31] It has been suggested that the abnormality in cutis laxa may be related to an increased destruction of elastic fibers by elastase (possibly due to low levels of elastase inhibitor) but this lacks confirmation.[39]

The abnormality generally begins at birth or shortly thereafter and is characterized by loose, inelastic redundant skin that sags and hangs in pendulous folds as if it were too large for the body. The drooping and ectropion of the eyelids, together with the sagging facial skin and accentuation of the nasal, labial, and other facial folds, help produce the "bloodhound" or aged appearance (Fig. 7–18). Although frequently prominent and, at times, almost grotesque in ap-

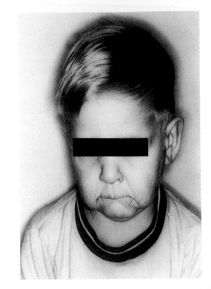

Figure 7–18 Sagging cheeks and bloodhound-like facies of a child with cutis laxa (Courtesy of Sidney Klaus, M.D., *In* Braverman IM: Skin Signs of Systemic Disease. W. B. Saunders Co., Philadelphia, 1970).

pearance, as the children grow older they often appear to grow into the skin abnormality and do not appear to be as severely affected in later life.

Cutis laxa affects the elastic fibers of the skin as well as those throughout the entire body. Although no histologic abnormality is demonstrable with hematoxylin and eosin stain, elastic tissue stains reveal a decreased number of elastic fibers throughout the entire dermis and electron microscopy reveals a granular degeneration of the elastic fibers. System manifestations due to weakened supportive tissue include pulmonary emphysema, diverticulae of the gastrointestinal tract or urinary bladder, rectal prolapse, and ventral, hiatal, or inguinal hernias. The disease is gradually progressive, and death from pulmonary complications related to emphysema may occur in the second to fourth decades of life.

The skin in cutis laxa is extensible but, in contrast to that of Ehlers-Danlos syndrome, does not spring back to place on release of tension. In Ehlers-Danlos syndrome the hyperextensibility of the joints and pseudotumors of the skin with large atrophic scars are diagnostic. In pseudoxanthoma elasticum the lax skin is covered with characteristic soft yellowish papules and plaques. In neurofibromatosis (von Recklinghausen's disease), the café au lait spots and fibrous tumors indicate the true nature of the disorder.

Therapy of cutis laxa is limited, and prognosis in general is poor. Surgery can correct diverticulae, rectal prolapse, or hernias; pulmonary function studies may aid in the early detection of emphysema; and plastic surgery can make a dramatic improvement in patients, inevitably with important psychological benefit.[34]

Pseudoxanthoma Elasticum

Pseudoxanthoma elasticum is a genetic disorder of the elastic tissue that involves the skin, eyes, and cardiovascular system. It is characterized by soft yellowish papules and polygonal plaques on the neck, below the clavicles, and in the axillae, antecubital fossae, periumbilical areas, perineum, and thighs (Fig. 7–19). There are two recessive and two dominant forms of this disorder. Most cases are autosomal recessive in nature.[31] Pathogenesis is controversial and appears to be related to an abnormal proliferation of elastic fibers that prematurely calcify and fragment.[39-42]

Skin lesions are a hallmark of this disorder. They are yellowish in color and xanthoma-like (hence the name pseudoxanthoma). They vary from several papules to linear plaques resembling plucked chicken skin, morocco leather, or orange skin (peau d'orange). Although lesions are seen in childhood, they may be overlooked because of their small size and the lack of symptomatology. As skin in affected areas becomes relatively inelastic, it may hang in lax redundant folds, especially on the neck.

Eye changes associated with this disorder are characteristic; they are slate-gray to brown linear bands (angioid streaks), caused by tears in Bruch's membrane and subsequent fibrosis, and are seen in 50 to 70 per cent of cases. The association of skin lesions with angioid streaks is known as the Grönblad-Strandberg syndrome. Loss of central vision is the most frequent disability and may develop in more than 70 per cent of cases with this complication. These retinal changes are not pathognomonic, as they may also be found in patients with sickle cell anemia and Paget's disease of the bone.

Significant cardiovascular changes include peripheral artery disease with easy fatigability and intermittent claudication, coronary artery involvement, and cerebral or gastrointestinal hemorrhage.

Histopathologic features of pseudoxanthoma elasticum include deposition of calcium in elastic tissue and basophilic degeneration of elastic tissue in the middle and deeper zones of the dermis. Elastic tissue degeneration also affects connective tissue elements of the aorta and medium-sized muscular arteries in coronary, renal, gastrointestinal, and other organs.

There is no specific therapy for this disorder. Removal of redundant skin by plastic surgery can improve the cosmetic appearance of affected individuals. Gastrointestinal hemorrhage can generally be managed by a conservative medical approach, but surgical intervention at times may be necessary. Since the disabling aspects of this disease are slow but progressive, a complete vascular survey and regular ophthalmologic examinations are important.

Progeria

Progeria (Hutchinson-Gilford syndrome) is a rare disease characterized by a combination of dwarfism, generalized atrophy of the subcutaneous tissue and muscle, a high incidence of generalized atherosclerosis, and early onset of progressive senile degenerative changes. Although its presence in siblings and examples of parental consanguinity have been reported, suggesting an autosomal recessive basis for this disorder, affected individuals do not reproduce and there are far too few familial cases to draw definitive conclusions as to the hereditability of this disorder.[31, 34, 43] There is no sex predilection, and rarely is more than one family member affected.

Affected children tend to have a reduced size and birth weight, but otherwise appear to be relatively normal during the first 6 to 12 months of life. The classical clinical picture consists of dwarfism; alopecia of the scalp, eyebrows, and lashes; prominent scalp veins; and generalized atrophy of muscle and subcutaneous tissue. Frequently there is nasolabial and circumoral cyanosis. The face is small, the chin is recessed, and the nose is thin and beaked, giving the face a bird-like appearance (Fig. 7–20).[43] Although the head is usually 2 to 4 cm smaller in circumference than average, severe growth retardation and alteration

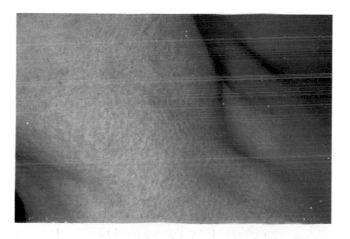

Figure 7 10 Soft yellowish papules and polygonal plaques in the axilla of a patient with pseudoxanthoma elasticum.

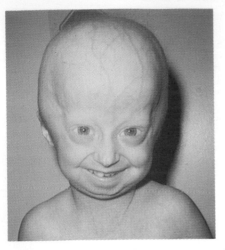

Figure 7–20 Progeria. Alopecia, subcutaneous atrophy, prominent scalp veins, and bird-like appearance. (Fleishmajer R and Nedwich A: Progeria (Hutchinson-Gilford). Arch. Dermatol. 107:253, 1973).

of the facial structures resulting in a disproportionately small face with frontal and parietal bossing give the head a hydrocephalic appearance.

The skin generally becomes thin (except for areas with sclerodermatous plaques), dry, and wrinkled, with mottled brownish-orange pigmentation. The underlying subcutaneous veins, especially those on the scalp and thighs, become plainly visible and more prominent in appearance. The nails become yellowish, thin, atrophic, and brittle, and resorption of bone leads to osteoporosis with a tendency to frequent fractures. The teeth become crowded, irregular in form or deficient in number, and deciduous dentition is often retained. Speech becomes high-pitched and squeaky, and intelligence is generally normal. The chest becomes narrow and the abdomen protuberant, and, owing to a mild flexion of the knees, a "horse-riding" stance becomes apparent.

Progeria should be distinguished from scleroderma, Werner's syndrome, Rothmund-Thomson syndrome, and anhidrotic ectodermal dysplasia. Atherosclerosis is early and severe. Cardiac murmurs frequently occur after the age of five years and are soon followed by hypertension, cardiomegaly, angina, myocardial infarction and congestive heart failure. Death usually occurs during the second decade of life.[43]

Werner's Syndrome

The Werner syndrome (progeria of the adult) is a rare autosomal recessive disorder characterized by premature graying of hair at the temples (which may develop as early as eight years of age but generally occurs between the ages of 14 and 18), progressive alopecia, shortness of stature due to arrest of growth at puberty, bird-like facies, cataracts, and an apparent aged appearance. Cutaneous features include sclerodermoid changes of the skin of the extremities and, to a lesser degree, the face and neck; telangiectases; mottled or diffuse pigmentation; keratoses; and indolent ulcers over pressure points, particularly on the soles and ankles.

Patients with adult progeria develop severe, often generalized vascular disease, diabetes mellitus (in 30 to 45 per cent of affected individuals), hypogonadism, and a predisposition to neoplastic disease (hepatoma, thyroid adenocarcinoma, osteosarcoma, and carcinoma of the breast).

Dyskeratosis Congenita

Dyskeratosis congenita is a rare genetic disorder characterized by atrophy and pigmentation of the skin, nail dystrophy, and leukoplakia. Almost all reported cases have been males, and available pedigrees suggest it to be autosomal recessive or X-linked in nature.

Nail changes are usually the first to make their appearance (Fig. 7–21). Between the ages of 5 and 13 they become thin and dystrophic. In mild cases they develop ridging and longitudinal grooving; in severe forms they are shortened and, at times, almost non-existent. Cutaneous changes may develop simultaneously or in a few years following the onset of nail changes and reach their full development within a subsequent period of three to five years. A fine reticulated grayish-brown hyperpigmentation (surrounding hypopigmented and atrophic patches of uninvolved skin) on the face, neck, shoulders, upper back, and thighs is

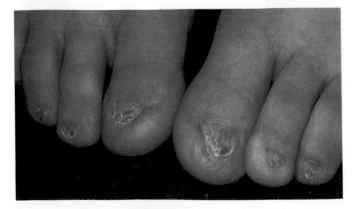

Figure 7–21 Dyskeratosis congenita. Thin dystrophic nails with longitudinal grooving.

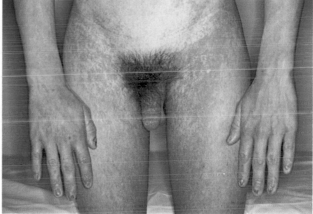

Figure 7–22 Dyskeratosis congenita. Fine reticulated grayish-brown hyperpigmentation of the thighs (Department of Dermatology, Yale University School of Medicine).

characteristic of this disorder (Fig. 7–22). Other cutaneous changes may include telangiectasia of the trunk (Fig. 7–23), redness and atrophy of the face with irregular macular hyperpigmentation, palmoplantar hyperkeratosis, hyperhidrosis of the palms and soles, and a diffuse atrophic, transparent, and shiny appearance on the dorsal aspects of the hands and feet.[44]

Mucous membrane changes consist of small blisters, erosions, and subsequent leukoplakia of the oral (see Fig. 8–26) and anal mucosa, esophagus, and urethra. Similar changes of the tarsal conjunctiva may result in atresia of the lacrimal ducts, excessive lacrimation, chronic blepharitis, conjunctivitis, and ectropion. The teeth tend to be defective and subject to early decay. Peridontitis may develop, and affected individuals have an increased incidence of cutaneous malignancy (predominantly epidermoid carcinoma) and a high incidence of carcinoma in the areas of leukoplakia.[45, 46]

In some patients a severe hematologic disease resembling Fanconi's anemia has been reported. In these patients there is severe anemia with leukopenia (especially neutropenia), splenomegaly, and hypoplastic bone marrow, and hemorrhagic diatheses are prominent.[45]

The management of patients with dyskerato-sis congenita consists of bougienage for esophageal stenosis, fulguration, curettage, and surgical excision of leukokeratosis of the buccal and anal mucosae, and regular supervision for early detection of mucosal or cutaneous carcinomata.

Focal Dermal Hypoplasia

Focal dermal hypoplasia (Goltz syndrome) is a rare hereditary disorder found only in girls and characterized by linear areas of dermal hypoplasia with herniation of underlying tissue, telangiectasia, linear or reticular areas of hyperpigmentation or hypopigmentation, localized superficial fatty deposits in the skin, red papillomas of mucous membranes of periorificial skin, and anomalies of the extremities, including syndactyly, adactyly, and oligodactyly. Available family histories suggested that this condition is caused by an X-linked dominant trait lethal in the male.[47]

Streaky pigmentation, atrophy, and telangiectasia are usually present at birth over the trunk and extremities. Yellowish-brown nodules of subcutaneous fat, red papillomatosis of the skin or mucosae of the oral, anal, or genital regions, hypohidrosis, and paper-thin nails have been associated with this syndrome. Other cutaneous abnormalities include sparseness of hair, lichenoid follicular hy-

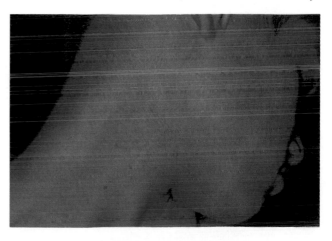

Figure 7–23 Dyskeratosis congenita. Telangiectasia and mottled pigmentation of the neck and face.

perkeratotic papules, and keratotic lesions on the palms and soles. Skeletal anomalies include syndactyly, polydactyly, absence or hypoplasia of a digit or hand bone, clinodactyly, vertebral anomalies, scoliosis, spina bifida, and aplasia or hypoplasia of the "right" clavicle. Other associated abnormalities include umbilical or inguinal hernia, strabismus, colobomata, microphthalmia, hypodontia and hypoplasia of the dental enamel, and, in some affected individuals, microcephaly and mental retardation.

Disorders included in the differential diagnosis of this condition include congenital ectodermal dysplasia, congenital poikiloderma (Rothmund-Thomson syndrome), incontinentia pigmenti, linear scleroderma, and nevus lipomatosus cutaneous superficialis of Hoffman and Zurhelle (an extremely rare cutaneous nevus of localized groups of soft papules or nodules manifested in the newborn).

When there is doubt, the diagnosis can be verified by biopsy of an affected area of the skin. Histopathologic features consist of absence or hypoplasia of dermal connective tissue with upward extension of the subcutaneous fat tissue almost to the normal epidermis.

Elastosis Perforans Serpiginosa

Elastosis perforans serpiginosa (perforating elastoma) is a disorder of elastic tissue characterized by an annular or linear arrangement of keratotic papules with a predilection for the posterolateral aspects of the neck and occasionally the chin, cheeks, and mandibular areas of the face, antecubital fossae, elbows, and knees. Affecting predominantly males, it appears to be a genetically determined disorder of particular significance in the fact that distinctive dermatosis may act as a cutaneous marker for systemic disease. Of the reported cases, up to 44 per cent have been seen in association with Down syndrome, osteogenesis imperfecta, Ehlers-Danlos syndrome, pseudoxanthoma elasticum, cutis laxa, Rothmund-Thomson syndrome, congenital berry aneurysms of the circle of Willis, acrogeria, and Marfan syndrome,[48]

and at times as a complication of penicillamine therapy.

This cutaneous disorder primarily affects young persons, especially those in the second decade of life, and generally disappears spontaneously within a period of five to ten years. Characteristic features consist of deep red conical papules, 2 to 4 mm in diameter, arranged in a linear, circinate, horseshoe, or serpiginous fashion, varying from 1.0 to 2.5 cm to as much as 15 to 20 cm in overall length. The papules are generally capped by a distinctive keratotic plug, which when forcibly dislodged reveals a bleeding crateriform lesion.

Diagnosis is dependent upon recognition of the characteristic keratotic plug–topped conicle papules in an arciform or linear arrangement and can be confirmed by histopathologic examination. The distinctive histopathologic features consist of elongated tortuous channels within the epidermis, which are perforated by abnormal and degenerated elastic tissue that is extruded from the dermis.[49]

The important feature of this disorder is recognition of the high incidence of associated systemic diseases. Although treatment, in most instances, is generally unsatisfactory and recurrences are common, stripping of the surface keratinous material by repeated application of Scotch tape has resulted in improvement of some lesions, and cryosurgical techniques may produce a satisfactory cosmetic result. Because of a high incidence of residual scar and keloid formation, removal by electrodesiccation and curettage or by surgical excision is not recommended.[48]

Keratosis Follicularis

Keratosis follicularis (Darier's disease, Darier-White disease) is an autosomal dominant defect characterized by greasy crusted papules on the scalp, face, neck, seborrheic areas of the trunk, and flexures of the extremities (Figs. 7–24, 7–25). Although there does not appear to be any specific predilection for a particular race or sex, many authorities suggest that it occurs more frequently in males.

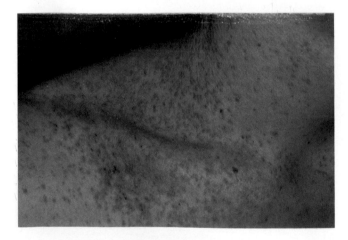

Figure 7–24 Greasy crusted papules of the neck and supraclavicular areas. Keratosis follicularis (Darier's disease).

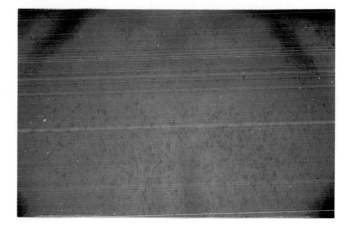

Figure 7-25 Keratosis follicularis (Darier's disease) on the upper chest in a 14-year-old male.

Lesions generally begin as pinhead to pea-sized flesh-colored papules. Most papules are perifollicular, which as the disorder progresses, coalesce to form plaques covered with flesh-colored to yellowish-brown greasy crusts that frequently tend to become purulent and malodorous. The sites of predilection are the seborrheic areas of the trunk, flanks, scalp, sides of the neck, and face (particularly the temples, forehead, ears, and nasolabial furrows). In 10 per cent of cases the lesions may occur in a zosteriform linear distribution confined to one side of the body.[49, 50] Exacerbations during summer months and following ultraviolet exposure suggest photosensitivity as a precipitating factor in the etiology of this disorder.

Lesions of the mucous membranes consist of small white papules or pebbly areas with verrucous white plaques simulating leukoplakia in up to 50 per cent of patients (particularly those with a familial history of the disorder). A generalized thickening of the palms and soles (palmoplantar hyperkeratosis) is present in about 10 per cent of affected individuals, and punctate keratoses or minute pits may be seen on the palms and soles.

Indolent papules resembling flat warts on the dorsal aspect of the hands and feet, with lesser involvement of the volar surfaces, wrists, and ankles (a disorder termed *acrokeratosis verruciformis of Hopf*), has been described in association with Darier's disease. Although initially viewed as distinct entities, these disorders have been linked together by a growing number of observers. In its mildest form acrodermatitis verruciformis may be manifested by white nails with subungual hyperkeratosis or by punctate keratoses of the palms or soles. In its more intense form it is expressed as the more widespread changes characteristic of Darier's disease.[51]

Significant complications, including bacterial and viral infections (Kaposi's varicelliform eruption due to herpesvirus hominis and Coxsackie virus type A16), suggest local factors or a basic immunologic abnormality as the genesis of increased susceptibility to infection seen in individuals with this disorder.[52, 53]

Warty *dyskeratomas* are benign keratotic lesions that occur as solitary verrucous nodules on the face, neck, scalp, mouth, or neck, or in the axillae. Seen primarily in adults, the lesions appear as brownish-red nodules that have a soft yellowish keratotic central plug. Although warty dyskeratomas are histologically indistinguishable from lesions of Darier's disease, warty dyskeratoma represents a distinct entity and there is no clinical resemblance between these two conditions.

The diagnosis of keratosis follicularis is dependent upon recognition of the characteristic appearance and distribution of the eruption and can be confirmed by histopathologic examination of affected areas. The histopathologic changes of Darier's disease (and warty dyskeratoma) consist of intraepidermal suprabasal clefts or lacunae, a peculiar form of dyskeratosis that results in the formation of corps ronds and grains, and irregular upward proliferation of villi (papillae lined with a single layer of basal cells) into the lacunae. "Corps ronds" are cells with a basophilic nucleus surrounded by a clear halo, and "grains" are small dark cells with a pyknotic nucleus, generally seen in the stratum corneum of the skin of affected individuals.

At present there is no satisfactory specific therapy for Darier's disease. Patients should be instructed to avoid excessive sun exposure, heat, and humidity, since this disorder is characteristically more severe during summer and is aggravated by sunlight or ultraviolet exposure, perspiration, heat, and humidity. Large doses of oral vitamin A (200,000 to 300,000 units per day for a period of months) have been used with variable results. Because of possible toxicity with such dosages, this is generally not recommended for children. Topical vitamin A acid, although potentially irritating, has been helpful (the irritation can be minimized by use of adequate yet threshold concentrations, or by the conjoint use of topical steroids).

Lipoid Proteinosis

Lipoid proteinosis (hyalinosis cutis et mucosae) is a rare chronic inherited disorder of lipid metabolism characterized by hoarseness and yellowish nodular infiltrates in the skin and mucous membranes. The exact cause of this disorder is unknown. It is an autosomal recessive trait and appears to be related to an abnormal deposition of hyaline material (believed to be a glycoprotein elaborated by fibrocytes) in the skin, mucous membranes, upper respiratory and gastrointestinal tracts, and other visceral organs, perhaps associated with an enzyme deficit of fibrocytes.[54, 55, 56]

Hoarseness secondary to vocal cord involvement is a clinical feature in virtually every case, and persons with this disorder can be recognized instantly because of their husky voice and thickened eyelids. The voice may be hoarse from birth or within the first few years of life and becomes progressively worse during early childhood. Further examination of such individuals commonly reveals hyperkeratotic plaques on elbows and knees, morphea-like plaques on the trunk, and papular infiltrates on the skin and mucous membranes.[56]

In a typical case the skin is yellow-white, resembling old ivory. Individual lesions, consisting of discrete or confluent 2 to 3 mm yellowish-white to yellowish-brown papules, are found most frequently on the face, eyelids, neck, and hands. In about 50 per cent of individuals a string of bead-like papules, often followed by a loss of cilia, appear on the free eyelid margins.[57] Also characteristic are eversion of the lips (with their surfaces studded with tiny yellow nodules), hypertrophic or vegetative lesions at the corners of the mouth, and round papules just below the lip on the midline of the chin. Skin lesions, particularly in children, may also occur as vesicles, pustules, or bullae. Ulcerations, atrophic or varioliform scars, plaques simulating localized scleroderma, radiating fissures at the corners of the mouth, alopecia of the scalp, eyebrows, eyelashes, or bearded area, impaired nail growth, and multiple confluent papules seen as verrucous plaques on the elbows, knees, hands, and feet help complete the picture.

The tongue tends to become thick, firm, woody, bound to the floor of the mouth, and difficult to extrude. Dysphagia caused by pharyngeal infiltration and respiratory obstruction as a result of severe laryngeal involvement can complicate the disorder. The abnormal glycoprotein has also been found in the stomach, intestine, trachea, lung, eye, pancreas, bladder, kidney, vagina, testis, lymph nodes, and striated muscle. A diabetic tendency has been stated to be part of the syndrome in 20 per cent of family members and affected individuals. This finding, however, requires further investigation and documentation. Central nervous system involvement has been associated with attacks of rage and psychomotor or grand mal epilepsy. Usually, however, the central nervous system involvement is restricted to asymptomatic calcification (seen in 70 per cent of patients above 10 years of age), which can be seen on radiographic examination as bilateral bean-shaped opacities above the sella turcica.

Diagnosis is aided by a history of hoarseness from early childhood; thickening, stiffening, and difficulty in extrusion of the tongue; an impaired ability to swallow; characteristic involvement of the skin and mucous membranes; and histopathologic examination of involved tissue. Histologic features consist of thick homogeneous bands of eosinophilic, PAS-positive, hyaline-like amorphous material in the upper dermis, with an associated patchy distribution surrounding blood vessels, sweat glands, and arrector pili muscles.

Lipoid proteinosis has a chronic but relatively benign course. Treatment is chiefly symptomatic and consists of surgical removal of laryngeal nodules or tracheostomy for laryngeal obstruction and cosmetic measures such as dermabrasion or electrodesiccation and curettage for unappealing cutaneous lesions on the face or other exposed surfaces.

ERRORS OF METABOLISM

The Hyperlipidemias

The hyperlipidemias (hyperlipoproteinemias) represent a group of metabolic diseases characterized by persistent elevation of plasma cholesterol, triglycerides, or both. Since plasma lipids circulate in the form of high molecular weight complexes bound to protein, the term hyperlipidemia also indicates an elevation of lipoproteins, hence justification for introduction of the term hyperlipoproteinemia for this group of disorders.

Plasma lipoproteins differ significantly in electrostatic charges, thus permitting their separation by electrophoretic techniques into four major fractions (chylomicrons and beta-, prebeta-, and alpha-lipoproteins). By means of ultracentrifugation it is also possible to separate the plasma lipoproteins into four major groups (chylomicrons and very low density, low density, and high density lipoproteins), which correlate well with those separated by electrophoresis. These recently introduced techniques allow reclassification of the familial hyperlipidemias into five groups, designated as hyperlipoproteinemias I through V, each with its own specific clinicopathologic, prognostic, and therapeutic features.[58, 59, 60]

CLINICAL MANIFESTATIONS

Xanthomas. Xanthomas are lipid-containing papules, nodules, or tumors that may be found anywhere on the skin and mucous membranes. Although the mechanism of their formation is not completely understood, it appears that serum lipids infiltrate the tissues where they are phagocytized by macrophages (histiocytes) and deposited, particularly in areas subjected to stress and pressure. Although they may suggest the presence of hyperlipidemia and can provide clues to the underlying disorder, when seen alone they are not diagnostic. Complete clinical and biochemical evaluations, therefore, are required before the true nature of the underlying disorder can be determined.[61]

Depending on their gross appearance, anatomic location, and mode of development, xanthomas can be categorized as *plane, eruptive* or *papuloeruptive, tendinous,* or *tuberous.*

Plane Xanthomas. Soft, flat, macular or slightly elevated yellow to orange or brownish-yellow intracutaneous plaques, plane xanthomas are generally seen on the face, sides of the neck, upper trunk, elbows, and knees, but may occur anywhere on the body and have a marked predilection for surgical or acne scars and the palmar creases. The most frequently seen xanthomas are those that occur on or near the eyelids during middle age. Termed *xanthelasmas* or *xanthoma palpebrarum,* they rarely occur in children or adolescents. When present, however, they require studies for diabetes mellitus, Hand-Schüller-Christian disease, myeloma, and hepatic or liver disorders; a search for xanthomas elsewhere on the body; and an investigation of plasma lipids for evidence of familial hyperlipidemia. Although approximately two thirds of individuals with xanthelasma may have normal lipid levels, these cutaneous lesions may prove to be the first clues to the presence of hyperlipoproteinemia type II disease. If the physician is to prevent the vascular consequences of type II disease, it is helpful if the disorder is detected early. Lesions that develop in palmar creases and flexural surfaces of the fingers, termed *xanthoma striatum planum,* generally portend the presence of hepatic disease or familial hyperlipidemia (types II and III).

Papulo-Eruptive Xanthomas. Small red to yellow papular lesions that have an erythematous base, these lipoidal lesions appear in crops and consist of multiple small red to yellow-orange raised solid papules, sometimes surrounded by an erythematous halo at the base of the lesion. Although they may involve the trunk and oral mucosa, they have a predilection for sites subjected to pressure or trauma, particularly the extensor surfaces of the arms, legs, and buttocks. Papulo-eruptive xanthomas are almost always associated with hypertriglyceridemia and are generally seen in patients with uncontrolled diabetes mellitus, in mild diabetics who are asymptomatic yet have high triglyceride levels, or in patients with hyperlipoproteinemia types I, III, IV, and V (see Fig. 7–26).

Tendon Xanthomas. Multiple skin-colored or yellowish, smooth, freely movable subcutaneous nodules and tumors, these xanthomas have a predilection for the extensor tendons of the elbows, knees, heels, hands, and feet. These nontender, firm nodules measure 1 cm or more in diameter and are best seen or palpated on the Achilles tendon and the tendons on the dorsal aspect of the hands.

Tuberous Xanthomas. Large, firm, nodular or tumorous, sessile or pedunculated, flesh-colored or yellowish, tuberous xanthomas are lipid deposits that occur on extensor surfaces subject to stress or trauma, particularly the elbows, knees, hands, and buttocks. Located in the dermis and subcutaneous layers, they can enlarge to 5 cm or more in diameter and, in contrast to tendon xanthomas, are not attached to underlying structures. Generally associated with increased serum triglycerides (either on an acquired or familial basis), tuberous xanthomas are most frequently seen in association with types II, III, and IV lipoproteinemia.

Tendinous Xanthomas. Firm, subcutaneous papules or nodules, tendinous xanthomas have a predilection for the extensor tendons of the fingers, patellae, and elbows. They frequently occur in association with xanthelasma, tuberous lesions, and coronary atherosclerosis. Although they may occur in patients with hypertriglyceridemia, they generally indicate the presence of hypercholesterolemia and appear almost exclusively in familial lipoproteinemia types II and III.

CLASSIFICATION OF THE HYPERLIPOPROTEINEMIAS. The classification of the hyperlipidemic disorders is based upon the classification by Fredrickson and Lees. Based upon electrophoretic and ultracentrifugal analyses of serum lipoproteins, they are designated as type I, hyperchylomicronemia; type II, increased betalipoprotein; type III, increased beta- and prebetalipoprotein; type IV, increased prebetalipoprotein; and type V, combined hyperchylomicronemia and hyperprebetalipoproteinemia (of these, types I and II are the most commonly seen in childhood (see table 7–6.)[60]

Type I Hyperlipoproteinemia (Bürger-Grütz Disease). A rare autosomal recessive disorder, type I hyperlipoproteinemia is characterized by an elevation of fasting serum triglycerides carried in the form of chylomicrons. The defect in type I disease, expressed as soon as the infant takes fat, probably lies in the faulty removal of normal chylomicrons from the serum because of a deficiency of lipoprotein lipase activity. Hyperlipemia is usually discovered accidentally because of lactescence (manifested by a creamy or chocolate appearance of whole blood), or because of the appearance of xanthomas, bouts of abdominal pain, or hepatic and splenic enlargements. Occasionally the disease may be noted for the first time during examination of a patient presenting with severe abdominal pain and signs of peritoneal irritation.

Episodic abdominal pain, seen in approximately one-half of affected children, is very common and frequently manifested by clinical signs of acute abdominal distress. General malaise and anorexia are common, and abdominal spasm, rigidity, rebound tenderness, leukocytosis, and fever may be present. Sometimes, particularly in patients under the age of six years, the pain is caused by lipid accumulations in the liver and spleen. In others it may be due to splenic infarct or pancreatitis associated with this disorder.

About two-thirds of children with type I disease are seen with xanthomas which, in almost all cases, are of the eruptive type. They may appear at any site, including the mucous membranes, and are most commonly seen on the buttocks, thighs, arms, forearms, chest, back, and face. Xanthelasmas and tendinous xanthomas account for less than 2 per cent of the lesions seen in such patients. Eruptive xanthomas usually occur suddenly when the hyperlipemia is severe and resolve rapidly when the chylomicrons decrease after institution of a low fat diet.

Type II Hyperlipoproteinemia (Familial Hypercholesterolemia). Best understood and most important from a pediatric point of view, type II hyperlipoproteinemia is an autosomal dominant disorder characterized by cutaneous xanthomas, increased concentrations of plasma cholesterol, and a high incidence of coronary artery disease.

Seen in approximately 1 in 250 to 500 persons in the general population, there are two groups of patients with type II disease. In patients homozygous for this disorder plasma cholesterol levels are extremely high (often reaching 700 to 1000 mg/100 ml). Cutaneous xanthomas usually develop during childhood, often in the first years of life, and affected individuals frequently die of ischemic heart disease in their twenties and thirties. In a second group, affected persons are presumably heterozygous for this disorder. They develop tendon xanthomas (usually after age 30), and even though serum cholesterol levels are markedly ele-

vated, patients have a normal longevity without a significant increase in atherosclerosis and coronary heart disease.

Although the exact defect in type II disease is as yet not completely understood, it appears to be related to a derangement of cholesterol metabolism. Recent studies suggest deficiency of hydroxymethylglutaryl coenzyme A reductase (HMG-CoA reductase) with an associated defect in fibroblast cell receptors that bind betalipoproteins, with a resulting elevation of plasma betalipoprotein and cholesterol.[62]

Cutaneous xanthomas reportedly occur in 40 to 50 per cent of patients with type II disease. These include tendinous xanthomas in 40 to 50 per cent of cases, xanthelasmas in 23 per cent, and tuberous lesions in 10 to 15 per cent of affected individuals. Large pendulous tuberous xanthomas may occur in children with this disorder; eruptive xanthomas, however, are unusual.

Arcus cornea (also termed arcus lipoides or arcus juvenilis), consisting of lipid deposits of cholesterol, triglycerides, and phospholipids around the edge of the cornea, is commonly seen in association with this disease. The significance of arcus cornea depends upon the age of the patient. When seen in childhood, it is almost always a sign of hyperlipoproteinemia.

Table 7–6 THE HYPERLIPOPROTEINEMIAS

Type	Clinical Features	Biochemical Features	Inheritance
I (Bürger-Grütz)	Common in infancy and early teens Episodic abdominal pain Eruptive xanthomas Lipemic plasma Lipemia retinalis	Exogenous fat-induced hyperlipemia	Autosomal recessive
II (Familial hypercholesterolemia)	Onset in childhood or adulthood Crops of eruptive xanthomas, tendinous and tuberous xanthomas Xanthelasma Atherosclerosis and coronary disease	High cholesterol levels	Autosomal dominant
III (Broad beta disease)	Onset in adulthood (uncommon in childhood) Plane xanthomas in palmar creases A high incidence of cardiovascular disease	Endogenous hyperlipemia Abnormal glucose tolerance Increased cholesterol, betalipoproteins, and triglycerides	Autosomal recessive
IV (Familial hyperbetalipoproteinemia)	Unusual before age 20 Eruptive tuberous xanthomas on elbows, knees, heels, and wrists Obesity Hepatosplenomegaly Abdominal pain Lipemia retinalis Premature cardiovascular disease	Endogenous carbohydrate-induced hyperlipidemia Laboratory findings similar to those in type III	Autosomal recessive
V (Familial hyperchylomicronemia with hyperbetalipoproteinemia)	Combination of types I and IV Rare in childhood Eruptive, tuberous, and xanthomas Obesity Hepatosplenomegaly Lipemia retinalis	Exogenous and endogenous Increase in both chylomicrons and prebetalipoproteins	(?) Recessive inheritance

Type III Hyperlipoproteinemia (Familial Hyperbeta- and Prebetalipoproteinemia). Often referred to as "broad beta disease," type III hyperlipoproteinemia is an autosomal recessive disorder characterized by xanthomas, a high incidence of cardiovascular disease, frequent abnormal tolerance to glucose, and an increase in serum levels of both cholesterol and triglycerides. The precise nature of type III disease is unknown, but it appears to be associated with a disturbance in the clearance of remnant lipoproteins, with accumulations of both cholesterol and triglycerides. It is uncommon in childhood and nearly always first diagnosed in adulthood (usually around middle-age) (Fig. 7–26).

Electrophoresis of plasma proteins shows a broad beta band. Seventy-five to 80 per cent of patients with this disorder have xanthomas. They may include the full range of xanthomatous lesions from eruptive xanthomas to tendinous nodules. Soft planar xanthomas (striatum palmare) in the palmar creases are a very common feature of familial type III hyperlipoproteinemia. However, since they may also be seen in individuals with the type II disorder and in patients with liver disease, they are not an exclusive feature of type III hyperlipoproteinemia. Atherosclerotic vascular complications are common in patients with type III disease. Although both coronary and peripheral artery diseases may occur, the latter are relatively more common in patients with type III as compared to type II forms of this disorder.

Type IV Disease (Familial Hyperbetalipoproteinemia). The most common form of familial hyperlipoproteinemia, type IV, is an endogenous carbohydrate-induced disorder (in contrast to type I, which is fat-induced). Characterized by obesity and elevation of serum prebetalipoproteins, type IV disease may be familial or acquired. The familial type appears to be inherited as an autosomal dominant disease. Usually not seen before the age of 20 years, type IV hyperlipoproteinemia may appear in children with renal disease or in diabetics who have become ketotic. The cutaneous lesions seen with this disorder are eruptive, tuberous, and palmar in distribution. Cardiovascular disease is extremely common and hepatosplenomegaly, abdominal pain, and lipemia retinalis may occur.[60]

Type V Disease (Familial Hyperchylomicronemia with Hyperprebetalipoproteinemia). A combination of type I and type IV disease, type V is a complex abnormality of both endogenous and exogenous origin characterized by increased concentrations of both chylomicrons and prebetalipoproteins. Although the exact mode of inheritance is still unclear, it appears to be a recessive disorder. Patients are usually obese, and their lipemia is often discovered in late adolescence or early adulthood because of the eruptive xanthomas, hepatosplenomegaly, and acute abdominal crises similar to those seen in individuals with type I disease. Although type V hyperlipoproteinemia may have its onset in adolescence, it has only rarely been reported in childhood.[63]

Tangier Disease

Tangier disease (familial high density lipoprotein deficiency) is a unique rare heritable disorder characterized by hypocholesterolemia, an almost complete absence of plasma high density lipoprotein (HDL), and storage of cholesterol esters in many tissues of the body. Seen in children as well as adults, it derives its name from the Chesapeake Bay Island home of the first two patients described with this disorder.

The biochemical defect of Tangier disease is uncertain but appears to be related to a defect in the synthesis of high density lipoprotein associated with a double dose of a rare mutant gene. The clinical manifestations include hypocholesterolemia (50 to 125 mg per 100 ml) and low phospholipid levels in association with normal or slightly elevated triglycerides (150 to 250 mg per 100 ml) and enlarged tonsils with distinctive alternating bands of red, orange, or yellowish-white striations overlying the normal red mucosa. Lipid deposits may be accompanied by a persistent maculopapular eruption over the trunk and abdomen, hepatosplenomegaly, lymph node enlargement, infiltration of the cornea in adults, and alterations in the intestinal and rectal mucosa. Several patients have had recurrent peripheral neuropathy.

The prognosis in Tangier disease is unknown. Children may have no detectable abnormality except in the tonsils and plasma. Adults, however,

Figure 7–26 Eruptive xanthomas on the knee in a 13-year old child with type III lipoproteinemia (Department of Dermatology, Yale University School of Medicine).

have shown more extensive cholesterol ester deposition in the rectal mucosa, skin, and cornea.[60]

The Mucopolysaccharidoses

The mucopolysaccharidoses are inherited disorders of mucopolysaccharide metabolism characterized by widespread accumulation of mucopolysaccharide (the major component in the ground substance of connective tissue) in tissues and cultured skin fibroblasts, with excessive excretion in the urine.[64] First described by Hunter in 1917 (and labeled "gargoylism" in 1936), these disorders can now be divided into at least six somewhat related clinical entities on the basis of their clinical features, their mode of inheritance, and the nature of the accumulated mucopolysaccharide.[64, 65, 66]

Although the precise biochemical defect is still not well understood, current evidence suggests a deficiency of beta-galactosidase, leading to abnormal accumulation of mucopolysaccharides in cells of the connective tissue and many organs.[66] The usual distinguishing features of the various syndromes of mucopolysaccharidosis (MPS), therefore, are based on the presence or degree of somatic and skeletal involvement, mental retardation, corneal clouding, cardiopulmonary changes, hepatosplenomegaly, and hearing loss, and on the mode of inheritance and the nature of their accumulated polysaccharides (Table 7-7). The Hunter syndrome (MPS II) is an X-linked recessive disorder; all others are autosomal recessive. They can be differentiated from the mucolipidoses, a group of disorders characterized by an accumulation of sphingolipids or glycolipids in the visceral and mesenchymal cells, which exhibit clinical and skeletal signs of the mucopolysaccharidoses but differ from them by the normal urinary excretion of uronic acid containing acid mucopolysaccharides (with the exception of mucosulfatidosis), and by the presence of clinical features usually seen in the sphingolipidoses (Niemann-Pick disease and Gaucher disease).[31]

The cutaneous changes of all six forms of mucopolysaccharidosis consist of pale, coarse, and dry skin with hirsutism, especially over the back and extremities, and thickened, roughened, taut inelastic skin, especially over the fingers.

Hurler Syndrome. The most common of the mucopolysaccharidoses, Hurler syndrome (mucopolysaccharidosis I-H, MPS I in McKusick's original classification), is the classic prototype of this group of disorders. Seen in approximately 1 out of 100,000 births, it appears in the first year of life and is a particularly grave disorder, with demise occurring in almost all cases before the age of 10 years. Death, when it occurs, is usually associated with cardiac failure or respiratory infection.

Cardinal features of the Hurler syndrome include coarsening of facial features; macrocephaly with frontal bulging; premature closure of the sutures, with hyperostosis frequently leading to a scaphocephalic skull; flattened nasal bridge with a saddle-shaped appearance; hypertelorism; protuberant tongue; short neck; protuberant abdomen

Table 7-7   THE MUCOPOLYSACCHARIDOSES

Syndromes	Clinical Features	Biochemical Features	Inheritance
Hurler (MPS I–H)	Severe retardation Corneal clouding Hepatosplenomegaly Chondrodystrophy Dwarfism Grave manifestations and early demise	Chondroitin sulfate B, heparan monosulfate Excessive urinary excretion of dermatan sulfate and heparan sulfate	Autosomal recessive
Scheie (MPS I–S; formerly MSP V)	Corneal clouding Severe osteochondro-dystrophy Aortic incompetence Retinitis pigmentosa	Keratosulfate Excessive urinary excretion of dermatan sulfate and heparan sulfate	Autosomal recessive
Hunter (MPS II)	Less severe than Hurler Longer survival Lack of corneal involvement Cutaneous markers over scapula, posterior axilla, or thigh Atypical retinitis pigmentosa	Chondroitin sulfate B, heparan monosulfate	X-linked recessive
Sanfilippo (MPS III)	Aggressive behavior Severe neurologic involvement Mild somatic changes	Heparitin monosulfate Excessive urinary excretion of heparan sulfate	Autosomal recessive
Morquio (MPS IV)	Normal intelligence Striking dwarfism Corneal opacity Severe osteoporosis and atlanto-axial dislocation	Chondroitin sulfate B Marked urinary excretion of keratin sulfate and chondroitin sulfate	Autosomal recessive
Maroteaux-Lamy (MPS VI)	Normal intelligence Dwarfism Severe corneal and bony lesions	Chondroitin sulfate B Increased urinary excretion of dermatan sulfate	Autosomal recessive

due to hepatic and splenic enlargement; deformity of the chest; shortness of the spine; laxity of the abdominal wall with inguinal and umbilical hernias; broad hands with stubby fingers; a claw hand due to stiffening of the phalangeal joints; and limitation of extensibility of the joints. Although the majority of infants are normal or above normal in length during the first year of life, growth rate decreases by two years of age. By age three almost all patients are below the 3rd percentile for stature. Clouding of the cornea develops in all patients with Hurler syndrome. On inspection this feature is most apparent if light is shone on the cornea from the side (slit lamp examination confirms the finding).[31, 34]

Diagnosis is based upon the clinical picture and identification of excessive mucopolysaccharides in the urine by the toluidine blue test and the gross albumin turbidity test. Routine histopathologic examination of the skin shows vacuolization of the cytoplasm in some of the epidermal cells (due to mucopolysaccharide), with displacement of the nucleus to one side, and occasional solitary swollen cells at all levels of the epidermis. Large vacuolated mononuclear cells ("gargoyle cells") are present beneath the basement membrane as well as in the periappendageal and perivascular areas.

As yet there is no effective definitive treatment of mucopolysaccharidosis. Although initial reports of beneficial effects from plasma infusions were exciting and promising, subsequent studies indicate no clinical or biochemical results from this technique.[67, 68] Prenatal diagnosis of the mucopolysaccharidoses is now possible through the study of cultured amniotic fluid cells and the amniotic fluid itself. The clinical course of patients is usually progressively downhill, with death in those with the fully expressed syndrome from either respiratory infection or cardiac failure, generally before the age of ten years.[34]

Scheie Syndrome. Originally considered to be a distinctive form of mucopolysaccharidosis, the Scheie syndrome (mucopolysaccharidosis I-S, formerly MPS V) now appears to represent a variant of the Hurler syndrome (MPS 1-H). It is characterized by stiff joints, coarse facies, corneal clouding, excessive body hair, retinitis pigmentosa, aortic regurgitation, few other somatic effects, and normal intellect. Patients with Scheie syndrome excrete excessive amounts of dermatan sulfate and heparan sulfate. The Hurler and Scheie syndromes, despite their striking clinical differences, are similar by fibroblast culture. They both are corrected by the Hurler factor and both show deficiency of the same enzyme, alpha-L-iduronidase.

Hunter Syndrome. The Hunter syndrome (mucopolysaccharidosis II, MPS II) is distinguished from the Hurler syndrome by an X-linked recessive inheritance, longer survival, lack of corneal clouding, characteristic cutaneous markers, and a different pattern of mucopolysaccharide excretion (chondroitin sulfate B and heparitin sul-

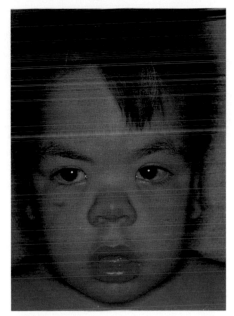

Figure 7–27 Coarse facial features in a child with Hunter syndrome (Mucopolysaccharidosis II).

fate). The clinical picture in all respects is generally less severe than that seen in the Hurler syndrome (Fig. 7–27). Mental retardation progresses at a slower rate, humping of the lumbar area (gibbus) does not occur, and progressive deafness is a frequent feature. Hearing loss is present in about 50 per cent of patients with Hunter syndrome, and children are often brought to a physician at about three years of age because of lack of speech. Although deafness also occurs in the Hurler syndrome (MPS I), severe mental retardation and death at an early age cause it to be a relatively inconspicuous feature of this disorder.

Distinctive cutaneous changes are highly characteristic of MPS II (Hunter syndrome) and probably represent a marker of this disorder. These pathognomonic lesions consist of firm flesh-colored to ivory-white papules and nodules that often coalesce to form ridges or a reticular pattern in symmetrical areas between the angles of the scapulae and posterior axillary lines, the pectoral ridges, the nape of the neck, and/or the lateral aspects of the upper arms and thighs (Fig. 7–28). They appear before age 10 and can spontaneously disappear. Although a reliable marker when present, the majority of cases reported with this syndrome fail to mention this finding, so the precise incidence of this cutaneous feature is unknown.[69]

Sanfilippo Syndrome. The Sanfilippo syndrome (MPS III) is an autosomal recessive disorder characterized by aggressive behavior, severe mental retardation, coarse hair, coarse immobile facies, and relatively less severe somatic changes than those seen in MPS I and MPS II. Thickening of the skin and subcutaneous tissues produces coarse features, with prominent eyebrows, thickened nares, thick lips, and a lack of

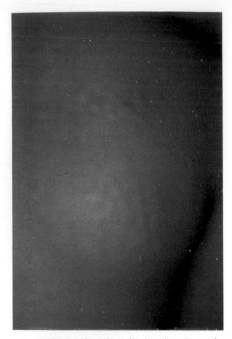

Figure 7–28 Distinctive, firm flesh-colored papules and nodules in a reticular pattern on the shoulder and scapular area (a cutaneous marker of Hunter syndrome, MPS II).

expressive facial movement.[70, 71] The hair is coarse and loss of extension of the interphalangeal joints of the hands develops, but not to a degree sufficient to cause the typical claw hand deformities seen in patients with Hurler and Hunter syndromes. When the diagnosis is indeterminate, examination of urinary mucopolysaccharides reveals excessive excretion of heparan sulfate (the only mucopolysaccharide excreted in excessive amounts in this disorder).[34]

Morquio Syndrome. The Morquio syndrome (MPS IV) is an autosomal recessive disorder characterized by normal intelligence, striking dwarfism (usually not apparent until the child reaches two or three years of age), and distinctive skeletal findings with marked osteoporosis of all bones. Usually the joints are not stiff. A barrel chest with pigeon breast (pectus carinatum) deformity, relatively short trunk and neck, an appearance of disproportionately long extremities, and looseness of some joints are characteristic features. Marked excretion of keratan sulfate and chondroitin sulfate A (about two or three times greater than normal) in the urine is a characteristic feature during childhood in patients with the Morquio syndrome. These findings, however, slowly decrease, reaching normal levels during adulthood.[31]

Maroteaux-Lamy Syndrome. Mucopolysaccharidosis VI (Maroteaux-Lamy syndrome) is an autosomal recessive disorder characterized by dwarfism, coarse facies, clouding of the corneas (frequently with severe impairment of vision), severe osseous changes, flexion contractures of the

hands, normal intellect, and increased urinary excretion of dermatan sulfate. No estimates as to its incidence exist (owing in part to the fact that this syndrome has only recently been delineated). Most authorities, however, consider this disorder to be extremely rare.[72]

The Mucolipidoses

The mucolipidoses are a group of disorders that exhibit clinical and skeletal signs of the mucopolysaccharidoses and clinical features seen in patients with sphingolipidoses. This group includes three disorders specifically termed mucolipidosis I, II, and III, gangliosidosis, juvenile sulfatidosis, fucosidosis, mannosidosis, and, perhaps, lipogranulomatosis.

Mucolipidosis I. Mucolipidosis I (lipomucopolysaccharidosis) is an autosomal recessive disorder characterized by mild Hurler-like clinical manifestations, moderate progressive mental retardation, skeletal changes of dysostosis multiplex, normal urinary mucopolysaccharide excretion, and coarse refringent inclusions in cultured fibroblasts similar to but without the clear perinuclear halo of those seen in mucolipidosis II.

Mucolipidosis II. Mucolipidosis II (MLII, I-cell disease) is an autosomal recessive Hurler-like disorder characterized by small orbits and prominent eyes, puffy and swollen eyelids, a pattern of tortuous veins around the orbits, fullness of the lower part of the face, full rounded cheeks that appear flushed because of many fine telangiectases, a prominent maxilla (which produces a fishmouth appearance), gingival hypertrophy, a severe type of dysostosis multiplex, short neck, thick and rigid skin (particularly on the ears and neck), stiffness of all joints with considerable reduction in range of motion, and death, usually due to severe respiratory infection and cardiac failure at about four years of age.

Mucolipidosis II can be distinguished from the Hurler syndrome by the presence of hypertrophic gums, vacuolated lymphocytes in the peripheral blood, striking inclusions ("I-cell disease" refers to these) in fibroblast cultures from cutaneous biopsy, normal urinary mucopolysaccharide excretion, and a 10- to 100-fold increase in the specific activity of several plasma acid hydrolases.[73, 74] Prenatal diagnosis of this disorder can be confirmed by enzyme assays of amniotic fluid.[75]

Mucolipidosis III. Mucolipidosis III (pseudo-Hurler polydystrophy) is an autosomal recessive disorder characterized by mental retardation, early restriction of joint mobility, and normal mucopolysacchariduria. Children with this disorder usually present at or about the age of three years, with stiffness of the joints as the main complaint.[75] The facies is variable, but most patients have coarse facies, short stature, fine ground-glass corneal clouding, and a moderate degree of mental retardation with I.Q.'s of 65 to 85. Aortic valve disease is present in most patients with this disorder.

GM₁ Gangliosidosis. GM₁ gangliosidosis, caused by generalized accumulation of GM₁ ganglioside due to a beta galactosidase deficiency, is characterized by coarse facies with depressed nasal bridge, full cheeks and puffy eyelids, corneal clouding, cherry-red macules, kyphoscoliosis, roentgenographic changes of dysostosis multiplex, hepatosplenomegaly, marked psychomotor retardation, progressive cerebral deterioration, and death usually before the age of two years. Features resembling the mucopolysaccharidoses include bone changes, hepatosplenomegaly, and corneal clouding. Those suggesting a sphingolipidosis include large head, cherry-red spot of the macula, and progressive neurologic deterioration.

Juvenile Sulfatidosis. Juvenile sulfatidosis with mucopolysacchariduria (also called the Austin type of leukodystrophy) is a very rare Hurler-like disorder characterized by mild Hurler-like features, slowly progressive neurologic deterioration that begins in the second year of life, and death, generally in the early teens.[20]

"Stiff Skin" Syndrome

A unique combination of skin and joint defects, presumably a form of focal mucopolysaccharidosis, termed the *stiff skin syndrome* has been reported in four patients.[76] This disorder is characterized by localized areas of stony-hard skin, mild hirsutism, limited mobility of various joints, and normal urinary mucopolysaccharide excretion. In one patient the areas of skin with less severe involvement had a cobblestone appearance suggestive of that occurring in patients with the Hunter type of mucopolysaccharidosis.

Although the exact nature of this disorder is unknown, the presence of abnormal amounts of hyaluronidase-digestible acid mucopolysaccharide in the dermis, as well as an increase in cytoplasmic metachromatic material in cultured fibroblasts, suggests a focal abnormality of mucopolysaccharide metabolism. The presence of this constellation of findings in a mother and her two children suggests a heritable disorder of the autosomal dominant type. The fact that the siblings were the progeny of a consanguineous marriage between cousins, however, cannot exclude an autosomal recessive pattern of inheritance.

Marfan Syndrome

The Marfan syndrome is a heritable disorder of connective tissue characterized by excessive length of long bones, ocular defects (particularly ectopia lentis), and cardiovascular defects. Inherited as an autosomal dominant trait with a high degree of penetrance and variable expressivity, it has an estimated prevalence of about 1.5 per 100,000 population. Although the nature of the basic defect is not known, increased urinary hydroxyproline excretion suggests a defect in the elastic tissue fiber of the connective tissue.[31, 91]

The chief manifestations of the Marfan syndrome are skeletal, ocular, and cardiovascular. Patients with this disorder are often tall, and the extremities are long (Fig. 7–29). The arm span characteristically is greater than the height, and after puberty the lower segment (pubis to sole) measurement is greater than that of the upper segment (vertex to pubis). Arachnodactyly, hyperextensible joints, kyphoscoliosis, pectus excavatus, and flat feet are commonly seen in patients with this disorder. At times the great toes are elongated out of proportion to the others; the skull and face are elongated; and dolichocephaly, frontal bossing, high arched palate, and large deformed ears are frequently seen.

Ocular abnormalities consist of ectopia lentis (the hallmark of ocular involvement seen in 50 to 70 per cent of patients), myopia, heterochromia iridis, and retinal detachment. Cardiovascular defects, due to a defect in the media of the great vessels, consist of aneurysmal dilatation of the ascending aorta, dilatation of the aortic rings with aortic insufficiency, and dilatation of the mitral rings with mitral regurgitation. Contrary to previous emphasis, mental retardation is not a component of this syndrome. Studies suggest that Abraham Lincoln had Marfan syndrome, and studies of some of his relatives show evidence of this disease or a form fruste of it.[77] Cutaneous changes include a pronounced sparsity of subcutaneous fat, striae (particularly over the pectoral and deltoid regions,

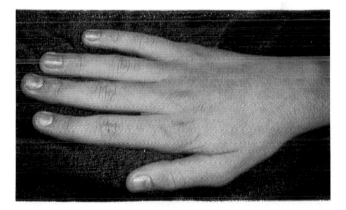

Figure 7–29 Arachnodactyly. Characteristic long fingers in a patient with marfanoid features. This patient had multiple mucosal neuroma syndrome (Chapter 18).

the thighs, and abdomen), and elastosis perforans serpiginosa.

The prognosis depends upon the extent and severity of cardiovascular defects. Dissection of the aorta, a frequent cause of death in children as well as adults, is common during the first decade of life and is most commonly seen during the thirties. Survival beyond the fifth decade is unusual. Although there is no specific treatment, propranolol (Inderal) has been shown to decrease myocardial contractility and to reduce the abruptness of ventricular ejection, thus limiting the progression of aortic dilatation. Surgical replacement of the aortic or mitral valve and excision of aortic aneurysms have been successful in some patients. Orthopedic surgery with casts and fusion have been beneficial for patients with kyphoscoliosis, and aspiration techniques appear to give improved results when lens extraction is necessary because of glaucoma or serious visual impairment.

Homocystinuria

Homocystinuria is an autosomal recessive disorder of methionine metabolism related to an absence or deficiency of hepatic cystathionine synthetase, the enzyme that catalyzes the formation of cystathionine from homocystine and serine. It is characterized by ectopia lentis, arachnodactyly, chest and spinal deformities as seen in the Marfan syndrome, seizures, developmental retardation, cerebrovascular accidents, and increased urinary excretion of homocystine.

The typical appearance of affected individuals usually develops during the first or second year of life. It consists of sparse, light or blond, easily friable hair; malar flush; a coarse, wide-pore appearance of the facial skin; and erythematous blotches on the skin of the face and extremities suggestive of livedo reticularis.

Mental retardation, generalized osteoporosis, and arterial and venous thromboses are features of homocystinuria not found in patients with the Marfan syndrome. Glaucoma is a frequent complication in patients with homocystinuria as well as in patients with the Marfan syndrome. Most homocystinuric patients are myopic, and ectopia lentis is seen in 90 per cent of patients. It has been recognized as early as eighteen months of age and is invariably present in older children. A curious difference between homocystinuria and the Marfan syndrome is the fact that the dislocation is generally congenital and upward in the Marfan syndrome, but acquired, downward, and progressive in patients with homocystinuria.

Presence of homocystinuria is suggested by the clinical features and may be confirmed by a urinary cyanide-nitroprusside test and by amino acid chromatography of the serum and urine. Therapy consists of a low methionine diet with cystine supplement and vitamin B_6 (pyridoxine, a cofactor for cystathionine synthetase) in dosages of 50 to 300 mg/day.[78, 79]

Phenylketonuria

Phenylketonuria (PKU, phenylpyruvic oligophrenia) is an autosomal recessive disorder characterized by mental retardation, diffuse hypopigmentation, seizures, an eczematoid dermatitis, and photosensitivity. A defect in phenylalanine hydroxylase, the enzyme that converts phenylalanine to tyrosine, is responsible for the disease.

Ninety per cent of affected infants are blond, blue eyed, and fair skinned. A peculiar musty odor, attributable to decomposition products (phenylacetic acid or phenylacetaldehyde) in the urine and sweat is characteristic and by itself often suggests the diagnosis. Infants appear to be normal at birth and develop the first manifestations of delayed intellectual development sometime between 4 and 24 months of age. Skeletal changes associated with this disorder include microcephaly, short stature, pes planus, and syndactyly. Eczematous dermatitis appears in 10 to 50 per cent of patients, and affected individuals may have sclerodermatous skin lesions. While many have a typical flexural distribution of atopic dermatitis, others have an ill-defined, poorly described eczematous dermatitis that follows no specific pattern.

The diagnosis of phenylketonuria depends upon the demonstration of elevated serum levels of phenylalanine (10 to 50 times that of normal) or elevated urinary levels of phenylpyruvic acid. The latter can be detected by a characteristic green or blue color that results when a few drops of urine are added to a 10 per cent solution of ferric chloride. False positive results and the technical difficulty occasionally associated with obtaining urine from infants have led to the Phenistix tape test, which utilizes a paper strip impregnated with buffered ferric ammonia sulfate.

Dietary management consists of a diet low in phenylalanine content. Appropriate diets should be started at as early an age as possible. This can be initiated by the use of Lofenalac (Mead-Johnson), a casein hydrolysate formula from which most of the phenylalanine has been removed. When kept on appropriate restriction of phenylalanine, the patient becomes free of seizures, the electroencephalogram reverts to normal, the eczema clears, and the skin and hair regain their normal color. The effect of treatment on intellectual function depends upon the age at which therapy is initiated. With initiation of appropriate therapy prior to six weeks to two months of age, normal mental development usually can be achieved. With delay in therapy beyond this period the beneficial effect is lessened and when initiated after $2\frac{1}{2}$ years of age, little benefit can be achieved.

Present evidence indicates that the final intelligence quotient is significantly higher if the average phenylalanine levels are kept in a range of 5 to 15 mg/ml. Since overtreatment with resulting phenylalanine deficiency is now a well-recognized hazard, blood phenylalanine levels should be determined at regular intervals — once or twice a week for the first months, perhaps every other week until six months of age, and, as the child's growth rate slows, monitoring at monthly intervals until the diet is discontinued.

As yet there is no agreement as to how long the low phenylalanine diet should be continued. In recent years many physicians have discontinued the diet when the patient reached 4 to 6 years of age. There is some evidence that after this age the intellectual level is maintained, presumably as a result of the fact that the brain has completed the critical growth phase during which it is sensitive to damage by elevated levels of phenylalanine and its metabolites. Long-term studies, however, are required in order to determine whether or not differences in intelligence quotients and behavior exist between groups whose treatment was terminated after the first four years of life and those on continued low phenylalanine diets.[80]

References

1. Wells RS, Kerr CB: Genetic classification of ichthyosis. Arch. Dermatol. 92:1–6, 1965.

   Genetic classification and a rational basis for the differentiation of various forms of ichthyosis.

2. Frost P, Van Scott EJ: Ichthyosiform dermatoses. Arch. Dermatol. 94:113–126, 1966.

   Separation of the ichthyoses on the basis of clinical and histologic features and observations of cellular kinetics.

3. Frost P, Weinstein GD, Bothwell JW, et al.: Ichthyosiform dermatoses, III. Studies of epidermal water loss. Arch. Dermatol. 98:230–233, 1968.

   Increased transepidermal water loss due to inefficient barrier function of the stratum corneum.

4. Lyon MF: Sex chromatin and genetic action in the mammalian X-chromosome. Am. J. Hum. Genet. 14:135–148, 1962.

   Formulation of an hypothesis that either of the two X chromosomes may be inactivated in different cells of the same animal early in the development, thus leading to partial phenotypic expression of an X-linked disorder.

5. Wells RS, Kerr CB: Clinical features of autosomal dominant and sex-linked ichthyosis in an English population. Brit. Med. J. 1:947–950, 1966.

   Separation of sex-linked ichthyosis from the autosomal dominant form of ichthyosis vulgaris.

6. Shapiro LJ, Weiss R, Webster D, et al.: X-linked ichthyosis due to steroid sulphatase deficiency. Lancet 1:70–74, 1978.

   An assay of cultured fibroblasts identified several individuals with 3 beta-hydroxysteroid-sulphatase deficiency. All patients with this inborn error of metabolism had clinically apparent ichthyosis and a family history of this skin disorder compatible with an X-linked inheritance.

7. Sever RJ, Frost P, Weinstein G: Eye changes in ichthyosis. JAMA 206:2283–2286, 1968.

   Corneal opacities on slit lamp examination of the eye help distinguish affected males and female carriers of X-linked ichthyosis.

8. Lentz CL, Altman J: Lamellar ichthyosis. The natural course of collodion baby. Arch. Dermatol. 97:3–13, 1968.

   Lamellar exfoliation of the newborn (the collodion baby) as an early stage of lamellar ichthyosis.

9. Mirrer E, McGuire JS: Lamellar ichthyosis — response to retinoic acid (tretinoin). A case report. Arch. Dermatol. 102:548–551, 1972.

   Dramatic response of lamellar ichthyosis to tretinoin (vitamin A acid).

10. Esterly NB: The ichthyosiform dermatoses. Pediatrics 42:990–1004, 1968.

    An overview of the ichthyoses.

11. Klaus S, Weinstein GD, Frost P: Localized epidermolytic hyperkeratosis. A form of keratoderma of the palms and soles. Arch. Dermatol. 101:272–275, 1970.

    A histopathologic relationship between epidermolytic hyperkeratosis and some forms of keratoderma.

12. Craig JM, Goldsmith LA, Baden H: An abnormality of keratin in the harlequin fetus. Pediatrics 46:437–440, 1970.

    X-ray diffraction analysis of the stratum corneum of a harlequin fetus revealed the presence of an unusual fibrous protein (cross-beta fibrous protein).

13. Buxbaum MM, Goodkin PE, Fahrenbach WH, et al.: Harlequin ichthyosis with epidermal lipid abnormality. Arch. Dermatol. 115:189–193, 1979.

    Histochemical, biochemical, and electron microscopic changes in the epidermis of a child with harlequin ichthyosis who survived for 9 months suggest a defect in epidermal lipid metabolism as the biochemical abnormality in the skin of patients with harlequin ichthyosis.

14. Esterly NB: Harlequin fetus. In Demis DJ, Dobson RL, McGuire J (eds.): Clinical Dermatology, Vol. 1. Harper and Row, Hagerstown, Md., 1977, 1:25, 1–3.

    In this severe form of congenital ichthyosis death usually occurs in utero or during the neonatal period.

15. Gewirtzman GB, Winkler NW, Dobson RL: Erythrokeratodermia variabilis. A family study. Arch. Dermatol. 114:259–261, 1978.

    Studies of erythrokeratodermia variabilis in a family with 12 involved members in five generations.

16. Hurwitz S, Kirsch N, McGuire J: Re-evaluation of ichthyosis and hair shaft abnormalities. Arch. Dermatol. 103:266–271, 1971.

    A patient with ichthyosis linearis circumflexa and a reappraisal of Netherton's syndrome, ichthyosis, and hair shaft abnormalities.

17. Herndon JH Jr, Steinberg D, Uhlendorf BS, et al.: Refsum's disease: characterization of the enzyme defect in cell culture. J. Clin. Invest. 48:1017–1032, 1969.

    Patients with Refsum's disease appear to be deficient in alpha-decarboxylase and therefore accumulate phytanic acid in their serum and tissues.

18. Ewing JA: The association of oligophrenia and dyskeratosis. A clinical investigation and an inquiry into its implications. Part III. The syndrome of Rud. Am. J. Ment. Defic. 10:575–581, 1955.

    A review of 6 cases in the literature and 5 personal cases of Rud's syndrome.

19. Sjögren T, Larsson T: A clinical and genetic study. Oligophrenia in combination with congenital ichthyosis and spastic disorders. Acta Psychiatr. Neurol. Scand. 32(Suppl. 113):9–112, 1957.

    All cases of this disorder appear to be explained by mutation of a recessive gene that occurred in a heterozygote in Nothern Sweden in the fourteenth century.

20. Bodian EL: Skin manifestations of Conradi's disease. Chondrodystrophia congenita punctata. Arch. Dermatol. 94:743–748, 1966.

    A review of Conradi's disease and report of a newborn with classic features of this disorder.

21. Spranger JW, Opitz JM, Bidder U: Heterogeneity of chondrodysplasia punctata. Humangenetik. 11:190–212, 1971.

    A review of reported cases of chondrodysplasia punctata and categorization of the disorder into two major forms with different modes of inheritance, radiologic changes, and prognosis.

22. Edidin DV, Esterly NB, Bamzai AK, et al.: Chondrodysplasia punctata. Conradi-Hünerman syndrome. Arch. Dermatol. *113*:1431–1434, 1977.

Report of a ten-year-old girl with chondrodysplasia punctata and a review of the characteristic findings seen in this disorder.

23. Baden HP, Alper JC: A keratolytic gel containing salicylic acid in propylene glycol. J. Invest. Dermatol. *61*:330–333, 1973.

A formulation of a gelling agent, propylene glycol, ethanol, and 6 per cent salicylic acid in distilled water is shown to be very effective in a variety of disorders with hyperkeratosis.

24. Van Scott J, Yu RJ: Control of keratinization with alpha-hydroxy acids and related compounds. 1. Topical treatment of ichthyotic disorders. Arch. Dermatol. *110*:586–590, 1974.

Topical preparations containing alpha-hydroxy acids and closely related compounds in the management of ichthyosiform dermatoses.

25. Frost, P, Weinstein GD: Topical administration of vitamin A acid for ichthyosiform dermatoses and psoriasis. JAMA *207*:1863–1868, 1969.

Topical vitamin A acid (tretinoin, retinoic acid) is helpful in the management of disorders associated with epidermal cell hyperplasia (psoriasis, lamellar ichthyosis, and epidermolytic hyperkeratosis).

26. Peck GL, Yoder FW: Treatment of lamellar ichthyosis and other keratinizing dermatoses with an oral synthetic retinoid. Lancet *2*:1172–1174, 1976.

Of 13 patients with various keratinizing dermatoses treated for 2 to 17 weeks with oral 13-*cis* retinoic acid, there was near complete clearing in all 5 patients with lamellar ichthyosis, in 2 of 3 patients with Darier's disease, and in 1 patient with pityriasis rubra pilaris.

27. Scriver CR, Solomons CC, Davies E, et al.: A molecular abnormality of keratin in ectodermal dysplasia. J. Pediatr. *67*:946, 1965.

Studies suggest a genetic mutation of keratin synthesis and abnormal S-S linkage as the cause of ectodermal dysplasia.

28. Reed WB, Lopez DA, Landing B: Clinical spectrum of anhidrotic ectodermal dysplasia. Arch. Dermatol. *102*:134–143, 1970.

Three patients and a review of anhidrotic ectodermal dysplasia.

29. Fisher M, Schneider R: Aplasia cutis congenita in three successive generations. Arch. Dermatol. *108*:252–253, 1973.

Three cases of aplasia cutis congenita in three successive generations of one family suggest an autosomal dominant mode of inheritance.

30. Hodgman JE, Mathies AW, Levan NE: Congenital scalp defects in twin sisters. Am. J. Dis. Child. *110*:293–294, 1965.

A defect in embryologic development is suggested as the cause of aplasia cutis congenita.

31. Gorlin RJ, Pindborg JJ, Cohen MM Jr: Syndromes of the Head and Neck, 2nd edition. McGraw-Hill, New York, 1976.

A complete compendium of syndromes and associated features involving the head and neck.

32. Hashimoto K, diBella RJ: Electron microscopic studies of normal and abnormal elastic fibers of the skin. J. Invest. Dermatol. *48*:405–423, 1967.

Ultrastructural studies of elastic tissue and collagen in pseudoxanthoma elasticum.

33. Jansen LH: The structure of connective tissue, an explanation of symptoms of Ehlers-Danlos syndrome. Dermatologica *110*:108–120, 1955.

Electron microscopy demonstrates the defect in Ehlers-Danlos syndrome to be due to a loose "wicker-work" weave of collagen.

34. McKusick VA: Heritable Disorders of Connective Tissue, 4th edition. C.V. Mosby Company, St. Louis, 1972.

A complete reference on connective tissue diseases and their genetic aspects.

35. Pope FM, Martin GR, McKusick VA: Inheritance of Ehlers-Danlos type IV syndrome. J. Med. Genet. *14*:200–204, 1977.

Biochemical studies of tissues from 5 patients with type IV Ehlers-Danlos syndrome reveal a lack of type III collagen in the tissues.

36. Pope FM, Martin GR, Lichtenstein JR, et al.: Patients with Ehlers-Danlos syndrome type IV lack type III collagen. Proc. Natl. Acad. Sci., U.S.A., 72:1314–1316, 1975.

Studies suggest that the fragile skin, blood vessels, and intestines of patients with type IV Ehlers-Danlos disease result from an absence of type III collagen.

37. Beighton P, Murdoch JL, Votteler T: Gastro-intestinal complications of the Ehlers-Danlos syndrome. Gut *10*:1004–1008, 1969.

Hernias, gastrointestinal bleeding, and rare bowel perforation are seen as complications in patients with Ehlers-Danlos syndrome.

38. Sulica VI, Cooper PH, Pope MF, et al.: Cutaneous histologic features in Ehlers-Danlos syndrome. Study of 21 patients. Arch. Dermatol. *115*:40–42, 1979.

On the basis of skin biopsies from 21 patients with Ehlers-Danlos syndrome it appears that histologic examination does not allow separation of the various types of this disorder.

39. Goltz RW, Hult AM, Goldfarb M, et al.: Cutis laxa: manifestations of generalized elastolysis. Arch. Dermatol. *92*:373–387, 1965.

A decrease in serum elastase inhibitor appears to cause increased fragmentation of elastic fibers in patients with cutis laxa.

40. Maxwell E, Esterly NB: Cutis laxa. Am. J. Dis. Child. *117*:479–482, 1969.

Differentiation of cutis laxa from Ehlers-Danlos syndrome and a review of the internal manifestations of cutis laxa.

41. Goodman RM, Smith EW, Paton D, et al.: Pseudoxanthoma elasticum: a clinical and histopathological study. Medicine *42*:297–334, 1963.

An exhaustive clinical and histopathologic study of 12 patients with pseudoxanthoma elasticum.

42. Eddy DD, Farber EM: Pseudoxanthoma elasticum. Internal manifestations with a report of cases and a statistical review of the literature. Arch. Dermatol. *86*:729–740, 1962.

A statistical review of 200 cases of pseudoxanthoma elasticum and presentation of four patients with this disorder.

43. Fleischmajer R, Nedwich A: Progeria (Hutchinson-Gilford). Arch. Dermatol. *107*:253–258, 1973.

A nine-year-old child with sclerodermatous lesions and typical features of progeria.

44. Rook A, Wilkinson DS, Ebling FJG: Textbook of Dermatology, 2nd edition. Blackwell Scientific Publications, London, 1972.

A complete textbook of dermatology with comprehensive analysis of cutaneous disorders.

45. Steier W, Van Voolen GA, Selmanowitz V: Dyskeratosis congenita: relationship to Fanconi's anemia. Blood 39:510–521, 1972.

Evaluation of two brothers and review of dyskeratosis congenita and Fanconi's anemia.

46. Carter DM, Gaynor A, McGuire J: Sister chromatid exchanges in dyskeratosis congenita after exposure to trimethyl psoralen and UV light. *In* Hanawalt PC, Friedberg EC,

Fox CF: DNA repair mechanisms. ICN-UCLA Symposium on Molecular and Cellular Biology, IX. Academic Press, Inc., New York, 1978, 671–674.

Studies suggest that dyskeratosis congenita is associated with a heritable defect in the repair of DNA cross-links.

47. Goltz RW, Henderson RR, Hitch JM, et al.: Focal dermal hypoplasia syndrome, a review of the literature and report of two cases. Arch. Dermatol. 101:1–11, 1970.

Report of two patients and a review of the distinguishing features of this disorder.

48. Christianson HB: Elastosis perforans serpiginosa: association with congenital anomalies. Report of 2 cases. Southern Med. J. 59:15–19, 1966.

Two patients with elastosis perforans serpiginosa (one of whom had a congenital berry aneurysm of the circle of Willis), and review of 66 patients, of whom 44 per cent had associated congenital defects or anomalies.

49. Mehregan HM: Elastosis perforans serpiginosa. A review of the literature and report of 11 cases. Arch. Dermatol. 97:381–393, 1968.

Pathologic changes of elastosis perforans serpiginosa, an attempt at transepidermal elimination of elastic tissue.

50. Leeming JAL: Acquired linear nevus showing histologic features of keratosis follicularis. Br. J. Dermatol. 81:128–131, 1969.

Linear and zosteriform configurations in Darier's disease.

51. Herndon JH Jr, Wilson JD: Acrokeratosis verruciformis (Hopf) and Darier's disease. Arch. Dermatol. 93:305–310, 1966.

A review of twelve members of a single family with acrokeratosis verruciformis, Darier's disease, and minor disturbances of keratinization supports the thesis that Darier's disease and acrokeratosis verruciformis result from a single dominant defect.

52. Goldsmith LA, Lazarus GS: Recurrent herpesvirus hominis infection in Darier's disease. Cutis 7:301–306, 1971.

Recurrent episodes of Kaposi's varicelliform eruption in a patient with Darier's disease suggest the presence of undetermined local factors in the genesis of increased susceptibility to herpetic infections in patients with this disorder.

53. Higgins PG, Crow KD: Recurrent Kaposi's varicelliform eruption in Darier's disease. Br. J. Dermatol. 88:391–394, 1973.

Kaposi's varicelliform eruption in a patient with Darier's disease attributed to infection with Coxackie virus type A 16.

54. Caplan RM: Visceral involvement in lipoid proteinosis. Arch. Dermatol. 95:149–155, 1967.

Lipoid proteinosis in the intestine, pancreas, lung, kidney, lymph nodes, and striated muscle confirm the systemic nature of this disorder.

55. Hashimoto K, Klingmüller G, Rodermund OE: Hyalinosis cutis et mucosae. Acta Dermatovener. 52:179–195, 1972.

Electron microscopic studies show the hyalin infiltrate to be an abnormal product of fibroblasts.

56. Shore RN, Howard BV, Howard WJ, et al.: Lipoid proteinosis. Demonstration of normal lipid metabolism in cultured cells. Arch. Dermatol. 110:591–594, 1974.

An assay of fibroblast lipids from tissues from a cutaneous lesion of a woman with lipoid proteinosis revealed normal quantities of all lipid fractions, apparently confirming the fact that the accumulation of lipid in lesions of this disorder is a secondary phenomenon, probably due to the affinity between lipoproteins and glycoproteins.

57. Parker F: Lipoid proteinosis (hyalinosis cutis et mucosae). In Demis DJ, Dobson RL, McGuire J (eds.): Clinical Dermatology, Vol. 2. Harper and Row, Hagerstown, Md, 1977, 12:2. 1–4.

A current review of the clinical and pathologic picture of lipoid proteinosis.

58. Fleischmajer R, Dowlati Y, Reeves JRT: Familial hyperlipidemias — diagnosis and treatment. Arch. Dermatol. 110:43–50, 1974.

A practical review of the clinical, biochemical, and therapeutic features of the hyperlipidemias.

59. Fredrickson DS, Levy RJ, Lees RS: Fat transport in lipoproteins: an integrated approach to mechanisms and disorders. N. Engl. J. Med. 276:32–44; 94–103; 148–156; 215–225; 273–281, 1967.

Analysis and classification of the hyperlipoproteinemic disorders.

60. Polano MK, Baes H, Hulsmans AM, et al.: Xanthomata in primary hyperlipoproteinemia — a classification based on the lipoprotein pattern of the blood. Arch. Dermatol. 100:387–400, 1969.

A review of the classification of hyperlipoproteinemia based upon analyses of the lipid and lipoprotein levels and cutaneous xanthomata of 23 patients.

61. Lloyd JK: Hyperlipoproteinemia in childhood. Aust. Paediatr. J. 8:264–272, 1972.

A review of hyperlipoproteinemia as seen in childhood.

62. Goldstein JL, Brown MS: Familial hypercholesterolemia: A genetic regulatory defect in cholesterol metabolism. Am. J. Med. 58:147–150, 1975.

HMG Co A reductase, a controlling enzyme in the synthesis of cholesterol.

63. Yeshuron D, Chung H, Gotto AM Jr, et al.: Primary type V hyperlipoproteinemia in childhood. JAMA 236:2518–2520, 1977.

A 9-year-old girl with type V disease.

64. McKusick VA, Kaplan D, Wise D, et al.: Genetic mucopolysaccharidoses. Medicine 44:445–483, 1965.

A critical review of the mucopolysaccharidoses.

65. Hunter C: A rare disease in two brothers. Proc. Roy. Soc. Med. 10:104–116, 1917.

A detailed report of two brothers with typical features of mucopolysaccharidosis I (the Hunter syndrome).

66. Gerich JE: Hunter's syndrome. Beta-galactosidase deficiency in the skin. N. Engl. J. Med. 280:799–802, 1969.

Deficient activity of beta galactosidase in the skin of two siblings with Hunter's syndrome and their mother, a carrier of the sex-linked disorder.

67. DiFerrante N, Nichols BL, Donnelly PV, et al.: Induced degradation of glycosaminoglycans in Hurler's and Hunter's syndromes by plasma infusion. Proc. Natl. Acad. Sci., U.S.A., 68:303–307, 1971.

Treatment of seven patients (two with the Hurler and five with the Hunter syndrome) with plasma infusions followed by decreased excretion of urinary acid mucopolysaccharides and an associated clinical improvement.

68. Dekaban AS, Holden KR, Constantopoulos G: Effects of fresh plasma or whole blood transfusions on patients with various types of mucopolysaccharidosis. Pediatrics 50:688–692, 1972.

Failure of fresh plasma and whole blood transfusions in the treatment of five children with mucopolysaccharidosis.

69. Prystkowsky SD, Maumanee IH, Freeman RG, et al.: A cutaneous marker in the Hunter syndrome. A report of four cases. Arch. Dermatol. 113:602–605, 1977.

Distinctive flesh-colored to ivory-white papules and nodules, characteristic of the Hunter syndrome, serve to separate this disorder from the other mucopolysaccharidoses.

70. Leroy JG, Crocker AC: Clinical definition of Hurler-Hunter phenotypes: review of 50 patients. Am. J. Dis. Child. 112:518–530, 1966.

A review of children with Hurler disease, Hunter syndrome, the Sanfilippo disorder, and the Scheie type of mucopolysaccharidosis.

71. Danks DM, Campbell PE, Cartwright E, et al.: Sanfilippo syndrome; clinical, biochemical, radiologic, hematologic, and pathologic features of nine cases. Aust. Paediatr. J. 8:174–186, 1972.

A large series of cases of the Sanfilippo form of mucopolysaccharidosis.

72. Spranger IW, Koch F, McKusick VA, et al.: Mucopolysaccharidosis VI (Maroteaux-Lamy disease). Helv. Paediatr. Acta 25:337–362, 1970.

Review of 19 patients with MPS VI.

73. Terashima Y, Katsuya T, Isomura S, et al.: I-cell disease, report of three cases. Am. J. Dis. Child. 129:1083–1090, 1975.

I-cell disease can be differentiated from Hurler syndrome (MPS I) by the presence of hypertrophied gums, vacuolated lymphocytes in the peripheral blood, and a normal level of urinary mucopolysaccharides.

74. Gellis S, Feingold M: Picture of the Month, I-cell disease (mucolipidosis II). Am. J. Dis. Child. 131:1137–1138, 1977.

Manifestations of a patient with I-cell disease.

75. Aula P, Rapola J, Antio S, et al.: Prenatal diagnosis and fetal pathology of I-cell disease (mucolipidosis II). J. Pediatr. 87:221–226, 1975.

Early prenatal diagnosis of I-cell disease can be confirmed by enzyme assays of lysosomal hydrolases in cell cultures of amniotic fluid and ultrastructural studies of fetal skin.

76. Esterly NB, McKusick VA: The stiff skin syndrome. Pediatrics 47:360–369, 1971.

Four patients with localized areas of stony-hard skin, mild hirsutism, and limitation of joint mobility — a connective tissue disorder possibly resulting from an abnormality of mucopolysaccharide metabolism.

77. Gordon AM: Abraham Lincoln — a medical appraisal. J. Kentucky Med. Assn. 60:249–253, 1962.

The Marfan syndrome is believed to explain Abraham Lincoln's tall stature, loose-jointedness, kyphoscoliosis, dolichocephaly, and unusually long thin arms and legs.

78. Schimke RN: Low-methionine diet of homocystinuria. Ann. Intern. Med. 70:642–643, 1969.

A low methionine diet supplemented with pyridoxine appears to be beneficial for patients with homocystinuria.

79. Carson NAJ, Carré IJ: Treatment of homocystinuria with pyridoxine. Arch. Dis. Child. 44:387–392, 1969.

Response of 6 of 11 patients to high dosages of oral pyridoxine suggests two basic defects in cystathionine synthetase: (1) a pyridoxine dependent syndrome and (2) a pyridoxine resistant disorder associated with deficiency of apoenzyme.

80. Holtzman NA, Welcher DW, Mellitis ED: Termination of restricted diet in children with phenylketonuria: randomized controlled study. N. Engl. J. Med. 293:1121–1124, 1975.

Children in whom phenylalanine restriction was terminated at age four revealed no significant loss of weight gain and physical growth.

CUTANEOUS TUMORS IN CHILDHOOD

Because of their frequency and an increasing public awareness of skin cancer, physicians are continuously consulted regarding tumors or tumor-like lesions of the skin. In children the vast majority of cutaneous tumors are benign, and their importance lies predominantly in the cosmetic defect they may create or in their occasional asso- ciation with systemic disease. Malignant lesions, however, despite their extreme rarity, cannot be disregarded or ignored. Each lesion, in children as well as adults, must be assessed individually, with particular emphasis as to its cosmetic effect, possi- ble association with systemic disease, and its ca- pacity for malignant degeneration.

Cutaneous tumors can be differentiated into those of the epidermal surface; those of epidermal appendages; those of fibrous, neural, vascular, fatty, muscular, and osseous tissues; those that are melanocytic; and those that are malignant. The term nevus has a broad meaning in dermatology. It refers to a circumscribed congenital abnormality of any cell type present at birth. When this term is used, therefore, it is appropriate to include a qualifying adjective (e.g., epidermal, melanocytic, pigmented, or vascular), thus specifying the particular cell of origin. Through common usage, however, this term is also used in a loose manner to refer to a benign tumor or pigment cells. In contrast to nevi, moles are pigmented cutaneous lesions *not* present at birth that are apparently hereditarily predetermined. Included in this group are pigmented nevocellular nevi and lentigines that develop after birth. In general, moles that appear during childhood and adolescence are flat or slightly elevated lesions. In adulthood they tend to be polypoid or dome-shaped, sessile, or papillomatous.

PIGMENTED MOLES AND NEVI

Pigmented moles and nevi are the most common neoplasms found in humans. Previous reviews suggest the incidence of moles and nevi to be 3 per cent in white and 16 per cent in black infants at birth. Although a recent study of 1058 newborn infants under 72 hours of age noted pigmented lesions in 4 per cent of infants, cutaneous biopsies revealed only one-third of these to be true melanocytic (nevus cell) nevi. This indicates that the incidence of melanocytic nevi in newborn infants is slightly more than 1 per cent.[2, 3] The incidence of melanocytic nevi increases throughout infancy and adulthood, reaching a peak at puberty and adolescence. The size and pigmentation of lesions also increase at puberty, during pregnancy, or following systemic estrogen or corticosteroid therapy. By 25 years of age most individuals acquire their maximum number of lesions, usually 20 to 40 per person; in later life most lesions tend to fade and eventually disappear.[4, 5]

Pigmented nevi and tumors may be composed of melanocytes or nevus cells. The melanocyte is a dendritic cell that produces melanin and transfers it to the keratinocytes and hair cells, thus supplying all the normal brown pigment to skin and hair. Both melanocytes and nevus cells are of neural origin. Melanocytes originate in the neural crest and early in fetal life migrate from there with the nerves to the skin. After birth melanocytes will occasionally remain in the dermis of certain races (Asiatics, Indians, Negroes and individuals from the Mediterranean area), where they usually appear as mongolian spots. Blue nevi and the nevi of Ota and Ito also represent examples of melanocytic migration in which the melanoblasts remain in the dermis.

There are, at present, two popular theories on the origin of pigment cell tumors. According to the

most popular concept, proposed by Masson in 1926, nevus cells have a dual derivation and develop from the melanocytes in the epidermis and Schwann cells of the neural sheath.[6] Schwann cells line the peripheral nerves and appear to form a pathway between the central nervous system and the skin. As peripheral nerves branch into cutaneous nerve twigs, Schwann cells migrate into the dermis and give rise to a number of dermal tumors. Nevus cells, therefore, may locate at the dermo-epidermal junction (where they appear clinically as junction nevi), within the dermis (as intradermal nevi), or a combination of both (compound nevi).

The contrasting theory of Mishima suggests that nevus cells arise from a bipotential precursor cell (nevoblast) capable of developing into a melanoblastic or Schwannian nevoblast.[7] In this theory the nevoblasts develop into epidermal nevus cells that give rise to the junction nevus and compound nevus; the Schwannian nevoblasts develop into neural nevus cells and the intradermal nevus.

Nevocellular Nevi

Lesions composed of nevus cells are termed nevocellular or pigmented nevi. Subdivided and described on the basis of the location of the nevus cells, they may be designated as junctional, intradermal, or compound lesions. Junctional nevi have nevus cell nests confined to the dermo-epidermal junction (above the basement membrane separating the epidermis from the dermis). Intradermal moles and nevi have these nests in the dermis alone, and compound nevi have nevus cells in both locations.

Pigmented moles and nevi have a wide range of clinical appearances. They may occur anywhere on the cutaneous or mucocutaneous surface and range from flat to slightly elevated or dome-shaped, nodular, verrucous, polypoid, or papillo-

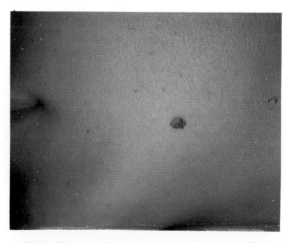

Figure 8–1 Junctional nevus. In contrast to a malignant melanoma, the skin surface is generally smooth and flat, and skin furrows are preserved.

Figure 8-2 Intradermal nevus. A dome-shaped, slightly elevated, irregularly pigmented nodular lesion.

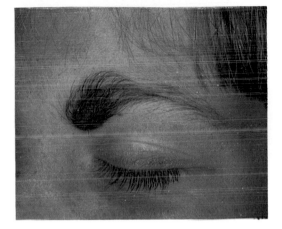

Figure 8-3 Compound nevus. Compound nevi tend to be more elevated, have a smooth or papillomatous surface, and, particularly when seen on the face, may contain dark coarse hairs.

matous configuration. Those that are flat (macular) in appearance are generally junctional (Fig. 8–1). Lesions with only slight elevation are usually compound, and those that are nodular, dome-shaped, polypoid, or papillomatous tend to be intradermal in nature (Fig. 8–2).

Junctional Nevi. Junctional nevi are generally hairless, light to dark brown or brownish-black macules. They range in size from 1 mm to 1 cm in diameter; their surface is smooth and flat; and skin furrows are preserved. Although most lesions are round, elliptical, or oval and show a relatively uniform pigmentation, some may be slightly irregular in configuration and color. Most junctional nevi represent a transient phase in the development of compound nevi and are found only in children. An exception to this rule, however, is seen on the palms, soles, and genitalia where the lesions generally retain their junctional appearance.

The nevus cell is the microscopic feature of all nevus cell nevi. In junctional nevi the cells are present as single cells or nests of nevus cells in the lower epidermis or immediately adjacent dermis. Those still in contact with the epidermis are said to be in the "dropping off" stage. Nevus cells are cuboidal, have a benign appearance without pleomorphism, and, when seen in nests, are characterized by an orderly arrangement and a central focus.

Compound Nevi. Although more common in older children and adults, compound nevi may also be present at birth.[2, 3] Often similar in appearance to junctional nevi, they tend to be more elevated and accordingly vary from a slightly raised plaque to a lesion of a somewhat more papillomatous nature. They are flesh-colored to brown, may have a smooth or warty surface, and, particularly when seen on the face, dark coarse hairs may be seen within the lesion (Fig. 8–3). In late childhood and adolescence, compound nevi frequently tend to increase in thickness and depth of pigmentation. It is at this stage that many children are brought to the physician for evaluation.

Compound nevi possess histologic features of both junctional and intradermal nevi. In this form, nevus cells are seen within the epidermis as well as in the dermis. The nevus cells in the lower part of the dermis frequently are spindle-shaped and may extend around appendages and neurovascular bundles.

Intradermal Nevi. The variety seen most frequently in adults, intradermal nevi, are usually dome-shaped, sessile (attached by a broad base), or pedunculated, and range in size from a few millimeters to a centimeter or more in diameter. Often clinically indistinguishable from compound nevi, they vary in color from non-pigmented lesions to those of varying shades of brown to black (Fig. 8–2). They may occur anywhere on the cutaneous surface and are frequently found on the head and neck; coarse hairs often are present. In older individuals intradermal nevi predominate. After the third decade of life, as maturation continues, there is often destruction and replacement of nevus cells by fibrous or fatty tissue, and by 70 years of age most individuals have few remaining moles or nevi.[5]

On histopathologic examination, intradermal nevi reveal nests and cords of nevus cells, little to no junctional activity, and spindle-shaped nevus cells in the lower dermis. Multinucleated giant cells, with rosettes or clumping of small dark-staining nuclei, may be seen within the nests or theques. These giant cells occur only in mature nevi, are indicative of the benign nature of the lesion, and should not be confused with the more irregularly shaped giant cells seen in malignant melanomas or benign spindle cell tumors of Spitz (benign juvenile melanoma).

For years it was presumed that malignant melanomas arise from pre-existing junctional nevi. It is now conceded, however, that junctional moles are no more precancerous than other pigmented lesions and that malignant melanomas may originate from melanocytes in normal skin as well as those of pigmented nevi. The increased frequency of malignant change in moles now appears to be related to an increased number of melanocytes in these lesions rather than an inherent predisposition to malignant change on the part of melanocytes in pigmented lesions.[8]

TREATMENT. The therapy of pigmented moles and nevi is usually related to their cosmetic appearance or the fear of potential malignant change. The majority of melanocytic lesions require no treatment; by careful clinical evaluation the patient can frequently be reassured as to their benign nature. Removal of nevi, when indicated, can be accomplished by shave excision techniques, shave excision and electrodesiccation,[9] or complete elliptical extirpation (depending upon the size, shape, and location of the lesion). Pedunculated tumors can be clipped off flush to the skin with scissors. Dome-shaped and other elevated nevi can be further elevated by injection of a local anesthetic beneath the lesion and the elevated portion then may be shaved or sliced off level with the skin.[4] Because of the mobility and muscularity of the upper arms, back, and shoulders, elliptical excision of moles in these areas often results in spreading of the scar and eventually a less cosmetically acceptable result.

Although some authorities suggest that simple shave excision with electrodesiccation of the underlying base may predispose to future malignant change, most lesions removed for cosmetic reasons or for reassurance can be shaved off flush with the surface under local anesthesia. Such a procedure often yields a superior cosmetic result and provides a specimen adequate for histopathologic examination.[8] No matter which of these methods is used, careful histopathologic examination of all of the specimen is imperative.

After superficial removal of pigmented lesions a certain number will show a recurrence, often causing anxiety to the patient, parent, and, at times, the physician. This is not necessarily an indication of malignancy but usually represents partial regrowth of nevus cells from the peripheral epidermis or hair root sheath.[4, 10]

In the past, many authors advocated routine excision of pigmented lesions in certain anatomic locations (the palms, soles, and genitalia), owing to the belief that the likelihood of malignant transformation was greater in these areas. Allyn and his associates reviewed the incidence of malignancy of pigmented lesions on the palms and soles. On the basis of these and other studies it now appears that prophylactic removal of all pigmented lesions in these areas is neither warranted nor feasible.[11] The role that trauma plays as a cause of malignant transformation also remains to be proved. Removal of lesions in areas of trauma, therefore, is probably more a matter of convenience than a bona fide prophylactic measure.

Malignant Melanoma

The incidence of malignant melanoma in childhood is extremely rare (less than 1 per cent of all melanomas arise prior to puberty). Despite this rarity, the course of melanoma, when it does occur, bears the same dismal prognosis as it does in adults.[1, 12] Many lesions previously thought to be melanomas of childhood are now recognized to be benign spindle cell tumors (Spitz tumors, benign juvenile melanomas). It now appears that malignant melanoma, when it occurs in childhood, is just as aggressive and potentially ominous as when seen in adults.[1, 13]

Melanoma accounts for 2 per cent of fatal malignant disease in the United States and historically has been associated with a mortality of 40 per cent.[14, 15] Malignant melanomas most commonly affect patients with fair skin, blue eyes, and red or blonde hair, particularly those of Celtic origin whose pigment cells have a limited capacity to synthesize melanin. Although melanomas may occur in blacks, the incidence, when compared to that of whites, is extremely low. In blacks, tumors usually arise in areas that are lightly pigmented, namely the mucous membranes (70 per cent), nail beds, or the sides of the palms and soles.[14] Reports of familial cases have been documented, suggesting a genetic basis (at least in some patients) with perhaps an autosomal dominant trait with reduced penetrance.[15]

Although statistics vary, it has been estimated that approximately 60 to 70 per cent of malignant melanomas arise from pre-existing nevi.[15] In the average pigmented mole, however, neoplastic transformation rarely occurs, with estimates of malignant transformation of pre-existing moles approaching one in 500,000 or one in one million lesions. The congenital pigmented nevus, however, present in 1 to 2.5 per cent of all newborns, appears to have a much greater malignant potential than that seen in pigmented lesions appearing later in life.[16, 17, 18]

CLINICAL MANIFESTATIONS. Although non-pigmented (amelanotic) melanomas can occur, most malignant melanomas present as irregularly pigmented nodules with various shades of red and blue haphazardly intermingled with black, white, and brown. They often appear as deeply pigmented nodules with an irregular shape, nodules dotting the surface, absence of overlying skin markings, and occasionally surrounding erythema (Fig. 8–4). Benign pigmented lesions show order in color, symmetry of border, and uniform surface characteristics. Malignant lesions often lack regularity of these features; their overall color pattern is often non-homogeneous, and their borders are frequently irregular or notched.[18] Danger signals in pigmented nevi suggesting abnormal activity or malignant change include changes of any type, particularly rapid growth, crusting, ulceration, bleeding, change in pigmentation, the development of inflammation, satellite lesions, the loss of normal skin lines, or subjective symptoms such as tenderness, pain, or itching.

Extremely malignant, the melanoma may proliferate locally, spread by satellite lesions, or

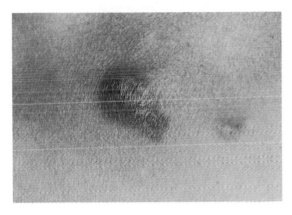

Figure 8–4   Malignant melanoma.

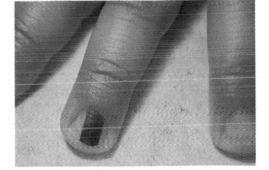

Figure 8–5   Intradermal nevus of nailbed with a broad pigmented band. Such lesions must be differentiated from melanotic whitlows (Courtesy of Thomas Hansen, M.D.).

extend via the lymphatics or blood stream, from which it may eventually invade any organ of the body. The prognosis is extremely poor, with 5 year survival rates between 20 and 38 per cent.[1, 19] Nodular melanomas, comprising 25 per cent of all pigment cell cancers, have the worst prognosis. They bypass the superficial spreading phase, immediately invade the dermis and subcutaneous fat, and soon metastasize to lymph nodes and distant sites. Survival rates with early diagnosis of patients with small superficial melanomas is materially higher (80 to 90 per cent) than those with large invasive lesions. The importance of early detection, therefore, is paramount.[19]

The question of whether or not biopsy is advisable in a lesion suspected of being a malignant melanoma has been widely discussed. There has been widespread belief (particularly in Europe) that cutting into a melanoma, as in performing a cutaneous biopsy, may induce lymphatic or hematogenous spread, or that incomplete removal can precipitate malignant degeneration in a premelanomatous junctional nevus. Many authors, however, refute this concept and feel that this procedure neither leads to spread nor alters the biologic behavior of the tumor.[20]

A melanoma that occurs beneath the nail fold is called a melanotic whitlow. The tumor begins as a brown or black discoloration, occasionally with mild deformity of the adjacent nail. Following the development of a pigmented band in the nail, granulation tissue may appear at the nail edge and the pigmented band frequently widens. If a melanoma is suspected, a biopsy (after a tourniquet has been placed on the finger) should be performed, frozen section should be carried out, and, if the diagnosis is confirmed, total amputation of the digit should be performed (Fig. 8–5).

Histopathologic examination of a typical malignant melanoma reveals irregular proliferations of melanoma cells from the dermo-epidermal junction into the dermis. These cells may vary considerably in appearance and mitotic activity. They may be cuboidal, with arrangement in irregular nests; loss of cohesiveness between cells may produce an alveolar appearance; or they may be composed primarily of spindle cells resembling those seen in fibrosarcoma.

In all malignant melanomas there is a direct correlation between the level of histologic invasion and prognosis.[21, 22] Level I refers to tumor confined above the basal lamina (in situ malignant melanoma). In Level II the tumor has penetrated the basal lamina and extends into the papillary layer of the dermis, but not into the reticular dermis. In Level III, the entire papillary region is occupied by neoplastic cells that impinge upon, but do not invade, the epidermis. Invasion of the reticular dermis by neoplastic cells constitutes Level IV, and in Level V, the invasion has extended into the subcutaneous tissue.[22]

TREATMENT.   The primary treatment of malignant melanoma is wide surgical excision with a 5 cm margin of normal skin, extension of the excision to include the deep fascia. In most cases this necessitates the application of a skin graft to cover the resulting defect. Regional lymph node dissection without evidence of lymph node involvement remains a subject of debate. Radiotherapy, although popular in Europe, generally has not met with enthusiasm in the United States. In patients with extensive or uncontrollable disease, regional limb perfusion chemotherapy with alkylating agents, immunotherapy with vaccinia or BCG vaccination of cutaneous lesions, and systemic administration of cytotoxic drugs have shown promising results. Although success of malignant melanoma therapy is usually measured by five-year survival, a significant number of patients will develop evidence of recurrent melanoma long after this five-year survival period has elapsed. Whereas patients with positive lymph node involvement seldom show five year survival rates exceeding 20 per cent, those without lymph node spread may have five year survival figures approaching 75 to 80 per cent or better.

Congenital Pigmented Nevi

Congenital giant pigmented nevi represent a special group of melanocytic lesions with a significant predisposition to malignant melanoma (2 to

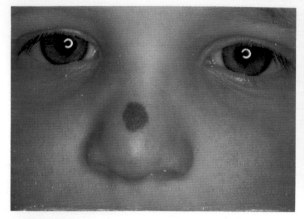

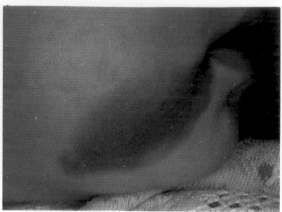

Figure 8–6 A 1.5 cm congenital pigmented nevus. Congenital nevi usually present as flat tan macules or papules with mottled freckling.

Figure 8–8 A 4 × 6 cm congenital pigmented nevus.

16 per cent or higher).[18, 22, 23] Although it has been suggested that the increased incidence of malignant melanoma in large garment-type nevi, as compared to that in small acquired nevi, may be related simply to the increased number of cells in larger lesions, recent studies suggest that small congenital pigmented nevi may be just as susceptible to malignant degeneration as the larger garment nevus.[22]

Most congenital nevi are larger than 1.5 cm in diameter and have a distinctive clinical appearance. Small congenital nevi usually present as flat, pale tan macules or papules (similar to café au lait spots) or tan, well-circumscribed lesions with mottled freckling (Figs. 8–6, 8–7, 8–8). With time they become elevated, and coarse dark brown hairs may or may not become prominent.

CLINICAL MANIFESTATIONS. The term giant congenital pigmented nevus refers to large garment-like congenital melanocytic lesions that lie in the distribution of a dermatome and vary in size to cover areas such as the scalp, buttock, large cutaneous surfaces of an arm or leg, or extensive regions of the trunk. Such lesions are frequently descriptively termed coat-sleeve, stocking, cape-like, bathing-trunk, or giant hairy nevi (Figs. 8–9, 8–10). These lesions are unevenly pigmented. Their color ranges from dark brown to black, and over 95 per cent have a hairy component consisting of large coarse terminal hairs. Giant pigmented nevi have an uneven verrucous or papillomatous surface and irregular margin. Almost invariably satellite nevi appear at the periphery of the lesion, and numerous other pigmented nevi and café au lait spots coexist elsewhere on the body. As the infant grows the involved areas become thicker and frequently darker; the surface becomes rugose; and verrucous nodules frequently develop.

Giant hairy nevi, particularly those on the scalp and neck, may be associated with leptomeningeal melanocytosis and neurologic disorders

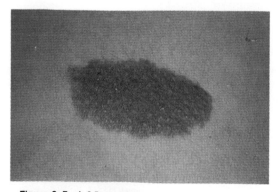

Figure 8–7 A 2.5 cm congenital pigmented nevus with a papular surface, uneven pigmentation, and irregular margin.

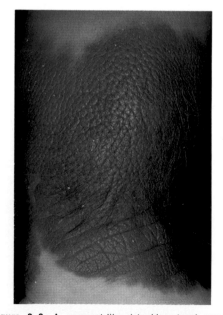

Figure 8–9 A garment-like (stocking type) congenital pigmented nevus on the skin of the ankle and lower aspect of the leg.

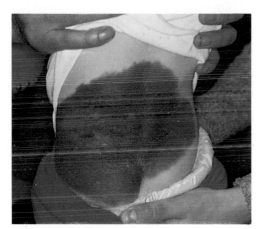

Figure 8-10 A bathing-trunk congenital pigmented nevus (Courtesy of Marvin Arons, M.D.).

such as epilepsy or other focal neurologic abnormality; those that overlie the vertebral column may be associated with spina bifida or meningomyelocele.[24]

On histopathologic examination the congenital nevus may appear as an intradermal or compound nevus, and is frequently characterized by nevus cells between the collagen bundles (as single cells or in Indian file) in the lower two-thirds of the dermis. In addition, the appendages, nerves, and vessels may also be invaded by nevus cells and at times, the melanocytic invasion may extend to involve subcutaneous tissue, fascia, lymphatic tissues, and underlying muscles or peritoneum.[25, 26]

PROGNOSIS. Unfortunately, there is no agreement as to how large a nevus must be before it can be classified as a giant nevus, exactly what size constitutes a risk, and when and if such nevi should be removed. Danger signals such as hemorrhage, crusting, erosion, friability, rapid growth, satellite lesions, and focal hypopigmentation or hyperpigmentation do not clearly distinguish malignant melanoma from benign congenital pigmented nevi.

A recent study by Trozak and others reviewed 68 cases of malignant melanoma in prepuberal children. Of 44 children with malignant melanoma before puberty (not including congenitally acquired metastatic melanoma or those arising from large congenital nevi), 11 had a primary lesion that had been present for two years or more before the melanoma was diagnosed. Of these, two-thirds were dead within five years. Of 21 patients in this study with giant pigmented nevi, 5 had proven malignancy before the age of two, all 21 had early and widely disseminated metastases, and none survived.[19]

The overall prognosis for individuals with giant congenital nevi is poor. Therefore it is no longer acceptable to consider such nevi as a problem only to be removed on the basis of cosmetic disfigurement. There is no documented explanation for the frequent occurrence of malignancy in large congenital nevi; is it due to the greater number of melanocytes in such lesions, or perhaps to a specific increased malignant potential in these nevus cells (Fig. 8–11A, B)?

On the basis of presently available data and until the true risk of congenital pigmented nevi is understood, it probably is best to remove congenital pigmented nevi whenever and as early as technically possible, with total excision, skin grafts when necessary, and careful examination of the histology of such lesions, without as much regard to the size of lesion and age of patient as heretofore has been the custom. This includes the removal of satellite lesions, which are also considered to be potentially malignant.

Spindle Cell Nevus (Benign Juvenile Melanoma)

Prior to 1948 when Sophie Spitz clearly delineated the concept of benign juvenile melanoma (spindle cell nevus, Spitz nevus), this lesion, which behaves in a benign fashion yet has certain histologic features resembling those of a malignant melanoma, was a great cause of concern to physicians and pathologists alike.[27] This tumor, a

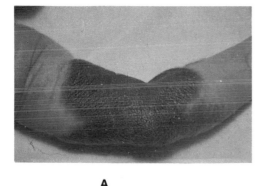

A

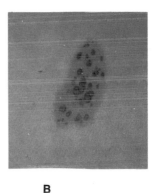

B

Figure 8-11 A. Malignant melanoma in a congenital pigmented nevus (Department of Dermatology, Yale University School of Medicine). B. Malignant melanoma in a congenital nevus overlying the scapular area of a 3½-month-old girl. Note the dark brown melanomas, which in this case appeared during the second week of life.

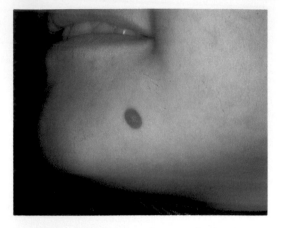

Figure 8–12 Spindle cell nevus (benign juvenile melanoma). A smooth-surfaced firm pink dome-shaped nodule on the face of a young child.

benign lesion of melanocytic origin, generally occurs on the face, usually the cheek, of children and adolescents (in about 15 per cent of cases) but may occur anywhere on the cutaneous surface.

The lesion is usually solitary and appears most frequently in children in the 3 to 13 year old age group. It generally presents as a firm smooth-surfaced dome-shaped nodule with a distinctive pink or reddish-brown color (Fig. 8–12). The lesion may vary in size from a few millimeters to three centimeters, although most spindle cell nevi range in size from 0.6 to 1 cm in diameter. Surface telangiectasia may be a prominent feature, and the characteristic pink to reddish color, when present, is correlated with the vascularity of the tumor. In some lesions, particularly those on the extremities, the reddish color is replaced by a mottled brown to tan or black appearance, often with a verrucous surface and irregular margin. Clinically it is this type of lesion that is most easily confused with malignant melanoma (Fig. 8–13).

Benign juvenile melanomas must be differentiated from intradermal nevi, pyogenic granulomas, juvenile xanthogranulomas, mastocytomas, and malignant melanomas. When the diagnosis is uncertain, the rapid onset of the lesion and expression of its vascularity by diascopy with a glass

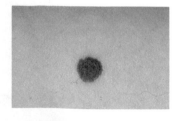

Figure 8–13 A mottled brownish black spindle cell nevus on the thigh. The reddish color may be replaced by a mottled brown, tan, or black appearance, often with a verrucous surface and irregular margin (this lesion may easily be confused with a malignant melanoma).

slide or hand lens can assist in its clinical differentiation.

The histologic pattern of this disorder appears to be a variant of the compound nevus. The nevus cells are pleomorphic and generally consist of spindle-shaped and less frequently polygon-shaped epithelioid cells. Multinucleated giant cells and mitotic figures complete the histopathologic picture. This benign tumor can be differentiated from malignant melanoma by the presence of spindle and giant cells, an absence or sparsity of melanin, edema and telangiectasia of the stroma, and increased maturation of the tumor cells in the deeper aspect of the dermis.

After the period of initial growth, spindle cell nevi of Spitz may remain static for years, may persist as such into adult life, or may develop into intradermal nevi. Once the diagnosis has been established conservative surgical excision is advisable. Biopsied lesions that leave a slight residual vascular component may be treated by cryosurgery with liquid nitrogen. This additional procedure may at times obviate the need for further surgery and frequently will result in an excellent cosmetic result.

Halo Nevus

A halo nevus is a unique cutaneous lesion in which a centrally placed, usually pigmented skin tumor becomes surrounded by a 1 to 5 mm halo of depigmentation. Termed Sutton's nevus or leukoderma acquisitum centrifugum, this relatively common disorder occurs in children and adults alike, generally those between 3 and 45, with late adolescence as the average age at time of onset (Fig. 8–14).

The cause of the spontaneous depigmentation is unknown but appears to be related to an immunologic destruction of melanocytes and nevus cells. Adding support to this hypothesis is the fact that 30 per cent of patients with halo nevi have a tendency to vitiligo. Although compound or intradermal nevi are the tumors most frequently associated with this disorder, this phenomenon may also occur around a blue nevus, neuroma, or malignant melanoma[28, 29, 30] and, at times, even giant pigmented nevi have been the sites of peripheral leukoderma, with self-destruction of the lesion.[31]

Halo nevi may appear on almost any cutaneous surface (except the palms, soles, nail beds, and mucous membranes), but the site of predilection for most halo nevi is the trunk, particularly the back. The course of halo nevi is variable, with a tendency toward spontaneous resolution, disappearance of the central lesion, and complete restitution of the site to normal appearing skin (generally over a period of five months to eight years) in about 50 per cent of affected lesions.

Histologic examination of halo nevi reveals reduction or absence of melanin and a dense inflammatory infiltrate composed primarily of lymphocytes with a few histiocytes and plasma cells

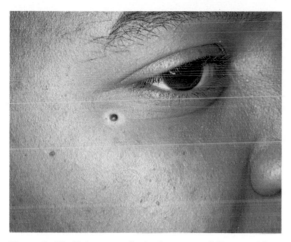

Figure 8–14 Halo nevus (leukoderma acquisitum centri-fugum). A halo of depigmentation surrounds a spontaneously regressing nevus.

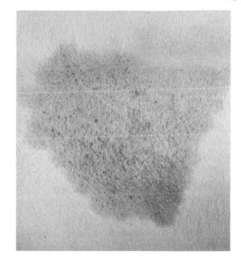

Figure 8–15 Nevus spilus. A solitary flat brown patch of melanization dotted by smaller dark brown to blackish-brown freckle-like areas of pigmentation.

around the central lesion. Electron microscopy may reveal complete absence of melanocytes and their replacement with Langerhans cells, ultra-structural findings identical to those seen in vitiligo.

Although the prognosis for benign halo nevi is excellent, attention must be focused on the rare instances in which a malignant melanoma can be the affected tumor[27] or cases in which halo nevi develop when a primary malignant melanoma is removed at a distant site.[32] The management of halo nevi, therefore, is dependent upon careful examination of the central pigmented tumor, its morphologic differentiation from malignant melanoma, and the exclusion of malignant melanoma on other parts of the cutaneous surface. If the central tumor has benign characteristics, the disorder need not be treated and the lesion may be observed at intervals until it has resolved. For lesions of unusual concern to the patient or physician, however, surgical excision, including the central tumor and its surrounding halo, with careful histologic examination is the method of choice.

Nevus Spilus

Nevus spilus is a solitary non-hairy flat, brown patch of melanization dotted by smaller dark brown to blackish-brown freckle-like areas of pigmentation (Fig. 8–15). This relatively common disorder may appear in infancy, in childhood, or at any age. It may vary from 1 to 20 cm in diameter and may occur on any area of the face, trunk, or extremities without relation to sun exposure.

Histologic examination of this disorder reveals the presence of nevus cells in a junctional or dermal location.[33] Nevus spilus accordingly should not be considered to be a form of café au lait spot, but should be considered to be a benign nevocellular nevus, with no greater potential for

neoplastic change than any other pigmented nevus.

EPIDERMAL MELANOCYTIC LESIONS

Becker's Nevus

In 1949 Becker described an irregular macular hyperpigmentation with hypertrichosis characteristically seen on the shoulders, anterior chest, or scapular region of adolescent males (Fig. 8–16).[34] This relatively common disorder, also known as pigmented hairy epidermal nevus or nevus spilus tardus, accordingly is classified as an epidermal rather than a melanocytic nevus.

Becker's nevus may begin in childhood, usually following exposure to sunlight in otherwise normal males (occasionally females), at or shortly after puberty. The first change generally appears as a grayish-brown pigmentation on the chest, back, or upper arm that spreads in an irregular fashion until it reaches an area 10 to 15 cm in diameter (about the size of a hand or larger). The outline is sharply demarcated, irregular, and often surrounded by islands of blotchy pigmentation. Although characteristically seen unilaterally on the upper half of the trunk, especially around the shoulder, it has also been reported in other areas on the trunk, forehead, cheeks, supraclavicular region, abdomen, forearm, wrist, buttocks, and shins.[35] After a period of time (often a year or two), coarse hairs appear in the region of, but not necessarily coinciding with, the pigmented area. Although the intensity of pigmentation may fade somewhat as the patient becomes older, the areas of hyperpigmentation and hypertrichosis tend to persist for life.

Histopathologic features reveal epidermal thickening, elongation of the rete ridges, and hyperpigmentation of the basal layer. There is no

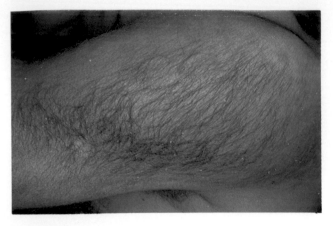

Figure 8–16   Becker's nevus (an irregular macular hyperpigmentation with hypertrichosis) on the shoulder of a 17-year-old male.

increase in the number of melanocytes, and since there are no nevus cells, malignant transformation does not occur.

Treatment of this disorder is purely cosmetic and consists of excision with split-thickness skin grafts. Unfortunately, this procedure is only partially satisfactory at best.

Freckles

Freckles (ephelides) are red or light brown well-circumscribed macules, usually less than 5 mm in diameter, which appear in childhood, especially on sun-exposed areas of the skin, and tend to fade during the winter and adult life (Fig. 8–17). They commonly arise in early childhood, generally between two and four years of age, but not in infancy, and appear to be inherited as an autosomal dominant trait linked with a tendency to fair skin and red or reddish-brown hair. Freckles are most common on the face (especially the nose), shoulders, and upper back. There is a seasonal variation in their appearance. They become darker and more confluent during the summer and are smaller, lighter, and fewer in number during the winter months. They bear cosmetic but no systemic significance, except perhaps when they occur in brunette patients, are of early onset, or persist throughout the winter (a marker of xeroderma pigmentosum trait).

Ephelides must be differentiated from lentigines (Fig. 8–18) (smooth, freckle-like pigmented macules that appear in childhood but may increase in number up to adult life). Lentigines are differentiated from freckles by their darker color, scattered distribution, comparative sparseness, and the fact that they do not darken or increase in number on sun exposure. Freckles become darker and more conspicuous after ultraviolet light exposure in the sunburn spectrum (290 to 320 nm) as well as in the long-wave ultraviolet range (320 to 400 nm). The long-wave spectrum is not blocked by window glass and sunscreen agents that filter out only the 290 to 320 nm sunburn spectrum.

Histopathologic features of ephelides include increased melanin pigmentation of the basal layer without an increase in the number of melanocytes. Ultrastructural studies reveal that the melanocytes in freckles produce increased numbers of large ellipsoid melanosomes, similar to those seen in blacks. The melanocytes are more highly arborized, react more intensely with dopa than those in normal adjacent skin, and contain more melanosomes in stages I through IV.

Treatment of freckles is best managed by avoidance of sun-exposure and appropriate covering makeup. Although sunscreens do not prevent freckle formation, they do permit a more uniform tan in which freckling is less pronounced. When

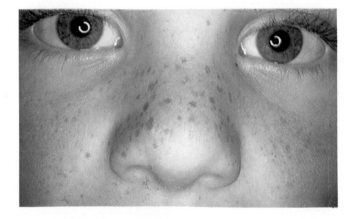

Figure 8–17   Freckles (ephelides). Red or light brown well-circumscribed macules that appear in childhood on sun-exposed areas of the skin.

desired, although seldom necessary, gentle peeling with 50 per cent trichloroacetic acid or cryotherapy with carbon dioxide slush or liquid nitrogen may remove the superficial pigmentation and make many of the freckles less conspicuous. Monobenzyl ether of hydroquinone (Benoquin or Eldoquin) may also be partially effective. Unfortunately, the possibility of contact dermatitis and occasional persistent hypopigmentation (leukoderma) suggests caution in the use of these physical or chemical methods.

Lentigines

Lentigines are small tan, dark brown, or black flat oval or circular lesions that usually appear in childhood and may increase in number up to adult life. They vary from 1 to 2 mm (occasionally up to 5 mm) in diameter and may occur on any cutaneous surface or, occasionally, on the mucous membrane or conjunctiva of the eyes. The pigmentation is uniform and darker than that seen in ephelides (freckles), and the color is unaffected by exposure to sunlight (Fig. 8–18). Adult forms of this disorder, termed senile lentigines or "liver" spots (due to their color and not their origin), are distinguished by their onset with advanced age and localization to the forearms, face, neck, and dorsal aspect of the hands.

Histopathologic features include elongated, often club-shaped rete ridges with small bud-like projections, an increase in the number of melanocytes just above the basal layer, and increased melanization of the keratinocytes of the basal layer.

Lentigines that appear early in life may fade or disappear; those appearing later in life tend to be permanent. Treatment other than for cosmetic purposes ordinarily is not indicated. When desired, however, excision by a small punch biopsy, by shaving, cryosurgery, or electrodesiccation may be beneficial.

LENTIGINOUS SYNDROMES

Several syndromes have lentigines as a major component. These include the *Peutz-Jeghers* and the *generalized* or *multiple lentigines (leopard)* syndromes.

Peutz-Jeghers Syndrome. The syndrome of mucocutaneous pigmentation and generalized intestinal polyposis constitutes a unique autosomal dominant disorder designated by the names of the authors, Peutz (Dutch) and Jeghers (American), who described it in 1921 and 1949 respectively.[36]

Characteristic bluish-brown to black spots, often apparent at birth or in early childhood, represent the cutaneous marker of this syndrome. These flat pigmented lesions are irregularly oval in shape and usually measure less than 5 mm in diameter. They are most commonly seen on the lips and buccal mucosa, nasal and periorbital regions, elbows, dorsal aspects of the fingers and toes, palms, soles, and perianal or labial regions; occasionally the gums and hard palate, and, on rare occasion, even the tongue may be involved. The pigmented lesions on the skin and lips frequently tend to fade after puberty; those on the buccal mucosa, palate, and tongue, however, persist.

Although some authors tend to classify the pigmentary lesions of Peutz-Jeghers syndrome with freckles, histologic demonstration of increased melanocytes in the basal layer of the skin and mucous membranes suggest them to be either lentigines or a separate and distinct form of melanosis.[37]

The gastrointestinal polyps seen in this disorder may be found from the gastroesophageal junction down to the anal canal; the small bowel represents the most frequently involved portion of the intestinal tract (96 per cent of cases).[37] The polyps represent benign hamartomas and, contrary to previous descriptions, have a low malignant potential. The polyps may vary in size from minute pinhead lesions to those measuring several centimeters in diameter. They may occur in early childhood, but frequently tend to develop during the second decade of life.

Symptoms in the pediatric patient frequently consist of abdominal pain, melena, or intussusception. The most common symptom, recurrent attacks of colicky abdominal pain, is believed to result from recurring transient episodes of incom-

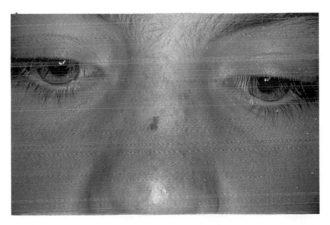

Figure 8–18 Lentigo. A smooth flat pigmented lesion on the nose in a child with ephelides. Note the generally uniform dark pigment in the lentigo. This is unaffected by exposure to sunlight.

plete intussusception. Hematemesis, although less common, may occur owing to involvement of the stomach, duodenum, or upper jejunum. Carcinoma rarely develops in the gross polyps of this disorder, but has been associated with micropolyposis of the mucosa of the colon or gastroduodenal area.[37-40]

Therapeutic management of polyposis in Peutz-Jeghers syndrome should be limited to relief of symptoms rather than radical multiple resections that may lead to malabsorption.[38, 39, 40] Multiple individual polypectomies are the treatment of choice when small bowel lesions become symptomatic, and elective major resection of benign polyps is not indicated. After initial evaluation such patients can be followed by barium contrast studies, gastroscopy, and gastric cytology. When the colon or rectum is involved, however, the possibility of an independently developing malignancy suggests careful inspection and prophylactic resection, just as if the Peutz-Jeghers syndrome did not exist.[38]

Multiple Lentigines Syndrome (Leopard Syndrome). In 1969 Gorlin and his associates published a review of an autosomal dominant disorder with high penetrance and variable expressivity characterized by striking cutaneous pigmentation.[41] The various aspects of this syndrome are best remembered by the term "leopard syndrome," a mnemonic device derived from an acronym that encompasses many of the protean manifestations of this disorder; *l*entigines, *e*lectrocardiographic conduction defects, *o*cular hypertelorism, *p*ulmonary stenosis, *a*bnormalities of genitalia, *r*etardation of growth, and *d*eafness.[42]

The cutaneous marker heralding this syndrome consists of small, dark, 1 to 5 mm lentigines, which are usually congenital in nature (but may appear soon after birth) and, with age, tend to increase in number, depth of color, and size (Fig. 8–19). Light and electron microscopy

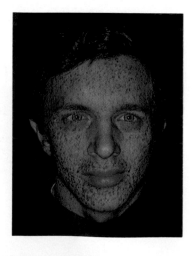

Figure 8–19 Multiple lentigines (Leopard) syndrome (Nordlund JJ, Lerner AB, Braverman IM, et al.: The multiple lentigines syndrome. Arch. Dermatol. 107:259–261, 1973).

confirm them to be lentigines with characteristic acanthosis, increase in melanocytes, and melanin deposition. The cutaneous lesions tend to be concentrated on the neck and upper trunk, but they may also appear on the skin of the face and scalp, arms, palms, soles, and genitalia. Occasionally formes frustes of this disorder occur in which the characteristic lentigines are absent.[43]

Skeletal aberrations may include retardation of growth (below the 25th percentile), hypertelorism, pectus deformities (carinatum or excavatum), dorsal kyphosis, winged scapulae, and prognathism. Cardiac abnormalities, commonly seen in this disorder, may consist of valvular pulmonary stenosis, subaortic stenosis, or cardiac conduction defects. Endocrine disorders include gonadal hypoplasia, hypospadias, undescended testicles, hypoplastic ovaries, and delayed puberty. Congenital neurosensory hearing loss, abnormal electroencephalograms, and slowed peripheral nerve conduction may complete the findings in this disorder.

Café au Lait Spots

Café au lait spots are large round or oval flat lesions of light brown pigmentation found in 10 to 20 per cent of normal individuals (Fig. 8–20). They are frequently present at birth, vary in size from 1.5 cm in their smallest diameter to much larger lesions that may measure up to 15 to 20 cm or more in diameter, often increase in number and size with age, and may occur anywhere on the body. Although most individuals with café au lait spots are normal, these pigmented macules may be a sign of neurofibromatosis and may be associated with other neurocutaneous disease.[44]

They occur in 90 per cent of patients with neurofibromatosis (von Recklinghausen disease) and tend to be more numerous and often larger in individuals affected with this disorder. Crowe has shown that the presence of six or more café au lait spots greater than 1.5 cm in diameter is presumptive evidence of neurofibromatosis, with 78 per cent of affected individuals manifesting this six or more café au lait spot rule.[45] This "six spot" criterion is particularly valuable in young children or adolescents before cutaneous neuromas make their appearance. In children five years of age or younger, however, lesions smaller than 1.5 cm in diameter may be significant in the diagnosis of this disorder. In this age group, five or more café au lait spots 0.5 cm or greater may indicate the presence of neurofibromatosis.[46] Smaller café au lait spots (1 to 4 mm in diameter) in the axillae, termed axillary freckling, may also serve as a valuable early diagnostic sign of neurofibromatosis. Seen in 20 per cent of patients with this disease, axillary pigmentation (Crowe's sign) is not seen in any other condition and, accordingly, is pathognomonic of this disorder.[47]

In addition it has been noted that frequently there is an increased incidence (26 per cent) of café au lait spots in patients with tuberous sclero-

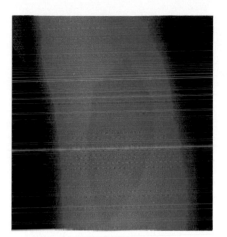

Figure 8–20   Café au lait spot. The presence of six or more café au lait macules with a diameter of 1.5 cm or more is diagnostic of neurofibromatosis.

sis.[44] Similar lesions with a more irregular border occur in 50 per cent of individuals with polyostotic fibrous dysplasia (Albright's syndrome), and café au lait spots may also be found in association with the epidermal nevus syndrome, Bloom's syndrome, ataxia-telangiectasia, pulmonary stenosis, temporal lobe dysrhythmias, and Silver's syndrome (a disorder of intrauterine growth retardation, hemihypertrophy, elevated gonadotropins giving rise to premature sexual development, inwardly curved fifth fingers, syndactylism of the toes, a triangular facies with turned-down corners of the mouth, and elongated arc or spike-shaped café au lait spots).

Histopathologic examination of café au lait spots reveals an increase in pigment in the basal layer of the epidermis. Ultrastructural examination may reveal giant pigment granules in the keratinocytes and melanocytes in café au lait spots, particularly in those of individuals with neurofibromatosis. These are not present in the café au lait spots of normal individuals.[48] The number of melanocytes per unit area in café au lait spots in patients with neurofibromatosis may be increased, decreased, or equal to the normal appearing surrounding skin. In individuals without neurofibromatosis, however, the café au lait spots have fewer dopa-positive melanocytes per unit area than the normal surrounding skin.[49, 50]

Treatment of café au lait spots per se is unnecessary. They do not have an increased tendency to neoplastic change, depigmenting agents are of no value, and surgical excision is generally impractical and unnecessary. In cases in which therapy is desirable for cosmetic appearance the most practical approach involves camouflage with appropriate cosmetics.

Albright's Syndrome

Albright's syndrome consists of polyostotic fibrous dysplasia, endocrine dysfunction, sexual precocity in females, and abnormal pigmentation of the skin. The bone changes appear roentgenographically as patchy areas of osteoporosis with a pseudocystic appearance (often with sclerosis, fractures, and skeletal deformities). The pigmentary lesions are frequently unilateral, with a predilection for areas with most bony involvement (the face, neck, thorax, sacral areas, and buttocks). Here again the cutaneous lesions with their irregularly jagged or serrated borders (described as resembling the "coast of Maine," in contrast to café au lait spots where the smooth borders are said to resemble the "coast of California") are present early in life and frequently are the first sign of this disorder.[51]

DERMAL MELANOCYTIC LESIONS

Mongolian Spots

Mongolian spots are flat, deep-brown to slate-gray or blue-black, often poorly circumscribed, large macular lesions generally located over the lumbosacral areas, buttocks, and occasionally the lower limbs, back, flanks, and shoulders of normal infants. Seen in over 90 per cent of Negro and American Indian, 81 per cent of Oriental, 70 per cent of Landino, and 9.6 per cent of Caucasoid infants, this disorder develops in utero, is present at birth, and often fades somewhat during the first year or two of life.[2] Occasionally, mongolian spots may persist into adulthood, but they usually disappear by 7 to 13 years of age.[52]

Mongolian spots may be single or multiple and vary in size from a few millimeters to 10 cm or more in diameter. They represent collections of spindle-shaped melanocytes located deep in the dermis, probably as the result of arrest during their embryonal migration from the neural crest to the epidermis. The slate-blue to blue-black color is dependent upon the Tyndall effect (a phenomenon in which light passing through a turbid medium such as the skin is scattered as it strikes particles of melanin). Long wavelength light rays (red, orange, and yellow) tend to be less scattered and therefore continue to pass downward into the lower levels of the skin; colors of shorter wavelengths (blue, indigo, and violet) are scattered to the side and backward to the skin surface, thus creating the blue-black or slate-gray discoloration.[53]

The diagnosis is based on the clinical morphology and, when in doubt, is confirmed by histopathologic examination of lesions. Microscopic features of mongolian spots include collections of greatly elongated slender spindle-shaped dopa-positive melanocytes that run parallel to the skin surface deep within the dermis or around the cutaneous appendages. Since this is a benign disorder, therapy is unnecessary.

Nevus of Ota and Nevus of Ito

The nevus of Ota (nevus fuscoceruleus ophthalmomaxillaris) represents a usually unilateral ir-

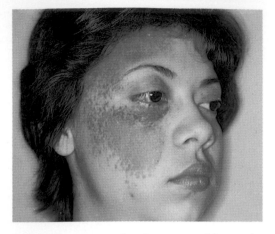

Figure 8-21 Nevus of Ota (Department of Dermatology, Yale University School of Medicine).

regularly patchy discoloration of the skin of the face supplied by the second division of the trigeminal nerve, particularly the periorbital region, the temple, the forehead, the malar area, and the nose (Fig. 8–21). About two-thirds of patients with this disorder have a patchy bluish discoloration of the sclera of the ipsilateral eye, and occasionally the conjunctiva, the cornea, and the retina.[53] In about 5 per cent of cases the nevus of Ota is bilateral rather than unilateral, and, in rare instances, the lips, palate, pharynx, and nasal mucosa are similarly affected.

Most commonly seen in Orientals, it has also been seen in Negroes, and 80 per cent of the total number of cases appear in females. Unlike mongolian spots, which tend to disappear with time, the nevus of Ota generally persists, although some have been observed to fade during the course of years. Approximately 50 per cent of lesions are congenital; the remainder generally appear during the second decade of life. Rarely the onset is later and may be associated with pregnancy. Nevus flammeus has been associated with this condition, and in a small percentage of cases, blotchy involvement (usually in association with persistent mongolian spots elsewhere) may be seen.

The nevus of Ito (nevus fuscoceruleus acromiodeltoideus) has the same features as the nevus of Ota, except that the pigmentary changes tend to involve the shoulder, supraclavicular areas, sides of the neck, and upper arm, scapular, and deltoid regions. It may occur alone or may be seen in conjunction with the nevus of Ota.

Histopathologic features of the nevus of Ota and nevus of Ito show, similar to mongolian spots, elongated dendritic melanocytes scattered among the collagen bundles. The melanocytes, however, frequently appear to be situated somewhat higher in the dermis than those seen in ordinary mongolian spots.

Although these lesions do not disappear spontaneously, changes in color do occur. Darkening of lesions has been noted during menses, and intensification of pigmentation after the age of 11 is common. These disorders are generally benign. Malignant transformation (malignant melanoma) and sensorineural deafness, however, have been reported in association with the nevus of Ota.[54] Except for such cases, no treatment other than cosmetic cover-up is necessary.

Blue Nevi

Blue nevi consist of two distinct types: the common and the cellular. The common blue nevus is a small, round or oval, dark blue or bluish-black smooth-surfaced, sharply circumscribed dome-shaped nodule (Fig. 8–22). Most common blue nevi range from 2 or 3 mm to 10 mm (less than 1 cm) in diameter. Although usually singular, they may be multiple in number. Lesions may be present at birth, but may appear at any age, and women are usually affected at least twice as frequently as men. Although ordinary blue nevi may occur on any part of the body, areas of predilection include the buttocks, dorsal aspect of the hands and feet, and the extensor surfaces of the forearms.[55] They also may occur on the face, bulbar conjunctiva, mucous membranes, and the hard and soft palates.

Once an ordinary blue nevus appears, it usually remains static and persists throughout life. Although fading of color and some degree of flattening may occur with time, malignant degeneration of this form of blue nevus is rare. When a diagnosis of malignant melanoma is considered, the common blue nevus can be differentiated from it by the presence of normal skin markings over the lesion, in contrast to the loss of such marking in lesions of malignant melanoma.

Cellular blue nevi are considerably less common than ordinary blue nevi and differ in several respects. They tend to be larger and generally measure more than 1 cm in diameter, and appear to have a relatively high incidence over the buttocks, sacrococcygeal areas, and occasionally the dorsal aspect of the hands and feet.

Although common blue nevi tend to remain benign, there is a low but distinct danger of malignant transformation in the cellular blue nevus.[56, 57] Malignant changes in cellular blue nevi are indicated by a sudden increase in size

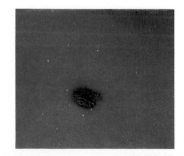

Figure 8-22 Blue nevus. An oval bluish-black smooth-surfaced, sharply circumscribed dome-shaped nodule.

and, at times, an associated tendency toward ulceration. Malignant blue nevi are locally aggressive and, in about 5 per cent of individuals, produce regional lymph node metastases. Although this malignant tumor, except for local spread, is often relatively innocuous, as with malignant melanoma, patients may be asymptomatic for many years after the primary tumor excision, only to die from sudden development of widespread metastases.[58]

Although the histogenesis of blue nevi has not been proved, it is assumed that the lesions represent hamartomas that result from the arrested embryonal migration of melanocytes bound for the dermal-epidermal junction. It would appear, therefore, that the blue nevus, mongolian spots, and the nevi of Ota and Ito are closely related and possibly represent different stages of the same physiologic process.[55]

Histopathologic examination of common blue nevi reveal compactly and loosely arranged, greatly elongated spindle-shaped, bipolar flattened or fusiform melanocytes. These cells have long, occasionally branching, dendritic processes, with their long axes parallel to the epidermis, and are grouped in irregular bundles, mainly in the middle and lower thirds of the dermis. The bundles of cells may be intimately mixed with the fibrous tissues of the upper reticular area of the dermis, or they may extend down into the subcutaneous layer. They often tend to aggregate about the adnexa, nerves, and blood vessels, and the normal dermal architecture (in contrast to that of mongolian spots) is frequently distorted.

In addition to spindle-shaped melanocytes, cellular blue nevi also have nodular islands composed of densely packed, rather large rounded or spindle-shaped cells with variously shaped nuclei and an abundant pale cytoplasm. Malignant cellular blue nevi, in addition, show mitotic figures, cellular pleomorphism, and evidence of invasion.

The treatment of choice for both types of blue nevus consists of conservative surgical excision with careful histologic examination of the lesion. Patients who have cellular blue nevi should be further examined for the presence of regional lymphadenopathy and, following surgery, should be studied at regular intervals for a period of five years for signs of recurrence or possible metastatic spread.[58]

TUMORS OF THE EPIDERMIS

Tumors of the epidermis range in severity from benign or nevoid lesions to those that are highly malignant. Benign tumors appear frequently; malignant tumors, rare in children, are often overlooked when they do occur.

Epidermal Nevi

Epidermal nevi represent a benign congenital disorder that is characterized by circumscribed

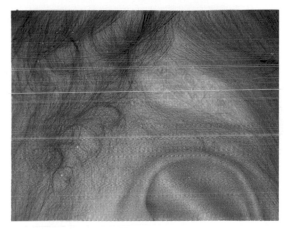

Figure 8–23 Epidermal nevus of the scalp in a newborn (this lesion must be differentiated from a nevus sebaceus of Jadassohn).

hyperkeratosis and hypertrophy of the epidermis (Fig. 8–23). This disorder, usually apparent at birth or in early childhood, affects both sexes equally and is known by several descriptive names: nevus verrucosus, nevus unius lateris, and ichthyosis hystrix. The lesions may be deeply or slightly pigmented, have either a unilateral or bilateral distribution, often favor the extremities in what appears to be a dermatomal distribution, but may occur anywhere on the cutaneous surface and, at times, appear on the oral mucosa and ocular conjunctiva. Although single lesions may occur, the disorder generally consists of multiple lesions arranged in a linear distribution.

The localized form (nevus verrucosus) usually consists of a solitary lesion. Generally present at birth, it may also appear in infancy, early childhood, and occasionally in adult life. Lesions may be grayish to yellow-brown in color, and velvety, granular, warty, or papillomatous in appearance. More often noted on the trunk or limb than on the head or neck, they may be single or multiple in number and round or oval in shape. They vary in size from 2 to 3 cm or more in diameter, and, when seen on the limbs, frequently appear in a linear distribution.

The term *nevus unius lateris* is used when lesions are extensive and systematized. Nevus unius lateris may present as a single linear or spiral warty lesion, or at times as an elaborate continuous or interrupted pattern affecting multiple sites, occasionally involving more than half of the body (Fig. 8–24). On the extremities lesions usually follow the long axis and on the trunk or extremities may be arranged in groups as spiral streaks (Fig. 8–25). On the trunk the lesions frequently tend to have a transverse orientation. If a large area of the body is affected, the term *systematized epidermal nevus* may be used. When the scalp, face, or neck is involved, adnexal tissues such as the sebaceous glands may be affected and become enlarged. For this form the term linear nevus sebaceus may be used. Linear nevus sebaceus should not be confused with *nevus seba-*

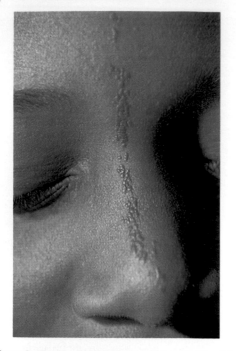

Figure 8–24 Linear epidermal nevus (nevus unius lateris). A linear arrangement of hypertrophic warty papules in an interrupted band (present since birth).

ceus (of Jadassohn), a distinct and unrelated disorder.

The term ichthyosis hystrix refers to widespread epidermal lesions, usually bilateral, arranged in irregular geometric patterns. This variant frequently consists of feather-like or marbled patterns, or sheets or whorls of hyperkeratosis.

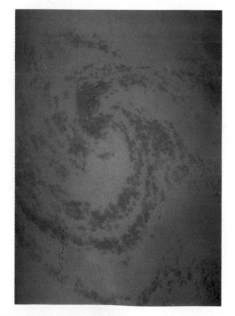

Figure 8–25 Nevus unius lateris in a whorled pattern (systematized epidermal nevus).

The predominant histologic features of epidermal nevi consist of hyperkeratosis, papillomatosis, and acanthosis. Nevus cells are absent, but in some cases, an increase in melanin pigment in the basal layer may be present. Hyperkeratosis, vacuolization (ballooning) of the cells, and microvesicles, as seen in epidermolytic hyperkeratosis, may be seen in some lesions, particularly in the ichthyosis hystrix form of the disorder. In some patients both histologic patterns may be noted in a single lesion or in lesions from different areas of the same patient.

The occurrence of malignant degeneration of epidermal nevi is unusual. When this does occur, however, it usually consists of a basal cell carcinoma rather than other neoplastic change.[59, 60] Therapy, accordingly, depends upon the site, the extent of the lesions, and the age of the patient. It is frequently wise, however, to delay surgery until the final extent of the process can be determined, as early excision may result in the appearance of new lesions in or adjacent to regions of previously treated areas. Excision by a plastic surgeon is the treatment of choice for lesions that are unsightly or uncomfortable, or when malignant change is suspected. Although cryosurgery (with liquid nitrogen), dermabrasion, or electrodesiccation and curettage may produce gratifying results initially, recurrences are common.

Epidermal Nevus Syndrome

Although there have been numerous isolated case reports of congenital anomalies associated with epidermal nevi, until recently little attention had been paid to them. The epidermal nevus syndrome is now delineated as a congenitally acquired syndrome consisting of deformities of the skin, the skeletal system, the central nervous system, and the cardiovascular system. Associated anomalies include cutaneous disorders (epidermal nevi, areas of hypopigmentation, other nevi, and café au lait spots), kyphoscoliosis, vertebral defects, hemihypertrophy, short limbs, phocomelia, angiomas of the skin, patent ductus arteriosus, coarctation and hypoplasia of the aorta, ocular abnormalities, and central nervous system involvement, with brain tumor, hydrocephaly, mental retardation, and convulsive disorders.[61-63] Although it appears that most cases of epidermal nevus syndrome occur sporadically, accumulated data suggest that, in some cases at least, an autosomal dominant transmission may be present.[63]

The nature of the verrucous lesions ranges from large unilateral hypertrophic deformities of the epidermis (nevus unius lateris) to whorled, brush stroke–like scaly lesions involving variable areas of the skin surface (ichthyosis hystrix) or large orange velvety changes of the scalp such as are seen in nevus sebaceus of Jadassohn.[62, 64, 65] It now appears that the linear nevus sebaceus syndrome and epidermal nevus syndrome are probably the same entity, the only difference being that of topography. Biopsies from patients with lesions in the sebaceous gland area (scalp, face, and ears) show sebaceous gland hyperplasia; those with lesions on the arms, legs, and trunk (where a sebaceous component is not prominent) show histopathologic features of epidermal nevi (nevus unius lateris).[64, 65]

Patients with large epidermal nevi require a careful family history and thorough physical evaluation, with particular emphasis on the affected individual's developmental pattern and musculo skeletal, nervous, ocular, and cardiovascular systems. Periodic electroencephalograms and radiologic examination of the long bones, pelvis, and vertebral column are also advisable.

Basal Cell Carcinoma

Basal cell carcinoma (often termed epithelioma) is a slow-growing, usually non-metastasizing but invasive malignant skin tumor with varying clinical patterns. This disorder arises from the basal cells of the epidermis or its appendages and is most commonly seen in persons of middle age. Although rarely seen in children, it can occur in childhood, and must be considered even in the very young. Occurrence in young adults and children in association with xeroderma pigmentosum, nevus sebaceus of Jadassohn, and nevoid basal cell carcinoma is well recognized. The spontaneous occurrence of childhood forms of this disorder, however, also requires the consideration of basal cell carcinoma in the differential diagnosis of cutaneous lesions, even in the young.[66, 67]

The majority of basal cell epitheliomas occur on the head and neck, with a predilection for the upper central part of the face. Although basal cell tumors may arise without apparent cause, prolonged exposure to the sun is a predisposing factor in individuals with fair skin. The tumor, the least aggressive neoplasm among cancers, is characterized by its capacity for local destruction. Several clinical forms of basal cell epithelioma occur.

Nodulo-ulcerative. The nodulo-ulcerative type (by far the most common) begins as a small elevated translucent nodule with telangiectatic vessels on its surface. The nodule often increases in size, undergoes central necrosis and results in an ulceration surrounded by a pearly rolled border. Although this form usually occurs as a single lesion, patients who develop this form of basal cell tumor frequently are likely to develop other such lesions. Basal cell epitheliomas enlarge more slowly than squamous cell carcinomas. In spite of the frequency of this disorder in adults, metastases are unusual and, when present, are usually associated with extremely aggressive primary lesions and repeated unsuccessful attempts at local treatment.

Pigmented. Pigmented basal cell carcinomas have all the features of the nodulo-ulcerative type, but also manifest an irregular dark pigmentation. The color may vary from light brown to dark black, and often simulates the color of malignant melanoma. Sclerosing or morphea-like basal carci-

nomas usually present on the head and the neck as elevated, firm, yellowish waxy plaques with an ill-defined border and absence of the translucent rolled edge. Tumors of this type have been known to arise in early childhood and may grow for years before attracting medical attention.

Superficial. Superficial basal cell tumors appear as psoriasiform, erythematous scaly flat or slightly infiltrated patches with superficial ulceration, crusting, and a fine thread-like pearly border. Often multiple, these lesions generally occur on the trunk or extremities, expand slowly, and are easily mistaken for lesions of psoriasis or tinea corporis.

Histopathologic features of basal cell carcinoma generally correspond to the clinical manifestations of the lesion and are characterized by masses of basal cells with large oval or elongated nuclei and relatively little cytoplasm. The nuclei resemble those of basal cells in the epidermis, generally have a uniform rather than anaplastic appearance, and do not show abnormal mitoses or pronounced variations in size or intensity of stain.[68]

No single method of therapy is applicable to all basal cell lesions. The goal, as with any skin tumor, is for permanent cure with the best functional and cosmetic result. Curettage and electrodesiccation is a simple office treatment most frequently used by dermatologists, and has a cure rate of over 95 per cent. Although cure rates are calculated in five-year periods, it is extremely rare to see recurrences one year or more after appropriate treatment. Large lesions are best treated by surgical excision, with grafting when necessary. Cryosurgery and Mohs' chemosurgery are particularly beneficial in recurrent basal cell carcinomas when other methods of therapy have proved unsatisfactory. Fractional doses of radiation therapy (used for large lesions in elderly patients in whom extensive surgical procedures are difficult) should be avoided whenever possible in the management of basal cell tumors in childhood.

Basal Cell Nevus Syndrome

The basal cell nevus syndrome (multiple nevoid basal cell carcinoma syndrome, Gorlin syndrome) is an autosomal dominant disorder characterized by childhood onset of multiple basal cell epitheliomas associated with other abnormalities such as odontogenic jaw cysts, bifid ribs, other abnormalities of the vertebrae, and intracranial calcification.[69, 70] The most obvious feature of the syndrome is the appearance of multiple basal cell epitheliomas early in life. These basal cell epitheliomas are indistinguishable on histopathologic examination from ordinary basal cell carcinomata.

The skin lesions of basal cell nevus syndrome may appear as early as the second year of life, frequently develop at puberty, and generally occur between puberty and 35 years of age. They involve, in decreasing order of frequency, the face, neck, back, thorax, abdomen, and upper extremities.[71] Lesions appear as flesh-colored to pale brown dome-shaped papules that measure 1 mm to 1 cm in diameter and tend to erupt in crops periodically throughout the lifetime of affected individuals. Secondary changes such as ulceration, crusting, and bleeding rarely occur before puberty, but if left untreated, these lesions can become extremely destructive. Unlike ordinary basal cell carcinomas, basal cell nevi are not induced by prolonged exposure to sunlight.[63]

In addition to nevoid basal cell carcinomas, affected individuals have other cutaneous stigmata. These include small milia on the face, numerous comedonal lesions, large epidermal cysts of the limbs, lipomas, fibromas, café au lait pigmentation, multiple pigmented nevi, and ectopic calcium deposits in the skin. Shallow 2 to 3 mm palmar and plantar pits, a characteristic feature of the syndrome, are seen in 60 per cent of affected individuals. These defective areas of keratinization usually first appear during the second decade of life or later. Palmar and plantar pits also frequently tend to have an underlying area of erythema, which on casual observation appears as multiple small red spots on the palms and soles.

Musculoskeletal anomalies, present in 60 to 75 per cent of patients, consist of frontal and temporoparietal bossing, prognathism, mandibular and maxillary bone cysts, splayed or bifid ribs, kyphoscoliosis, cervical or upper thoracic vertebral fusion, spina bifida, a marfanoid build, pectus excavatum and carinatum, and shortened fourth metacarpals (seen in 10 per cent of affected individuals).

Neurologic abnormalities include mental retardation, electroencephalographic abnormalities, a peculiar calcification of the dura and falx cerebri, seizures, congenital communicating hydrocephalus, nerve deafness, and, in some patients, medulloblastomas, which generally appear during the first two years of life.[69]

Ophthalmic abnormalities, documented in approximately one-third of patients with this disorder, include hypertelorism and lateral displacement of the medial canthi (dystopia canthorum), congenital blindness due to corneal opacities, cataracts, strabismus, glaucoma, and colobomas of the retina and iris. Associated endocrine findings include ovarian fibromas and calcifications, pseudohypoparathyroidism, hypogonadism, cryptorchism or testicular agenesis, and adrenal cortical adenomas.

The relatively benign course of these lesions suggests a non-radical therapeutic approach such as simple surgical excision or electrodesiccation and curettage. Radiotherapy, however, particularly in childhood, is not recommended in the management of this disorder.

Squamous Cell Carcinoma

Squamous cell carcinoma (epidermoid carcinoma) is a malignant tumor of the epidermis rarely seen in children. Occasionally it may arise in normal skin, but generally is seen in skin that has been injured by sunlight, trauma, thermal burn, or chronic irritation. In highly susceptible subjects, however, such as patients with xeroderma pigmentosum, squamous cell carcinoma may also occur in childhood or early adult life.

The most common sites for this tumor are the face (in particular the lower lip and pinna of the ear) and the dorsal aspect of the hands and forearms. Lesions are generally dull red in color, frequently contain telangiectasias, and appear as indurated plaque-like nodules with shallow, centrally crusted ulcerations surrounded by wide elevated and indurated borders. Lesions that arise de novo usually appear as solitary, slowly enlarging firm nodules with central crusting, underlying ulceration, and an indurated base.

Histopathologic examination of squamous cell carcinoma is characterized by irregular nests of epidermal cells that proliferate downward and invade the epidermis. The tumor masses are composed of varying proportions of differentiated squamous cells, keratinized cells, and anaplastic squamous cells. Of prognostic significance are the depth of the lesion and the histologic classification of squamous cell carcinomas into grades I to IV. In grade I, most cells are differentiated, and the tumor has not penetrated beyond the level of the eccrine glands. In grade IV most of the cells are atypical and undifferentiated; the greater the number of atypical cells and depth of invasion, the higher the degree of malignancy.

Because of the tendency toward deep invasion of the tissues and the possibility of metastases, treatment by electrodesiccation may not be effective. This approach, however, may be of value for small lesions one centimeter or less in diameter, particularly when present on the head and neck or other areas where mutilating surgery is particularly undesirable. Excisional surgery may be used for lesions where primary closure or simple grafting is possible, and radiation therapy is often preferred for the treatment of large carcinomas. When properly executed, a five-year cure rate of about 90 per cent can be attained for patients with this disorder.

Keratoacanthoma

Keratoacanthomas are benign self-limiting epithelial tumors resembling squamous cell carcinoma in their gross appearance, histopathologic structure, and predilection to sun-exposed areas. Multiple keratoacanthomas characteristically have their onset in adolescence or early adult life. Although this tumor has been reported during childhood and even in infancy, it is rarely seen in individuals under twenty years of age. Solitary keratoacanthomas appear primarily in adults over age 45, with approximately half of all such lesions occurring during the sixth and seventh decades of life.

The lesion consists of a firm dome-shaped nodule that generally measures 1 to 3 cm or more in diameter. The center contains a horny plug or is covered by a crust that conceals a central keratin-filled crater. The nodule generally reaches its full size within a period of two to eight weeks. Following a period of quiescence, which may last for periods of two to eight weeks, lesions heal spontaneously within a few months (frequently in less than six months) and resolve with only a slightly depressed somewhat cribriform scar in the previously affected area.

The main problem in the diagnosis of this disorder is its differentiation from squamous cell carcinoma. In most cases the rapid evolution to a relatively large size and its crateriform shape with a keratotic plug help to establish the correct diagnosis. Inasmuch as the architecture of the lesion is as important as the cellular characteristics, elliptical excisional biopsy, including both edges and the center of the lesion, is important for proper histopathologic diagnosis of this disorder. The characteristic microscopic features include a central invagination of the epidermis from which strands protrude into the dermis. The central crater is filled with eosinophilic keratin and a buttress or lip of epidermis overlaps the sides of the keratin-filled crater. Aside from the architecture, a high degree of keratinization, manifested by the eosinophilic glassy appearance of many cells, is an important diagnostic feature.

The treatment of keratoacanthoma is usually approached with a view toward its spontaneous resolution. Its close resemblance to squamous cell carcinoma, however, frequently dictates excisional biopsy. Treatment, when indicated, generally consists of surgical excision, electrodesiccation and curettage, topical application of 5-fluorouracil alone or under occlusion, and, at times, x-ray therapy. Again, in treatment of children, radiation therapy is best avoided whenever possible.

TUMORS OF THE ORAL MUCOSA

White Sponge Nevus

White sponge nevus is an exuberant, extensive, and asymptomatic white spongy plaque on the oral mucosa, which may be present at birth or may appear in early childhood, and usually does not reach maximal severity until adolescence or early adulthood. Both sexes are equally affected and the condition is inherited as an autosomal dominant trait.

The lesions are symptomless, hence often discovered by accident. They appear as soft, gray-white, somewhat friable plaques with fissures, corrugations, and folds. The superficial keratin has a tendency to desquamate, at times leaving a raw mucosal surface. The disorder is differentiated from leukoplakia, pachyonychia congenita, and cheek-biting by its history, diffuseness, and soft spongy feel. Histologic alterations are characterized by marked spongiosis of the epithelium, parakeratosis, and vacuolization of cells.

The disorder is benign and requires no specific therapy.

Leukoplakia

Leukoplakia is a term used to describe a somewhat variable whitish thickening of the epithelium of the lower lip, oral mucosa, and the vulva of older women.

Usually seen in older individuals over age 40, it may also be seen in children in association with dyskeratosis congenita (Fig. 8–26). When seen in older individuals, it is frequently associated with chronic irritation (cheilitis, pipe-smoking, biting of the lips, dentures, tobacco, and, in vulvar leukoplakia, involutional atrophy of the mucosa after menopause).

The clinical appearance and extent of lesions are variable. They generally consist of well-demarcated and irregularly outlined white patches resembling drops of candle-wax, extensive thick leathery plaques, or fine opalescent patches. The histopathologic features of leukoplakia include hyperkeratosis, individual cell dyskeratosis, and cellular atypism. Since 10 per cent of lesions of leukoplakia may eventuate in squamous cell carcinoma unless treated, therapy includes removal of the source of irritation, improvement of dental hygiene, surgical removal in the form of "shaving" or "stripping" techniques, cryosurgery with liquid nitrogen, electrodesiccation and curettage, radiation therapy (in adults), and surgical excision.

TUMORS OF THE EPIDERMAL APPENDAGES

Nevus Sebaceus

Nevus sebaceus of Jadassohn is a well-circumscribed hairless plaque that is usually solitary. It is generally present at birth or in early childhood, but at times it may arise in adult life. These nevi are not inherited and occur with equal frequency in males and females and in all races. In young individuals it is yellow or yellow-brown to

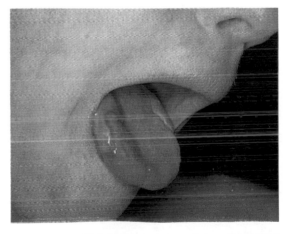

Figure 8–26 Well-demarcated, irregularly outlined thick white plaques (leukoplakia) on the tongue of a patient with dyskeratosis congenita.

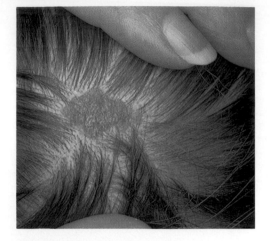

Figure 8–27 Nevus sebaceus. A yellowish-brown, orange, or pink velvet-like plaque on the scalp.

orange or pink in color and has a flat, velvet-like appearance (Fig. 8–27). The lesion is generally solitary; is round, oval, or linear; and varies in size from a few millimeters to several centimeters in diameter. On occasion, multiple and extensive lesions have been reported. Lesions often enlarge gradually, but, on occasion, have been seen to grow with rapidity.[72] With puberty, lesions of nevus sebaceus become raised, thickened, and nodular, with closely set papillomatous projections.

Of particular significance is the fact that secondary neoplastic changes occur in 10 to 15 per cent or more of lesions, generally during adolescence or in adult life. On occasion this change has occurred in children less than five years of age.[72] The most common neoplasm arising from this

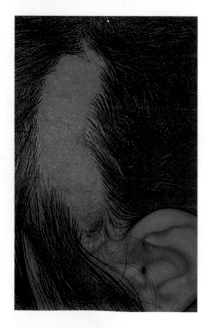

Figure 8–28 Nevus sebaceus with syringocystadenoma papilliferum.

disorder is a basal cell carcinoma (epithelioma). Frequently the individual is a teen-ager or in the early twenties when the basal cell tumor appears. The second most common tumor is a *syringocystadenoma papilliferum* (a disorder derived from apocrine sweat glands) (Fig. 8–28). Ulceration or rapid enlargement of lesions of nevus sebaceus may indicate malignant change, usually the basal-cell type, but occasionally squamous cell carcinoma with metastasis. Other tumors arising from lesions of nevus sebaceus include squamous cell carcinoma (2 per cent of cases), keratoacanthoma, hidradenoma, and apocrine cystadenoma.

On occasion, large lesions may be associated with ocular dermoids, mental retardation, pigmentary and skeletal abnormalities, and seizure disorders. Although characterized by a predominance of sebaceous gland elements, this disorder (nevus sebaceus syndrome) probably represents a variant of the epidermal nevus syndrome. Malignant degeneration is heralded, usually, by the appearance of a discrete nodule (often with superficial ulceration) on or within the lesion. At times the onset is insidious, and the clinical diagnosis of a carcinoma arising from a nevus sebaceus may be most difficult.

Early in life, histopathologic examination of the sebaceous nevus reveals large numbers of immature sebaceous glands and incompletely formed hair follicles. At puberty papillomatous hyperplasia in association with hyperkeratosis and hypergranulosis takes place, and apocrine glands frequently are seen deep in the dermis beneath masses of sebaceous gland lobules.

The recognition of this lesion and its potential for neoplastic change is critical. Local excision when the patient is prepubertal, preferably before enlargement of the sebaceous elements, is recommended. Since electrodesiccation and curettage may result in recurrences, deep full-thickness surgical excision, preferably by a plastic surgeon, is generally recommended.

Nevus Comedonicus

The comedo nevus (nevus comedonicus) is a circumscribed or systematized disorder in which grouped hair follicles filled with horny plugs constitute a prominent and histologic feature. The disorder, a developmental or nevoid condition, is rarely seen. There is no racial or sexual predisposition, and approximately half the cases are present at birth. The remainder generally appear before 10 to 15 years of age.

The disorder is manifested by groups of comedones (20 to 50 or more) in a linear or band-like distribution on any part of the body, with the face, neck, upper arm, chest, and abdomen as areas of predilection. The lesions tend to grow as the child matures, and large lesions extending above the surrounding cutaneous surface give a nutmeg grater–like feeling to the skin.

Histopathologic examination of lesions reveals a thickened epidermis with hyperkeratosis and acanthosis and large keratinous cysts with patulous openings extending into the cutaneous surface. Although lesions show little tendency to extension, secondary infection and abscess formation occasionally may prove to be troublesome. Management includes appropriate antibiotics for secondary infection, when present, and when lesions are particularly troublesome, surgical excision of involved areas is frequently beneficial.

Trichoepithelioma

Trichoepitheliomas may occur as a benign dominantly inherited disorder characterized by the presence of multiple small tumors, usually appearing on the face, or by a solitary nonhereditary tumor usually seen in early adult life, occasionally in childhood (Fig. 8–29). The terms epithelioma adenoides cysticum and multiple benign cystic epithelioma denote the hereditary disorder with a multiplicity of lesions, and the term trichoepithelioma may indicate either single or multiple lesions.

Multiple trichoepitheliomas (epithelioma adenoides cysticum) generally begin during early childhood or at puberty as small firm skin-colored papules and nodules on the face, particularly on the nasolabial folds and over the nose, forehead, upper lip, and eyelids. The lesions usually measure 2 to 5 mm in diameter, are firm, and have a translucent sheen. Occasionally telangiectatic vessels are present over the rounded translucent surface of larger lesions. Trichoepitheliomas may enlarge slowly, reaching a size of 5 mm in diameter on the face and ears and up to 2 to 3 cm in diameter in other sites, often coalesce to form nodular aggregates, and then remain static.

The single non-hereditary trichoepithelioma usually appears during the second or third decade of life and generally appears on the face. In 20 per cent of individuals it may be found on the scalp, neck, trunk, upper arms, or thighs. Solitary lesions

usually appear as firm flesh-colored tumors and generally reach a size of 5 mm or slightly larger in diameter.

The gross and microscopic appearances of solitary trichoepithelioma and epithelioma adenoides cysticum are similar. Histologically these lesions are characterized by horn cysts surrounded by solid nests and lace-like strands of epithelial cells (basalioma cells). The latter show peripheral palisading of cells and, but for the characteristic horn cysts, are frequently indistinguishable from basal cell epitheliomas.

Simple surgical excision or electrodesiccation and curettage is the treatment of choice for solitary lesions. Surgical removal by electrodesiccation and curettage, dermabrasion, or cryosurgery with liquid nitrogen (for multiple trichoepitheliomas) frequently presents a problem, since attempts at removal are often followed by regrowth. Whatever the method of removal, microscopic examination to rule out the possibility of basal cell carcinoma is recommended.

Trichofolliculoma

Trichofolliculomas occur as benign solitary lesions. Usually seen on the face of adults, they may occur at any age and occasionally can be seen in childhood. The lesion presents as a small skin-colored or pearly papule or dome-shaped nodule with a smooth surface. Frequently there is a central pore with a protruding woolly or cotton-like tuft of hair (a highly diagnostic clinical feature). On occasion the protruding hairs may be so fine that a magnifying lens may be required in order to detect their presence.

Since this is an adnexal tumor of the hair follicle, histologic examination of lesions reveals large keratinous sinuses that contain horny material and fragments of birefringent hairshafts.

Treatment of trichofolliculoma by local surgical excision generally produces a good cosmetic result.

Pilomatrixoma

An uncommon lesion, pilomatrixoma (calcifying epithelioma of Malherbe) is a benign tumor of hair structures. It usually develops before the age of 21 and manifests itself clinically as a solitary calcified deep-seated nodule on the face, neck, or upper extremities of children or young adults. More than 50 per cent of lesions appear on the head and neck. The overlying skin may be normal or slightly discolored with a reddish-blue tint, and although larger lesions may be encountered, the disorder generally measures 0.5 to 2 cm in diameter. Females are affected more often than males, and lesions are characterized by a stony-hard lobular consistency.

Microscopic examination of lesions reveals sheets of epithelial cells with two patterns. Some sheets consist of compact basal cells resembling those seen in basal cell epithelioma. Adjacent

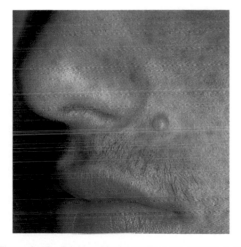

Figure 8–29 Trichoepithelioma (Brooke's tumor). A round translucent nodule with fine telangiectasia. Multiple trichoepitheliomas (epithelioma adenoides cysticum) is a disorder inherited as an autosomal dominant trait.

cells devoid of basophilic material are seen as ghost cells or shadow cells, with transitional areas showing evolution of basaloid into shadow cells. A frequent but not constant feature, particularly in older lesions, is the presence of calcification within the areas of shadow cells, where it may occur either as fine granules within the cytoplasm of the shadow cells or as large sheets of calcification replacing these cells.

Lesions of pilomatrixoma may be subject to periodic inflammation or granulomatous swelling, but they do not become malignant. Treatment (for cosmetic purposes) consists of surgical excision by a plastic surgeon, and recurrences are uncommon.

Syringoma

Syringomas represent benign tumors of eccrine structures and are predominantly seen in females (2:1). The lesions occur at any age but frequently make their first appearance during puberty or adolescence as small firm, translucent to skin-colored or somewhat yellowish 1 to 3 mm papules or nodules. In more than half the patients the lesions are located on the lower eyelids. Other common locations include the sides of the neck and upper thorax (especially the anterior aspect of the trunk), the abdomen, back, upper arms, thighs, and genitalia.

Children with Down's syndrome have an incidence of 19 to 37 per cent (30 times greater than that seen in other individuals).[73] In addition to their greater incidence in females and their tendency to proliferate at puberty, syringomas appear to be influenced by hormones, as evidenced by premenstrual swelling, enlargement in individuals on estrogenic hormones, and an increase in the size of lesions during pregnancy.

Histologic examination of lesions reveals dilated cystic eccrine ducts, some of which possess small comma-like tails of epithelial cells, with a resulting tadpole-like appearance.

Syringomas gradually enlarge until they attain their full size and then persist, with little tendency for spontaneous resolution. They are considered benign in nature, and treatment, when desired for cosmetic reasons, consists of destruction by electrodesiccation, cryosurgery with liquid nitrogen, or local surgical excision. When lesions are multiple and relatively unsightly, avoidance of therapy is often recommended.

Eccrine Poroma

Eccrine poromas are benign cutaneous tumors that generally arise from the intraepidermal sweat duct unit. Generally seen in individuals of middle-age or older, they have also been noted to develop as early as 15 years of age. The disorder is manifested by firm, sometimes lobulated, reddish nodules that may be sessile or slightly pedunculated. Eccrine poromas generally appear as solitary lesions (2 to 12 mm in diameter) on the non-hairy surface of the foot, occasionally the palm, and, at times, on other areas such as the neck, chest, or back. Although lesions tend to occur singly, multiple lesions may also occur. The disorder often has a vascular component, and the clinical appearance may, at times, suggest a pyogenic granuloma. A striking clinical feature is the frequent presence of a cup-shaped shallow depression from which the tumor grows and protrudes.

The histologic appearance of eccrine poromas is distinctive and consists of well-circumscribed, non-encapsulated tumor masses made up of broad anastomosing bands of basophilic epithelial cells that are connected by intracellular bridges and have a uniform cuboidal appearance with oval nuclei.

Since lesions may recur following incomplete removal, surgical excision appears to be the treatment of choice for this tumor.

DERMAL TUMORS

Angiofibroma

Angiofibromas may occur as isolated lesions or multiple lesions on the face. When seen as multiple lesions, they form an essential component (in 80 to 90 per cent) of the tuberous sclerosis complex. Angiofibromas (previously incorrectly termed adenoma sebaceum) represent hamartomas of fibrous and vascular tissue. They begin in childhood, only rarely are present at birth, generally appear between two and five years of age, and often do not occur until puberty.

Characteristically they are seen as small, 1 to 4 mm, firm, pink or flesh-colored dome-shaped tumors arranged in a symmetrical distribution in the nasolabial folds, on the cheeks or chin, and occasionally elsewhere on the face and scalp (Fig. 8–30). They are rarely found on the upper lip except for the central area immediately below the

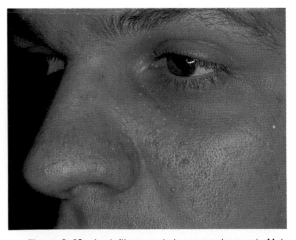

Figure 8–30 Angiofibromas (adenoma sebaceum). Multiple firm pink or flesh-colored dome-shaped tumors in a symmetrical distribution on the face of a patient with tuberous sclerosis.

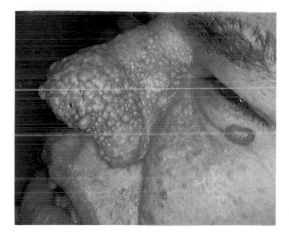

Figure 8-31 Florid adenoma sebaceum in an older individual with tuberous sclerosis.

Figure 8-32 Connective tissue nevus. Slightly elevated flesh-colored collagenous plaques (shagreen patches) on the lower aspect of the back of a child with tuberous sclerosis.

nose.[44, 74] The lesions persist indefinitely and genally increase in size and number. Fully developed angiofibromas often appear as verrucous or polypoid growths, with or without the angiomatous hue (Fig. 8-31).

Histopathologic examination of angiofibromas reveals a proliferation of fibrous and vascular tissues. As the lesions mature, dermal fibrosis is more marked, plump spindle-shaped and stellate-shaped cells (some of which contain melanin) are loosely scattered in the areas of fibrosis, and the overlying epidermis reveals atrophy or acanthosis, effacement of the rete ridges, and increased melanocytic activity.

These skin tumors require no treatment except for cosmetic reasons. Best results are seen following cryosurgery, electrodesiccation and curettage, or dermabrasion, but some lesions tend to recur following superficial removal.

Connective Tissue Nevi

Connective tissue nevi represent localized malformation of either or both dermal collagen and elastic fibers. These benign skin lesions, often hereditary, are usually seen in young children as firm, clustered, slightly raised, pea-sized, skin-colored oval lesions, distributed symmetrically over the abdomen, back, buttocks, arms, or thighs.

Early descriptions emphasized alterations in either elastic tissue (hence the term nevus elasticus, or juvenile elastoma) or collagen (collagenoma). More recently these distinctions have been obscured by a similarity in the appearance of all lesions and by the recognition of alteration of both collagen and elastic tissue. Microscopic examination of connective tissue nevi, accordingly, reveals disorganization of collagen fibers, elastic fibers, or both.

Connective tissue nevi may be familial and connected with other diseases. The collagenous plaques (shagreen patches of tuberous sclerosis)

are flat, slightly elevated, flesh-colored collagenous plaques varying from 1 to 8 cm in diameter, with a wrinkled "pig-skin" appearance, possibly due to indentation by the cutaneous appendages (Fig. 8-32).

Another form of connective tissue nevus, dermatofibrosis lenticularis disseminata, has been reported with osteopoikilosis (Albers-Schönberg disease, Buschke-Ollendorf syndrome), a hereditary dysplasia of bone affecting the long bones, pelvis, hands, and feet. The cutaneous changes usually first appear in adult life, but their onset in the second decade has been reported.[75]

Nevus lipomatosis superficialis of Hoffman-Zurhelle is a rare connective tissue nevus that is usually present at birth. The buttocks, sacrococcygeal areas, and thighs are the most frequent sites of involvement. The lesions appear as soft, skin-colored to yellowish papules, nodules, and plaques. Microscopic examination of lesions of nevus lipomatosus reveals groups of ectopic mature fat cells lying within the collagen fibers.

The management of connective tissue nevi consists of biopsy, when indicated, for diagnostic purposes. Otherwise treatment is unsatisfactory and accordingly not indicated.

Neurofibroma

Neurofibromas may appear as isolated, usually single, lesions in a healthy individual or as a cutaneous marker of dominantly inherited neurofibromatosis (von Recklinghausen disease) (Chapter 18). Tumors usually appear first in childhood or adolescence and gradually increase in size and, in neurofibromatosis, in number. They may occur anywhere on the body, with no specific site of predilection other than that they usually avoid the palms and soles.

Solitary cutaneous neurofibromas are smooth, polypoid, and soft or firm. Although generally flesh-colored, they tend to have a distinctive violaceus hue when small and, as they enlarge, they tend to become pink, blue, or pigmented. They may appear as superficial tumors, varying in size from one or two millimeters to several centimeters in diameter, or as discrete beaded, nodular, elongated masses (plexiform neuromas) along the course of nerves, usually the trigeminal or upper cervical nerves. Small tumors may be deep-seated, sessile, or dome-shaped. As they become larger they become globular, pear-shaped, pedunculated, or pendulous. With moderate digital pressure the smaller lesions may be invaginated into an underlying dermal defect, an almost pathognomonic maneuver termed "buttonholing."

In addition to solitary neurofibromas and the florid forms of neurofibromatosis, there are incomplete forms (formes frustes) of von Recklinghausen disease in which only a few manifestations occur. The presence of café au lait spots, axillary freckling, scoliosis, and bilateral acoustic neuromas suggest formes frustes or minor manifestations of this disorder.

Histopathologic features consist of fine wavy fibrils of connective tissue and nerve fibers. The nuclei tend to parallel one another and at times may be arranged in whorl-like formations. Remnants of nerve bundles usually appear within the tumor. If nerve bundles are not seen, the distinction between neurofibroma and an ordinary fibroma may be difficult.

Treatment of cutaneous neurofibromas consists of surgical excision of tumors that are disfiguring, interfere with function, or are subject to irritation, trauma, or infection. Large plexiform neurofibromas have a small but definite incidence of fibrosarcoma in later life. Excision, accordingly, should be performed prophylactically when feasible. Although malignant degeneration of lesions is rare before age 40, complete surgical excision with histopathologic examination is required if cutaneous neurofibromas become painful or show signs of rapid enlargement.

Dermatofibroma

Dermatofibromas (histiocytoma cutis) are benign growths of connective tissue generally seen in adults; occasionally they are seen in children. They appear as small, well-defined dermal nodules, firmly fixed to the skin but freely movable over the subcutaneous fat. Nodules may be found on any part of the body and are common on the extremities, particularly the anterior surface of the leg.

Their size varies from 1 mm to 3 cm in diameter, and their color may range from a flesh-color to red-brown, tan, or black. The majority of lesions are dome-shaped, but occasionally they will be depressed below the cutaneous surface. Usually lesions attain their maximum size and then remain stationary for years.

Generalized eruptive histiocytomas are characterized by symmetrical, discrete flesh-colored or bluish-red papules or papulonodules with no ten-

dency to grouping. These lesions are more closely related to juvenile xanthogranuloma (nevoxanthoendothelioma), histiocytosis X, and xanthoma disseminatum than to the classical solitary histiocytoma. These lesions tend to develop in crops and often involute spontaneously.[76]

Dermatofibromas vary in their microscopic appearance. Some lesions show a well-circumscribed but encapsulated proliferation of fibroblasts and young collagen fibers, while in others histiocytes predominate. Lesions contain varying numbers of cells with small spindle-shaped nuclei which represent the fibroblasts. The collagen appears irregularly arranged in intertwining and anastomosing bands, and a significant acanthosis of the epidermis in the center of the lesion is of considerable diagnostic value. Histiocytic lesions are composed of histiocytes that show evidence of phagocytosis of lipid and hemosiderin. At times, multinucleated giant cells of the Touton type may be observed.

Although treatment of dermatofibromas or eruptive histiocytomas is unnecessary, surgical excision may be done for cosmetic or diagnostic purposes.

Recurring Digital Fibroma of Childhood

Recurring digital fibroma of childhood is a benign, asymptomatic swelling that appears on the distal phalanges during infancy or early childhood (Fig. 8–33). Eighty-six per cent of cases occur during the first years of life.[77] The fingers and toes are about equally affected in this disorder, but the thumb and great toe are spared. The tumor presents a smooth, dome-shaped, tense elevation up to 1 cm in diameter on the tips, sides, or dorsa of affected digits. The overlying cutaneous surface is smooth, shiny, and erythematous.

The lesion affects both sexes equally and, although the etiology is unknown, the appearance of virus-like cytoplasmic inclusion bodies in the dermis suggests a viral infection as the cause of this disorder. Electron microscopic examinations, however, are equivocal and accordingly have not confirmed this hypothesis.[78]

Histopathologic features include interdigitat-

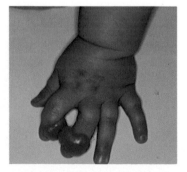

Figure 8–33 Digital fibroma of childhood (Department of Dermatology, Yale University School of Medicine).

ing sheets of spindle-shaped fibroblasts and collagen fibers. Although nuclear atypia and the occasional presence of mitotic figures have been described, such features are not regularly present.

Despite the apparent benignity of this disorder, because of its high recurrence rate (60 per cent), either amputation of the digit or wide surgical excision with dissection down to the periosteum, with grafting when necessary, has generally been recommended. However, the fact that the tumor is benign and that, at least in some cases, spontaneous resolution has been reported suggests observation as a reasonable alternate to radical surgery once the diagnosis has been made. When functional impairment or deformity of the affected digit occurs, however, appropriate surgery appears to be warranted.[77]

Epidermal Cysts

Epidermal cysts (epithelial, sebaceous, or pilar cysts) are discrete slow-growing, elevated, round, firm, slightly compressible 0.5 to 5.0 cm nodules that may appear at any time after puberty and most commonly occur on the face, scalp, nape of the neck, back, or scrotum. Although it has been well established that true sebaceous cysts do occur, most differentiate toward hair keratin and not sebaceous material. Accordingly, the term sebaceous cyst is frequently incorrectly applied to these common tumors.

Epidermal cysts are generally unilocular and result from the proliferation of surface epidermal cells situated within the dermis. Production of keratin and lack of communication with the surface are responsible for cyst formation. Most epidermal cysts arise from occluded pilosebaceous follicles. Some, however, arise from traumatic displacement of epidermal cells into the dermis, or from entrapment of epidermal cells along embryonic lines of closure (dermal cysts).

Milia (small multiple inclusion cysts within the dermis) differ from epidermal cysts only in size. They are multiple, 1 to 2 mm, whitish, hard

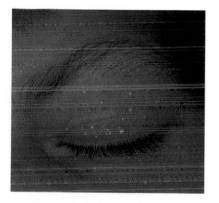

Figure 8–34 Multiple milia. One to two millimeter whitish firm globoid lesions of the eyelids and upper cheek.

globoid lesions that arise spontaneously on the face (Fig. 8–34). They occur as congenital lesions in newborns. In older individuals, they also may arise as a result of trauma, such as may be seen following dermabrasion, or in the course of bullous disorders such as epidermolysis bullosa and porphyria.

Pilar cysts (wens) are epidermal cysts that occur on the scalp, and chalazions represent analogous cystic tumors of the eyelids that develop from meibomian glands. In Gardner's syndrome (a dominantly transmitted disorder characterized by premalignant colonic and rectal polyps and osseous and dental lesions) large disfiguring cysts may be found on the face, scalp, trunk, scrotum, or extremities. In Oldfield's syndrome premalignant polyposis of the colon may also be seen in association with multiple sebaceous cysts.

Histopathologic examination of epidermal cysts reveals a wall of flattened or atrophic squamous and granular cells enclosing a keratin-filled cystic area. When the cyst ruptures and the contents are released into the dermis, a foreign body reaction with foreign-body giant cells may be noted.

Malignant degeneration (squamous cell or basal cell epithelioma) of epidermal and pilar cysts is rare. The treatment of epidermal cysts consists of local excision and suturing of the remaining cutaneous defect, or a small puncture at the dome of the tumor with expression of the contents and removal of the cystic sac through the surgical opening. In treatment of epidermal cysts it is essential that the entire epidermal lining be removed or destroyed; otherwise small numbers of cells left behind may be responsible for recurrence.

Steatocystoma Multiplex

Steatocystoma multiplex is a disorder characterized by numerous small 2 to 4 mm rounded, moderately firm, yellowish cutaneous cystic nodules located primarily on the chest and occasionally on the face, arms, and thighs of affected individuals. The disorder has a high familial tendency and is often dominantly inherited, and an occasional concomitant occurrence with pachyonychia congenita has been recognized.

Although lesions were formerly regarded as sebaceous or keratin-inclusion cysts, it now seems clear that they represent hamartomas and are a histologic variant of dermoid cysts.[79] They usually appear or become larger at puberty. No punctum is apparent, and the more superficial lesions may have a yellowish color. On puncturing the cystic lesions, a syrup-like odorless liquid and, in some instances, small hairs may be noted.

On histopathologic examination the lesions have an intricately folded thin epidermal lining. The cyst wall incorporates abortive hair follicles and, at times, sebaceous, eccrine, or apocrine structures.

Because of the large number of lesions involved, treatment is generally not recommended. When desired, however, individual lesions can be excised, electrodesiccated, or incised and drained, and on occasion, dermabrasion of multiple lesions of the face may be cosmetically acceptable.

Keloids

Keloids represent an exaggerated connective tissue response to skin injury. Rare in infancy, their incidence increases throughout childhood, reaching a maximum between puberty and thirty years of age. Blacks and other deeply pigmented individuals are more susceptible to keloids than individuals with fair skin, and the tendency often runs in families. Early growing lesions are pink, smooth, and rubbery, and often tender, with surfaces extending beyond the area of the original wound (see Fig. 6–8). Hypertrophic scars, conversely, tend to stay within the margins of the lesion.

Microscopic examination of keloids reveals dense and sharply defined connective tissue in the dermis composed of whorl-like arrangements of hyalinized bundles of collagen. The superficial collagen bundles lie parallel to the epidermis, but those lower down interlace in all directions.

Elective cosmetic procedures in persons who have a tendency to form keloids should be avoided. Keloids less than 5 cm in diameter may respond to intralesional injections of long-acting corticosteroids (10 to 40 mg per cc of triamcinolone acetonide) with concomitant cryosurgery with liquid nitrogen. The use of intralesional steroid or x-ray therapy in conjunction with careful plastic surgery is helpful for larger lesions.

TUMORS OF FAT, MUSCLES, AND BONE

Lipomas

A lipoma, one of the most common benign tumors, is composed of mature fat cells. It can be seen at any age but usually occurs from puberty on. Lesions may be present on any part of the body but predominantly appear in the subcutaneous tissues of the neck, shoulders, back, and abdominal wall. They may be single or multiple, of variable size, with a characteristic soft, often lobulated rubbery, putty-like consistency.

A rare nevoid variety, nevus lipomatodes cutaneous superficialis, may present as groups of non-tender papules and nodules in the buttocks or sacral or coccygeal regions, or as a vascular variant, angiolipoma, clinically indistinguishable except for the elicitation of pain on direct pressure or palpation.

Microscopic examination of lipomas reveals encapsulated tumors composed of adipose tissue, with essentially the same appearance as normal subcutaneous fat.

Lipomas may be left untreated unless they become painful, increase in size, or are large enough to be objectionable. Malignant change is very rare except in lesions of 10 cm or more in diameter, particularly on the thighs. These should be investigated for malignancy, and surgical excision is the treatment of choice.

Leiomyomas

Leiomyomas represent benign tumors principally derived from cutaneous smooth muscle. The majority of these lesions arise from arrector pili muscles, the media of blood vessels, or smooth muscle of the scrotum, labia majora, or nipples. Although found among all age groups, leiomyomas generally occur during the third decade of life and are relatively uncommon in childhood.

Cutaneous leiomyomas may be solitary or multiple and generally present as pink, red, or dusky brown firm dermal nodules of varying size (Fig. 8–35). The lesions generally are subject to episodes of paroxysmal, often spontaneous, pain. Multiple cutaneous leiomyomas are reddish-brown to blue, firm elevated intradermal nodules, often with a translucent or waxy appearance. They tend to occur on the back, face, or extensor surfaces of the extremities, and are usually arranged in groups.

Enlarging lesions often coalesce to form plaques with an arciform or linear configuration. Solitary leiomyomas have their onset at a later age than multiple lesions. They are generally somewhat larger but, although lesions as large as 10 cm in diameter have been described, seldom grow to more than 1.5 to 2 cm in diameter. Solitary leiomyomas are generally found on the extensor surface of the lower extremities, the scrotum, labia majora, and the breasts.

Leiomyomas are characterized by unencapsulated tumors of smooth muscle bundles and masses with an irregular arrangement. Although the smooth muscle cells of the tumor resemble normal smooth muscle, they are generally somewhat larger.

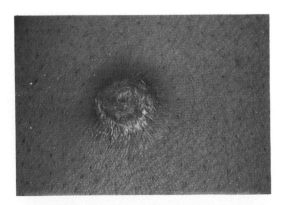

Figure 8–35 Solitary leiomyoma. An elevated flesh-colored, pink, red, or dusky brown firm dermal nodule on the extensor aspect of the arm.

Angiomyomas are a variety of leiomyoma arising from the tunica media of the blood vessels and embryonic muscle rests. Most often found on the lower leg, they are made of smooth muscle bundles derived from the arrector pili muscles. Leiomyosarcomas seldom arise in the skin, but when they do they have the same general age distribution as leiomyomas but are more widely distributed and do not tend to favor the extensor surfaces. Clinically they are larger than leiomyomas and present as nondescript subcutaneous masses. Metastases, when they occur, generally spread through the blood stream and lymphatics, and lung involvement is a common complication. Their microscopic appearance varies from a pattern closely resembling leiomyoma to a highly malignant appearance with an atypical cellular pattern and frequent mitotic figures.

Leiomyomas are benign but have a high incidence of recurrence (up to 50 per cent) following removal. Surgical excision is the treatment of choice with wide surgical excision and skin grafting, if necessary, for lesions of leiomyosarcoma.

Calcinosis Cutis

Cutaneous calcification can be either focal or widespread and can be the consequence of cutaneous injury, secondary to metabolic alteration of calcium and phosphorus, or of unknown cause.

Solitary Nodular Calcification. Occasionally solitary small raised verrucous nodular calcifications of the skin may be seen in infants and small children (Fig. 8–36).[80] Originally described as "solitary congenital nodular calcification of the skin," they are not always solitary, frequently are not congenital, and generally measure some 3 to 11 mm in diameter. Histologically they consist of a subepidermal mass of calcified materials.[81] Treatment consists of surgical excision or electrodesication and curettage.

Calcinosis Universalis and Calcinosis Cutis Circumscripta. Calcinosis universalis and calcinosis cutis circumscripta may be idiopathic or secondary to tissue damage or connective tissue or metabolic disorders. They are characterized by papules, plaques, or tumors; are often purple-red in color; and are firm or stony to palpation.

Lesions of calcinosis circumscripta vary in size from 2 to 30 mm in diameter and occur chiefly on the upper extremities (particularly the fingers or the wrists) and have a tendency to be situated in locations subject to frequent motion or trauma, namely the flexor tendons of the hands and the extensor tendons of the elbows and knees. Lesions consist of creamy material containing small gritty particles of calcium and are generally seen in patients with dermatomyositis or CRST syndrome (calcinosis cutis, Raynaud's phenomenon, scleroderma, and telangiectasia).

Calcinosis universalis is a generalized disorder usually seen in girls. Although the etiology of this disorder is unknown, a local factor controlling calcification in the tissues is postulated. In this disorder, nodules or plaques 0.5 to 5 cm in size are distributed symmetrically over the extremities and, less commonly, the trunk.

Metastatic Calcinosis Cutis. This rare entity is characterized by metastatic calcifications to the skin, hyperphosphatemia, and elevated serum calcium. The cutaneous manifestations consist of small firm white papules 1 to 4 mm in diameter surrounded by slight edema. Occurring symmetrically in the popliteal fossae and over the iliac crests and posterior axillary lines, this type of calcinosis is seen in disorders such as parathyroid neoplasms, hypervitaminosis D, and diseases associated with excessive destruction of bone (severe osteomyelitis, Paget's disease, chronic renal disease, or metastatic carcinoma).

Treatment of calcinosis cutis consists of correction of the underlying disorder whenever possible, surgical removal of painful deposits, and, in some instances, administration of oral aluminum hydroxide antacids and a diet low in phosphorus and calcium.[82, 83]

Osteoma Cutis

Osseous formation in the skin may be primary or secondary. The term osteoma cutis generally refers to the primary type, which represents spontaneous new bone formation in the skin. Secondary ossification occurs in areas of tissue degeneration caused by irritation, trauma, or various granulomatous disorders.

Cutaneous osteomas are usually multiple but may be solitary. Lesions may be present at birth or may arise at any age and occasionally have a familial pattern. Lesions generally occur over the face (especially the forehead, cheeks, and chin), are hard, raised, sharply defined, and range in size from 1 to 5 mm in diameter. Lesions may be painful and tender, and the overlying skin may be normal, erythematous, pigmented, ulcerated, or atrophic.

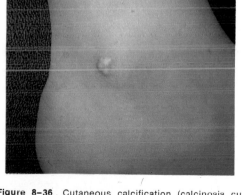

Figure 8–36 Cutaneous calcification (calcinosis cutis). Firm nodular flesh-colored deposition of calcium in the skin overlying the lateral malleolus of the ankle.

Secondary osteomas of the skin can develop in pigmented nevi, fibromas, basal cell epitheliomas, tricholemmal cysts, lesions of acne vulgaris, folliculitis, scleroderma, and areas of scar tissue.

Histopathologic examination of lesions reveals proliferation of normal bone tissue in the dermis or subcutis. Osteoblasts and osteoclasts are also present on the periphery of these lesions.

Treatment, when necessary, consists of surgical excision of involved tissues.

Subungual Exostosis

Subungual exostosis is a solitary fibrous nodule on the terminal border of the distal phalanx of a finger or toe. Although the great toe reputedly has been described as the most commonly afflicted, this disorder may involve any of the toes and, on occasion, even a finger may be affected.[84]

Although trauma has frequently been described as a precipitating factor, lesions commonly evolve spontaneously without a history of previous injury or trauma. Lesions are invariably solitary and unilateral, usually develop in older children, adolescents, or young adults between 12 and 30 years of age, and appear twice as often in females than males.

The first appearance is a small pink or flesh-colored growth that develops beneath and projects slightly beyond the free edge of the nail. The portion of the nail overlying the lesion is lifted and becomes detached, or may be removed by the patient or a parent in an effort to relieve the pain that frequently is associated with this disorder. The tumor then mushrooms upward, often above the nail as a mass of dense fibrous tissue, and generally attains a size of 8 to 10 mm in diameter.

The differential diagnosis of subungual exostoses includes verrucae, pyogenic granuloma, glomus tumor, epidermoid carcinoma, or melanoma. When the diagnosis is in doubt, the firm, often stony nature of the disorder may suggest, and x-ray generally will confirm, the diagnosis.

Once the diagnosis of subungual exostosis is established, total excision, preferably by an orthopedic surgeon under aseptic conditions, such as afforded by a hospital operating room, is the proper method of treatment. Complete excision with actual sauceration is generally required, since incomplete excision frequently results in recurrence of the disorder.

References

1. Skov-Jensen T, Hastrup J, Lambrethesen E: Malignant melanoma in children. Cancer 19:620–626, 1966.

   A survey of 45 cases of malignant melanoma in children confirms the aggressive course and poor prognosis of this tumor in childhood.

2. Jacobs AH, Walton RG: The incidence of birthmarks in the neonate. Pediatrics 58:218–222, 1976.

   A study of the various types of birthmarks in 1058 newborn infants under 72 hours of age.

3. Walton RG, Jacobs AH, Cox AJ: Pigmented lesions in newborn infants. Br. J. Dermatol. 95:389–396, 1976.

   Clinical and pathologic evaluation of pigmented lesions in 1058 newborn infants emphasizes the importance of pathologic examination in order to determine the true nature of various pigmented lesions.

4. Stegmaier OC: Cosmetic management of nevi. JAMA 199:917–919, 1967.

   A review of the pigmented nevus and its management.

5. Walton RG: Pigmented nevi. Pediat. Clin. North Am. 18:897–923, 1971.

   A comprehensive review of histogenesis, clinical description, and management of pigmented cutaneous lesions.

6. Masson P: My conception of cellular nevi. Cancer 4:9–38, 1951.

   The neural theory of the origin of nevi.

7. Mishima Y: Macromolecular changes in pigmentary disorders. Arch. Dermatol. 91:519–557, 1965.

   Light microscopic, electron microscopic, and histochemical studies of various pigmentary disorders suggests a working hypothesis for the origin and pathogenesis of various cellular nevi and melanotic tumors.

8. Clark WH, From L, Bernardino EA, et al.: The histogenesis and biologic behavior of primary human malignant melanomas of the skin. Cancer Res. 29:705–726, 1969.

   Melanoma may develop regardless of where the melanocytes are located; junction nevi, therefore, have no formal predisposition to malignant melanoma.

9. Walton RG, Cox AJ: Electrodesiccation of pigmented nevi. Arch. Dermatol. 87:342–349, 1963.

   There are innumerable opinions regarding the proper therapy of pigmented lesions; this study suggests that shave biopsy and electrodesiccation are safe and cosmetically effective.

10. Schoenfeld RJ, Pinkus H: The recurrence of nevi after incomplete removal. Arch. Dermatol. 78:30–35, 1958.

    Recurrence of nevi by nevus cells from the periphery and hair root sheaths of the original lesion is common and does not imply malignant potential.

11. Allyn B, Kopf AW, Kahn M, et al.: Incidence of pigmented nevi. JAMA 186:890–893, 1963.

    Routine excision of pigmented nevi on palms and soles is unnecessary.

12. McGovern VJ, Goulston E: Malignant moles in childhood. Med. J. Aust. 1:181–182, 1963.

    Of 8 children with malignant melanoma (ages 2 to 12) four died from the disease, and survival times of the remaining children were too short to be reassuring.

13. McWhorter HE, Woolner LB: Pigmented nevi, juvenile melanomas, and malignant melanomas in children. Cancer 7:564–585, 1954.

    Review of 172 cases of pigmented lesions (moles and melanomas) in prepuberal children.

14. Nordlund JJ, Lerner AB: Melanomas: fascinating tumors. Conn. Med. 41:414–417, 1977.

    A review of the pathophysiology, diagnosis, and therapeutic problems of melanoma.

15. Kirkwood JM, Tonkonow B, Nordlund JJ, et al.: Melanoma: a multidisciplinary overview of current concepts and management. Conn. Med. 44:21–26, 1980.

    A multidisciplinary approach to the classification, diagnosis, and treatment of malignant melanoma.

16. Anderson DE, Smith JL Jr, McBride CM: Hereditary aspects of malignant melanoma. JAMA 200:741–746, 1967.

    Data in 22 families, with particular emphasis on one kindred in whom malignant melanoma developed in a total of 15 individuals, demonstrates an autosomal genetic basis for some individuals with this disorder.

17. Greeley PW, Middleton AG, Curtin JW: Incidence of malignancy in giant pigmented nevi. Plastic Reconst. Surg. 36:26–37, 1965.

The incidence of malignant change in giant pigmented nevi is greater than generally realized; although the majority of cases occur after puberty, malignant melanoma can occur in such lesions during infancy and early childhood.

18. Mark GJ, Mihm MC, Liteplo MG, et al.: Congenital melanocytic nevi of the small and garment type. Human Path. 4:395–418, 1973.

Small congenital nevi may share the same propensity for malignant degeneration as large garment nevi.

19. Trozak DJ, Rowland WD, Hu F: Metastatic malignant melanoma in prepuberal children. Pediatrics 55:191–203, 1975.

Review of 68 prepuberal cases of malignant melanoma with proven metastases suggest that there is no safe waiting period and suspicious cases be removed as soon as technically feasible.

20. Epstein E, Bragg K, Linden G: Biopsy and prognosis of malignant melanoma. JAMA 208:1369–1371, 1969.

A series of 155 patients supports the feeling that biopsy can be performed safely when the clinical diagnosis of malignant melanoma is indeterminate.

21. Clark WH Jr, From L, Bernardino EA, et al.: The histogenesis and biologic behavior of primary human malignant melanomas of the skin. Cancer Res. 29:705–727, 1969.

The relationship between prognosis and depth of invasion of primary malignant melanoma.

22. Mihm MC Jr, Clark WH Jr, From L: Current concepts. The clinical diagnosis, classification and histogenetic concepts of the early stages of cutaneous malignant melanomas. N. Engl. J. Med. 284:1078–1082, 1971.

Review of histopathologic features of malignant melanomas, levels of invasion of the primary tumor, and their relation to survival data.

23. Kaplan EN: The risk of malignancy in large congenital nevi. Plast. Reconst. Surg. 53:421–428, 1974.

In a review of 7 patients (and 49 cases from the literature) of melanoma that arose in large congenital nevi, nearly 60 per cent developed during the first decade of life.

24. Reed WB, Becker SW Sr, Becker SW Jr, et al.: Giant pigmented nevi, melanomas and leptomeningeal melanocytosis. Arch. Dermatol. 91:101–119, 1965.

Epilepsy, hydrocephalus, and other mental and neurologic changes associated with giant pigmented nevi.

25. Dellon AL, Edelson RL, Chretien PB: Defining the malignant potential of the giant pigmented nevus. Plast. Reconst. Surg. 57:611–618, 1976.

Report of a giant pigmented nevus with lymphocytic infiltrates and apparent muscle invasion without melanoma.

26. Solomon LM, Altman AT, Bader K: Management of giant nevus. Cutis 4:434–437, 1968.

Giant pigmented nevi may show melanocytic invasion to subcutaneous tissue, fascia, and even underlying muscle.

27. Spitz S: Melanomas of childhood. Am. J. Path. 24:591–602, 1948.

Clinical and histologic features of 13 patients (aged 18 months to 12 years) with benign juvenile melanoma.

28. Frank SB, Cohen HJ: The halo nevus. Arch. Dermatol. 89:367–373, 1964.

Fourteen patients with a total of 34 halo nevi observed for periods of up to 17 years confirm previous reports of a self-destructive process that results in a patch of depigmentation, which itself may disappear over a period of four months to several years.

29. Stegmaier OC, Becker SW Jr, Medenica M: Multiple halo nevi. Histopathologic findings in a 14-year-old boy. Arch. Dermatol. 99:180–189, 1969.

A patient with nine halo nevi (seven on the trunk, one on the neck, and one on the deltoid area) and histopathologic features of this disorder.

30. Kopf AW, Morrill SC, Silberberg I: Broad spectrum of leukoderma acquisitum centrifugum. Arch. Dermatol. 92:14–35, 1965.

A review of clinical and histologic features of 35 patients with 59 halo nevi.

31. Ridley CM: Giant halo nevus with spontaneous resolution. Trans. St. John's Hosp. Dermatol. Soc. 60:54–58, 1974.

The inflammatory response associated with a halo nevus was capable of destroying a giant congenital pigmented nevus in a 3-year-old child.

32. Epstein WL, Sagebeil R, Spitler L, et al.: Halo nevi and melanoma. JAMA 225:373–377, 1973.

Five patients with halo nevi associated with the removal of a primary malignant melanoma.

33. Cohen HJ, Minkin W, Frank SB: Nevus spilus. Arch. Dermatol. 102:433–437, 1970.

Review of 17 patients with nevus spilus suggests its classification as a nevus cell nevus.

34. Becker SW: Concurrent melanosis and hypertrichosis in the distribution of nevus unius lateris. Arch. Derm. Syph. 60:155–160, 1949.

The original description of a unique epidermal hairy nevus (Becker's nevus).

35. Copeman PWM, Wilson Jones E: Pigmented hairy epidermal nevus (Becker). Arch. Dermatol. 92:249–251, 1965.

Report of 24 patients with Becker's nevus, a common disorder particularly of young men, classified (despite its features of pigmentation and hairiness) as an epidermal nevus.

36. Jeghers H, McKusick VA, Katz KH: Localized intestinal polyposis and melanin spots of the oral mucosa, lips and digits. N. Engl. J. Med. 241:993–1005, 1031–1033, 1946.

The classic description of a syndrome of intestinal polyposis and perioral pigmentation.

37. Dormandy TL: Peutz-Jeghers syndrome. N. Engl. J. Med. 256:1093–1102, 1141–1146, 1186–1190, 1957.

Although true malignant transformation in polyps of the small intestine rarely occurs, 4 of 21 patients with this disorder died of rectal or colonic cancer.

38. McKittrick JE, Lewis WM, Doane WA, et al.: The Peutz-Jeghers syndrome. Arch. Surg. 103:57–62, 1971.

When polyps are symptomatic, individual polypectomies are preferable to resection in Peutz-Jeghers syndrome.

39. Beck AR, Jewett TC: Surgical implications of the Peutz-Jeghers syndrome. Ann. Surg. 165:299–302, 1967.

Surgical intervention in the Peutz-Jeghers syndrome should be limited to relief of intestinal obstruction or resection of polyps of the stomach, duodenum, or colon.

40. Wenzl JE, Bartholomew LG, Hallenbeck GA, et al.: Gastrointestinal polyposis with mucocutaneous pigmentation in children (Peutz-Jeghers syndrome). Pediatrics 28:655–661, 1961.

In order to avoid unnecessary loss of intestine and possible malabsorption states, conservative surgical treatment of Peutz-Jeghers syndrome is advocated.

41. Gorlin RJ, Anderson RC, Blaw M: Multiple lentigines syndrome. Amer. J. Dis. Child. 117:652–662, 1969.

Six family members with this syndrome demonstrate autosomal dominant inheritance with variable expressivity of the gene.

42. Gorlin RJ, Anderson RC, Moller JH: Leopard (multiple lentigines) syndrome revisited. Laryngoscope 81:1674–1681, 1971.

Despite personal preference for the "leopard syndrome," the authors were prevailed upon to call it "the multiple lentigines syndrome."

43. Nordlund JJ, Lerner AB, Braverman IM, et al.: The multiple lentigines syndrome. Arch. Dermatol. 107:259–261, 1973.

The basic genetic defect appears to be neuroectodermal in origin with associated changes in organs derived from mesoderm.

44. Hurwitz S, Braverman IM: White spots in tuberous sclerosis. J. Pediatr. 77:587–594, 1970.

The increased incidence of cutaneous aberration in patients with neurologic disorders such as tuberous sclerosis appears to be associated with the neural crest derivation of pigment cells.

45. Crowe FW, Schull WJ, Noel JV: A Clinical, Pathologic and Genetic Study of Multiple Neurofibromatosis. Publication 281. Springfield, Illinois, Charles C Thomas, 1956.

A comprehensive monographic survey of 223 patients with neurofibromatosis.

46. Whitehouse D: Diagnostic value of the café-au-lait spot in children. Arch. Dis. Child. 41:316–319, 1966.

Five café au lait spots 0.5 cm or more in diameter are diagnostic of neurofibromatosis in children five years of age or under.

47. Crowe FW: Axillary freckling as a diagnostic aid in neurofibromatosis. Ann. Intern. Med. 61:1142–1143, 1962.

Twenty per cent of patients with neurofibromatosis present axillary freckling as a pathognomonic feature of von Recklinghausen disease.

48. Benedict PH, Szabo G, Fitzpatrick TB, et al.: Melanotic macules in Albright's syndrome and in neurofibromatosis. JAMA 25:618–626, 1968.

Studies of 27 patients with Albright's syndrome and of 19 patients with neurofibromatosis revealed that melanocytes in café au lait spots have distinctive giant melanocytic granules not present in the pigmented lesions of patients with Albright's syndrome.

49. Jimbow K, Szabo G, Fitzpatrick TB: Ultrastructure of giant pigment granules (macromelanosomes) in cutaneous pigmented macules of neurofibromatosis. J. Invest. Dermatol. 61:300–309, 1973.

Giant pigment granules in melanocytes and keratinocytes in café au lait spots of patients with neurofibromatosis not found in café au lait macules of normal individuals.

50. Johnson BL, Charneco DR: Café au lait spots in neurofibromatosis and in normal individuals. Arch. Dermatol. 102:442–446, 1970.

Giant melanin granules and increased numbers of melanocytes in café au lait spots and axillary freckles diagnostic of neurofibromatosis.

51. Albright I, Butler AM, Hampton AO, et al.: Syndrome characterized by osteitis fibrosa disseminata, areas of pigmentation, and endocrine dysfunction, with precocious puberty in females. N. Engl. J. Med. 216:727–746, 1937.

A review of 5 patients and 13 cases from the literature with peculiar pigmentation, multiple bone cysts, and precocious puberty in females.

52. Cole HN Jr, Hubler WR, Lund HZ: Persistent, aberrant mongolian spots. Arch. Derm. Syph. 61:244–260, 1950.

Four patients with dermal and ocular melanosis (hypermelanosis of the nevi of Ota and Ito).

53. Kopf AW, Weidman AI: Nevus of Ota. Arch. Dermatol. 85:195–208, 1962.

Clinical and histologic features of the nevus of Ota suggest a variant of the mongolian spot–blue nevus complex.

54. Jay B: Malignant melanoma of the orbit in a case of oculodermal melanocytosis (nevus of Ota). Br. J. Ophthal. 49:359–363, 1965.

A 64-year-old woman with melanoma of the orbit associated with the nevus of Ota.

55. Dorsey CS, Montgomery H: Blue nevus and its distinction from Mongolian spot and the nevus of Ota. J. Invest. Dermatol. 22:225–236, 1954.

Clinical and histologic study of 200 patients with blue nevi.

56. Kwittken J, Negri L: Malignant blue nevus. Arch. Dermatol. 94:64–69, 1966.

A patient with malignant blue nevus on the foot, with death due to subsequent neoplastic spread.

57. Rodriguez HA, Ackerman LV: Cellular blue nevus. Clinicopathologic study of forty-five cases. Cancer 21:393–405, 1968.

Study of pathologic features of 45 cellular blue nevi and 147 blue nevi, with comprehensive criteria for the differential diagnosis of cellular blue nevus and malignant melanoma.

58. Silverberg GD, Kadin ME, Dorfman RF, et al.: Invasion of the brain by a cellular nevus of the scalp. Cancer 27:349–355, 1971.

A 3-year-old boy with a large cellular blue nevus of the left frontoparietal scalp with focal invasion of the underlying skull, meninges, and brain.

59. Litzow TJ, Engel S: Multiple basal cell epitheliomas arising in a linear nevus. Report of a case. Am. J. Surg. 101:378–379, 1961.

A 50-year-old man with four basal cell epitheliomas in a linear nevus on his neck and ear (the lower half of the lesion had been excised when he was 3 years of age).

60. Wechsler HL, Fisher ER: A combined polymorphic epidermal adnexal tumor in nevus unius lateris. Dermatologica 130:158, 1965.

A linear epidermal nevus of the ear containing elements of basal cell carcinoma as well as sebaceous cell hyperplasia, syringocystadenoma papilliferum, and myoepitheliomas.

61. Solomon LM, Fretzin DF, Dewald RL: The epidermal nevus syndrome. Arch. Dermatol. 97:273–285, 1968.

Review of the literature and report of findings in 23 patients with the epidermal nevus syndrome.

62. Solomon LM: Epidermal nevus syndrome. Mod. Probl. Paediatr. 17:27–30, 1975.

Review of a congenitally acquired syndrome consisting of deformities involving the skin, skeletal system, central nervous system, and peripheral vasculature based upon findings in 44 patients (71 per cent had skeletal anomalies, 46 per cent had CNS abnormalities, and 38 per cent had both).

63. Solomon LM, Esterly NB: Epidermal and other congenital organoid nevi. In Current Problems in Pediatrics. Vol. VI, No. 1. Year Book Medical Publishers, Chicago, 1975, 3–56.

A review of epidermal and organoid nevi in childhood.

64. Lovejoy FH Jr, Boyle WE: Linear nevus sebaceous syndrome: report of two cases and review of the literature. Pediatrics 52:382–387, 1973.

Review of two patients and 11 cases from the literature with the "linear sebaceous form" of epidermal nevus syndrome.

65. Holden KR, DeKaban AS: Neurologic involvement in nevus unius lateris and nevus linearis sebaceus. Neurology 22:879–887, 1972.

Three patients with extensive skin lesions and neurologic complications.

66. Murray JE, Cannon B: Basal-cell cancer in children and young adults. N. Engl. J. Med. 262:440–443, 1960.

The diagnosis and course of basal cell carcinoma in 41 children and young adults.

67. Milstone EB, Helwig EB: Basal cell carcinoma in children. Arch. Dermatol. 108:523–527, 1973.

Clinical and pathologic features of 22 children with basal cell carcinoma and review of 25 previously cited cases in the literature.

68. Lever WF: Basal cell epithelioma. *In* Histopathology of the Skin, 4th edition, J. P. Lippincott Co, Philadelphia, 1967, 576–593.

A review of the clinical and histologic features of basal cell epithelioma.

69. Howell JB, Caro MR: Basal-cell nevus: its relationship to multiple cutaneous cancers and associated anomalies of development. Arch. Dermatol. 79:67–80, 1959.

Diagnosis, treatment, and review of four patients with basal cell nevus syndrome.

70. Gorlin RJ, Goltz RW: Multiple nevoid basal-cell epithelioma, jaw cysts, and bifid rib syndrome. N. Engl. J. Med. 262:908–912, 1960.

Case reports of two patients and review of the literature.

71. Gorlin RJ, Pindborg JJ, Cohen MM Jr: Multiple nevoid basal cell carcinoma syndrome. *In* Syndromes of the Head and Neck, 2nd ed. McGraw-Hill Book Co., New York, 1976, 520–526.

The basal cell nevus syndrome is well described in an encyclopedic compendium of syndromes of the head and neck.

72. Constant E, David DG: The premalignant nature of the sebaceous nevus of Jadassohn. Plastic Reconst. Surg. 50:257–259, 1972.

Report of two patients with nevus sebaceus, one of whom had rapid growth of the lesion during the fourth and fifth months of life.

73. Butterworth T, Strean LP, Beerman H, et al.: Syringoma and mongolism. Arch. Dermatol. 90:483–487, 1964.

Of 200 patients with Down's syndrome, 37 per cent had syringomas.

74. Fitzpatrick TB, Szabo G, Hori Y, et al.: White leaf-shaped macules: earliest visible sign of tuberous sclerosis. Arch. Dermatol. 98:1–6, 1976.

Of 31 patients with tuberous sclerosis, 10 had white macules as the only visible manifestations of this disorder.

75. Racque CJ, Wood MG: Connective tissue nevus. Dermatofibrosis lenticularis disseminata with osteopoikilosis. Arch. Dermatol. 112:390–396, 1970.

Three patients demonstrate a familial incidence of osteopoikilosis with connective tissue nevi in dermatofibrosis lenticularis disseminata.

76. Muller SA, Wolff K, Winkelman RK: Generalized eruptive histiocytoma. Enzyme chemistry and electron microscopy. Arch. Dermatol. 96:11–17, 1967.

Histochemical and ultrastructural study of generalized eruptive histiocytomas, a disorder consisting of multiple widespread 2 to 10 mm flesh-colored to bluish-red lesions.

77. Beckett JH, Jacobs AH: Recurring digital fibrous tumors of childhood: a review. Pediatrics 59:401–406, 1977.

Review of the literature and two new cases reveal a tendency toward local recurrence in 61 per cent of patients with digital fibroma of childhood.

78. Mehregan AH, Nabai H, Matthews JE: Recurring digital fibrous tumor of childhood. Arch. Dermatol. 106:375–378, 1972.

Histopathologic and ultramicroscopic review of two cases fails to support a viral etiology for this disorder.

79. Kligman AM, Kirschbaum JD: Steatocystoma multiplex: a dermoid tumor. J. Invest. Dermatol. 42:383–388, 1964.

Lesions of steatocystoma multiplex containing hair follicles and sebaceous glands regarded as a variety of dermoid cyst.

80. Winer L: Solitary congenital nodular calcification of the skin. Arch. Dermatol. 66:204–211, 1967.

Description of localized areas of calcinosis (believed to be congenital hamartomas of childhood).

81. Woods B, Kellaway TD: Cutaneous calculi. Subepidermal calcified nodules. Brit. J. Dermatol. 75:1–11, 1963.

Review of 20 patients with cutaneous calculi.

82. Nassim JR, Connolly CK: Treatment of calcinosis universalis with aluminum hydroxide. Arch. Dis. Child. 45:118–121, 1970.

Calcinosis universalis (due to dermatomyositis in a 9-year-old boy) successfully treated with oral administration of aluminum hydroxide, 15 ml of Aludrox (Wyeth) four times a day.

83. Mozzafarian G, Lafferty FW, Pearson OH: Treatment of tumoral calcinosis with phosphorus deprivation. Ann. Intern. Med. 77:741–745, 1972.

A 16-year-old boy with a seven-year history of calcinosis of the hips and scapulae successfully treated with aluminum hydroxide suspension.

84. Zimmerman EH: Subungual exostosis. Cutis 19:185–188, 1977.

Subungual tumors should not be confused with subungual verrucae.

9

VASCULAR DISORDERS OF INFANCY AND CHILDHOOD

VASCULAR NEVI

Congenital vascular malformations occur in 20 to 40 per cent of newborn infants and accordingly comprise the largest single group of neoplasms in infancy and childhood. These disorders are of developmental origin and arise when islands of angioblastic tissue fail to restablish normal communication with the adjacent vascular system. The rapid enlargement of certain capillary hemangiomas results from canalization and establishment of blood flow in fresh areas of the angioblastic tissue. Benign tumors derived from and composed of endothelium-lined vascular spaces are classified as hemangiomas or lymphangiomas, or a combination of the two, and are distinguished

190

Table 9–1   INCIDENCE OF VASCULAR NEVI*

1. 10 per cent of infants
   a. Salmon patches (40%)
   b. Strawberry hemangiomas (2.6%)
   c. Nevus flammeus (0.3%)
2. Somewhat more common in prematures
3. More common in girls than boys (60–70%)

*Based on Jacobs A H, Watson R G: The incidence of birthmarks in the neonate. Pediatrics 58:218, 1976.

from telangiectases by a collection of vessels in a fibrous or mucinous matrix that surrounds the vessels and replaces the normal connective tissue in the area of involvement.[1]

Although hemangiomata have been observed in several members of a family, there is no evidence of genetic predisposition. They are seen in about 10 per cent of infants, with a higher frequency in girls (60 to 70 per cent) than in boys, and they appear to be somewhat more common in premature infants (Table 9–1). In a study of over 1000 newborns seen in the first 48 hours of life, strawberry hemangiomas were noted in 2.6 per cent, port-wine stains (nevus flammeus) in 0.3 per cent, and salmon patches in 40 per cent.[2]

STRAWBERRY AND CAVERNOUS HEMANGIOMAS

Strawberry Hemangiomas

The term capillary hemangioma has been used for both strawberry hemangiomas and port-wine stains (nevus flammeus). This term, however, is not entirely satisfactory since cavernous spaces may also be present in such lesions.

Strawberry hemangiomas (circumscribed capillary hemangiomas) may be present at birth but generally develop during the first few postnatal weeks. Although the majority are not seen at birth, 90 per cent are detected during the first month of

Figure 9–2 Strawberry hemangioma. A purplish-red raised lobulated vascular tumor with well-defined borders and minute capillaries that protrude from its surface (hence its strawberry-like appearance).

life. It must be noted that most reports of the onset of strawberry marks "at birth" as described by many authors are based upon the statements of mothers. Most evidence suggests that these lesions make their appearance during the third and fifth weeks of life.[3] Eighty per cent are seen as single lesions, 20 per cent of individuals have more than one, and, in exceptional cases, there may be many hundreds. Strawberry hemangiomas may occur on any area of the body but are most commonly seen on the head and neck (38 per cent) and trunk (29 per cent) of affected individuals.[4]

Strawberry nevi initially appear as small well-demarcated telangiectatic macules or papules, as clusters of closely packed pinhead lesions, as telangiectatic patches, or as bright punctate stippling or fine thread-like telangiectases surrounded by an area of localized pallor (Fig. 9–1).[3] During the first five weeks of life these lesions become vascularized and grow to present the strawberry type lesion. The classic strawberry hemangioma is a raised bright or purplish-red lobulated tumor (Fig. 9–2) with well-defined borders and minute capillaries protruding from its surface, hence its "strawberry"-like appearance. Although it is compressible, it seldom blanches completely on pressure.

Cavernous Hemangiomas

Cavernous hemangiomas represent basically the same pathologic process as strawberry nevi but are composed of larger mature vascular elements (primarily dilated, well differentiated vessels or sinusoidal blood spaces lined by a single layer of endothelial cells) in a delicate fibrous stroma that involves the dermis and subcutaneous tissues. Individual lesions occur chiefly on the head and neck, but are found in other regions as well. They are present at birth, grow in proportion to the growth of the individual, and are generally seen as bluish-red masses with less distinct borders (Fig. 9–3). If the lesion is deeply situated, the overlying skin may appear normal or show only a blue discoloration. Occasionally a combination of strawberry and cavernous hemangioma may occur. In mixed forms the deep component may be

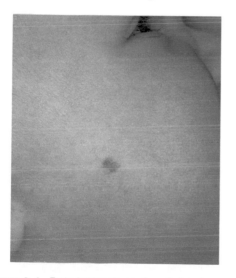

Figure 9–1 Early hemangioma. A well-demarcated vascular lesion surrounded by an area of pallor. During the first few weeks of life this area becomes vascularized and progresses into the classic strawberry hemangioma.

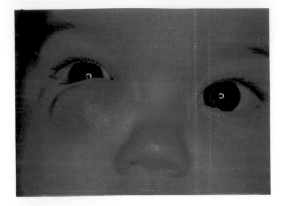

Figure 9–3 Cavernous hemangioma. Soft bluish-red vascular tumor with a poorly circumscribed border.

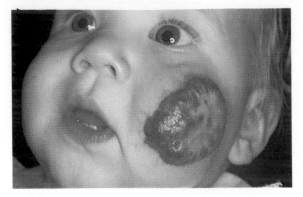

Figure 9–4 Mixed strawberry-cavernous hemangioma. A strawberry nevus overlying a bluish cavernous hemangioma.

visible or palpable beneath a typical strawberry nevus (Fig. 9–4), or the entire lesion may consist of an irregularly bluish-red mass, sometimes lobulated, involving the subcutaneous tissue.

COURSE. Strawberry hemangiomas grow rapidly during the first six months of life. The majority reach their maximal growth by the first year of life and although the majority of lesions average 2 to 5 cm in diameter, the ultimate size ranges from 2 to 3 mm to 20 cm or more in diameter. In a study of 340 lesions, 80 per cent showed maximal increase in size (less than double their original size) during the first two years of observation, less than 5 per cent tripled their size, and 2 per cent quadrupled in size.[5] Following their initial growth phase, most strawberry angiomas remain stationary and do not increase in size after the infant reaches 12 months of age. This stationary phase is soon followed by a period of involution, generally during the subsequent 6 to 12-month period (Fig. 9–5). This involutional period is variable; many lesions show complete involution by the time the child is two or three years of age.

During the first year of involution the strawberry hemangioma becomes dull-red, and small foci of gray appear on the surface. These foci increase in size, coalesce, and gradually the entire lesion becomes pink-gray or gray in color (Fig. 9–6).

At least 90 per cent of strawberry and cavernous angiomata undergo complete or partial resolution (Fig. 9–7). Superficial lesions generally resolve completely without trace or only with slight atrophy of the area of involvement. Cavernous and mixed angiomatous lesions with a deep component also resolve (Figs. 9–8 and 9–9). Accordingly, fewer than 10 per cent of hemangiomas, whether they are strawberry, cavernous, or mixed, constitute any cosmetic handicap, and less than 2 per cent require active therapy.[5, 6] In 50 per cent of cases the hemangiomas disappear by five years, in 70 per cent they disappear by seven years, and in 90 per cent they disappear by age nine years without leaving any scars or evidence that they ever existed.[7]

Cavernous-type hemangiomas generally tend to soften and, although little change occurs in their surface area, usually demonstrate a gradual decrease in thickness or volume during the second or

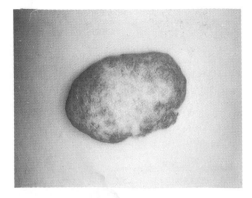

Figure 9–5 Strawberry hemangioma with focal areas of involution. Most strawberry hemangiomas begin to show signs of involution between the ages of 12 and 24 months.

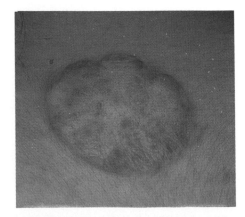

Figure 9–6 An involuting strawberry hemangioma in a 5-year-old child.

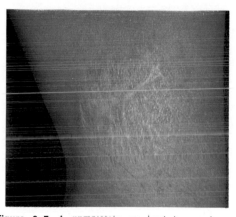

Figure 9-7 A completely resolved hemangioma with slight atrophy. In 90 per cent of cases the hemangioma (whether strawberry, cavernous, or mixed) will disappear by the age of 9 years without leaving any scar or cosmetic handicap; less than 2 per cent require therapy.

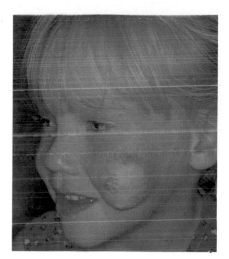

Figure 9-9 Further resolution at 5 years of age.

third years of life. Although the natural history of cavernous hemangiomas parallels that of strawberry hemangiomas, cavernous lesions generally are less active. They have a lesser growth rate than capillary hemangiomas, and although 90 per cent also improve by the time the child is nine years of age, regression of cavernous lesions is often not as complete but generally results in a satisfactory cosmetic appearance.

MANAGEMENT. Because of the tendency for most hemangiomas to regress completely, or almost completely, most cases require no therapy and the final result in untreated lesions is generally far superior to that obtained from most forms of therapeutic intervention. In general, the end results of seven years of observation of 210 children with 336 hemangiomata, were cosmetically excellent and complications uncommon (5 per cent). This was in sharp contrast to a tenfold increase in

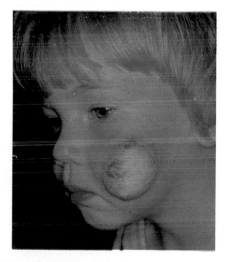

Figure 9-8 Partial resolution of a mixed strawberry-cavernous hemangioma at age 3 years (this is the same patient depicted in Figure 9-4).

complications (56 per cent) in the group that was actively treated.[4] Office management, accordingly, consists of judicious observation; avoidance, whenever possible, of active therapy; and constant reassurance to the parents of affected infants. For parents who find it difficult to accept the concept of conservative neglect, careful measurement and serial photographs of lesions, photographs of other typical cases, and discussion with parents of children who had similar lesions will usually help gain confidence and cooperation.[4]

Hemangiomas that require intervention are those that by their size and growth compromise vital structures such as the eyes (Fig. 9-10),[8] nares, auditory canals, pharynx, or larynx; those that have an alarming rate of growth, tripling or quadrupling in size within a period of a few weeks; large, usually cavernous lesions that have an associated thrombocytopenia (Kasabach-Merritt syndrome); or lesions that by their size or location are particularly susceptible to trauma, hemorrhage, or secondary infection. Unfortunately, no method of treatment is entirely satisfactory, and all forms of therapy may present significant complications.

In general, lesions permitted to undergo spontaneous resolution result in a far better cosmetic result than those treated by sclerosing agents, radiation, or surgery. Light applications of liquid nitrogen or dry ice may be beneficial, particularly in small or early lesions, but, if done too vigorously, may result in scarring or atrophy. Irradiation is not advisable and may result in serious sequelae.

Complications during spontaneous involution (ulceration, bleeding, or infection) fortunately are relatively infrequent. Therapy for ulceration and infection consists of open wet compresses, gentle cleansing with an antibacterial soap, and application of topical antibacterial agents. Bleeding and ulceration frequently hasten spontaneous involution, and residual scarring after complete involution is uncommon and rarely unsightly. Most ooz-

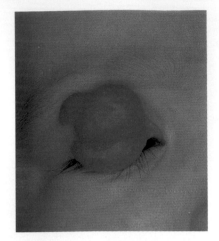

Figure 9–10 Strawberry hemangioma of the upper eyelid with obstruction of vision.

ing and crusting lesions do better when left open to the air. When topical dressings are required, however, topical antibacterial agents and sterile Telfa dressings are preferable to gauze or occlusive adhesive bandages.

When intervention is required, intralesional injection of sterile triamcinolone acetonide suspension (Kenalog-10 Injection, Squibb), in a dosage of 1 to 3 mg/kg two or three times at three-week intervals, may result in involution within a period of several months,[9] or a course of oral prednisone may be used in a dosage of 2 to 3 mg/kg per day (or its equivalent) for four weeks, followed by alternate day therapy using the same or doubled dosage for periods of four to six weeks, with gradual tapering of the dosage as the condition warrants (Fig. 9–11). Involution usually begins about the second or third week and continues during the second month. If rebound occurs, a second or third course may be necessary.[10, 11]

SALMON PATCHES AND NEVUS FLAMMEUS

Salmon Patches

The salmon patch (nevus simplex, telangiectatic nevus) is the most common vascular lesion of infancy. It occurs in 40 per cent of newborn infants and appears as a flat dull pink macular lesion (often with telangiectasia) on the nape of the neck, glabella, forehead (Fig. 9–12), upper eyelids, and nasolabial regions. When seen on the nape of the neck, it is frequently referred to as a "stork bite" (Fig. 9–13). Twenty-two per cent of infants have salmon patches only on the nape of the neck, 5 per cent have them either on the eyelids or on the glabella, and almost 20 per cent have them on both the glabella and the eyelids.

Histopathologic examination of salmon patches reveals distended dermal capillaries that represent the persistence of fetal circulation rather than newly formed capillaries. No treatment is necessary, since 95 per cent of salmon patches (with the exception of those on the nuchal region) fade, generally within the first year of life (unlike the true nevus flammeus, which is permanent). It should be noted, however, that a slight erythematous color may be more persistent or may reappear in salmon patches of fair-skinned children during episodes of crying, breath holding, or physical exertion. Those on the nuchal region (known as nuchal or Unna's nevus) persist in up to 50 per cent of individuals (Fig. 9–13). Since they are usually covered by hair, nuchal lesions do not generally present a cosmetic problem.

Nevus Flammeus

Port-wine stains (nevus flammeus), in contrast to strawberry hemangiomata, represent a congenital vascular malformation involving mature capillaries. Such lesions are generally present at birth and usually do not grow out of relation to the growth of the child (Figs. 9–14 and 9–15). On

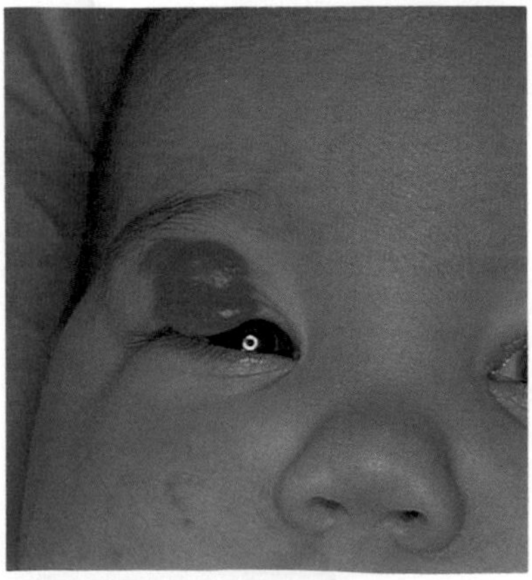

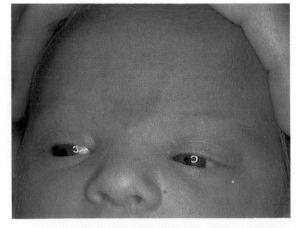

Figure 9–11 Partial resolution following 7 weeks of systemic steroid therapy.

Figure 9–12 Salmon patch (nevus simplex). A dull pink macular lesion on the forehead of a 9-month-old infant.

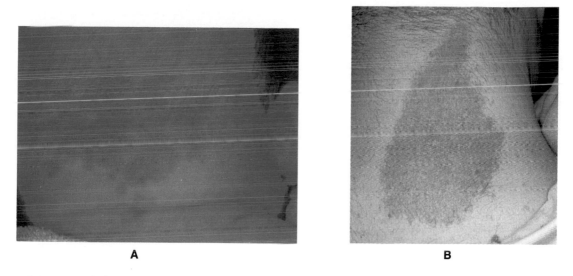

Figure 9–13 A. Salmon patch on the nape of the neck in a 3-month-old infant. B. Unna's nevus. A persistent salmon patch on the nucha (nape of the neck) of an adult.

histopathologic examination numerous dilated capillaries without endothelial proliferation are found in the dermis. Lesions are reddish-purple, flat or barely elevated above the surface of the surrounding skin, do not fade appreciably with age, and, although benign, may be associated with other syndromes. Their color ranges from pale pink to bright red or bluish purple and, although initially flat, as the patient grows the areas may develop angiomatous papules and overgrowth of tissue. Port-wine stains are generally, but not necessarily, unilateral. Although they most commonly involve the face, they actually may occur on any cutaneous surface.

Lesions of nevus flammeus show little tendency toward involution, and treatment heretofore has generally been unsatisfactory. Treatments with thorium X, cryosurgery, and Grenz rays have been disappointing. Tattooing with skin-colored pigment is tedious, and since the secondary skin color changes with age, seasons, and tanning, results generally have not been very successful. The use of Covermark, a tinted opaque waterproof cream (manufactured by Lydia O'Leary, New York City), however, is useful and can do much to alleviate the cosmetic appearance of such lesions.

Of recent interest are encouraging studies on

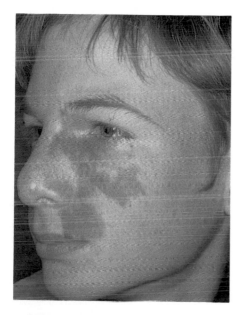

Figure 9–14 Port-wine stain (nevus flammeus), a diffuse capillary hemangioma on the left side of the face of a 16-year-old male.

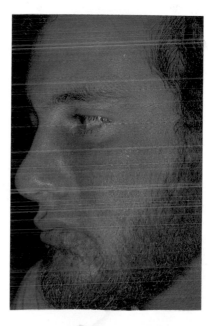

Figure 9–15 Bluish-purple nevus flammeus with angiomatous papules on the lower lip in a 21-year-old male.

the use of argon laser beam therapy. Hemoglobin's red color selectively absorbs the blue-green light of the argon laser and transforms the radiant energy into intense heat that coagulates small blood vessels up to 0.5 mm in diameter. Although this technique may not completely eliminate the lesion, it can induce lightening of the hemangioma. Those that are deep purple may become light violet; those that are deep red become light pink; and the sponginess and irregularity of the skin that may appear during later life is frequently improved to a significant degree, thus allowing easier application of readily available makeups. Although results to date remain preliminary and future clinical and laboratory investigation will be necessary before argon laser therapy can be recommended as the treatment of choice for all such vascular deformities, it appears that this approach allows a more optimistic outlook for the future management of such disorders.[12, 13] At present argon therapy is not recommended for children under 9 years of age.

ASSOCIATED SYNDROMES

Kasabach-Merritt Syndrome

The Kasabach-Merritt syndrome (thrombocytopenia reputedly caused by platelet sequestration in giant cavernous hemangiomas) is a disorder that generally affects infants three months of age or younger. Although most cavernous hemangiomata associated with thrombocytopenia are exceedingly large, excessive size is not necessarily a prerequisite of this disorder. Lesions as small as 5 or 6 cm in diameter have had confirmed thrombocytopenia.[14] Thrombocytopenia, frequently with blood platelet levels as low as 10,000 to 40,000, may be detected during the first few days of life. Children with rapidly expanding cavernous lesions (with or without ecchymoses) accordingly should be checked for platelet entrapment and incipient thrombocytopenia.

The danger of the Kasabach-Merritt syndrome is the development of acute hemorrhage or possible compression of vital structures during a period of rapid growth. Nearly one-fourth of reported infants with this complication died from bleeding disorders, respiratory distress, infection, or malignant transformation. Hence, infants with large cavernous hemangiomas and thrombocytopenia should be hospitalized and promptly treated.

Treatment consists of fresh whole-blood or platelet transfusions as needed, compression bandages over the hemangioma site whenever possible, a short intensive course of systemic steroids, cautious use of anticoagulants in the presence of disseminated intravascular coagulopathy, and surgical removal of the hemangiomatous lesion whenever feasible. Although surgery is relatively safe (if fresh whole-blood transfusions are used and the surgeon is experienced), surgical excision is almost never justified unless the characteristics of the hemangioma itself warrant

this approach.[15, 16] Although this procedure can at times be successfully accomplished, the hazards are often great, and most patients require treatment with corticosteroids or judicious radiation because of poor surgical risk or the size of the hemangioma.

Sturge-Weber Syndrome

The Sturge-Weber syndrome (encephalofacial or encephalotrigeminal angiomatosis) is a syndrome characterized by a nevus flammeus (port-wine stain) in the distribution of the first branch of the trigeminal nerve associated with a vascular malformation of the ipsilateral meninges and cerebral cortex (Table 9–2 and Fig. 9–16). Although there have been reports of Sturge-Weber syndrome in the absence of a facial nevus, these do not fulfill the criteria for Sturge-Weber syndrome and are termed meningeal angiomatosis.[17, 18]

Alexander and Norman, in their survey of 787 cases of nevus flammeus reported in the literature, found 257 cases of Sturge-Weber syndrome. All cases showed part of the facial nevus involving the forehead and upper eyelid to some extent. When the nevus occurred exclusively below the palpebral fissure, the cerebral angiomatosis was not found.[17] From this observation it may be inferred that if the vascular nevus does not involve the upper eyelid or forehead, one need not worry about the possible association of central nervous system involvement.

The oral mucous membranes may show telangiectatic hypertrophy, and ocular involvement occurs in 40 to 50 per cent of patients with Sturge-Weber syndrome. Studies suggest that if the vascular nevus involves both the ophthalmic and maxillary divisions of the sensory branch of the trigeminal nerve, childhood glaucoma appears in 45 per cent of patients; involvement of one branch alone does not seem to be associated with glaucoma.[19]

In 50 per cent of patients, the earliest symptoms of the intracranial lesions of Sturge-Weber syndrome develop during the first year. Although extensive meningeal lesions may remain silent throughout life, onset of symptoms after age 20 is unusual. Seizures, reported in 80 per cent of affected individuals, often as early as three months of age, frequently present as the initial symptom of this disorder. Hemiplegia has been reported in up

Table 9–2   STURGE-WEBER SYNDROME*

1. First branch of trigeminal nerve.
2. Ipsilateral meninges and cerebral cortex.
3. All involve forehead and upper eyelid.
4. Seizures (80%), retardation (60%), hemiplegia (30%).
5. 45% with glaucoma (with involvement of both ophthalmic and maxillary divisions of trigeminal).

*Based on Alexander G L, Norman R M: The Sturge-Weber Syndrome. John Wright & Sons, Ltd, Bristol, 1960; and Stevenson R F, et al.: Unrecognized ocular problems associated with port-wine stain of the face in children. Can. Med. Assoc. J. *111*:953, 1974.

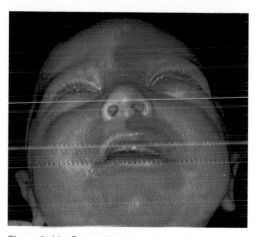

Figure 9–16 Sturge-Weber syndrome. Nevus flammeus in the distribution of the fifth (trigeminal) nerve. It should be noted that Sturge-Weber syndrome is unlikely when the vascular nevus occurs exclusively below the palpebral fissure.

to 30 per cent, and mental retardation may be seen in 60 per cent of affected individuals.[20]

The association of a conspicuous nevus flammeus with epilepsy or hemiplegia establishes the diagnosis. If the port-wine stain does not involve the upper eyelid or forehead, then Sturge-Weber syndrome is not present. Electroencephelography shows unilateral depression of cortical activity with or without spike discharges.[14] X-ray of the skull reveals characteristic calcifications in two-thirds of patients. These calcifications follow the convolutions of the cerebral cortex and are characterized by sinuous parallel streaks (called "tram-lines"). Calcifications can be detected after the first or second year of life and become more extensive up to the second decade, after which time they remain stable.

Surgical treatment of the intracranial lesion is occasionally successful. Accordingly, neurosurgical consultation should be sought as soon as the diagnosis has been established, preferably, if possible, before the onset of seizures. Palliative measures for the control of gingival overgrowth include surgical excision of excess tissue, injection of sclerosing solutions, and radiation therapy.[14] Reg-

ular supervision by an ophthalmologist and control of glaucoma by goniotomy is an important aspect of therapy. For management of the vascular lesions, refer to the preceding discussion on treatment of nevus flammeus.

Klippel-Trenaunay-Parkes-Weber Syndrome

The Klippel-Trenaunay-Parkes-Weber syndrome (nevus vasculosus hypertrophicus) is a vascular malformation characterized by local overgrowth of bone and soft tissue of an extremity or portion of the trunk associated with phlebectasia, arteriovenous aneurysms, and cutaneous telangiectasia resembling a port-wine stain. More often of an upper rather than a lower extremity and on the left rather than the right side of the body, the hypertrophy involves the length as well as the circumference of the extremity, and boys are more frequently affected than girls (Fig. 9–17).

The hemangioma may be capillary or cavernous in nature and is often complicated by arteriovenous shunts and lymphangiomatous anomalies. Treatment is generally unsatisfactory. Compression of dilated veins by support bandages has some merit, and surgery may be effective in the prevention of severe limb hypertrophy in occasional patients. Surgery is not indicated for superficial venous varicosities resulting from hypoplasia or atresia of the deep venous system and can produce disastrous results. Appropriate radiographic studies, therefore, are advisable prior to any attempts at surgical correction.[21] Although radiation therapy has been advocated for some individuals, to date this approach has not met with enthusiastic support and should be used judiciously or rarely, if at all.

Maffucci's Syndrome

Maffucci's syndrome (dyschondroplasia with hemangiomata) is characterized by vascular hamartomas (hemangiomas, phlebectasias, and lymphangiomas) and associated dyschondroplasia. Two thirds of reported patients have been males.

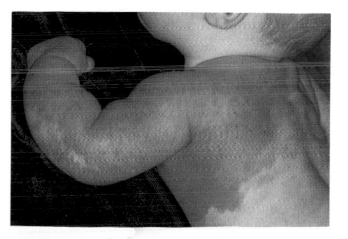

Figure 9–17 Klippel Trenaunay-Parkes-Weber syndrome. Local hypertrophy of the bone and soft tissue associated with a port-wine stain in a 3-month-old infant.

Individuals with this disorder are usually normal at birth (only rarely are they born with visible hemangiomas or skeletal nodules). During the prepubertal years (the first twelve years of life) the multiple hemangiomata and dyschondroplasias, usually manifested clinically by hard nodules on the fingers or toes followed by other nodular lesions elsewhere on the extremities, become apparent. Subsequently other progressive skeletal abnormalities due to defects of ossification (marked bony deformities complicated by pathologic fractures) may be seen.

The vascular lesions consist of dilated veins and soft bluish cavernous hemangiomata, which occur on the affected limb or elsewhere. The distribution of vascular lesions does not correspond to that of the skeletal lesions. Of particular significance is the fact that some 30 per cent of patients with this disorder develop some type of associated malignant disease (chondrosarcoma or angiosarcoma). The management of this disorder, accordingly, consists of surgery, when indicated, and periodic evaluation to detect and extirpate any lesions suggestive of neoplastic degeneration.

Blue Rubber-bleb Nevus Syndrome

The blue rubber-bleb nevus is a variant of a cavernous hemangioma that presents as a soft compressible blue to purple rubbery protuberance of the dermis and subcutaneous tissue. Some lesions may be spontaneously painful and tender to palpation. In this syndrome the vascular lesions are sometimes present at birth and, with time, frequently tend to increase in size or number. The importance of this type of lesion lies in its frequent association with angiomas of the gastrointestinal tract. The gastrointestinal hemangiomas most frequently are found in the small intestine or colon but may occur anywhere throughout the gastrointestinal tract. They tend to bleed readily and frequently cause anemia.

The cutaneous lesions are blue and raised, their surfaces are wrinkled, and they vary in size from 0.1 to 5.0 cm in diameter. They may present as large cavernous hemangiomas, blue rubber blebs, or irregular blue marks on the cutaneous surface. They may be solitary or may number in the hundreds and can occur anywhere on the cutaneous surface (usually the trunk or arms) or the mucous membranes of the nose and mouth. One of the diagnostic features is the fact that blood can be expressed from the lesions with pressure, leaving an empty wrinkled sac. The treatment of this disorder is mainly symptomatic with resection of bowel, when indicated, to control excessive bleeding and anemia.[22, 23]

Diffuse Neonatal Hemangiomatosis

A number of infants have been reported with multiple hemangiomas of the visceral organs, the gastrointestinal tract, liver, central nervous system, and lungs. Although on occasion such infants have no cutaneous involvement, most affected children display widely disseminated small, red to bluish-black papular cutaneous hemangiomata (usually present at birth or developing during the first few weeks of life) numbering in the hundreds (diffuse neonatal hemangiomatosis, multinodular hemangiomatosis). Despite supportive therapy affected infants often die of high output cardiac failure, from hepatic complications, gastrointestinal hemorrhage, respiratory tract obstruction, or severe neurologic deficit due to compression of neural tissue.

When seen in association with multinodular hemangiomatosis, cardiac failure is believed to be the result of arteriovenous shunts in hepatic hemangiomas, which ultimately lead to increased venous return and increased cardiac output. When present, this complication occurs early in life (usually at 2 to 9 weeks of age). Hepatic hemangiomas, when present, may be delineated by liver and spleen scan or hepatic angiography or both. Recognition of the cutaneous component, which may be minimal in some infants, will permit correct early diagnosis and help prevent confusion with cardiac failure seen in association with congenital heart disease. Surgical management of this complication, by lobectomy or selective ligation of hepatic vessels, can frequently be avoided by therapy with systemic corticosteroids and digitalis (particularly when initiated early).[24, 25]

Gorham's Syndrome

Gorham's syndrome (disappearing bones, vanishing bone disease, angiomatous nevi with osteolysis) is an extremely uncommon disorder that consists of cutaneous hemangiomas in association with massive osteolysis and complete or partial replacement of bone by extensive fibrosis. The skin and soft tissue involvement in this disorder is usually confined to areas near the bony lesions. Although the cause of increased bone resorption is not known, it has been theorized that this phenomenon may be due to localized hyperemia associated with the hemangiomas.

Usually a disorder of young children, involving single or multiple bones, Gorham's disease is believed to be a slowly developing, probably self-limiting, condition and does not progress to neoplastic formation. Numerous methods of therapy have been employed, but not one has proved of value. The only reported deaths associated with this disorder are those that resulted from hemorrhage into serous cavities.[26, 27]

Riley-Smith Syndrome

The Riley-Smith syndrome (macrocephaly with unusual cutaneous angiomatosis) is presumably an autosomal dominant disorder characterized by multiple cavernous hemangiomata, macrocephaly, and pseudopapillomata. Recently this disorder has been expanded to include individuals with the Klippel-Trenaunay-Parkes-Weber syndrome, a combination of Sturge-Weber and the Klippel-Trenaunay-Parkes-Weber syndrome, cutis marmorata telangiectatica congenita, and macrocephaly with multiple lipomas and hemangiomas.[28, 29] Because normal central nervous system function is frequently seen in association with this syndrome, awareness of the benign nature of the macrocephaly should help avoid unnecessary concern or intervention, except in patients who also manifest signs of increased intracranial pressure or central nervous system dysfunction.

The Cobb Syndrome

The Cobb syndrome consists of a cutaneous vascular nevus (angiolipoma, cavernous hemangioma, port-wine stain, or angiokeratoma) and an associated angioma in the spinal cord corresponding within a segment or two to the involved dermatome.[30] Males slightly outnumber females in most cases reported to date, and in the majority of patients, the neurologic problems occur during childhood or adolescence. In most patients, lateral thoracic and lumbar spine radiograms may show early bone erosion.

Treatment, as well as diagnosis, may be aided by spinal angiography. Spinal angiomas fed by the posterior spinal artery are often juxtamedullary and can be extirpated surgically without appreciable damage to the spinal cord. Those fed by the anterior spinal artery, however, are often intramedullary and supply critical motor pathways and neurons. Surgical removal of such lesions, therefore, is frequently technically impossible.

VASCULAR TUMORS

Verrucous Hemangioma

A verrucous hemangioma is an uncommon variant of a capillary, cavernous, or mixed hemangioma that develops secondary proliferative epidermal change. Easily mistaken for verrucae, pigmented tumors, or angiokeratomas, they are vascular lesions that generally occur on the lower extremities, occasionally the chest and forearms. Most are present at birth or appear during early childhood. Initially they are soft, bluish-red, well demarcated, and range in size from 4 mm to as much as 5 to 7 cm in diameter. As the patient grows the lesions enlarge and frequently develop a brown or bluish-black color with keratotic and verrucous features, which tend to obscure the true vascular nature of this disorder. When the diagnosis remains in doubt, histopathologic examination will reveal a capillary or cavernous hemangioma with overlying epidermal hyperkeratosis, irregular acanthosis, and papillomatosis.

Since verrucous hemangiomas do not regress spontaneously and tend to enlarge in proportion to the growth of the body, early excision generally is advisable. Smaller lesions (1 to 2 cm in diameter) are frequently amenable to local excision or electrocautery. Larger lesions, however, often extend into the subcutaneous fat and tend to recur (particularly when subjected to secondary infection or trauma). Such lesions are probably best treated by wide excision and subsequent skin graft.[31]

Pyogenic Granuloma

Pyogenic granuloma (granuloma pyogenicum, granuloma telangiectaticum) is a common vascular lesion, which in most instances consists of a bright red to reddish-brown, soft or moderately firm, raised, usually slightly pedunculated nodule (Fig. 9–18). The mechanism that brings about the formation of a pyogenic granuloma is unknown. It is thought to be caused by a reactive proliferative vascular process, possibly associated with trauma and the presence of a pyogenic bacteria. Although there may indeed be an association with bacteria, pyogenic granuloma does not appear to be an infectious process. Affecting individuals of all ages, it occurs frequently in children and young adults but is unusual in older persons.

Lesions are solitary and develop rapidly. Although they may occur on any cutaneous surface, they most commonly appear in areas subject to trauma, namely the hands (particularly the fingers), the forearms, the face, and occasionally the mucosal surfaces of the mouth. Pyogenic granulomas are vascular, range in size from 5 mm to 1 or 2 cm in diameter, and bleed easily, even on the slightest trauma. In most cases the history and clinical appearance are highly characteristic, and the correct diagnosis is easily established. The histologic picture is that of a well-circumscribed capillary hemangioma embedded in a loose edematous stroma and covered by a flattened epidermis.

Treatment consists of destruction of the lesion by electrodesiccation and curettage, with coagulation of the base. A number of pyogenic granulomas recur after such treatment, however, because the proliferating vessels in the base extend in a conical manner into the deeper dermis. In such instances repeat electrodesiccation, cryosurgery

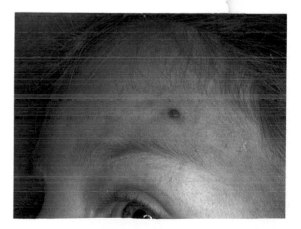

Figure 9–18 Pyogenic granuloma. A benign bright red elevated vascular nodule on the forehead of a young child.

with liquid nitrogen, or surgical excision are generally effective.

Glomus Tumor

Glomus tumors are relatively uncommon hamartomas of the glomus body, a special temperature-regulating arteriovenous shunt which bypasses the usual capillary bed of the dermis. Rarely seen in infants, the lesions may be solitary or multiple in number and occur in children as well as adults.

Solitary glomus tumors, the more common form of this disorder do not appear to have a familial tendency. They usually occur as extremely tender bluish-red cutaneous nodules that vary from one millimeter to several centimeters in size. Lesions usually appear on the upper extremities, particularly the nail beds, occasionally the lower extremities, the head, neck, or penis. They are extremely tender and frequently give rise to paroxysms of pain. Although the etiology is unknown, some lesions appear to be associated with previous trauma to the involved area.

In contrast to the solitary type, multiple glomus tumors are dominantly transmitted, may be painful or painless, and vary from a few lesions to several hundred in number. They are relatively more common in children than adults, and the majority of lesions involve the lower extremities and only sometimes the upper extremities. The face, neck, and subungual areas generally are spared. Multiple glomus tumors appear as flesh-colored to bluish-red, flat to dome-shaped papules that vary in size from a few millimeters to several centimeters in diameter and blanch completely on diascopy.

Solitary glomus tumors must be differentiated from neurofibromas, dermatofibromas, melanomas, blue nevi, and leiomyomas; multiple lesions must be differentiated from leiomyomas and cavernous hemangiomas. When the diagnosis remains in doubt, the true nature of the disorder may be verified by cutaneous biopsy.

On histopathologic examination solitary glomus tumors are surrounded by a fibrous capsule and contain numerous small vascular lumina lined by a single layer of glomus cells that have a faintly eosinophilic cytoplasm and a large, oval or cuboidal pale nucleus. Multiple glomus tumors possess no capsules and are much more vascular than the solitary type. They are lined by a single layer of flat endothelial cells, and glomus cells are seen peripheral to the endothelial cells as a narrow rim of only one to three layers.

Glomus tumors are not radiosensitive, and electrocoagulation is frequently followed by recurrence. Surgical excision is the best method of treatment, but recurrences, particularly in the subungual region, are common.

Hemangiopericytoma

Hemangiopericytomas are very rare tumors of the skin, subcutaneous, and muscular tissues and may appear on any part of the body. Derived from pericytes (smooth muscle cells that surround small blood vessels), these usually solitary firm nodules have been reported in individuals from birth to 93 years of age but usually appear shortly after birth, during early childhood, or in middle life.[32, 33] Their clinical appearance is not distinctive, and their course is highly variable. Lesions are painless, often well circumscribed, vary in size from 1 to 8 cm or more in diameter, and are flesh-colored to reddish-blue. Some lesions are benign and remain quiescent. Others show rapid growth and an incidence of neoplastic change estimated at 20 per cent, with a predilection for the musculoskeletal system. In children, those that are superficial or located in the subcutis generally tend to remain benign, however.

Histologically, hemangiopericytomas often resemble glomus tumors and may indeed be related to them. They are characterized by branching capillaries surrounded by closely packed cells with oval or spindle-shaped nuclei (pericytes) embedded in a network of reticulum fibers.

Since hemangiopericytomas are unpredictable and have a high incidence of neoplastic change (generally during the second or third decades of life), wide local excision is the treatment of choice.

ANGIOKERATOMAS

The term angiokeratoma is applied to a group of disorders characterized by ectasia (dilatation of the superficial vessels of the dermis) and hyperkeratosis of the overlying epidermis. All have in common the presence of asymptomatic vascular lesions, seen as firm dark-red to black papules that measure from 1 to 10 mm in size with varying degrees of secondary hyperkeratosis (Figs. 9–19 and 9–20).

At least six forms of angiokeratoma have been recognized. Four represent cosmetic problems only. These include solitary or multiple angiokeratomas, angiokeratoma circumscriptum, angiokeratoma of Mibelli, and angiokeratoma of the scrotum and vulva (angiokeratoma of Fordyce). The fifth and sixth forms are diffuse diseases of

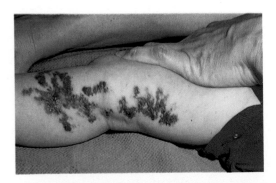

Figure 9–19 Angiokeratoma circumscriptum on the leg of a 15-year-old child (Department of Dermatology, Yale University School of Medicine).

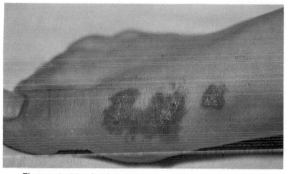

Figure 9-20 Angiokeratoma of Mibelli. Hyperkeratotic vascular lesions over the bony prominences of the foot (Courtesy of Hillard H. Pearlstein, M.D.).

systemic significance. They are known as angiokeratoma corporis diffusum or Fabry's disease (a sex-linked disorder characterized by storage of a neutral glycolipid, ceramidetrihexoside, in many types of cells in the body) and fucosidosis (an autosomal recessive disease characterized by the abnormal intracellular accumulation of a fucose-containing glycosphingolipid).

Solitary or Multiple Angiokeratomas

Solitary or multiple angiokeratomas represent a group of individual lesions generally seen on the lower extremities. They appear to follow trauma and begin as an area of telangiectasia followed by hyperkeratosis and angiokeratoma formation. Although they may be seen in childhood, these lesions are not congenital in nature but appear to be acquired as a result of injury to the papillary vessels, with resultant dilatation and impaired contractility of the capillary wall. Single angiokeratomas may be mistaken for nevi or malignant melanoma, but can be differentiated on the basis of histopathologic examination.

Microscopic features include groups of dilated papillary blood vessels, acanthosis and hyperkeratosis of the epidermis, and elongation of the rete ridges, which often tend to enclose the underlying capillary spaces. Treatment of asymptomatic angiokeratomas is usually unnecessary. When desired, however, because of trauma or for cosmetic purposes, local excision or electrodesiccation generally gives a good cosmetic result.[34]

Angiokeratoma Circumscriptum

Angiokeratoma circumscriptum is a rare disorder usually seen as a solitary large hyperkeratotic plaque or nodule. In half of the reported cases the lesion begins in infancy or early childhood, with females reportedly affected three times as frequently as males. Usually deep red or blue-black in color, lesions are seen as localized unilateral papules, nodules, or plaques, often arranged in streaks or bands, with an uneven verrucous surface. Although they may occur on the back,

forearm, or penis, the thighs, lower legs, and buttocks are the more typical areas of involvement. Lesions usually increase in size only in proportion to general body growth but may go on to enlarge during adolescence or early adult life, and in several instances, extensive lesions covering as much as one-quarter of the body have been reported.

Angiokeratoma circumscriptum does not show a tendency to spontaneous involution. Small lesions may be removed by electrodesiccation and curettage; in larger lesions extensive surgical excision appears to be the treatment of choice.[35]

Angiokeratoma of Mibelli

Angiokeratoma of Mibelli is a rare disorder first described by Mibelli in 1889. It is characterized by hyperkeratotic vascular lesions that occur over the bony prominences of the extremities of children, usually girls, during late childhood or early adolescence. Since it has been described in siblings and children with an affected parent, a dominant mode of inheritance with variable penetrance has been suggested.[36, 37]

Lesions usually occur over the dorsal and lateral aspects of the fingers and toes, but may also involve the ears, knees, ankles, elbows, palms, soles, and backs of the hands and feet. This distribution and the frequent association of lesions with acrocyanosis, chilblains, and frostbite suggest cold-sensitivity as the precipitating factor of this disorder.

Early lesions are minute reddish to purple macules or soft papules. With time they increase in size to 5 to 8 mm or more in diameter and become elevated, verrucous, and darker in color. Although often numerous and disfiguring, lesions are generally asymptomatic. They do, however, bleed easily and, at times, may involute spontaneously following trauma. In patients with associated acrocyanosis and chilblains there may be abnormalities of immunoglobulin levels, with elevations of IgG, IgA, and IgM. One patient, an 11-year-old mentally retarded spastic girl, also had oral ulcerations and bony and soft tissue necrosis of the fingertips.[38]

Treatment of this disorder consists of cryosurgery with solid carbon dioxide or liquid nitrogen, electrocautery, or surgical excision.

Angiokeratoma of Fordyce (angiokeratoma of the scrotum and vulva)

Angiokeratoma of the scrotum is a relatively common disorder first described by Fordyce in 1896. It occasionally appears in adolescents but most commonly occurs in males over the age of 30, with an increasing incidence with age.[39] Clinically and histologically similar lesions may also appear on the labia of older women.

Lesions are distributed along the superficial vessels of the scrotum in a linear configuration, generally perpendicular to the scrotal raphe. Oc-

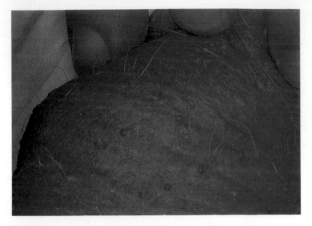

Figure 9–21 Angiokeratoma of the scrotum (Angiokeratoma of Fordyce).

casionally they may appear on the glans or shaft of the penis, and rarely they may be noted on the upper thigh or inguinal area.

Scrotal angiokeratomas are seen as multiple small 1 to 4 mm reddish-purple to black dome-shaped vascular-appearing papules (Fig. 9–21). With increase in the age of the patient they become larger, darker, more numerous, nodular, and keratotic in appearance. The etiology of these papules is unknown. Some investigators believe them to be neoplastic in origin. Others consider them to be venous telangiectases, possibly associated with venous obstruction. In support of the latter hypothesis is a frequent associated finding of varicocele, hernia, prostatitis, tumors of the bladder or epididymis, lymphogranuloma venereum, or thrombophlebitis in patients with this disorder.

Although angiokeratomas of the scrotum generally tend to be asymptomatic, they may become pruritic and tend to bleed when traumatized. Treatment, when desired, consists of electrocoagulation or cryosurgery with solid carbon dioxide or liquid nitrogen.

Angiokeratoma Corporis Diffusum

In 1898 Fabry in Germany and Anderson in England independently described a form of angiokeratoma now known as angiokeratoma corporis diffusum or Fabry syndrome. The disorder appears to be an X-linked recessive disease with complete penetrance and variable clinical expressivity in homozygous males and occasional mild penetrance in the heterozygous female.[40-42] The disorder is characterized by systemic intracellular accumulation of glycophingolipid (trihexosyl ceramide) in the skin and viscera, particularly in the cardiovascular-renal system. The primary metabolic defect is the deficient activity of a specific alpha-galactosidase (ceramide trihexosidase) which normally catabolizes the accumulated glycosphingolipid.

The cutaneous vascular lesions characteristic of this disorder are telangiectases. They usually appear before puberty, generally between 5 and 13 years of age. Occasionally they may occur during infancy. The lesions generally appear as clusters of individual punctate macular or papular dark red angiectases that do not blanch with pressure. The eruption is usually symmetrical, and the lesions generally increase progressively in size and number with age. Despite their name, they generally show little to no hyperkeratosis.

Angiokeratomas of Fabry usually appear in the area between the umbilicus and knees. They may number into the thousands and tend to cluster in the ileosacral areas, about the umbilicus, and over the scrotum, buttocks, posterior thorax, and thighs. The first lesions frequently appear in the scrotum and must be differentiated from angiokeratoma of Fordyce. Lesions seldom occur on the hands or feet, have not been reported on the scalp, ears, or face, except for a small area on the chin, and are permanent unless they become thrombosed, after which they may disappear (which is rare). A majority of patients have pinpoint macular purplish spots on the lips, particularly near the vermilion border of the lower lip. These lesions are smaller than those on the skin. The tongue is not affected, but hemoptysis and epistaxis have been reported with involvement of the buccal and nasal mucosae. In addition to the typical cutaneous lesions, fine telangiectases have been described in the axillae on the upper chest. In heterozygous females angiomas appear in only 20 per cent of cases and, when present, are less numerous and more limited in extent than in males.[43]

Attacks of pain and paresthesias of the hands and feet often accompany the eruption. Although often spontaneous or elicited by exertion, they are apparently associated with vasomotor disturbances and usually occur subsequent to temperature changes. Edema of the ankles, paralyses, scant body hair, and hypohidrosis are often present. Pedal and ankle edema are present in most cases and may result in stasis ulcers. Edema, when present, is presumably due to increased vascular permeability and is more prominent in summer than winter.

Patients with angiokeratoma corporis diffusum are often hypertensive and, with advancing age, are particularly susceptible to cerebrovascular accidents, coronary artery disease, and renal disease. Neurologic complications are common and include aphasia, paresis, tremors, paralyses, loss of consciousness, and psychotic disturbances. Other systemic manifestations include diarrhea, colitis and proctitis, an unusual arthritis of the distal interphalangeal joints with some loss of motion, cataracts, corneal opacities, and tortuosity of the conjunctival blood vessels with characteristic sausage-like constriction and dilatation.

The corneal opacities are usually present during childhood; they are found in all affected males as well as most female carriers with this disorder. Of particular diagnostic importance is the fact that the posterior capsular cataracts have a characteristic spoke-like appearance. This spoke-like feature, when present, is pathognomonic of this disorder.

Most men with angiokeratoma of Fabry die in their thirties as a result of renal failure with uremia and hypertension. Others succumb to cerebrovascular accidents and congestive heart failure.

The course in female heterozygotes is more benign. Afflicted women have skin lesions (in 20 per cent of cases), cataracts, and relatively normal longevity. Although the disorder is generally asymptomatic in women, some have hypohidrosis, attacks of pain in the extremities, arthritis, urinary tract infection, and renal failure.

The diagnosis of angiokeratoma corporis diffusum is made by the presence of cutaneous angiomas, a positive family history, corneal opacities on slit-lamp examination, and the presence of trihexosyl ceramide in the urine, plasma, or cultured fibroblasts. Hemizygotes and heterozygotes may also be diagnosed by hair root analysis.[44] Early in the course of the disease, casts, red cells, fat-laden epithelial cells (mulberry cells), and lipid inclusions with characteristic birefringent "Maltese crosses" appear in the urinary sediment. Proteinuria, gradual deterioration of renal function, and azotemia occur in the second to fourth decade of life. Biopsy of the skin or kidney is confirmatory if intracellular birefringent lipoid deposits can be demonstrated, and prenatal detection can be accomplished by the demonstration of deficient alpha galactosidase in cultured cells obtained by amniocentesis.[45]

Unfortunately, there is no specific therapy to correct the biochemical defect of Fabry's disease. Treatment, therefore, is generally supportive in nature. Replacement transfusion and periodic infusion with normal plasma have been suggested in an attempt to provide ceramidetrihexosidase to patients with this inherited metabolic disease.[46]

Fucosidosis

Disseminated angiokeratomas may also be seen in patients with fucosidosis, an autosomal recessive disease characterized by absence or deficiency of the lysosomal enzyme alpha-L-fucosi-

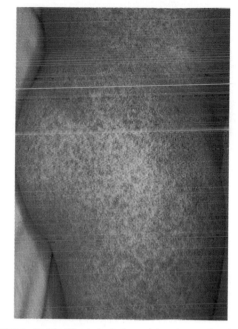

Figure 9–22 Disseminated angiokeratomas in a child with fucosidosis (Courtesy of Benjamin K. Fisher, M.D.).

dase (Figs. 9–22 and 9–23). This disorder, first described by Durand in 1966, is associated with tissue accumulation of polysaccharides, mucopolysaccharides, and glycolipids and is characterized by mental retardation, weakness, spasticity, and retardation, with or without angiokeratomas.[47, 48]

Three variants of fucosidosis have been described. The first occurs in infancy and is characterized by progressive neurologic degeneration, mental retardation, weakness, spasticity, marked growth retardation, enlarged heart, repeated respiratory infection, hypoplastic lumbar vertebrae, and death generally within the first few years of life. Cutaneous signs of this variant include hyperhidrosis and thickening of the skin.

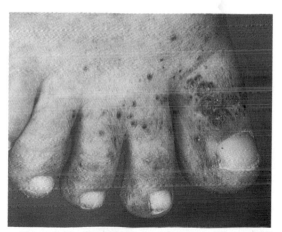

Figure 9–23 Fucosidosis. Angiokeratoma diffusum of the foot (Courtesy of Benjamin K. Fisher, M.D.).

The second, a milder form of fucosidosis described in 1971, is referred to as lysosomal bone disease. This unusual form is associated with normal intelligence, moderate growth retardation, and spondyloepiphyseal dysplasia.[49]

The third type of fucosidosis is compatible with life, at least until adolescence. It is associated with central nervous system involvement (mental retardation, weakness, spasticity, and, at times, seizures), coarse facies, mild spondyloepiphyseal dysplasia, retardation of growth, frequent respiratory infections, decreased sweating, purple nail bands in some patients, and cutaneous lesions of angiokeratoma corporis diffusum.[50]

Patients with all three types of fucosidosis have markedly decreased or absent alpha-L-fucosidase activity, which results in increased levels of fucose-containing compounds in all tissues. Asymptomatic carriers of this autosomal recessive trait have also been found to have abnormally low alpha-L-fucosidase activity in cells and serum. Patients with Fabry disease may be confused with those with the third variant of fucosidosis. Those with fucosidosis, however, do not have hypertensive cardiovascular disease, cerebral hemorrhage, or renal failure, and fat stains of histologic material from patients with fucosidosis do not show lipids, as seen in the cytoplasmic inclusions of Fabry disease.

There is, to date, no effective form of therapy for fucosidosis. Efforts at enzyme replacement, as in other lysosomal diseases, however, show promise.

DISORDERS ASSOCIATED WITH VASCULAR DILATATION

Livedo Reticularis

Livedo reticularis is a mottled or reticulated bluish-red discoloration of the skin that occurs chiefly on the trunk, legs, and forearms of children and adults. The etiology of livedo reticularis is not completely understood, but exposure to cold usually intensifies the vascular pattern of this disorder. Most investigators attribute its reticulated appearance to vasospasm of the arterioles in response to cold, with subsequent hypoxia and dilatation of capillaries and venules. This results in sluggish blood flow through the subpapillary venous plexuses and a mottled livid or cyanotic appearance to the involved areas.

The blotchy pattern of livedo reticularis, in contrast to that of cutis marmorata, persists even when the skin is rewarmed. Livedo is usually normal when it affects the trunk or limbs of girls and young women in a continuous or persistent pattern. When livedo reticularis develops in a blotchy or interrupted asymmetrical distribution, it often represents an early sign of systemic disease, such as rheumatoid arthritis, rheumatic fever, lupus erythematosus, idiopathic thrombocytopenia, thrombotic thrombocytopenic purpura, leukemia, neurologic disorders (cerebrovascular accidents), and cryoglobulinemia.[51] In rare cases, recurrent small ulcerations may develop on the lower legs and feet in adults with idiopathic livedo reticularis. Mild hypertension and edema of the skin of the ankles, feet, and legs have been described in such cases. Although there is no specific treatment for livedo reticularis, vasodilating and anticoagulant drugs have been used with moderate success in patients with severe ulceration.[52]

Congenital Generalized Phlebectasia

Cutis marmorata telangiectatica congenita (congenital generalized phlebectasia) is a relatively uncommon disorder of infants and children characterized by a reticulated bluish mottling of the skin that resembles an exaggerated form of cutis marmorata. Seen in males as well as females (contrary to many statements in current textbooks and literature), the disorder is seen as dilated reticulated venous and capillary channels measuring 3 to 4 mm or more in diameter (Fig. 9–24). Usually present at birth, the vascular pattern generally extends somewhat during the first few weeks of life and, in most patients, eventually improves substantially during childhood. In some cases the cutaneous marbling pattern persists on into adulthood.[53, 54, 55] In most patients the vascular pattern of cutis marmorata telangiectatica congenita is distributed in a generalized manner over the trunk and extremities. In some, however, the involvement may be segmental or localized to one extremity or a limited portion of the trunk.

The etiology is unknown, but it appears to represent a developmental ectasia involving both capillaries and veins. In some patients little or no histopathologic abnormality can be seen. In others, however, microscopic examination of a cutaneous biopsy may reveal dilated capillaries, capillary and venous lakes, and large dilated veins in all layers of the dermis and subcutaneous tis-

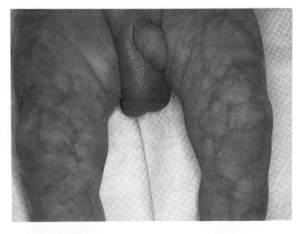

Figure 9–24 Congenital generalized phlebectasia (cutis marmorata telangiectatica congenita). This disorder must be differentiated from cutis marmorata.

sue.[53, 55] Since histopathologic features are variable, diagnosis is best made on clinical criteria.

Ulcerations over the reticulated vascular pattern have been seen in a few patients with this disorder. In general, however, cutis marmorata telangiectatica congenita has a benign course and requires no specific therapy. Other defects in association with this disorder have been reported. These include hemangiomatous abnormalities and varicosities, telangiectatic capillary nevi, patent ductus arteriosus, congenital glaucoma with mental retardation, branchial cleft cysts, and atrophy or hypertrophy of soft tissue or bone, suggesting a possible developmental defect of the mesoderm. It therefore is suggested that patients with this disorder be followed carefully for the possibility of other associated malformations.[54, 55]

Diffuse Phlebectasia

Diffuse phlebectasia (Brockenheimer syndrome) is a rare hemartomatous malformation involving the deeper venous channels of a limb or part of a limb. This disorder is characterized by gradual onset during infancy, childhood, adolescence, or early adult life. It consists of multiple spongy irregular venous sinusoids and dilated veins that assume bizarre patterns, with tumor-like vascular swelling of the involved area. The overlying skin may be atrophic, and secondary complications consisting of thromboses and phleboliths, with resultant bleeding, ulceration, or infection of the affected limb, may occur. The name *congenital phlebectasia* has been used as synonym for *cutis marmorata telangiectatic congenita*. Although the latter is more cumbersome, it is probably more accurate and helps avoid confusion between the congenital and diffuse forms of phlebectasia.

TELANGIECTASES

Telangiectases are permanent dilatations of capillaries, venules, or arterioles in the skin that may or may not disappear on diascopy (gentle pressure with a microscope slide or hand lens). Many processes affecting the blood vessel endothelium and its supporting structure can lead to the development of this common vascular lesion. Some of these are primary disorders of the blood vessels themselves for which the cause is unknown. Others are secondary in nature and are related to some other known disturbances, such as aging, light exposure, x-ray, or systemic disorders for which they may serve as useful diagnostic clues.[51]

Spider Angioma

The spider angioma (nevus araneus) is the best known type of telangiectasia. It is characterized by a central, occasionally elevated, vascular punctum with symmetrically radiating thin

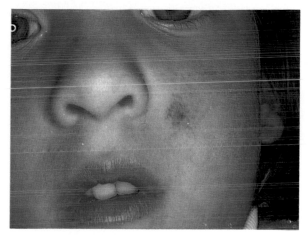

Figure 9–25 Spider angioma (nevus araneus). A central vascular body with radiating vascular legs and a surrounding flush. Diagnosis can be confirmed by blanching the legs and demonstration of pulsations of the central vessel by gentle pressure with a glass slide (diascopy).

branches (legs). Spider angiomas appear most commonly on exposed areas of the face, upper trunk, arms, hands, and fingers, and occasionally on the mucous membranes of the lip and nose. The central body is an arteriole (which at times can be shown to pulsate by gentle diascopy) (Fig. 9–25).

Although spider angiomas can be associated with liver disease, pregnancy, and estrogen therapy, they are frequently idiopathic and occur in 15 per cent of normal children and young adults. A small proportion of spider nevi regress spontaneously. The majority of such lesions, particularly in children, however, tend to persist indefinitely.

Diagnosis of spider angioma depends upon recognition of the typical morphology of the lesion, demonstration of the central pulsating vessel, and blanching of the surrounding legs with diascopy of the central body. Therapy, when desired, consists of gentle electrodesiccation, electrocoagulation, or cryosurgery with solid carbon dioxide or liquid nitrogen, and usually results in a good cosmetic result.

Angioma Serpiginosum

Angioma serpiginosum is a rare nevoid disorder of the small vessels of the dermis that occurs predominantly in females (90 per cent) and usually has its onset during childhood.[20] Lesions may affect any part of the body but generally are seen on the lower limbs and buttocks of affected individuals. They are characterized by minute copper-colored to red or purple angiomatous puncta with a background of diffuse erythema, which often measures a centimeter or more in diameter. The condition generally begins as one or more small lesions and characteristically extends slowly over a period of months or years. Individual puncta often disappear, and although complete clearing of lesions may occur at times, the prognosis for complete spontaneous resolution is generally poor.

Histopathologic characteristics include dilated and tortuous capillaries (ectasia), acanthosis, scattered parakeratosis and hyperkeratosis, occasional atrophy of the epidermis, and varying degrees of liquefaction necrosis of the basal layer.

Although electrocoagulation and electrodesiccation of individual puncta may give partial resolution, treatment of this disorder is unsatisfactory and generally not recommended.

Hereditary Hemorrhagic Telangiectasia

Hereditary hemorrhagic telangiectasia (Osler's disease, Osler-Rendu-Weber disease) is an autosomal dominant disorder characterized by the presence of numerous telangiectases on the skin and mucous membranes of the nose and mouth, recurrent nosebleeds, and a family history of the disorder (Fig. 9–26). Recurrent epistaxis, the usual presenting symptom of this disorder, may begin in early childhood (generally at about 8 or 10 years), or early in infancy, but more commonly does not begin until puberty or adult life. The characteristic mucocutaneous lesions, however, are rarely observed in children and generally do not become evident until the third decade of life, or later.

True lesions of this disorder tend to be "slightly elevated with an ill-defined border and one or more legs radiating from an eccentrically placed border."[51] They develop primarily on the lips, tongue, palate, nasal mucosa, conjunctiva, ears, palms, under the nails, on the plantar surfaces of the feet, and occasionally the trunk and toes. Similar lesions may also occur in the pharynx, larynx, bronchi, liver, brain, retina, urinary

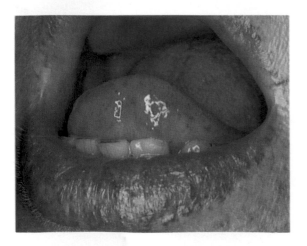

Figure 9–26 Hereditary hemorrhagic telangiectasia (Osler's disease, Osler-Weber-Rendu disease). Cutaneous manifestations usually appear after puberty and are characterized by 1 to 4 mm slightly elevated bright red to purple telangiectatic vessels with one or more legs radiating from an eccentrically placed punctum.

bladder, and gastrointestinal tract. Hemorrhages may occur from any site, and their severity and frequency determine the clinical manifestations and course of the disorder.[20] Pulmonary arteriovenous fistulae are present in some cases and tend to occur in certain families, but are rare in children. When present, associated signs and symptoms include dyspnea, cyanosis, polycythemia, and clubbing of the fingers and toes in adolescence.

Diagnosis is dependent upon the history and morphologic configuration of individual telangiectatic lesions. Microscopic examination reveals a subepidermal tortuous mass of dilated vessels with a markedly thin wall composed almost entirely of a single layer of endothelium.

Treatment of mild cases is not necessary. Individual lesions may be cauterized, and iron supplements may help control secondary anemia. In severe disorders, systemic estrogens have been advocated but, when used in small dosages (as in contraceptive pills) actually may aggravate the disorder. Resection of pulmonary arteriovenous shunts and involved segments of the gastrointestinal tract may be necessary, and for severe epistaxis, dermoplasty may be beneficial for some individuals.

Ataxia Telangiectasia

Ataxia telangiectasia (Louis-Bar syndrome) is an autosomal recessive multifaceted syndrome characterized by progressive cerebellar ataxia, oculocutaneous telangiectasia, and frequent severe respiratory tract infections. An associated thymic defect and immunologic defect in some cases has led some to classify this as a disturbance of defective thymic development, generalized lymphoreticular abnormalities, immunologic deficiency, and unusual susceptibility to lymphoreticular malignancy.[56]

Children affected with this disorder are usually small and appear to be normal until the ataxia and clumsiness become apparent during the second year of life. In association with the ataxia affected individuals develop choreoathetosis, drooling, peculiar ocular movements, and a sad mask-like facies. By age 12 the ataxia becomes so severe that patients are unable to walk without assistance.

Ataxia telangiectasia usually develops between the ages of three and five years (occasionally as early as the second year of life). Fine symmetrical bright red telangiectases are generally first noted in the temporal and nasal areas of the bulbar conjunctiva, and subsequently the cutaneous telangiectases appear on the ears, eyelids, butterfly areas of the cheeks, the neck, and the V area of the upper chest (areas receiving the greatest sun exposure). With time they extend to the popliteal and antecubital fossae and the dorsal aspect of the hands and feet. With continued sun exposure and aging, the skin tends to become sclerodermatous, with a mottled pattern of hyperpigmentation and hypopigmentation. Other cutaneous findings include café au lait spots, diffuse graying of the scalp hair, seborrheic dermatitis, follicular hyperkeratosis, excessive dryness of the skin and hair, eczema (in 40 to 60 per cent of patients), and hirsutism of the arms and legs.

Recurrent sinopulmonary infections, varying from acute rhinitis with infections of the ears to chronic bronchitis, recurrent pneumonia, and bronchiectasis, occur in 75 to 80 per cent of affected patients. Death, when it occurs, is generally associated with bronchiectasis and pneumonia. Among the immunologic defects seen in association with this disorder are deficiencies of immunoglobulin A (IgA) and immunoglobulin E (IgE), structural anomalies of the thymus and lymph nodes, impaired lymphocyte transformation, and lymphopenia.[56, 57]

No specific therapy is known, and patients with this disorder generally go progressively downhill, with death usually occurring in the second decade of life. Antibiotic therapy of the recurrent sinopulmonary infections is only of temporary benefit, and long-term prophylaxis is generally ineffective. Of those individuals who survive to the late teens, about 10 per cent develop lymphoreticular malignancy (lymphosarcoma, Hodgkin's disease, reticular cell sarcoma, or leukemia). Other neoplastic disorders include ovarian dysgerminoma, medulloblastoma, glioma, and adenocarcinoma.[41]

Generalized Essential Telangiectasia

Generalized essential telangiectasia is a benign cutaneous disorder generally seen in females (2:1), which frequently has its onset in late childhood or early adult life but most frequently develops in the fourth and fifth decades. The etiology of this disorder is unknown.

Essential telangiectasia may be generalized or segmented and usually begins on the legs and slowly spreads to involve the thighs, lower abdomen, and occasionally the arms or face (Fig. 9–27).

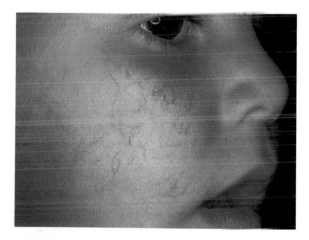

Figure 9–27   Essential telangiectasia on the face in a 3-year-old girl.

Two varieties of telangiectases are present: (1) large venous stars consisting of superficial varicosities and (2) bright red blotchy erythema produced by many fine wiry vessels. Although the disorder is usually slowly progressive and asymptomatic for many years, it can subside spontaneously. Regression of lesions, however, is rare and this basically cosmetic defect is not associated with any systemic disorder.[51]

There is no effective treatment for this condition. If lesions are cosmetically significant, however, cover makeups and electrodesiccation or electrocoagulation may help to a limited degree.

PIGMENTED PURPURIC ERUPTIONS

The pigmented purpuric eruptions consist of a group of related benign dermatoses of unknown etiology characterized by increased capillary fragility or permeability. The primary lesion, related to a lymphocytic vasculitis, results in pinhead-sized reddish puncta occurring in irregularly shaped dusky red or yellowish-brown patches of purpura, with secondary pigmentation from hemosiderin deposition. Four dermatoses are included in this group of disorders. Whether they are separate entities or expressions of the same pathologic process remains controversial.

Schamberg's Disease

Schamberg's disease (progressive pigmented purpuric dermatosis) is an uncommon asymptomatic disorder of the lower extremities that may

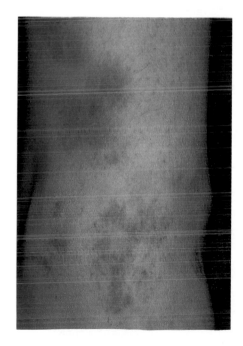

Figure 9–28   Schamberg's disease (progressive pigmented purpuric dermatosis). Discrete reddish-brown patches with pinpoint-sized cayenne pepper spots on the lower leg and ankle of an 11-year-old girl).

occur in childhood (Fig. 9–28) but generally is seen in adolescent and young adult males. Typical lesions are discrete brown or yellow patches with red or reddish-brown pinpoint-sized spots representing freshly extravasated erythrocytes and hemosiderin deposition (Cayenne pepper spots) in the center or on the periphery of the lesions. This disorder begins on the lower legs, generally the shins, ankles, and dorsa of the feet and toes, and only occasionally involves the trunk or upper limbs. Its course is chronic and may persist for years.

The histopathologic picture of Schamberg's disease, as with the other pigmented purpuric eruptions, consists of a lymphocytic vasculitis with extravasation of erythrocytes and hemosiderin deposition.

Itching Purpura

Itching purpura appears to represent a generalized form of Schamberg's disease except that the disorder is extremely pruritic and occasionally lichenified owing to persistent scratching. The histopathologic picture consists of spongiosis and inflammation of the epidermis in association with the usual vasculitic pattern. Eczematoid-like purpura of Doucas and Kapetenakis probably represents the same condition. Itching purpura is generally localized to the legs, with dissemination to the thighs, trunk, and upper extremities, and is more pronounced at the sites of friction. The disorder persists for months with marked fluctuations and episodic recurrences and may remit spontaneously or improve with the use of topical corticosteroids.

Lichenoid Dermatitis of Gougerot and Blum; Majocchi's Disease

Pigmented purpuric lichenoid dermatosis of Gougerot and Blum and purpura annularis telangiectodes (Majocchi's disease) also probably represent variants of the same disorder. The former, however, favors older men (between 40 and 60 years of age). Majocchi's disease generally occurs in adolescents and young adults of either sex, but may occur at any age. The eruption generally begins symmetrically on the lower extremities and may extend on to the trunk and arms. Lesions may be few or numerous in number and consist of small plaques 1 to 3 cm in diameter that are usually annular in configuration, often with clearing or atrophy in the center of some lesions. Treatment is generally ineffective, and the eruption usually persists for months to years.

PURPURA FULMINANS (DISSEMINATED INTRAVASCULAR COAGULATION)

Purpura fulminans and disseminated intravascular coagulation are terms used to describe a relatively uncommon form of non-thrombocytic

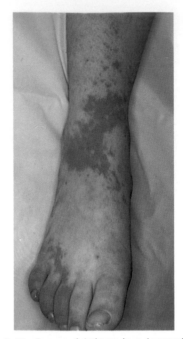

Figure 9–29 Purpura fulminans in a 4-year-old boy with Rocky Mountain spotted fever.

purpura characterized by an acute, severe, often rapidly fatal hemorrhagic infarction and necrosis of the skin. Usually occurring in children, the disease is triggered by a preceding infectious process such as scarlet fever or other streptococcal infection, meningococcal and other septicemias, chickenpox, measles, vaccinia, or rickettsial disorders such as Rocky Mountain spotted fever (Fig. 9–29).

The etiology has not been firmly established, but purpura fulminans usually has its onset within 3 to 30 days after a resolving infection. The cause appears to represent a non-immunologic hypersensitivity reaction similar to that of an induced Schwartzman phenomenon. The primary pathology is a consumptive coagulopathy (disseminated intravascular coagulation) characterized by intravascular consumption of plasma coagulation factors (fibrinogen, factors II, V, and VIII), with low-normal to severely reduced platelet counts, hypofibrinogenemia, and hypoprothrombinemia associated with microthrombosis and a hemorrhagic diathesis.[58, 59]

The disorder is characterized by symmetrically distributed localized cutaneous ecchymoses, often with sharp irregular borders on the extremities, particularly in the areas of pressure. Lesions are tender, enlarge rapidly, coalesce, and develop central necrosis, with hemorrhagic blebs and a raised edge with surrounding erythema. They spread to the trunk and occasionally may involve the lips, ears, and nose. Chills, fever, tachycardia, anemia, and prostration are common. Visceral involvement with hematuria or gastrointestinal bleeding may occur, and shock, coma, and death frequently develop. When hemorrhage and necrosis of the adrenal glands are present the designation Waterhouse–Friderichsen syndrome has been applied to this disorder.

Since current studies support the concept that purpura fulminans is usually the result of disseminated intravascular coagulation, the presence of a consumptive coagulopathy should be confirmed prior to the institution of therapy.[60] The number of platelets is commonly markedly reduced, coagulation factors I (fibrinogen), II (prothrombin), V, and VIII are usually decreased in number, and histopathologic studies show small vessel occlusion and hemorrhagic necrosis of the skin, subcutaneous tissue, and often the underlying fascia and muscle.

Although the outlook is grave and death frequently occurs within 48 to 72 hours (until recently the mortality was over 90 per cent), prompt initiation of therapy improves the prognosis for most patients. Treatment consists of early recognition of this disorder, prompt identification and therapy of any associated infection, correction of clotting factor deficiencies due to intravascular coagulation, and general supportive measures. It should be noted, however, that disseminated intravascular coagulation is more difficult to diagnose in premature infants because of the normal prolonged coagulation value in prematures.[61] In view of its rapid onset of action, heparin, 50 to 150 units (0.5 to 1.5 mg) per kg of body weight, intravenously immediately and repeated every four hours, with periodic adjustment according to clinical progress is generally the treatment of choice. Dextran, 6 per cent solution in saline or water (600 mg/kg over a period of two to four days and then every two or three days), or low molecular weight dextran (Dextran 40), 10 ml of the 10 per cent solution per kg every 12 hours for the first 2 days and then daily until adequate healing has occurred, and the replacement of the consumed clotting factors with fresh whole blood or frozen plasma is often necessary. General supportive measures, treatment of shock, anemia, infection, renal failure, debridement, skin grafting, and, on occasion, amputation may also be performed, if necessary, depending upon the clinical picture.[62]

PERIARTERITIS NODOSA

Periarteritis nodosa (polyarteritis nodosa) is a rare systemic disorder characterized by a necrotizing arteritis of the small and medium-sized muscular-type arteries generally affecting those of the gastrointestinal tract, pancreas, kidney, heart, muscles, and, in 25 to 50 per cent of affected individuals, the skin. Cutaneous manifestations, seen in one-third of cases, range from livedo reticularis, purpura, and bullae to maculopapular eruptions, necrotic vesicles or pustules, urticaria, and tender subcutaneous nodules or ulcerations that follow the course of medium-sized arteries.

The disorder that affects infants 1 year old or less often begins with a febrile illness suggesting a virus, and differs from the disorder seen in older patients. In older persons, the lesions consist of crops of subcutaneous nodules along the course of the superficial arteries of the trunk and extremities. They vary in size from 0.5 to 1.0 cm, are tender on palpation, and usually red to purple in color. Nodules may persist for days or months, may disappear spontaneously, or may result in ulceration and scar formation depending upon the degree of necrosis. Other cutaneous manifestations include ecchymoses and peripheral gangrene of fingers or toes.

Histologic examination of cutaneous lesions reveals a necrotizing pancreatitis with fibrinoid necrosis of the media, endothelial proliferation, and predominantly polymorphonuclear leukocytic infiltration of the vessel wall.

Coronary arteritis may lead to aneurysms and infarction, producing cardiomegaly and congestive heart failure. Kidney, peripheral artery, and nervous system involvement may result in hypertension, abnormal urinary sediment, peripheral ischemia, paralysis, and convulsions. Death, when it occurs, is usually associated with renal failure, intracranial or intra-abdominal hemorrhage, hypertensive heart failure, myocardial involvement, and cardiac decompensation.

Polyarteritis in older children behaves similarly to that seen in adults, with fever, calf pain, painful subcutaneous nodules, arthritis, abdominal pain, Raynaud's phenomenon, hypertension, peripheral neuropathy, and myocardial infarction.

Management of periarteritis nodosa consists of general supportive therapy and the use of corticosteroids (1 to 2 mgm/kg per day of prednisone or its equivalent). Prognosis in the infantile form of this disorder is poor; that in older childhood forms, however, generally is better, and complete recovery may occur.[63]

DISORDERS OF LYMPHATIC VESSELS

Tumors of lymphatic origin are classified as hamartomas of the lymphatic system. They consist of dilated lymph channels lined by normal flat or cuboidal lymphatic endothelium. They may be superficial or subcutaneous and, at times, may extend into the underlying muscle tissue. Lymphangiomas are generally slow-growing, and their clinical appearance is dependent upon their size, depth, and location. Four major forms of lymphangioma (lymphangioma simplex, lymphangioma circumscriptum, cavernous lymphangioma, and cystic hygroma) have been described. Of these, 70 to 90 per cent are present at birth or develop within the first two years of life. They rarely appear after the age of five years.

Lymphangioma Simplex

Simple lymphangiomas appear in infancy as solitary well-circumscribed flesh-colored dermal or subcutaneous tumors. They may occur anywhere on the subcutaneous or mucosal surface and are most often seen on the neck, upper trunk, proximal extremities, and tongue. Their surface is generally smooth, but on occasion they may be verruciform in character. Simple lymphangiomas either remain stable or grow quickly. Uncomplicated tumors can be removed easily by simple excision. For those that are more widespread, however, simple excision is not always satisfactory.

Lymphangioma Circumscriptum

This is the most common form of lymphangioma. Present at birth or appearing in early childhood, it is characterized by groups of deep-seated thick-walled vesicles that have the appearance of frog spawn. Common sites of involvement include the proximal limbs, shoulders, neck, axillae and adjacent chest wall, perineum, tongue, and mucous membranes. Frequently there also is a hemangiomatous component (hemangiolymphoma) so that some of the vesicles are filled with fresh or altered blood (Figs. 9–30, 9–31). Mixed lesions may increase rather suddenly because of bleeding into the lymphatic spaces. Although usually localized, these lesions may be quite extensive. If therapy is desired, such lesions require deep and extensive surgery (down to the fascial plane), and recurrences are common.

Cavernous Lymphangioma

Cavernous lymphangiomas consist of diffuse soft tissue masses of large cystic dilatations of lymphatic vessels in the dermis, subcutaneous tissue, and intermuscular septae. These lesions are ill-defined and frequently involve large areas of the face, trunk, and extremities. They may appear in childhood or adult life. Surgical excision may be effective for local lesions, but extensive cavernous lesions require full-thickness skin grafts and recurrences are common.

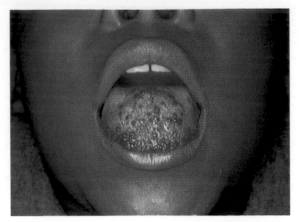

Figure 9–31 Hemangiolymphoma of the tongue.

Cystic Hygroma

Cystic hygromas are benign, unilocular or multilocular lymphatic tumors (Fig. 9–32). These lesions are often found in the neck region (hygroma colli) and occasionally in the axillae, groin, or popliteal fossae. Cystic hygromas may on rare occasion undergo spontaneous regression. The majority, however, tend to increase in size and frequently infiltrate adjacent vessels and nerves. In general, when surgery is considered, the earlier the lesions can be removed the better the clinical result. In contrast to cavernous lymphangiomas, however, recurrences following surgical removal of cystic hygromas are uncommon.[64, 65]

Lymphedema

Lymphedema is a term used to describe a diffuse soft-tissue swelling caused by increased accumulation of lymph due to inadequate lym-

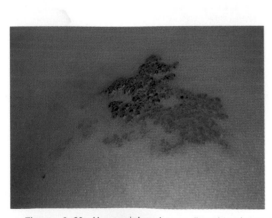

Figure 9–30 Hemangiolymphoma (lymphangioma circumscriptum with a hemangiomatous component).

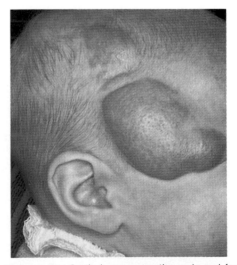

Figure 9–32 Cystic hygroma on the scalp and face of a 2-month-old infant.

phatic drainage. It may be divided into primary and secondary forms.

Primary lymphedema may be subdivided into congenital (13 per cent of patients), lymphedema praecox (that appearing after birth and before age 35), and lymphedema tarda (that appearing after age 35).

Secondary lymphedema is due to obstruction of lymphatic pathways by some pathologic process (following surgery, from recurrent lymphangitis or cellulitis, or from filariasis) or by some extralymphatic process, such as compression by direct invasion of lymphatics or lymph nodes by neoplasms, or by fibrosis resulting from radiation therapy and scar formation. Secondary lymphedema is generally a disorder of adults and is relatively uncommon in childhood.

In congenital lymphedema the involved area is swollen at birth. The swelling is firm and is characterized by pitting on pressure. In lymphedema praecox, females are primarily affected, and the swelling appears spontaneously, generally between the ages of 9 and 25 years.

The term Milroy's disease refers to a familial disorder with autosomal dominant transmission in which the edema is almost always confined to the legs and feet. This disorder may be present at birth but usually appears during adolescence or the early twenties. The age of onset and severity tend to be similar in affected members in a family. Hot weather, menses, and gestation may accentuate the edema, and serum proteins, hepatic, cardiac, and renal function studies are normal. In some affected individuals, aldosterone levels have been found to be abnormal.

The pathogenesis of Milroy's disease is unknown. Treatment consisting of trial on a low sodium diet, elastic stockings or bandages, and systemic diuretics may be helpful but is not curative. In children with moderate to severe lymphedema praecox, subcutaneous lymphangiectomy may be performed. This reduces the swelling of the extremity but, unfortunately, generally results in unsightly scars.

References

1. Reed, RJ, O'Quinn SE: Vascular neoplasms. In Fitzpatrick TB, et al.: Dermatology in General Medicine. McGraw-Hill Book Co, New York, 1971, 533–556.

   A review of the classification, clinical manifestations, pathology, and management of vascular malformations.

2. Jacobs AH, Walton RG: The incidence of birthmarks in the neonate. Pediatrics 58:218–222, 1976.

   A statistical study of birthmarks in 1058 infants under 72 hours of age.

3. Hidano A, Nakajima S: Earliest features of the strawberry mark in the newborn. Br. J. Dermatol. 87:138–144, 1972.

   The majority of strawberry angiomata are not detectable at birth, but a few are apparent as telangiectatic lesions surrounded by a pale halo.

4. Margileth AM, Museles M: Cutaneous hemangiomas in children. JAMA 194:523–526, 1965.

   Evaluation of the course of 366 hemangiomas in 210 patients reveals that conservative management results in spontaneous involution in the majority of lesions.

5. Margileth AM, Museles M: Current concepts in diagnosis and management of congenital cutaneous hemangiomas. Pediatrics 36:410–416, 1965.

   Observations in over 200 children confirm previous studies in which over 90 per cent of congenital cutaneous hemangiomas involute spontaneously.

6. Illingworth RS: Thoughts on the treatment of vascular nevi. Arch. Dis. Child. 51:138–140, 1976.

   A review of several studies discussing the clinical course of strawberry hemangiomas reveals that less than 2 per cent require active treatment.

7. Bowers RE, Graham EA, Tomlinson KM: The natural history of the strawberry nevus: Arch. Dermatol. 82:667–680, 1960.

   A study of 169 untreated cases of strawberry nevi: 50 per cent had complete resolution by age 5, 70 per cent by age 7, and, of those that did not resolve, only 6 per cent had a cosmetic handicap.

8. Robb, R. M.: Refractive errors associated with hemangiomas of the eyelids and orbit in infancy. 83:52–58, 1977.

   Astigmatic and myopic errors in 46 per cent of 37 patients who had hemangiomas with extensive involvement of the upper eyelids.

9. Moschella S: Capillary and cavernous hemangioma. Transactions of the Philadelphia Dermatologic Society (discussion). Arch. Dermatol. 113:1308, 1977.

   Intralesional steroids in five patients with hemangiomas.

10. Fost NC, Esterly NB: Successful treatment of juvenile hemangiomas with prednisone. J. Pediatr. 72:351–357, 1968.

   Of six children with extensive hemangiomata treated with oral prednisone, all except one showed dramatic regression of the lesion within two weeks of therapy.

11. Zarem, HA, Edgerton MT: Cavernous hemangiomas and prednisolone therapy. Plast. Reconstr. Surg. 39:76–83, 1976.

   Both cavernous and strawberry hemangiomas treated with oral prednisolone (20 mg daily with gradual reduction to 2.5 mg daily) gave rapid cessation of growth in four patients, and partial cessation in three, within two weeks of the start of therapy.

12. Goldman L: Laser treatment of extensive mixed cavernous and port-wine stains. Arch. Dermatol. 113:504–505, 1977.

   Treatment of an extensive disfiguring mixed nodular cutaneous and port-wine stain treated with ruby and argon lasers with substantial cosmetic improvement.

13. Apfelberg DB, Maser MR, Lash H: Argon laser treatment of cutaneous vascular abnormalities. Ann. Plast. Surg. 1:14–18, 1978.

   Of 106 cutaneous vascular abnormalities treated over a three-year period by argon laser, patients with port-wine hemangiomas, capillary/cavernous hemangiomas, and telangiectases showed good response.

14. Solomon LM, Esterly NB: Vascular disorders and malformations. In Neonatal Dermatology. W.B. Saunders Co., Philadelphia, 1973, 68–80.

   A review of vascular disorders of the newborn infant.

15. Martins AG: Hemangioma and thrombocytopenia, J. Pediatr. Surg. 5:641–640, 1970.

   Review of 19 of 94 patients with Kasabach-Merritt syndrome who died (6 added to 88 previously reported cases); 10 deaths were unavoidable, 4 were from unnecessarily aggressive therapy; and 5 probably could have been avoided.

16. Hagerman LJ, Czapek EE, Donellan WL, et al.: Giant hemangioma with consumption coagulopathy. J. Pediatr. 87:766–768, 1965.

   Report of excision of a large cavernous hemangioma in an 8-week-old infant with Kasabach-Merritt syndrome treated with heparin in an attempt to obtain optimal coagulation capacity prior to surgical excision.

17. Alexander GL, Norman RM: The Sturge-Weber syndrome. John Wright and Sons, Ltd., Bristol, 1960.

An extensive monograph on the problem of Sturge-Weber syndrome and report of seven cases in detail; in all of 257 cases at least part of the facial nevus involved the forehead and upper eyelids.

18. Jacobs AH: Response to a letter. Sturge-Weber syndrome without port-wine nevus. Pediatrics 60:785, 1977.

By definition, Sturge-Weber syndrome consists of a combination of facial port-wine nevus, vascular malformations of the meninges, and cerebral cortex; those without facial nevus represent cases of meningeal angiomatosis.

19. Stevenson RF, Thomson HG, Marin JD: Unrecognized ocular problems associated with port-wine stain of the face in children. Can. Med. Assoc. J. 111:953–954, 1974.

Of fifty children with port-wine stains, glaucoma was present in 45 per cent of those with vascular lesions involving areas of skin supplied by both ophthalmic and maxillary divisions of the sensory branch of the trigeminal nerve. Those with involvement of only one of the above areas did not manifest glaucoma.

20. Rook A: Naevi and other developmental defects. In Rook A, Wilkinson DS, Ebling FJG: Textbook of Dermatology, 2nd dition. Blackwell Scientific Publications, London, 1972, 126–167.

An in-depth review of developmental defects and nevi as related to the skin.

21. Phillips GN, Gordon DH, Martin EC, et al.: The Klippel-Trenaunay syndrome: clinical radiologic aspects. Radiology 128:428–434, 1978.

Radiologic techniques available for study of patients with Klippel-Trenaunay-Parkes-Weber syndrome.

22. Fine RM, Derbes VJ, Clark WH Jr: Blue rubber bleb nevus. Arch. Dermatol. 84:802–805, 1961.

A 15-year-old boy with multiple blue rubber-bleb nevi.

23. Morris SJ, Kaplan SR, Ballan K, et al.: Blue rubber-bleb nevus syndrome. JAMA 239:1887, 1978.

A 23-year-old man with several blue rubber-bleb nevi on the neck, arms, abdomen, and feet, melena, and a vascular lesion on the greater curvature of the gastric antrum.

24. Wishnick MM: Multinodular hemangiomatosis with partial biliary obstruction. J. Pediatr. 92:960–962, 1978.

Report of an infant with multiple cutaneous hemangiomas, congestive heart failure, and evidence of biliary obstruction (biliary obstruction, as observed in this infant, is a rare complication).

25. Keller L, Bluhm JF III: Diffuse neonatal hemangiomatosis. A case with heart failure and thrombocytopenia. Cutis 23:295–297, 1979.

A review of diffuse neonatal hemangiomatosis and its therapy.

26. Frost JI, Caplan RM: Cutaneous hemangiomas and disappearing bones with a review of cutaneo-visceral hemangiomatosis. Arch. Dermatol. 92:501–508, 1965.

A 15-year-old boy with multiple hemangiomas, massive osteolysis of the left side of the pelvis, lumbar vertebrae, "soap-bubble" osteolysis of the skull and humerus, and massive osteolysis of the bones of the left lower extremity, necessitating partial amputation of the left lower extremity because of multiple recurrent fractures.

27. Gellis SS, Feingold M: Picture of the month. Contributed by Ryan ME, Spahr RC: Hemangioma with osteolysis (Gorham's disease, vanishing bone disease). Am. J. Dis. Child. 132:715–716, 1978.

A patient with hemangiomas involving mainly the skin of the back and left femur with osteolytic areas of the left pelvis and femur.

28. Stephan MJ, Hall BD, Smith DW, et al.: Macrocephaly in association with unusual cutaneous angiomatosis. J. Pediatr. 87:353–359, 1975.

Ten patients with macrocephaly, unusual angiomatosis, and limb asymmetry.

29. Zonana J, Rimoin DL, David DC: Macrocephaly with multiple lipomas and hemangiomas. J. Pediatr. 89:600–603, 1976.

A family of three individuals with an apparent autosomal dominant disorder consisting of macrocephaly with multiple hemangiomas and lipomas.

30. Jessen RT, Thompson S, Smith EB: Cobb syndrome. Arch. Dermatol 113:1587–1590, 1977.

The combination of a cutaneous angioma in a dermatomal distribution and spinal cord angioma comprises a rare but potentially crippling or fatal syndrome.

31. Imperial R, Helwig EB: Verrucous hemangioma — a clinicopathologic study of 21 cases. Arch. Dermatol. 96:247–253, 1967.

Verrucous hemangiomas (variants of capillary or cavernous hemangiomas with secondary epidermal change) often misdiagnosed as nevi, pigmented tumors, verrucae, or angiokeratomas.

32. Kaufman SL, Stout AP: Hemangiopericytoma in children. Cancer 13:695–710, 1960.

Thirty-one children with hemangiopericytoma.

33. Beckwinkel KD, Diddams JA: Hemangiopericytoma. Report of a case and comprehensive review of the literature. Cancer 25:896–901, 1970.

Report of a hemangiopericytoma in a 42-year-old woman with a review of the literature.

34. Imperial R, Helwig EB: Angiokeratoma. Arch. Dermatol. 95:166–175, 1967.

Analyses of 116 examples of angiokeratoma support the concept of solitary and multiple angiokeratomas.

35. Lynch PJ, Kosanovich M: Angiokeratoma circumscriptum. Arch. Dermatol. 96:665–668, 1967.

A description of a 20-year-old Negro man with angiokeratoma circumscriptum of the right forearm and review of the literature.

36. Pringle JJ: Four cases of angiokeratoma from one family. Br. J. Dermatol. 25:40–53, 1913.

An early description of angiokeratoma.

37. Smith RBW, Prior IAM, Park RG: Angiokeratoma of Mibelli: a family with nodular lesions of the legs. Aust. J. Dermatol. 9:329–334, 1968.

Four sisters and a female cousin with angiokeratomas confirm a genetic basis for this disorder.

38. Dave VK, Main RA: Angiokeratoma of Mibelli with necrosis of the fingertips. Arch. Dermatol. 106:726–728, 1972.

A case of angiokeratoma of Mibelli in an 11-year-old girl with elevated IgG, IgA, and IgM, oral ulcerations, and necrosis of the fingertips.

39. Imperial R, Helwig EB: Angiokeratoma of the scrotum (Fordyce type). J. Urol. 95:379–387, 1967.

One hundred thirty-five patients with angiokeratoma of the scrotum.

40. Danehower CC, Moyer DGM: Angiokeratoma corporis diffusum. Arch. Dermatol. 94:628–631, 1966.

Diagnosis prior to onset of the rash can be aided by demonstration of mulberry cells on urinalysis and ophthalmologic examination.

41. Gorlin RH, Pindborg JJ, Cohen MM Jr: Fabry Syndrome. In Syndromes of the Head and Neck. McGraw-Hill Book Co., New York, 1976, 295–299.

An exceptional compendium of syndromology covering all known features of each disorder, not just those pertaining to the head and neck.

42. von Gemmingen G, Kierland RR, Opitz JM: Angiokeratoma corporis diffusum (Fabry's disease). Arch. Dermatol. 91:206–218, 1965.

A description of a pedigree that includes five males and one female with clinical evidence of Fabry's disease.

43. Burda CD, Winder PR: Angiokeratoma corporis diffusum universale (Fabry's disease) in female subjects. Am. J. Med. 42:293–301, 1967.

A report of a case of Fabry's disease in a 47-year-old woman with review of 12 living women with manifestations of the disease, and six women, including the propositus, who died of the disease.

44. Beaudet AL, Caskey CT: Detection of Fabry's disease heterozygotes by hair root analysis. Clin. Genet. 13:251–258, 1978.

Measurement of enzyme ratios in individual hair roots appears to be an accurate technique for the detection of carriers of this disorder.

45. Brady RO: Fabry's disease. Science 172:174–175, 1971.

Enzyme assays performed on extracts of cells obtained by transabdominal amniocentesis confirmed the diagnosis of a hemizygous male with Fabry disease in a fetus during the 17th week of pregnancy.

46. Mapes CA, Anderson RL, Sweeley CC: Enzyme replacement in Fabry's disease, an inborn error of metabolism. Science 169:987–989, 1970.

Studies describe the treatment of Fabry's disease by infusion with normal human plasma.

47. Durand P, Borrone C, Della Cella G: A new mucopolysaccharide lipid-storage disease? Lancet II:1313–1314, 1966.

Clinical, histochemical, and microscopic findings in two brothers suggest a distinct autosomal recessive mucopolysaccharide/lipid complex disease.

48. Smith EB, Graham JL, Ledman JA, et al.: Fucosidosis. Cutis 19:195–198, 1977.

Three children with mental retardation, retarded growth, corneal opacities, dilated and tortuous conjunctival and retinal vessels, and angiokeratomas with low or absent alpha-L-fucosidase activity.

49. Schafer IA, Powell DW, Sullivan JC: Lysosomal bone disease. Pediatr. Res. 5:391–392, 1971.

Deficiency of lysosomal hydrolase, alpha-L-fucosidase, hypothesized as the cause of bone disease in a 9-year-old dwarf.

50. Epinette WW, Norins AL, Drew AL, et al.: Angiokeratoma corporis diffusum with alpha-L-fucosidase deficiency. Arch. Dermatol. 107:755–757, 1973.

Report of a case of a 21-year-old mentally and physically retarded male who first developed angiokeratoma corporis diffusum at the age of four years, with normal alpha-galactosidase activity and reduced alpha-L-fucosidase activity (alpha-fucosidosis).

51. Braverman IM: Blood vessels. In Skin Signs of Systemic Disease. W.B. Saunders Co., Philadelphia, 1970, 287–311.

The value of skin lesions in the recognition of systemic disease.

52. Feldaker M, Hines EA Jr, Kierland RR: Livedo reticularis with summer ulcerations. Arch. Dermatol. 72:31–42, 1975.

Twelve patients with a syndrome of edema and ulcerations of the legs and feet.

53. Lynch PJ, Zelickson AS: Congenital phlebectasia — a histopathologic study. Arch. Dermatol. 95:98–101, 1967.

Electron microscopic examination of the cutaneous vascular system of a patient with a segmental pattern of cutis marmorata telangiectatica congenita.

54. Miller JQ: Cutis marmorata telangiectactica congenita. J. Assoc. Milit. Dermatol. 1(2):33–35, 1975.

A case of cutis marmorata congenita telangiectatica in a 21-year-old male associated with branchial cleft cyst and chronic skin ulceration.

55. Petrozzi JW, Rahn EK, et al.: Cutis marmorata telangiectatica congenita. Arch. Derm. 101:74–77, 1970.

A case of cutis marmorata telangiectatica congenita combined with other defects (Sturge-Weber disease and patent ductus arteriosus) suggests that this disorder should be considered with other diseases manifesting vascular nevi with developmental defects.

56. Peterson RDA, Cooper MD, Good RA: Lymphoid tissue abnormalities associated with ataxia-telangiectasia. Am. J. Med. 41:342–359, 1966.

Detailed analysis of the immunologic capacity of eight patients and review of cases reported by other clinical investigators clearly define an abnormality of lymphoid tissue as a major component of ataxia-telangiectasia.

57. Amman AJ, Cain WA, Ishizaka K, et al.: Immunoglobulin E deficiency in ataxia-telangiectasia. N. Engl. J. Med. 281:469–472, 1969.

Eleven of sixteen patients with ataxia telangiectasia had a deficiency of immunoglobulin E (IgE), suggesting that IgA and IgE may be linked with one another and with the production of cell-mediated immune responses.

58. Dudgeon DL, Kellogg DR, Gilchrist GS, et al.: Purpura fulminans. Arch. Surg. 103:351–358, 1971.

A clinical description of purpura fulminans, its diagnosis, and management.

59. Antley RM, McMillan CW: Sequential coagulation studies in purpura fulminans. N. Engl. J. Med. 276:1287–1290, 1967.

Sequential coagulation studies in a child treated with heparin suggest that purpura fulminans is a manifestation of intravascular coagulation and confirm the value of heparin in the treatment of this disorder.

60. Esterly NB: Purpura fulminans. In Demis DJ, Dobson RL, McGuire J (Eds.): Clinical Dermatology, Vol. 2. Harper and Row, Hagerstown, Md., 1977, 7–24, 1–3.

A clinical review of purpura fulminans, its pathology, diagnosis, and management.

61. Woods WG, Corman Lubin NL, Hilgartner MG, et al.: Disseminated intravascular coagulation in the newborn. Am. J. Dis. Child. 133:44–46, 1979.

Disseminated intravascular coagulation in newborns is frequently more difficult to diagnose because of normal prolonged coagulation values in premature infants.

62. Corrigan JJ, Jr: Disseminated intravascular coagulation and purpura fulminans. In Gellis SS, Kagan BM (Eds.): Current Pediatric Therapy 8. W.B. Saunders Co., Philadelphia, 1978, 162–163.

Review of present concepts and treatment of disseminated intravascular coagulation and purpura fulminans.

63. Landing BH, Larson EJ: Are infantile periarteritis nodosa with coronary involvement and fatal mucocutaneous lymph node syndrome the same? Comparison of twenty patients from North America with patients from Hawaii and Japan. Pediatr. 59:651–662, 1977.

Clinical and pathologic data on patients with infantile periarteritis nodosa (IPN) with coronary involvement and fatal cases of mucocutaneous lymph node syndrome (MCLS, MLNS) appear to justify the opinion that these two entities are clinically and pathologically identical. It should be noted, however, that classic periarteritis nodosa differs both clinically and pathologically from IPN and MCLS (MLNS) and may have a different etiology.

64. Saijo M, Munro IR, Mancer K: Lymphangioma: long term follow-up study. Plast. Reconst. Surg. 56:642–651, 1975.

A review of resections of lymphangioma or lymphangiohemangioma in 164 patients.

65. Barrand KC, Freeman NV: Massive infiltrating cystic hygroma of the head and neck in infancy. Arch. Dis. Child. 58:523, 1973.

Followup studies on children with cystic hygroma, with and without surgery, revealed several patients who had spontaneous regrowth of their lesions.

10

BACTERIAL AND PROTOZOAL INFECTIONS OF THE SKIN

The normal skin of healthy infants and children is resistant to invasion by most bacteria, the cutaneous surface providing a dry mechanical barrier from which contaminating organisms are constantly removed by desquamation. Under normal conditions the skin is sterile at delivery and for a short period thereafter. During the process of vaginal birth it picks up organisms from the birth canal, which gradually increase in number during the first ten days of life. If the neonate is delivered by cesarean section, however, the cutaneous surface remains sterile until after delivery but soon becomes exposed to bacteria from human contactants and fomites.

Almost any organism may live on the cutaneous surface under appropriate conditions. A complete list of transient organisms accordingly would include virtually all microorganisms found in the human environment. The number of species comprising the resident flora, however, is relatively small. It consists predominantly of gram-positive organisms and a few gram-negative species and includes *Propionibacterium acnes* (normally found in high concentrations about the pilosebaceous follicles of the face and less commonly in areas such as the axillae and forearms), aerobic diphtheroids (*Corynebacterium minutissimum* and *C. tenius*), *Staphylococcus epidermidis* (formerly termed *S. epidermidis albus*), micrococci, anaerobic gram-positive cocci, and gram-negative bacilli found uncommonly on normal skin except about the moist intertriginous areas of the groin, axillae, and toe webs (*Escherichia coli*, *Proteus*, *Enterobacter*, *Alcaligenes*, *Pseudomonas*, *Actinetobacter calcoaceticus*, *A. lwoffi*), and *Staphylococcus aureus*. The organisms of *S. aureus*, a common pathogen, appear to be seeded from a carrier state in the anterior nares.

Since the cutaneous surface is continuously exposed to microorganisms, it is most helpful to be able to distinguish between transient, resident, and pathogenic flora. The transient flora consists of a multiplicity of organisms that are deposited on the skin from the environment, presumably do not proliferate, and are removed easily by washing or scrubbing of the affected area. The resident flora consists of a smaller number of organisms that are found more or less regularly in appreci-

214

able numbers on the skin of normal individuals, multiply on the skin, form stable communities on the cutaneous surface, and are not easily dislodged. Pathogenic bacteria, not ordinarily a regular part of this flora, persist on the skin if there is continuous replacement from some internal or external source, or if the integrity of the skin is disrupted by injury or disease. It should be noted that the mere presence of potentially pathogenic bacteria in a cutaneous lesion does not necessarily prove the demonstrable organism to be a cause of bacterial infection.[1, 2]

The skin provides a dry mechanical barrier from which contaminating organisms are constantly being removed by desquamation. In the past it was believed that a low pH on the cutaneous surface limited proliferation of skin flora. This "acid mantle" theory, however, has currently fallen into disrepute. It now appears that the relative dryness, rather than the pH, constitutes the major factor in the retardation of growth of gram-negative bacteria with high moisture requirements.[3] Accordingly, it is not the acidity or fatty acids that protect the skin. It is a combination of normal epidermal shedding; dryness of the cutaneous surface; the virulence of the organisms; the presence of normal flora, which contributes to host defenses; and the host response that determines the clinical picture.

Children have a more varied cutaneous flora than adults and often harbor soil bacteria on their skin. Prepuberal children lack sebum and accordingly have less diphtheroid organisms than adults. It is estimated that 20 per cent of individuals are persistent nasal carriers of *Staphylococcus aureus*, that 60 per cent are intermittent carriers, and that 20 per cent of individuals are resistant to nasal colonization. Coagulase-positive staphylococci (S. *aureus*) are not considered part of the normal cutaneous flora of glabrous skin in adults but are frequent transients acquired from carrier sites such as the anterior nares and perineum.

Many individuals carry *Staphylococcus aureus* in the nose without skin colonization, and, with certain virulent strains, colonization of staphylococci of the axilla and groin, in addition to the nose, is common. Colonization with staphylococci, therefore, may not necessarily be related to a process of seeding from a carrier state, but, may be due to the acquisition of an outside organism which, once acquired, persists in a tenacious manner.

Pathogenic streptococci are usually not found on the skin of normal individuals, and impetigo occurs in a high percentage of patients after cutaneous contamination. This is particularly important as a source of disease in children in warm moist climates where the infection rate during the summer may exceed 50 per cent, the streptococci invading damaged skin with resultant pyoderma.[3] The nasopharynx is probably contaminated from this site, and isolation of streptococci from this mucous membrane area is common even though clinical pharyngitis does not occur.

The introduction of a vast array of specific antibiotics and chemotherapeutic agents has affected striking changes in the management of bacterial infection. With the availability of these agents the focus of attention is directed to determination of the specific bacterial cause and its sensitivity, when indicated, so that a proper choice of antibacterial agents can be made. In purulent infections of the skin it is easy to obtain adequate specimens for microscopic examination and culture. When the lesion is dry or crusted, however, the superficial area must be cleansed with an antiseptic solution (alcohol, providine-iodide, or clorhexidine gluconate) to prevent contamination of the specimen. The crusted lesion is then gently lifted off and cultures obtained from the moist underlying surface. In non-purulent infections (erysipelis or cellulitis) a diagnostic specimen may be obtained by aspiration of the most active area (not the surrounding area of erythema) with a 25-gauge needle attached to a syringe containing 2.0 ml of sterile saline without added preservatives. A drop of this specimen may be stained with Gram stain for microscopic examination, and the remainder may be cultured in blood agar and thioglycollate broth.

BACTERIAL INFECTIONS

Impetigo

The primary bacterial infections of the skin are impetigo and folliculitis. Impetigo is a contagious superficial infection of the skin by streptococci, staphylococci, or both. Although seen in all age groups, the disease is most common in infants and children. Lesions may involve any body surface, but occur most frequently on the exposed parts of the body, especially the face, hands, neck, and extremities.

CLINICAL MANIFESTATIONS. The disease begins with 1 or 2 mm erythematous macules, which soon develop into thin-roofed vesicles or bullae surrounded by narrow areolae of erythema.

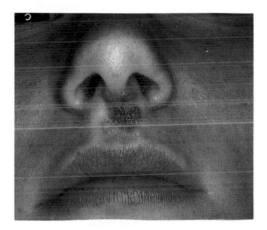

Figure 10–1 Impetigo. Moist thin-roofed vesicles and honey-colored crusts surrounded by an areola of erythema.

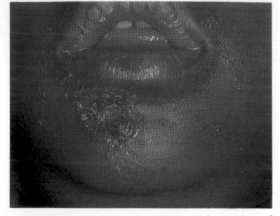

Figure 10–2 Impetigo. Red weeping surface with overlying encrustation.

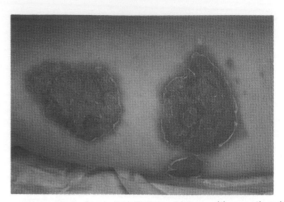

Figure 10–4 Large impetiginous lesions with smooth red weeping surfaces.

The vesicles rupture easily, with release of a thin cloudy yellow fluid. The serous discharge subsequently dries, with formation of thick, soft honey-colored crusts, the hallmark of impetigo (Fig. 10–1). Crusts can be removed easily, leaving a smooth, red, weeping surface, which rapidly becomes encrusted again (Fig. 10–2). The exudate is easily spread by autoinoculation by fingers, towels, or clothing, with resultant satellite lesions to adjacent areas or other parts of the body. Individual lesions sometimes extend peripherally, with central clearing, and frequently eventuate in annular, circinate, or gyrate lesions (Figs. 10–3 and 10–4).

Impetigo is seen in two forms: (1) a bullous impetigo associated with phage group II staphylo-cocci (Fig. 10–5), and (2) a vesiculo-pustular form with resulting thick crusted lesions due to beta hemolytic streptococci (alone or in combination with staphylococci). Lesions of impetigo due to S. *aureus* generally affect the face, trunk, and extremities; do not appear to have a seasonal predilection; and consist of superficial blisters that rupture and leave a "scalded skin"-like appearance. Fever and lymphadenopathy appear late in the course of the disorder. Those due to streptococci frequently affect the lower extremities; appear in the hot, muggy summer months; and often consist of punched-out ulcers on the legs with superimposed crusts. Fever and lymphadenopathy are early prominent features of this disorder.

Current information suggests that the reservoir for staphylococci is the upper respiratory tract (particularly the nose) of asymptomatic persons. These carriers spread the agent to the skin of infants, probably with their hands. The reservoir for streptococci responsible for cutaneous infection appears to be cutaneous lesions of other individuals, not the respiratory tract of affected or

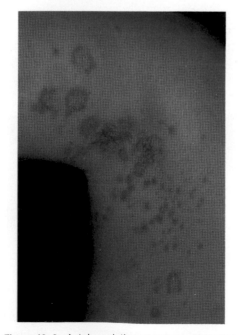

Figure 10–3 Autoinoculation of lesions of impetigo in the axillary region with multiple gyrate and circinate lesions due to peripheral extension and central clearing.

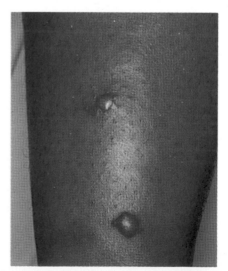

Figure 10–5 Bullous impetigo. Characteristic of group II staphylococcal infection. *Use Diclox or Erythromycin*

asymptomatic individuals.[4] The presence of streptococci on normal skin does not seem to be the only factor responsible for cutaneous infection. Factors such as trauma and insect bites probably contribute to the pathogenesis of this disorder. Staphylococci, when seen, are late colonists and accordingly play no role in the pathogenesis of streptococcal pyoderma.

TREATMENT. Although appropriate management of impetigo is generally prompt and highly effective, untreated impetigo may last for two to three weeks, with continuous spread and development of new lesions. In severe neglected cases there may be large crusted vegetations with deep extension and ulcerative lesions. Simple uncomplicated lesions, however, ordinarily do not produce ulceration or deep infiltration and heal without scarring or atrophy. Gentle washing of lesions, removal of crusts, and drainage of blisters and pustules help prevent local spread and reaccumulation of crusts. If crusts are firmly adherent, warm soaks or compresses are useful. Topical antibiotics, if used properly, are frequently highly effective in the treatment of early superficial pyoderma due to *Staphylococcus aureus*. In cutaneous infection due to beta hemolytic streptococcus or persistent staphylococcal infection, however, systemic antibiotics produce a swifter response and fewer failures.[5]   *Bullous impetigo*

Owing to changing patterns and increasing resistance to penicillin, penicillin G is generally not recommended for the treatment of *Staphylococcus aureus* infection.[5] Patients with impetigo caused by *Staphylococcus aureus* may be treated with erythromycin, 30 to 50 mg/kg/day (up to 250 mg four times a day) for seven to ten days. For those acutely ill or with severe forms of bullous impetigo, however, dicloxacillin should be administered (12.5 to 25 mg/kg/day given at 6 hour intervals) for seven to ten days.

Bacitracin, polymyxin, gramicidin, and erythromycin are effective topical agents and are relatively non-allergenic. Although a high incidence of allergenicity has been attributed to the topical use of neomycin, this has probably been exaggerated. The majority of contact allergies to this agent follow prolonged use on chronically inflamed skin. When that group is excluded, the incidence of neomycin allergy falls drastically, with an estimated incidence of 1 in 100,000 usages.[6]

Acute glomerulonephritis is the most significant complication of streptococcal impetigo. As in the case of nephritis following streptococcal infection of the throat, only certain serological types, different from those producing nephritis as a sequel of streptococcal pharyngitis, appear to result in this complication of cutaneous infection.[7] Clinical glomerulonephritis secondary to impetigo is uncommon, except for certain epidemics due to nephritogenic strains of streptococci. The risk of developing nephritis following skin infection with a nephritogenic strain of streptococcus, however, is high (12 to 28 per cent).[8] It must be emphasized that although systemic antibiotics help eliminate cutaneous streptococci, they do not appear to prevent glomerulonephritis due to streptococcal impetigo.[9] In areas where nephritogenic M-strains of streptococci are endemic urinalysis should be performed and patients should be watched for signs of glomerulonephritis for at least seven weeks after the cutaneous streptococcal infection.

Folliculitis

The term folliculitis refers to a superficial or deep infection of hair follicles. The clinical appearance varies according to the location and depth of follicular involvement. Superficial folliculitis (Bockhart's impetigo), an infection of the follicular ostium, begins with superficial small dome-shaped, thin-walled yellow pustules, often with a narrow red areola and a hair shaft in the center of the lesion. It is seen most commonly in children and usually occurs on the scalp, face, buttocks, and extremities. Most lesions are painless, occur in crops, and generally heal in a period of seven to ten days. Coagulase-positive *Staphylococcus aureus* is the most common pathogen; occasionally other organisms (streptococcus, proteus, pseudomonas, or coliform bacilli) may be responsible for the infection. Superficial folliculitis is not always primarily or exclusively infectious in origin. Occupational contact with oil, occupational or therapeutic contact with tar and tar products, and occlusive dressings with polyethylene or adhesive may cause obstruction of pilosebaceous follicles, resulting in follicular plugging and inflammation. Although those lesions are usually sterile, *Staphylococcus epidermidis* may occasionally be isolated from them.

Superficial folliculitis usually responds to gentle cleansing and the application of topical antibiotics. Occasionally systemic antibiotics (penicillin or erythromycin) may be required for persistent or recurrent folliculitis. In such instances, bacterial culture should be obtained prior to the initiation of systemic therapy.

Folliculitis Barbae. Folliculitis barbae (sycosis barbae) is a term used to describe a deep-seated folliculitis of the bearded area involving the entire depth of the follicle and perifollicular region (Fig. 10–6). A pruritic follicular or perifollicular infection is usually the initial lesion, with the process spreading from one follicle to another by trauma from scratching, shaving, or impetiginization. Sycosis barbae is characterized by follicular papules and pustules and, as the condition progresses, by erythema, crusting, and boggy infiltration of the skin. Although occasionally, other bacteria may be isolated, the infection is usually of staphylococcal origin. Care in the technique of shaving should be taken, and the use of an electric rather than safety razor is sometimes helpful in the prevention and treatment of this disorder. Although relapses are common, warm compresses and topical antibiotics are often sufficient to con-

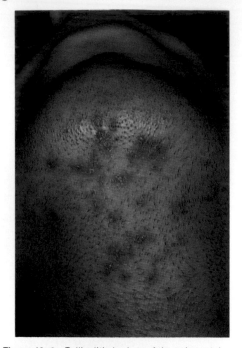

Figure 10–6 Folliculitis barbae of the submental area and upper aspect of the anterior neck. Follicular papules, pustules, boggy erythema and crusting with spread from one follicle to another due to shaving and impetiginization.

trol minor forms of sycosis barbae. If the condition is chronic, severe, or recurrent, however, several weeks of systemic antibiotics are after required.

Pseudofolliculitis Barbae. Pseudofolliculitis barbae is a common and troublesome inflammatory disorder of the pilosebaceous follicles of the beard caused by shaved hairs that curve inward with resultant repenetration of the skin, seen particularly in blacks and in people with curly hair. Upon re-entry into the epidermis, the hairs grow in a curved or arcuate path, with the creation of an inflammatory foreign body reaction. Although cocci, particularly *Staphylococcus epidermidis*, can be cultured from lesions at times, pathogenic bacteria seem to play little role in this type of folliculitis. Mild cases may be managed by careful shaving and occasionally by changing from a safety razor to an electric razor, or vice versa. Since close shaving promotes oblique penetrations of hairs into the skin, this should be avoided whenever possible. A chemical depilatory alternating with careful shaving will often help control this disorder to a moderate degree, and the topical use of vitamin A acid (Retin-A), as in the treatment of acne vulgaris, is often helpful in the prevention of this disorder.

Folliculitis Keloidalis Nuchae. Folliculitis keloidalis nuchae (acne keloidalis) represents a chronic perifollicular infection of the nape of the neck seen in men. Early cases are characterized by follicular papules, pustules, and occasionally abscesses. The lesions are gradually replaced by fibrous nodules and, in some individuals, by keloidal scarring. The condition usually occurs in

males after puberty and is most commonly seen between the ages of 15 and 25, especially in blacks. Seen most frequently, but not exclusively, in those with a tendency toward acne vulgaris, the condition is extremely chronic and new lesions may continue to form at intervals for years.

The bacteriology varies from case to case and at different time intervals. Although pathogenic staphylococci are often found, they appear to be secondary invaders. Treatment consists of long-term antibiotic therapy, as in the treatment of severe acne and chronic folliculitis, with intralesional triamcinolone in an effort to minimize keloid formation and incision and drainage of lesions. In severe cases, excision and plastic surgical repair may be necessary.

Ecthyma

Ecthyma is a deep or ulcerative type of pyoderma commonly seen on the lower extremities and buttocks of children. It may occur as either a small punched-out ulcer (ecthyma minor) or a deep spreading ulcerative process (ecthyma major). The disorder begins in the same manner as impetigo, often following infected insect bites or minor trauma, but penetrates through the epidermis to produce a shallow ulcer. The initial lesion is a vesicle or vesiculopustule with an erythematous base, surrounding halo, and firmly adherent crust. Removal of the crust reveals a deeper lesion than that seen in impetigo, with an underlying saucer-shaped ulcer and raised margin (Fig. 10–7). Lesions are painful, slow growing, and chronic; healing occurs after a few weeks, often with scar formation. Scratching and a lack of appropriate hygienic measures may lead to progression and autoinoculation of the disease. Lesions are usually initiated by beta hemolytic streptococci, although in later stages, other organisms are frequently isolated. Treatment, as in impetigo, consists of warm compresses with gentle removal

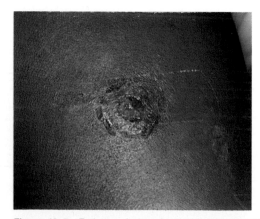

Figure 10–7 Ecthyma. A deep form of pyoderma with a saucer-shaped erythematous ulcer and raised margin associated with occlusion of the infection by an adhesive dressing.

of crusts bacterial cultures, and appropriate systemic antibiotics.

Furuncles and Carbuncles

Furuncles or boils are painful circumscribed perifollicular staphylococcal abscesses that have a tendency to central necrosis and suppuration. Seen most frequently in older children and adults, they usually develop from a preceding folliculitis with deeper extension into the dermis and subcutaneous tissue. They generally occur in areas of the skin that are unusually hairy and subject to friction and maceration, particularly the face, back of the neck, scalp, axillae, breasts, thighs, buttocks, and perineum. Clinically they appear as red tender nodules, which enlarge to a diameter of 1 to 5 cm. They gradually become boggy and fluctuant and, if untreated, often suppurate with release of a purulent blood-tinged discharge. There is a high rate of contagion in patients with deep angry boils and Group I phage type 80-81 and certain other Group I and II strains are re-emerging as the cause of small epidemics of furunculosis.

The treatment of boils depends largely upon the extent and location of lesions. Simple furunculosis may respond to warm moist compresses. Severe or persistent infections require systemic antibiotics, with incision and drainage after they have softened and become fluctuant. Since penicillin-resistant staphylococci are commonly seen as pathogens, cultures and sensitivity tests should be performed. Oral beta-lactimase-resistant antibiotics such as dicloxacillin, cloxacillin, nafcillin, or cephalexin are usually the antibiotics of choice. If the patient is allergic to penicillin or its derivatives, erythromycin or clindamycin may be administered.

Carbuncles may be considered as large deep-seated staphylococcal abscesses composed of aggregates of interconnected furuncles that drain at multiple points on the cutaneous surface. Usually seen in men on the back of the neck, shoulders, buttocks, and outer aspect of the hip joints and thighs, they extend into the deeper dermis and subcutaneous tissues, reach a larger size than furuncles (3 to 10 cm in diameter), and undergo necrosis and suppuration more slowly than furuncles (usually 7 to 14 days are required before fluctuation becomes apparent). Because of the delay in suppuration and the larger size of lesions, patients may present with extreme pain and constitutional symptoms (fever, chills, malaise, and, in extreme situations, even prostration).

Carbuncles should be treated with appropriate antibiotics and incision and drainage of large lesions, preferably after appropriate antibiotics have been initiated and lesions have become fluctuant.

Cellulitis and Erysipelas

Cellulitis. Cellulitis is an accute suppurative inflammation of the skin, particularly the deeper subcutaneous tissues. It is characterized by erythema, swelling, and tenderness of the affected area. The borders of cellulitis are not elevated or sharply defined. This is in contrast to erysipelas, a more superficial form of cellulitis with a well-demarcated border, which is due to group A (or uncommonly group G) streptococci (Fig. 10–8).

Cellulitis usually occurs as a complication of a wound or trauma, which is followed within a day or two by markedly red, tender, warm swelling with an edematous infiltrated appearance. Although group A beta-hemolytic streptococci and *Staphylococcus aureus* are the most common etiologic agents, occasionally other bacteria may be implicated. In young children, however, particularly those under two years of age, *Hemophilus influenzae* should be considered as a cause of cellulitis (in young children this agent is probably more common than either streptococcus or staphylococcus). Children with *H. influenzae* cellulitis may be extremely ill and toxic, often with accompanying upper respiratory symptoms and an associated bacteremia or septicemia.[10] In approximately 50 per cent of instances of *H. influenzae* cellulitis, the lesion has a peculiar dusky red, bluish, or purplish-red discoloration. It should be noted, however, that bluish-purple discoloration can also occur with cellulitis due to other organisms, such as *Streptococcus pneumoniae*.[11]

The treatment of cellulitis is dependent upon identification of the affecting organism whenever possible and use of appropriate antibotics. Most cases of cellulitis should be needle-aspirated for Gram stain and bacterial culture. Patients with cellulitis due to *H. influenzae* should be treated with ampicillin (ampicillin and chloramphenicol for very severe cases); penicillinase-resistant penicillins should be used for patients with cellulitis due to staphylococci; and penicillin should be utilized for those individuals with streptococcal cellulitis. For patients in whom needle-aspiration and bacterial culture do not reveal the organism, therapy with both a penicillinase-resistant penicillin and ampicillin is recommended (a one-drug alternative is cephazolin). For those allergic to penicillin, erythromycin or clindamycin is indicated; for patients with penicillin-resistant staphylococci, a semisynthetic penicillinase-resistant penicillin (methicillin, nafcillin, oxacillin, dicloxacillin, cephalothin, or cefazolin) will generally result in a rapid clinical response. The dosage of ampicillin is 200 mg/kg/day and that of chloramphenicol is 100 mg/kg/day. Aplastic anemia, however must be considered as a possible complication of chloramphenicol administration.

Erysipelas. Erysipelas occurs most frequently in infants, very young children, and older adults as a superficial cellulitis of the skin, with marked lymphatic vessel involvement, due to group A beta-streptococci. In most cases the organism gains access by direct inoculation through a break in the skin, but occasionally hematogenous infection may occur. After an incubation period of two to five days, the initial lesion begins as a small area

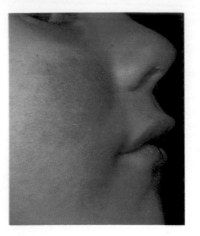

Figure 10–8 Erysipelas. Superficial streptococcal cellulitis with a distinct and well-marginated border.

of redness that gradually enlarges to reveal a characteristic tense, hot, painful, shiny bright-red brawny infiltrated plaque with a distinct and well-marginated border (Fig. 10–8). The periphery of the lesion may appear irregular because of projections of the inflammatory process. Although the face and scalp are favorite sites of involvement, the infection may appear anywhere on the cutaneous surface. The most common location of erysipelas, however, is the face, with involvement of the bridge of the nose and one or both cheeks.

Penicillin is the drug of choice for the treatment of erysipelas. For individuals allergic to penicillin, erythromycin or clindamycin is recommended. Penicillin-resistant staphylococci often coexist in chronic or persistent cases. For such individuals a semisynthetic penicillinase-resistant penicillin, such as methicillin, nafcillin, oxacillin, cephalothin, or cefazolin, is recommended.

Meningococcemia

During meningococcemia or meningococcal meninigitis approximately two-thirds of patients will develop skin lesions. Acute meningococcemia may present as an influenza-like illness associated with fever, malaise, myalgia, and arthralgias, followed by macular, morbilliform, urticarial, petechial, or purpuric lesions and profound hypotension. The petechiae are usually small and somewhat irregular, measure 1 to 2 mm in diameter, have a smudged appearance, and may have a slightly raised, pale-grayish vesicular or pustular center. The trunk and lower extremities are the most common sites, but lesions may also appear on the face, palms, and soles, and the conjunctivae and other mucous membranes may have similar petechiae. More extensive hemorrhagic lesions are seen in fulminant meningococcal infections, and a progressive increase on all areas of the body may be followed by coalescence of lesions to form large ecchymotic areas with sharply marginated

borders. In overwhelming disease, necrotic bullae may advance to ischemic necrosis with sloughing, the skin frequently becoming gangrenous in areas of extensive involvement.

Chronic meningococcemia is rare in children. When it occurs, it is characterized by showers of erythematous macules and papules in association with fever, joint pain, and myalgia. Cutaneous lesions, seen in more than 90 per cent of cases, appear in crops coincident with or after a rise in fever. Lesions vary in character and size, are usually distributed on the trunk or the extremities, about one or more painful joints, or on areas of pressure. They generally appear as red macules and may evolve into tender papules or nodules with bluish or purpuric centers, often with ulceration.

Meningococcemia must be differentiated from gonococcemia, Henoch-Schoenlein purpura, typhoid fever, rickettsial disease, erythema multiforme, purpura fulminans, and other bacterial septicemias. The cutaneous and visceral lesions in acute meningococcemia result from direct damage to capillaries and postcapillary venules; the purpura is caused by an acute vasculitis.

Diagnosis is suggested by a careful history and physical examination and can be confirmed by culture of the blood and cerebrospinal fluid. Isolation of meningococci from the nasopharynx is presumptive, but not diagnostic. Petechial lesions can be smeared and examined for the presence of gram-negative diplococci and may be cultured for organisms. On histopathologic examination the walls of vessels may show necrosis, endothelial cells are swollen, lumina are often occluded by thrombi composed to platelets, erythrocytes, and fibrin, and meningococcal organisms may be demonstrated in the lumina of vessels, within thrombi, in neutrophils, in perivascular spaces, and in the cytoplasm of endothelial cells.

The course of meningococcal infection is variable. In untreated cases the temperature is erratic, the symptoms of infection persistent, and death nearly always occurs. Crystalline sodium penicillin G, in dosages of 100,000 to 400,000 units/kg/day administered intravenously in six divided doses is the treatment of choice. Chloramphenicol (100 mg/kg per 24 hours given every 6 hours intravenously, with a maximum dose of 4 gm per day) is an adequate alternative if the patient is allergic to penicillin. Antibiotic therapy should be continued for about 7 days for children with meningococcemia and for at least 10 days for those patients with meningococcal meningitis.

Shock frequently occurs in patients with meningococcemia. When circulatory failure occurs, every effort should be made to ensure an adequate circulating blood volume. This requires the rapid infusion of osmotically active fluids such as 5 per cent dextrose in Ringer's lactate solution, 5 per cent dextrose in normal saline, colloids, or whole blood. Fresh whole blood may be particularly helpful for patients who also have disseminated intravenous coagulopathy. If circulatory failure

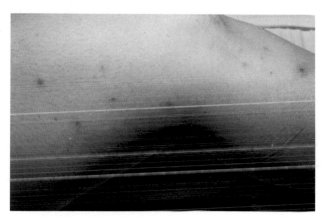

Figure 10-9 Gonococcemia. Small erythematous papules and vesiculopustules on a hemorrhagic base (Department of Dermatology, Yale University School of Medicine).

occurs, digitalization may be necessary and, if persistent, isoproterenol, 0.2 mg (200 μg) in 200 ml of 0.25 per cent normal saline (1 μg per ml) should be infused at a rate of 1 to 5 μg per minute (this rate may be doubled if there is no response). In patients with meningococcal meningitis who develop hypotension every effort must be made to minimize the development of cerebral edema.[12]

The rate of meningococcal disease among household contacts and in the military is greater than that in the general community. For this reason, such contacts should be examined and nasopharyngeal cultures obtained. Treatment may be initiated for prophylaxis or elimination of the carrier state in institutional or military populations. Prophylaxis against meningococcal infection consists of the use of rifampin (20 mg/kg/day in two divided oral doses) for two days for children between 1 and 12 years of age. For infants between three months and one year of age, rifampin may be given in a dose of 5 mg/kg/day. Sulfonamides are not indicated unless sensitivity of the meningococcal organisms has been ascertained. Sulfonamides (150 mg/kg, up to 1 to 2 gm of sulfadiazine per day for two days) accordingly may be administered prophylactically to individuals when such sensitivity of the meningococcus to sulfa has been established.

Gonococcemia

Gonococcemia is associated with lesions similar to those of meningococcemia and appears with bouts of fever, chills, arthralgia, and myalgia in patients with gonococcal septicemia. Skin lesions, usually appear within 3 to 21 days of contact, are located principally on joints of the distal portions of the extremities, and usually appear as small erythematous or hemorrhagic papules, petechiae, or vesicopustules on a hemorrhagic and, at times, necrotic base (Fig. 10-9). Lesions usually heal spontaneously in a period of four to six days.

The causative agent, *Neisseria gonorrheae*, may be demonstrated by smear or culture of early skin lesions, by specific immunofluorescent staining of vesiculopustular lesions, or by culture of the blood, genitourinary tract, or joint fluid on Thayer-

Martin medium (chocolate agar with the addition of antibiotics to inhibit normal flora and nonpathogenic neisseria).

The treatment of choice is parenteral penicillin G in high doses (150,000 units per kg per day up to 10 million units of aqueous penicillin G daily) for 10 days. For patients sensitive to penicillin, the alternate drug of choice is tetracycline, 0.5 gm every 6 hours for at least 7 days. Spectinomycin (Trobicin), the treatment of choice for individuals with gonorrhea who fail to respond to treatment with other antibiotics, is not recommended for the treatment of bacteremia due to this organism.

Toxic Epidermal Necrolysis

Toxic epidermal necrolysis due to staphylococci, staphylococcal scalded skin syndrome (SSSS), is a distinctive dermatitis caused by an exfoliative toxin termed "exfoliatin," generally elaborated by coagulase-positive Group II staphylococci, usually but not necessarily phage-type 55 or 71 (Figs. 10-10, and 10-11), occasionally Group I, type 52.[13, 14, 15] Although staphylococcal scalded

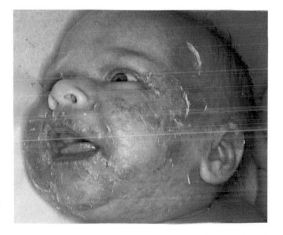

Figure 10-10 Toxic epidermal necrolysis in an infant due to infection with coagulase positive group II phage-type 71 staphylococci: (staphylococcal scalded skin syndrome, SSSS).

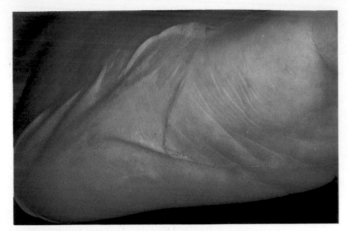

Figure 10–11 Tissue paper-like exfoliation in staphylococcal-induced toxic epidermal necrolysis (staphylococcal scaled skin syndrome).

skin syndrome is primarily a disorder seen in children under 10 years of age and toxic epidermal necrolysis, when seen in adults, is usually a drug-induced disorder, on occasion the staphylococcal form of this disease has been reported in adults and drug-induced toxic epidermal necrolysis can occur in childhood.

The reason for the lowered incidence of staphylococcal scalded skin syndrome in adults appears to be related to the fact that 85 per cent of children over 10 years of age and adults have specific antistaphylococcal antibody and are better able to metabolize and excrete the toxin,[16] thus allowing the development of localized impetigo while limiting the dissemination of toxin in older children (personal communication, Marion E. Melish). The reason for the decreased incidence of drug-induced toxic epidermal necrolysis in infants and young children, however, remains unknown.

In staphylococcal scalded skin syndrome three phases are generally recognized: erythematous, exfoliative, and desquamative. It often begins with a prodromal period of malaise, fever, irritability, and generalized erythema with a fine, stippled, sandpaper appearance and exquisite tenderness of the skin. From the intertriginous and periorificial areas and trunk, the erythema and tenderness spread over the entire body, usually sparing the hairy parts. Affected children are extemely irritable, uncomfortable, and difficult to hold because of the extreme tenderness of the skin.

The exfoliative phase is heralded by exudation and crusting around the mouth and sometimes the orbits. Large fragments of crust often become separated, leaving radial fissures surrounding the mouth, which give this disorder its characteristic and diagnostic appearance. Within two or three days, frequently in a few hours, the upper layer of the epidermis may become wrinkled or may be removed by light stroking (often peeling off like a wet tissue paper), the characteristic Nikolsky sign. Shortly thereafter the patient develops flaccid bullae and eventual exfoliation of the skin. (For further discussion and photographs of toxic epidermal necrolysis please refer to Chapter 18).

Diagnosis of staphylococcal scalded skin syndrome can be verified by isolation of coagulase-positive *Staphylococcus aureus*. In patients with this disorder the exfoliative toxin is disseminated from a primary infection site, usually in the nose or around the eyes. The organism may be recovered from pyogenic foci on the skin, conjunctivae, ala nasi, nasopharynx, stools, and occasionally the blood; it is important to note that the organism is usually not recovered from blisters or areas of exfoliation. When the diagnosis is indeterminate, differentiation of staphylococcal from drug-induced disease can be made by cutaneous biopsy. The histologic picture reveals cleavage in the epidermis in SSSS; in drug-induced toxic epidermal necrolysis, the separation occurs in the upper dermis (below the dermal-epidermal junction). Treatment requires prompt initiation of antistaphylococcal therapy to eradicate the focus of infection and eliminate further toxin production. Topical antibiotics are ineffective, and since most of the staphylococcal organisms are resistant to penicillin and some are resistant to erythromycin, penicillinase-resistant antistaphylococcal agents are preferred. Dicloxacillin, 12.5 to 25 mg per kg per day in four equal doses, is given to children weighing less than 40 kg (88 lbs); for adults and children weighing 40 kg or more, 250 mg every 6 hours is usually an adequate dose.

Chronic Granulomatous Disease of Childhood

Chronic granulomatous disease of childhood is an X-linked disorder predominantly affecting young males during the first year of life and, prior to the availability of prophylactic antibiotics, generally resulted in death during early childhood.[17, 18] A few families have been described in which females were affected, probably as a result of an autosomal recessive type of inheritance.[19, 20, 21] Male patients with chronic granulomatous disease seem to be more severely affected and outnumber females by approximately seven to one.

Chronic granulomatous disease consists of severe, recurrent, and chronic granulomatous reac-

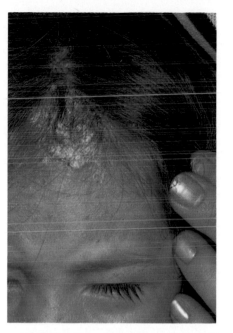

Figure 10–12 Chronic granulomatous disease with recurrent candidal granuloma of upper forehead and scalp.

tions to a number of common bacteria of low virulence that require phagocytic production of hydrogen peroxide for death. The organisms usually associated with this disease are *Staphylococcus aurerus, Klebsiella, Enterobacter aerogenes, Salmonella,* and *Serratia*. The earliest characteristic feature of the disease is an eczematous reaction in infancy. Patients often have infectious eczematoid dermatitis, purulent miliaria, frequent pustules, paronychia, and granulomatous lesions, particularly about the nares, the postauricular and periobital areas, the scalp, the axillae, and the inguinal region (Fig. 10–12).[19] Organs other than the skin which are infected include lymph nodes with chronic draining lymphadenitis, particularly in the cervical and inguinal regions; abscesses or interstitial infiltrative granulomatous processes of the lungs, bone marrow, pericardium, and gastrointestinal tract also occur. Other clinical manifestations include pyoderma, stomatitis, conjunctivitis, osteomyelitis, meningitis, pneumonia, peritonitis, and septicemia.

The primary disorder of chronic granulomatous disease (formerly termed fatal granulomatous disease) of childhood is a defect in the ability of peripheral leukocytes (both neutrophils and monocytes) to kill bacteria. This defect is not a failure of the cells to phagocytize organisms, but a defect in the intracellular killing processes of the phagocytic cells. The leukocyte defect is detectable by use of the nitro blue tetrazolium (NBT) slide test. Whereas leukocytes from normal individuals reduce nitro-blue tetrazolium dye during phagocytosis, cells from patients with this disorder have an inability or marked decrease in the ability to reduce the dye from a colorless to deep blue state during phagocytosis.[20, 21, 22]

Treatment of children with chronic granulomatous disease has, in general, been frustrating. Genetic counseling, including carrier states in sisters of affected males, is recommended in all cases, and although the value of continuous courses of antibiotics remains questionable, treatment with a bactericidal antibiotic specific for the patient's infecting organism for long periods of time appears to prolong symptom-free intervals in patients.[22]

Job Syndrome

Job syndrome appears to be an autosomal recessive variant of chronic granulomatous disease.[23] In this disorder there is also a defect in polymorphonuclear function in which certain species of bacteria are ingested but not destroyed. The granulomatous reactions seen in X-linked chronic granulomatous disease of childhood, however, do not occur.

The few patients described with this condition are young and fair-haired girls. Symptoms generally begin in the first year of life with a persistent seborrheic form of eczema of the scalp, ears, periorbital areas, and inguinal regions. Scalp folliculitis and subcutaneous abscesses, usually of staphylococcal origin are prominent features, and recurrent upper respiratory infection, otitis media, pneumonia, and abscesses of the lung and liver are commonly seen in this disease. Studies by Hill suggest that the chemical mediators released by interaction of leukocytes, IgE, and specific antigen are responsible for the leukocyte dysfunction seen in this disorder.[24]

Erythrasma

Erythrasma is a superficial bacterial infection of the skin caused by *Corynebacterium minitussimum*. It is characterized by well-demarcated, reddish-brown, slightly scaly to smooth shiny patches in the groin or axillae, or by maceration and scaling in the interdigital spaces of the toes. Fifteen per cent of cases occur in children between 5 and 14 years of age. The incidence, however, increases with age and is noted most frequently during adolescence and adulthood.[25, 26] The most common sites of involvement are the genitocrural region and interdigital spaces, where the disorder may coexist with tinea cruris and tinea pedis. The disorder can also be found in intertriginous areas and, particularly in institutionalized individuals or diabetics, may be widely disseminated.[25]

Although erythrasma is frequently confused with a dermatophyte infection, with which it may co-exist, it does not elicit an inflammatory response and does not progress to vesiculation. Erythrasma can often be differentiated from tinea infection by a characteristic coral-red fluorescence under Wood's light (due to the production of porphyrins by the corynebacteria organisms in the stratum corneum). Since erythrasma may coexist with or may precede candidiasis, particularly in intertriginous regions, examination of the lesions for fungi is important.

Without treatment the disorder tends to persist indefinitely. Antibacterial soaps may help prevent recurrences of this disorder, and less restrictive clothing or other means to reduce friction and sweating may be helpful, particularly in the groin. Although tetracycline is frequently effective, the treatment of choice is oral erythromycin, 250 mg 4 times a day for 7 to 14 days (30 to 50 mg/kg/day in equally divided doses for young children).

Trichomycosis Axillaris

Trichomycosis axillaris is a relatively innocuous superficial infection of the axillary and, less commonly, pubic hairs that results in adherent white or yellow (occasionally red or black) concretions distributed irregularly along the hair shafts (Fig. 10–13). A diphtheroid organism (*Corynebacterium tenuis*) is believed to be the causative agent for this condition. The name trichomycosis axillaris, which implies a fungal etiology, accordingly is actually a misnomer.[27]

The disorder occurs only after puberty, owing to its association with axillary and pubic hair, but then occurs with equal frequency in all postpuberal age groups. It is common in adult males, but owing to the female practice of shaving axillary hair, is relatively uncommon in females. The most frequent sign of trichomycosis axillaris is the presence of red-stained perspiration on the clothing, and individuals with hyperhidrosis frequently complain of a particularly offensive axillary odor. The nodules of trichomycosis axillaris consist of bacterial elements embedded in an amorphous matrix and, except for the red form, produce a yellow or blue-white fluorescence under Wood's light examination.

Treatment consists of shaving the hairs of the affected areas, using deodorants (which decrease hyperhidrosis and growth of gram-positive bacterial flora) and frequent washing with germicidal soaps.

Atypical Mycobacterial Infections (Swimming Pool or Fish-tank Granulomas)

Abrasions sustained in swimming pools or fish tanks may become infected with atypical mycobacteria (*Mycobacterium marinum,* formerly known as *M. balnei*) and possibly other unclassified mycobacteria. Most lesions are seen as solitary (occasionally multiple) subcutaneous nodules, ulcers, or abscesses at points of trauma, usually on the elbows (in 70 to 88 per cent of cases), knees, hands, feet, and, sometimes, the nose.

The classic clinical picture is characterized by the appearance of reddish papules or pustules at a point of trauma that grow to be the size of a pea in about three weeks and tend to break down to form a crusted ulcer, reddish-brown papules, or suppurative ulcerations. Lesions tend to be solitary (multiple lesions are infrequent). They may remain in groups at the site of the abrasion or may ascend proximally from the point of trauma. Although they may at times resemble a sporotrichoid infection, lymphangitis and lymphadenitis do not appear. Healing usually occurs spontaneously in a few months, and although exceptional cases may persist for many years, almost all cases heal spontaneously within a period of one or two years.

Mycobacterium marinum is an acid-fast nonmotile bacillus that often has transverse bands and is longer and wider than *M. tuberculosis*. The differential diagnosis of this disorder includes cutaneous tuberculosis, sporotrichosis, syphilis, cat-scratch disease, neoplastic skin tumors, and deep mycotic infections. The histologic changes resemble those of tuberculous granulation tissue, with a diffuse epithelioid-cell reaction, tubercle formation without caseation, and, at times, scattered giant cells of the Langerhans type. Cultures on Löwenstein-Jensen medium can help clarify the diagnosis; the greatest yield of positive cultures is obtained by direct inoculation of freshly biopsied material.

In all cases, a careful epidemiologic study should be performed to locate and eliminate the source of infection. Tetracycline and minocycline

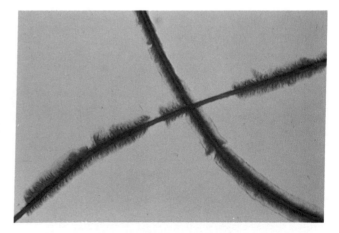

Figure 10–13 Trichomycosis axillaris with adherent concretions irregularly distributed along the hair shaft (Courtesy of Joseph McGuire, M.D.).

have been used with varying degrees of success, and the use of hot soaks on the affected area twice daily for 30 minutes is helpful, but there is, to date, no completely satisfactory treatment for this disorder.[28] Electrodesiccation and curettage, cryosurgery with liquid nitrogen, or surgical excision may be satisfactory for early or small lesions, but recurrences are common.

Tuberculosis of the Skin

The incidence of cutaneous tuberculosis, which is already rare in the United States, is declining the world over owing to the availability of effective antitubercular drugs, elimination of infected herds of cows that give milk, improvement in living standards, and vigorous preventive and therapeutic programs. However, it still occurs in some countries, and in epidemic regions, it is usually first contracted in childhood.

Primary Tuberculous Complex. Primary tuberculous complex (tuberculous chancre) develops as a result of inoculation of tuberculous organisms into the skin (occasionally into the mucosa) of an individual who has not previously been infected or who has not acquired natural or artificial immunity to the tubercle bacillus. Since tubercle bacilli cannot penetrate intact skin, this disorder occurs on exposed surfaces (the hands, most often the radial border of the dorsal aspect, the fingers, and, particularly in children, the lower extremities) through a small abrasion, insect bite, or cutaneous infection. After the bacteria have gained entry into the tissue, they remain at the site of infection, multiply, and, after two to four weeks, produce cutaneous lesions.

The earliest lesion is a brownish-red papule that develops into an indurated plaque that may ulcerate or scab over and is frequently associated with prominent regional lymphadenopathy.[29] The ulcer may be quite insignificant or may enlarge to a diameter of up to 5 cm or more. The ragged reddish-blue edges are undermined, and as they become older, they become more indurated. Thick adherent crusts and "apple-jelly" nodules (lesions that on gentle pressure with a glass slide or hand lens [diascopy] result in a yellowish-brown or "apple-jelly" color) may arise at the periphery of lesions. Healing generally takes place within a period of several weeks, with the regional lymphadenopathy remaining as the only indication of previous infection. This regional lymphadenopathy develops three to eight weeks after the infection. The glands enlarge slowly and harden, are usually painless, and, after weeks or months, may soften and form "cold" abscesses, which form sinuses and perforate to the overlying cutaneous surfaces. With healing, scars may mark the sites of previous sinuses.

The histologic picture of tuberculous chancre (primary cutaneous tuberculosis) is that of an acute inflammatory reaction with numerous bacilli, epithelioid cells, and areas of necrosis and ulceration. After three to six weeks a more specific histologic picture, with caseation necrosis, epithelioid cells, lymphocytes, and Langhans giant cells, appears. During this stage the number of tubercle bacilli decreases, and organisms may no longer be demonstrable.

Lupus Vulgaris. Lupus vulgaris is the most common form of cutaneous tuberculosis. An extremely chronic, serious, and progressive disorder, it usually occurs in individuals with a high degree of sensitivity. Earlier studies suggested that it was essentially a disorder of childhood, but this predisposition has been overemphasized.

Although lupus vulgaris can arise at the site of a primary inoculation, in the scar of scrofuloderma, or at the site of a B.C.G. vaccination, it generally appears in previously normal areas of skin. The disorder may affect any cutaneous surface, but over 90 per cent of lesions appear on the head and neck, usually originating on the nose or cheek as tiny brownish-red papules with a soft consistency. As the disorder progresses, larger patches are formed by peripheral enlargement and coalescence of papules, with elevation of lesions and intensification of their brownish color (Fig. 10–14). As in tuberculous chancre, the infiltrate exhibits a characteristic apple-jelly color on diascopy.

The course of lupus vulgaris is slow, and lesions frequently remain limited to small areas for years, occasionally decades. Areas of involvement often tend to ulcerate, frequently healing by atrophic or hypertrophic scarring with gross disfigurement. This is especially prominent when nasal cartilages or eyelids are involved; the destruction of soft tissues, cartilage, and subsequent cicatricial changes frequently result in a "parrot-beaked" or "werewolf" appearance.

Lesions of lupus vulgaris must be differentiated from those of sarcoidosis, lymphocytoma cutis, lupus erythematosus, halogenoderma, leishmaniasis, leprosy, blastomycosis, coccidiomycosis, and cutaneous malignancy. The histopathologic features consist of tubercles with epithelioid cells,

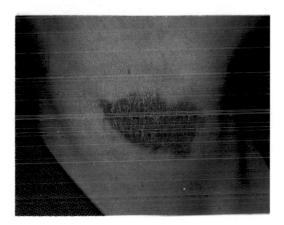

Figure 10–14 Lupus vulgaris, the most common form of cutaneous tuberculosis. An elevated brownish-red plaque formed by coalescence of papular lesions (Department of Dermatology, Yale University School of Medicine).

Langhans giant cells, and a peripheral zone of lymphocytes. Caseation necrosis may be slight or absent, and tubercle bacilli are present, but in such small numbers that their demonstration is frequently difficult or impossible.

Scrofuloderma. The terms scrofuloderma and scrofula refer to tuberculous involvement of the skin by direct extension from underlying tuberculous lymph nodes or bones. A disorder of children and young adults infected from drinking milk containing tubercle bacilli, it has become exceedingly rare as a result of the routine pasteurization of milk in the United States and Western Europe. While scrofula from *M. tuberculosis* is rare today, draining lesions from atypical mycobacteria are not that uncommon.

Tuberculous scrofuloderma is seen most frequently over cervical lymph nodes, bones, and joints. Clinical manifestations include painless swelling in the parotid, submandibular, subclavicular, and lateral regions of the neck (Fig. 10–15). On the extremities and trunk the lesions may represent hematogenous spread or they may accompany tuberculous disease of the phalanges, joints, sternum, and ribs. The overlying skin is stretched, purplish, and depressed because of fixation to infected nodes, and, with time, ulcerations and draining fistulous sinuses develop. Untreated lesions of scrofuloderma may persist with little change for years, and when healing occurs, cord-like cicatricial bands overlying ulcerated regions or areas of otherwise normal-appearing skin may appear.

The histologic features of scrofuloderma consist of ulceration or abscess formation and tubercles, with caseation necrosis at the periphery and massive necrosis and abscess formation in the center of lesions. Plasma cells may be quite numerous in the surrounding inflammatory infiltrate, and tubercle bacilli may be detected by Ziehl-Neelsen stain.

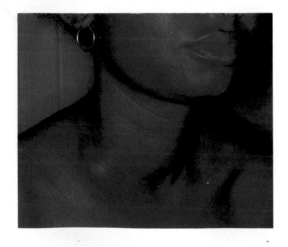

Figure 10–15 Scrofula (scrofuloderma). A painless tuberculous swelling due to breakdown of tuberculous cervical nodes in the neck (Department of Dermatology, Yale University School of Medicine).

Tuberculosis Verrucosa Cutis. Tuberculosis verrucosa cutis (warty tuberculosis) is an externally acquired, relatively uncommon inoculation type of tuberculosis in individuals who have had previous contact with *M. tuberculosis* and have thus acquired a degree of immunity and cutaneous hypersensitivity. The inoculation of tubercle bacilli occurs at sites of minor wounds or abrasions and generally appears in young or middle-aged individuals whose occupations require the handling of tuberculous patients or tissues (physicians, laboratory attendants, veterinarians, medical students, nurses, butchers, or farmers) or by auto-inoculation from sputum of a patient with active tuberculosis.

Lesions usually occur on the dorsal surfaces of the hands, on the fingers, and, in children, on the buttocks or lower extremities. Asymptomatic, they begin as small papules or papulo-pustules with a purple inflammatory halo. With time, they tend to become hyperkeratotic and wart-like and, with slow extension and growth, form a single verrucous plaque with an inflammatory border, papillomatous horny surface, and areas of pustule formation and suppuration. Multiple lesions may occur, but most areas of tuberculosis verrucosa are solitary, and although uncommon, tuberculous involvement of regional glands has been described.

Warty tuberculosis must be differentiated from viral warts, bromoderma, blastomycosis, chromoblastomycosis, actinomycosis, sporotrichosis, lieshmaniasis, chronic vegetating pyoderma, and atypical mycobacterial infection (swimming pool granuloma). The histologic picture shows acanthosis, hyperkeratosis, pseudoepitheliomatous hyperplasia of the epidermis, dense inflammatory dermal infiltrates, and abscesses consisting of polymorphonuclear leukocytes and lymphocytes. Epithelioid cells and giant cells are found in the dermis, but typical tubercle formation and caseation are uncommon. Although tubercle bacilli are not commonly found, they are more numerous than in lupus vulgaris and, occasionally, can be demonstrated.

Orificial Tuberculosis. Orificial tuberculosis (tuberculosis cutis orificialis) is a tuberculous disorder of the mucocutaneous junctions of the orifices (the nose, mouth, anus, urinary meatus, and genital orifices) due to autoinoculation of tubercle bacilli from tuberculosis of internal organs. A rare disorder, it affects males more frequently than females, and although it may occur in practically all age groups, it is relatively rare in childhood and most commonly seen in debilitated middle-aged or elderly individuals.

Lesions appear as shallow oval painful ulcers with a granulating base and undermined edges, with swelling, edema, and inflammation of the surrounding mucosa. Lesions are particularly painful, spontaneous healing is rare, and lesions often extend from the mucous membranes into contiguous cutaneous surfaces.

Painful ulcers of the mouth or other mucosal

membranes in patients with visceral tuberculosis should arouse suspicion of this disorder. The histopathologic picture is not diagnostic and may merely reveal an ulcer surrounded by a non-specific inflammatory infiltrate. The demonstration of tuberculous bacilli in cultures or histopathologic examination of material taken from clinically active mucosal ulcers is diagnostic.

Miliary Tuberculosis. Miliary tuberculosis (disseminated tuberculosis, tuberculosis cutis miliaris disseminata) is an extremely rare manifestation of fulminating pulmonary or meningeal tuberculosis. Cutaneous lesions are uncommon in infants and younger children, and are seen even less frequently in adults. When present, the eruption is due to hematogenous spread in gravely ill individuals and is characterized by minute, symmetrically distributed erythematous, ulcerated reddish-brown macules, papules, vesiculopustules, or purpuric lesions. Children usually run a progressively downhill course, and the prognosis of this disorder is poor.

In miliary tuberculosis, the tuberculin test is usually negative, either because it is administered too early in the disease or because overwhelming infection prevents a positive reaction. Early histologic changes are non-specific and often consist of necrosis, inflammation, and extravasation of red blood cells. Numerous acid-fast bacilli are present, and if the patient survives, classic tuberculoid architecture with caseation eventually becomes apparent.

TREATMENT. The treatment of all forms of cutaneous tuberculosis is similar to that used for active pulmonary tuberculosis. Chemotherapy, to be adequate, must be continued without interruption for a minimum of one year or more depending on the bacteriologic and clinical findings. Isoniazid, para-aminosalicylic acid, streptomycin, ethambutol, ethionamide, and rifampin are currently the most effective antituberculous agents.

Isoniazid. Isoniazid (INH) has a combined bactericidal and bacteriostatic action and readily penetrates caseous material. The dosage for children is 10 to 20 mg/kg daily, with a maximum of 300 to 500 mg per day, depending on the severity of infection, given in a single daily dose. Para-aminosalicylic acid (PAS), a relatively weak drug, is valuable as a secondary therapeutic agent in combination with isoniazid or streptomycin. Never given as the sole agent, when combined with INH or streptomycin the addition of PAS helps prevent the emergence of bacilli resistant to the primary chemotherapeutic agent. A drug available as an alternative to PAS in young children is ethionamide (Trecator-SC, Ives Laboratories). This preparation, as with PAS, should not be given alone but should be administered in conjunction with other effective antituberculous therapy. Optimum dosage for children has not been established.

Streptomycin is still an effective drug for multiple therapy although tubercle bacilli rapidly develop resistance to streptomycin when this preparation is used alone. It is usually used as a third drug for a short period of time in adults with extensive disease, or in children with severe tuberculous meningitis and miliary dissemination. It is given intramuscularly in doses of 20 to 40 mg/kg daily (with a maximum of 1 gm per day). Streptomycin has adverse neurotoxic effects, and the development of vertigo, tinnitus, or loss of hearing (especially to high frequency levels) should lead to re-evaluation of therapy and, usually, withdrawal of streptomycin therapy.

Ethambutol. Ethambutol (EMB), available as Myambutol (Lederle), is a highly effective first-line antituberculous drug. Frequently used in place of PAS in the treatment of adults, ethambutol is not recommended for use in young children under 5 years of age who cannot be tested for visual acuity, color blindness, and visual fields. It acts by delaying the multiplication of bacteria through interference with RNA synthesis. Resistance develops slowly, and when given in combination with other drugs, ethambutol delays the emergence of bacterial resistance. Available in tablets of 100 to 400 mg, EMB may be given in a dosage of 15 mg/kg daily. Because this drug may have adverse effects on vision, periodic evaluation of individuals on this agent should include ophthalmoscopy, finger perimetry, and testing for color discrimination.

Rifampin, a derivative of *Streptomycin mediterranei*, has been used with excellent results in patients with tuberculosis. When used alone as a single antituberculous agent, however, resistance rapidly develops. Therefore rifampin must always be given in combination with other antimycobacterial agents, usually isoniazid (with or without streptomycin). The most common side effects are gastrointestinal disturbances (abdominal pain, nausea, vomiting, and diarrhea) and nervous system effects (headache, drowsiness, dizziness, and depression). Other side effects include hepatitis or a shock-like syndrome with hepatic involvement and abnormal liver function tests (due to a primary tissue toxicity on the liver), skin rash, pruritus, urticaria, purpura, and a "flu-like" syndrome.

Indications for the use of rifampin are treatment failures, infections due to bacilli resistant to other therapeutic agents, and extensive severe disease in which immediate control of infection is essential. Available in 300 mg capsules, rifampin may be given once daily, preferably one hour before or two hours after a meal. The pediatric dosage is 10 to 20 mg/kg per day up to a maximum daily dose of 600 mg. Data are not available, however, for determination of the dosage for children under the age of five years.[30]

The Tuberculid Disorders

The term tuberculid is used to described a group of recurrent cutaneous eruptions of unknown etiology. Originally considered to be related to toxins or possibly to an allergic response to tubercle bacilli, they are currently believed to be the result of hematogenous dissemination of mycobacteria from an internal focus into the skin, where they are destroyed by cutaneous defense mechanisms. Although the existence and pathogenesis of tuberculids is presently uncertain, most textbooks describe the following four "tuberculid" disorders: erythema induratum, papulonecrotic tuberculid, lichen scrofulosorum, and lupus miliaris disseminatus faciei.

Erythema Induratum. Erythema induratum (Bazin's disease) is a chronic benign tuberculous vasculitis that typically occurs on the calves and occasionally thighs or heels of girls and young women. Lesions consist of symmetrical chronic, painless but tender deep-seated subcutaneous infiltrations that begin as subcutaneous plaques and nodules that eventuate in red or purple tender indurated masses that tend to ulcerate. The ulcers are irregular and shallow, have a bluish margin, rarely exceed 3 to 4 cm in size, and heal with an atrophic scar. The disease is chronic and recurrent, and in the majority of patients, a personal or family history of tuberculosis is reported. Patients have a positive tuberculin skin test, but mycobacteria are seldom recovered from lesions and there is no clinical or radiologic evidence of tuberculosis. The disease typically persists for years, with slow progression, relapses, and remissions.

Recurring bilaterally symmetrical nodules and ulcerations on the lower legs of young women are characteristic of this disorder. Histologic features include a tuberculoid infiltrate, inflammation of arteries and veins, and areas of caseation necrosis. Vascular changes consist of endothelial swelling, edema, and hypertrophy of the vessel wall, occlusion of the lumen, fibrinoid necrosis, and vasculitis.

Many eruptions of erythema induratum undergo involution over a period of years simply as the result of supportive therapy, rest, careful bandaging, and elevation of the involved limbs. In cases in which active tuberculosis is considered present, chemotherapy should be carried out in the same manner as for other forms of tuberculosis.

Papulonecrotic Tuberculid. Papulonecrotic tuberculid, an eruption primarily seen in children and young adults, is characterized by symmetric crops of indolent dusky-red pear-sized papules and small nodules with central necrosis that heal spontaneously, with superficially depressed scars. Sites of predilection are the extensor aspects of the extremities, particularly the knees and elbows, the buttocks, and the lower trunk.

The histologic findings consist of small areas of necrosis in the upper dermis with extension into the epidermis. The inflammatory infiltrate surrounding the necrotic areas may be nonspecific but usually exhibits tuberculoid features. As a rule, bacteria cannot be demonstrated in the lesions. Epithelioid cells and occasional Langhans giant cells are present, and obliterative endarteritis and endophlebitis leading to thrombosis and occlusion of the vascular channels complete the picture.

The response of this disorder to antituberculous therapy appears to support a tuberculid nature.

Lichen Scrofulosorum. Lichen scrofulosorum is a disorder characterized by clusters of lichenoid papules on the trunk of children or young adults, with caseous tuberculous lymph nodes or bone or joint tuberculosis. Lesions are firm, pinhead-sized 1 to 5 mm or smaller, and skin-colored or reddish-brown. They are flat-topped follicular lichenoid papules. Asymptomatic, they are arranged in nummular groups, usually on the trunk, where they persist for months and slowly undergo spontaneous involution. Histopathologic examination reveals small tubercles that may show caseation, just below the epidermis, usually in relation to hair follicles or eccrine ducts. Since sensitivity to tuberculin is often extreme, tuberculin tests, should be performed only with high dilutions.

Spontaneous healing is the rule for this disorder.

Lupus Miliaris Disseminata Faciei. Lupus miliaris disseminata faciei is a self-limiting papular eruption of adolescents and adults that involves the central portion of the face. It is characterized by asymptomatic, raised, moderately firm, small millet seed or larger-sized papules arranged more or less symmetrically on the central area of the face that later turn brown and reveal an apple-jelly color on diascopy. The papules appear singly or in groups about the eyelids, cheeks, angles of the mouth, paranasal and mental areas, and occasionally spread to involve the neck and adjacent mucous membranes of the nose and lips. They disappear spontaneously, often leaving small pitted scars.

Although the histologic picture of lupus miliaris disseminatus faciei features typical tubercles, patients as a rule have no history of tuberculosis and often have a negative tuberculin test. The disorder has been seen in adults as a variant of "lupoid" rosacea or as a tuberculid dermatitis of unknown cause.

Miliary lupus faciei does not respond to antituberculous therapy. Systemic corticosteroids or superficial x-ray therapy are occasionally effective but not generally indicated, since the process usually resolves spontaneously within a period of 12 to 18 months.

Leprosy

Leprosy (Hansen disease) is a chronic infectious disorder of worldwide distribution in which the acid-fast bacillus *Mycobacterium leprae* has a special predilection for the skin and nervous system. The disorder is generally classified into three types: (1) lepromatous, (2) tuberculoid, and (3) intermediate (borderline or mixed). Lepromatous leprosy, the disfiguring disease familiar to the public, is usually manifested by numerous symmetrically arranged lesions, which although macular at first, develop nodules or diffuse infiltrates, especially on the eyebrow and ears, resulting in a leonine facies. Patients with lepromatous leprosy are usually more infectious than those with other forms of the disease, presumably because bacteria are more numerous in their skin and respiratory secretions.[31] Tuberculoid leprosy often shows only a single or, occasionally, a few cutaneous lesions. They are large, well-defined macules that show hypopigmentation and loss of sensation. The peripheral nerves are often thickened and palpable, and as in the lipromatous type, anesthesia, trophic disturbances, and paralyses occur. Intermediate leprosy represents an early stage of this disorder and generally shows one or a few macules or edematous papules that are erythematous and may show loss of pigment.

Leprosy affects children as well as adults. The incubation period is typically very long, two to six years, and incubation periods up to 40 years have been reported. Early childhood forms reveal solitary lesions, which may occur on any exposed area of the skin. They appear as small, slightly raised hyperemic macules or groups of tiny papules surrounded by a blanched halo. Lesions are asymptomatic, tend to heal spontaneously after a period of 18 to 24 months, and leave a thin wrinkled hypopigmented scar. This is followed by a period of quiescence until puberty or early life when the condition may erupt into the more easily recognized forms of the disorder.

Leprosy should be suspected whenever a patient from a leprosy-endemic area presents with chronic skin lesions, skin anesthesia, thickened nerves, or eye complaints. The diagnosis is confirmed by the finding of acid-fast bacilli in skin smears or biopsy material.[31] The histologic picture of leprosy features a granulomatous infiltrate containg large foamy histiocytes (lepra cells) in the epidermis. Acid-fast strains reveal the presence of the lepra bacilli, which frequently lie in bundles (like packs of cigars).

Sulfones are the treatment of choice for leprosy if there is no deficiency of glucose-6-phosphate dehydrogenase. Dapsone (4,4'-diaminodiphenylsulfone, Avlosulfon, DDS) is given in dosages of 50 to 150 mg daily for adults, with children receiving dosages in proportion to their weight. Patients should be started on small doses and increased slowly in an effort to reduce possible acute reactions which might aggravate existing damage to vital areas such as motor nerves, eyes, or testes. In the intermediate form, treatment should be given for at least two years or for at least one year after all clinical signs of activity have disappeared. In the lepromatous form, treatment should be continued for a period of at least four years, or for at least two years after all clinical signs of activity have ceased and cutaneous smears no longer show evidence of acid-fast lepra bacilli. Borderline cases require treatment periods of 5 to 10 years. For individuals with Dapsone-resistant strains of the lepra bacillus and

for patients with complications of leprosy, rifampin (150 mg/day for 6 to 18 months) may be given.

Disorders Due to Fungus-like Bacteria

Actinomycosis and nocradiosis are disorders caused by actinomycetes, gram-positive organisms once thought to be closely related to fungi because of their tendency to grow in branches or mycelia in culture and infected tissue. Although these disorders can occur at any age and have been seen as early as the first month of life, most reported cases are seen in adults. Primary cutaneous infection is rare, and involvement of the skin and subcutaneous tissues is generally a result of contiguous spread from other sites or of secondary infection of injured skin and subcutaneous tissue, particularly in individuals who are debilitated or immunodeficient.[32]

Actinomycosis. Actinomycosis (lumpy jaw) is a chronic granulomatous disorder caused by *Actinomyces israeli,* an anaerobic gram-positive saprophyte of the tonsillar crypts or carious teeth, and rarely by *Actinomyces bovis* or other species. It is characterized by suppuration, painful induration, and the formation of multiple draining sinuses.

The disorder generally occurs at three sites: the cervicofacial area, the lungs, and the intestinal tract; two-thirds of all human cases occur in the cervicofacial area. Cervicofacial actinomycosis, generally seen in individuals with poor oral hygiene and carious teeth, begins when the infecting organism invades a traumatized mucous membrane in the oral cavity. The primary lesion commonly develops as a swelling over the mandibular area and increases in size to form a brawny, erythematous lesion that breaks down to discharge serosanguineous or purulent material through multiple sinus tracts, from which the characteristic sulfur-yellow granules consisting of masses of actinomycetes can be demonstrated. Destruction of bone, with periostitis and osteomyelitis, is common, and absence of regional lymph node involvement is characteristic.

Aspiration of the organism causes pulmonary infection, which progresses through the pleura, causing draining sinus tracts of the chest wall. The abdominal form develops in a similar fashion from the ileum, cecum, or appendix (via the gastrointestinal tract) and is seen as draining sinuses, tracts, or subcutaneous abscesses, extending to either the abdominal wall or the perineum. As in the skin and lungs, the disease progresses slowly, producing localized, granulomatous lesions, which may spread to involve adjacent soft tissue and bone, eventually presenting on the abdominal wall as a brawny erythematous mass with draining sinuses, from which the organism can be recovered.

Primary infection of other body sites may affect the urinary tract, central nervous system, bones, and joints. A localized form, known as mycetoma, occurs most frequently on the feet or ankles of individuals who walk around barefoot (see Chapter 13).

The diagnosis of actinomycosis is established by isolation and identification of the causative organism by strict anaerobic culture from tissue exudate of lesions. The diagnosis may also be confirmed by observation of the highly characteristic "sulfur" granules (groups of delicate filaments, frequently with club-shaped ends) in purulent or biopsied materials.

The course of the disease is prolonged, indolent, and characterized by closure of one sinus tract and the opening of another. Treatment consists of surgical incision and drainage of abscesses, excision of chronic, fibrotic, avascular tissue, and chemotherapy, primarily with aqueous penicillin G, 150,000 up to 300,000 units/kg/day, administered intravenously for a period of approximately four weeks, followed by oral penicillin until all lesions have cleared completely or until they have been stable for a period of six weeks. Alternate antibiotics for patients who are allergic to penicillin include tetracycline, erythromycin, and chloramphenicol.[32]

Nocardiosis. Nocardiosis is a severe acute or subacute frequently fatal, primary pulmonary infection caused by an aerobic gram-positive partially acid-fast fungus-like organism, *Nocardia asteroides*. Acquired by the respiratory route with a focal infection in the lungs and frequent hematogenous dissemination, *nocardiosis* may be found in any organ of the body. Worldwide in distribution, the organism infects men more frequently than women (in a ratio of three to one). The disease generally appears in individuals between 20 and 50 years of age, and although uncommon, it has been increasingly recognized in infants and children and is no longer considered a rarity.[33]

Nocardiosis generally occurs through inhalation of contaminated dust, and the clinical picture is usually that of a primary pulmonary disease that resembles tuberculosis in its clinical and x-ray findings. In those instances in which the skin is involved (less than 15 per cent of cases) the most common lesions are abscesses of the chest wall with granulomatous lesions surrounding draining sinuses.[33] Although the disease is respiratory in origin, there may be dissemination to the brain, heart, spleen, and other organs, and lymphocutaneous infection with a typical chancriform syndrome, although relatively uncommon, has been described at the site of injury by a thorn or splinter.[32]

Nocardiosis should be considered in obscure pulmonary and meningeal syndromes and chronic suppurative disorders of the bones or skin. The diagnosis is established by the presence of organisms in smears or cultures of sputum, aspirated material collected from lesions, or biopsied material. Unfortunately, the diagnosis is seldom established until the disease is far advanced. Accordingly, the prognosis is generally poor and mortality remains high.

Treatment consists of surgical incision and drainage of abscesses, excision and debridement of localized tissue, and sulfonamide therapy, up to 4 to 6 gm per day in older children and adults, with blood levels maintained at 10 mg/100 ml for a period of two to three months. Even today, with such therapy, fatality rates are high (approximately 50 per cent).

TREPONEMAL INFECTIONS

Syphilis

Syphilis is a contagious disease caused by the spirochetal organism *Treponema pallidum*. Transmitted principally through intimate contact with infectious lesions of the skin or mucous membranes, *T. pallidum* enters the body by the penetration of intact mucous membranes or minute abrasions of the stratum corneum. In congenital infection (prenatal syphilis) the fetus is infected by way of placental transmission from an untreated mother generally after the 16th week of pregnancy (for a discussion of neonatal syphilis, see Chapter 2).

Untreated acquired syphilis consists of the following five stages: (1) an incubation period of approximately three to four weeks (outside limits 9 to 90 days); (2) a primary stage at the site of penetration by the treponemes, usually manifested by an initial syphilitic lesion or chancre, which lasts for a period of one to six weeks; (3) a secondary stage two to ten weeks later manifested by widespread cutaneous lesions and systemic symptoms, which last for a period of two to ten weeks; (4) a subclinical latent stage, with no symptoms or signs of the disease, that follows the disappearance of the eruption of the secondary stage, lasts for a period of 1 to 40 years or more, and is diagnosable only by the presence of a reactive serologic test for syphilis; and (5) a tertiary or late stage (seen in about one-third of cases) characterized by mucocutaneous, osseous, visceral, cardiovascular, and central nervous system lesions with, at times, debilitation and death.[34, 35]

Early syphilis (primary, secondary, and the first two to four years of latent syphilis) is infectious, tends to relapse, and seldom leads to scarring. The late latent (after the first 2 to 4 years of latent syphilis) and late stages, conversely, are considered non-infectious, rarely relapse, and often tend to be destructive and scarring.

Primary Syphilis. The initial lesion of syphilis appears at the site of penetration of the treponemes after an incubation period of three to four weeks following infection. The primary syphilitic lesion or chancre begins as a small red papule or crusted erosion, which in the course of a few weeks becomes round or oval, firm and indurated, and develops a button-like papule or plaque a few millimeters to one or two centimeters in diameter with an erosive rather than ulcerative surface that is raw and exudes a serous fluid (Fig. 10–16). Since 95 per cent of all cases of syphilis are transmitted sexually, most syphilitic chancres appear on the

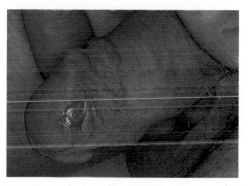

Figure 10-16 A chancriform plaque with an erosive surface as seen in primary syphilis

genitals. The are painless if free of secondary infection. They may occasionally be multiple, but traditionally have been described as solitary lesions. In women, genital chancres are less commonly observed, because of their painless nature and frequent location on the cervix, and are generally detected only on intravaginal speculum examination.

Extragenital chancres may occur on any region of the body, but most commonly occur about the anus or mouth, in the axillae or rectum, and on the lips, tongue, tonsils, eyelids, breasts, umbilicus, fingers, and toes.[34] These may be single or multiple, and in the male homosexual, any anal lesion, even the smallest fissure or ulceration must be viewed with suspicion. Regional lymphadenopathy usually accompanies primary syphilis. This may be unilateral or bilateral and is characterized by discrete, non-suppurative, firm, freely movable painless nodes without overlying cutaneous change.

If left untreated, healing of the chancre generally occurs, and the lesion tends to disappear spontaneously after an interval of three to six weeks. The diagnosis of primary syphilis depends upon the clinical picture, identification of *Treponema pallidum* by darkfield microscopy of serum from the lesion or fluid from an aspirated lymph node, by immunofluorescent staining of *T. pallidum* in serum from the lesion, by blood serologic tests, or by findings on cutaneous biopsy.

After the appearance of the chancre, the fluorescent treponemal antibody absorption (FTA-ABS) test is usually the first to become positive, followed shortly by the reagin plasma rapid (RPR) circle test. Both are usually reactive in primary syphilis within a week or two after the appearance of the lesion. The venereal disease research laboratory (VDRL) test becomes reactive soon thereafter, and the *Treponema pallidum* hemagglutination (TPHA) and *Treponema pallidum* immobilization (TPI) tests generally become positive slightly later.[35]

Secondary Syphilis. Manifestations of secondary syphilis generally appear six to eight weeks (occasionally up to six months) after the appearance of the primary lesion and, in almost one-third of patients, the primary lesion is still present when the secondary eruption appears. The exanthem of secondary syphilis extends rapidly and it is usually pronounced a few days after onset. It may be evanescent, lasting only a few hours or days, or, at times, it may persist for a period of several months.

This stage is characterized by a generalized cutaneous eruption usually composed of brownish dull-red macules or papules (in dark skinned individuals the lesions tend to be hyperpigmented). Lesions vary in size from a few millimeters to a centimeter in diameter; they are generally discrete and symmetrically distributed, and, particularly over the trunk, they tend to follow the lines of cleavage, often suggesting a diagnosis of pityriasis rosea. Papular lesions over the palms which, because of the thickness of the stratum corneum, appear as macular or hyperkeratotic reddish-brown hyperpigmented lesions, are often of help in the differentiation of these two disorders (Fig. 10–17). Papular lesions occasionally spread peripherally with central clearing to form ringed or arciform papulosquamous eruptions. These so-called annular syphilids are commonly seen on the face of dark-skinned individuals (Fig. 10–18).

Of particular diagnostic significance is the presence of constitutional symptoms, namely gen-

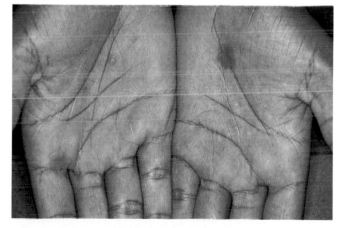

Figure 10-17 Secondary syphilis. Reddish-brown hyperpigmented macules on the palms (Department of Dermatology, Yale University School of Medicine).

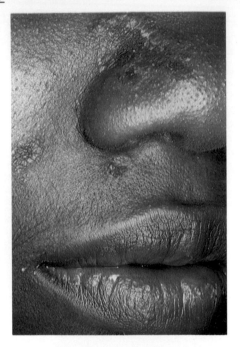

Figure 10–18 Arciform papulosquamous eruption (annular syphilids) as seen on the face of dark-skinned individuals with secondary syphilis (Department of Dermatology, Yale University School of Medicine).

eral tiredness, a grippe-like syndrome consisting of headaches that are characteristically worse at night, sore throat, nasal discharge, lacrimation, arthralgia, generalized lymphadenopathy, and an associated anemia, leukocytosis with relative lymphocytosis, an increased sedimentation rate, and, at times, elevated alkaline phosphatase (with little to no jaundice). Particularly significant is swelling of lymph nodes that are otherwise seldom swollen, namely those of the posterior triangle of the neck and the occipital, auricular, paramammary, axillary, and supratrochlear nodes.

Other features of secondary syphilis include a patchy "moth-eaten" type of alopecia and mucous membrane lesions (mucous patches) that appear as slightly raised grayish-white round or oval 5 to 10 mm plaques with central erosions and dull-red areolae. Mucous patches are painless, may occur on the buccal, labial, and lingual mucosae, the palate and tonsils, cervical and vaginal mucosae, labia minora, and the glans and corona of the penis. On the tongue the lesions are usually not eroded but appear as reddish flat papules with surfaces devoid of lingual papillae.[35]

Condylomata lata are cutaneous lesions of secondary syphilis that occur in moist areas of the body, the folds of the genitalia, gluteal cleft, and medial thighs. They are highly infectious and must be differentiated from venereal warts (condylomata acuminata) that occur around mucocutaneous junctions and intertriginous areas. Syphilitic condylomata lata are highly infectious. They appear as smooth, moist, grayish-pink 1 to 3 cm round or oval wide-based, often mushroom-like or lobulated, papules or nodules and, unlike condylomata acuminata, are never covered by digitate vegetations.

Cutaneous lesions of secondary syphilis usually heal without scarring, whether treated or not, within a period of two to ten weeks. Residual hyperpigmentation or hypopigmentation at sites of healed lesions may occur. Residual hypopigmentation on the skin of the neck has been termed "the necklace of Venus" (leukoderma colli).

The cutaneous manifestations of secondary syphilis must be differentiated from pityriasis rosea, drug eruption, lichen planus, acute exanthemata, tinea versicolor, sarcoidosis, infectious mononucleosis, scabies, Mucha-Habermann disease (pityriasis lichenoides), urticaria pigmentosa, leprosy, and psoriasis.

Treponema pallidum are present in large numbers in the cutaneous and mucous membrane lesions of secondary syphilis. Early diagnosis and treatment, accordingly, is important to prevent progression of the disease and infection of contacts.

Latent Syphilis. Latent syphilis is that stage of the disease during which there are no clinical signs or symptoms of the disease, or during which there are mild but generally unrecognized symptoms such as malaise, anorexia, headache, sore throat, arthralgia, and low-grade fever.[34] A diagnosis of latent syphilis is usually established on the basis of a positive serologic test after other stages of syphilis have been ruled out by physical and cerebrospinal fluid examination.

Late Tertiary Syphilis. Late syphilis is divided into benign tertiary syphilis (Gumma), neurosyphilis, and cardiovascular syphilis. It appears after a latent period of 3 to 12 years (often much longer) and is seen primarily in older individuals rather than children.

The cutaneous lesions of tertiary syphilis may appear as superficial nodules or deep granulomatous lesions that break down to form punched-out ulcers. Cutaneous nodular lesions can occur anywhere on the body but tend to favor the extensor surfaces of the arms, the face, and the back of the trunk. Characteristically they are asymptomatic and slow growing, and consist of rounded, red to flesh-colored nodules that tend to be grouped in a rounded or polycyclic arrangement. These lesions may ulcerate, producing noduloulcerative lesions, and after healing, hyperpigmentation and atrophic scars may persist. Ulcerative lesions appear primarily on the face, scalp, arms, and presternal region. They begin as painless subcutaneous tumors, which may be single or multiple, and as the lesions increase in size, they eventuate in dull-red lesions with punched-out ulcers.

Gummas may appear anywhere on the skin but most commonly appear on the scalp, the face (particularly the forehead, nose, and lips), the skin over the sternum, the thick portion of the calves, and the sternoclavicular joints. They usually develop at points of trauma, are almost always painless, and begin as soft cutaneous or subcutaneous swellings that tend to necrose at the center, forming one or more punched-out ulcers with a granulomatous base. When the hard or soft palate or nasal mucosa are affected, destruction is often pronounced and may lead to perforation of the affected areas. Large gummas may have several perforations and, as the intervening bridges of skin break down and necrose, lesions tend to produce arched or scalloped margins with arciform and geographic patterns.

DIAGNOSIS. The diagnosis of syphilis depends upon the history, clinical features, histopathologic findings, serologic studies, and in primary and secondary lesions, darkfield examination. The fundamental histopathologic change consists of a predominantly perivascular infiltrate composed of lymphocytes and many plasma cells, endarteritis, and endophlebitis. On special staining of primary lesions with Levaditi's stain, spirochetes can usually be found in the dermis and in and around the walls of capillaries and lymphatics. In secondary syphilis, the number of spirochetes varies with the type of lesions. In papular and condylomatous lesions they are almost always present in sufficient numbers to be found in the dermis and usually between epidermal cells. In macular lesions, spirochetes are few and generally cannot be found. In cutaneous lesions of tertiary syphilis, spirochetes may be demonstrated in early nodules or ulcerations, but usually cannot be found in older gummatous lesions.

TREATMENT. The treatment of choice for all forms of syphilis (except congenital syphilis or neurosyphilis) is benzathine penicillin, 2.4 million units (1.2 million units in each buttock) intramuscularly, repeated in one week for a total of 4.8 million units, or aqueous procaine penicillin G, 600,000 units by intramuscularly injection daily for eight days (for a total of 4.8 million units). For patients allergic to penicillin, erythromycin (2 gm daily for 15 days), tetracycline hydrochloride (2 gm daily for 15 days), or minocycline (200 mg daily for 12 to 15 days) may be prescribed. Because of potential side effects, erythromycin estolate should not be used for syphilitic infection in pregnant women and tetracycline should not be given to children under 12 years of age or pregnant women after the first trimester.

Patients with early syphilis and congenital syphilis should have repeat quantitative, nontreponemal tests three, six, and twelve months after treatment. Patients with syphilis of more than one year's duration should also have a serologic test 24 months after therapy has been completed.

Pregnant patients should be treated with 10 million units of aqueous penicillin intravenously daily for three days (if hospitalization is possible), or with 2.4 million units of benzathine penicillin G in addition to an equal dose of aqueous penicillin intramuscularly. Infants born to women who have been treated for syphilis should be treated at birth if maternal treatment was inadequate, indeterminate, consisted of agents other than penicillin, or if adequate followup of the infant cannot be assured (treatment of congenital syphilis is discussed in Chapter 2).[36]

Pinta

Pinta, a non-venereal treponemal infection caused by *Treponema carateum,* is seen almost exclusively among the colored population of Central and South America and Cuba. It is transmitted by direct contact and frequently is seen in children of parents afflicted with this disorder. Although transmission by insects is possible, this mode of exposure is considered to be exceedingly rare.

There are three basic forms of this disease, termed primary, secondary, and late. The primary stage, seen on uncovered areas such as the face, arms and legs, begins seven to ten days after inoculation as red papules, which, by proliferal extension, grow into oval or rounded erythematous squamous patches that measure up to 10 cm or more in diameter. Small papules frequently tend to become surrounded by satellite macules or papules that coalesce to form configurate patterns.

After a lapse of months or even years, secondary lesions appear. Clinically these lesions are hypochromic, pigmented, and erythematosquamous. In this secondary stage disseminated lesions appear. They, too, show proliferative enlargement, may coalesce, and are often covered with scales frequently suggesting a diagnosis of psoriasis, eczema, tinea corporis, syphilis, or leprosy. The lesions always retain their tendency to merge and eventually become hypochromic, thus leading to the third or late phase of this disorder.

The late phase takes two to five years to develop and is characterized by irregular pigmentation with a range of different shades according to the site of deposition of melanin in the dermis. The pigmentary changes present a spotted and highly characteristic appearance. These lesions have an insidious onset, usually during adolescence or young adulthood. After a period of years hyperpigmented lesions become more widespread and are replaced by depigmented spots resembling vitiligo. The hypopigmented patches of pinta are located chiefly on the face, waist, and areas close to bony protruberances such as elbows, knees, malleoli, wrists, and backs of hands. Hyperkeratosis frequently develops on the legs, forearms, elbows, knees, and ankles, and the skin becomes thick and often scaly. Atrophy is the final stage of this disorder and is generally localized in the vicinity of the large joints.

Histopathologic lesions of the primary form of pinta show migration of lymphocytes through an edematous and slightly acanthotic epidermis. The basal layer shows loss of melanin and liquefactive degeneration. Numerous melanophores are found in the upper dermis, and a moderately dense infiltrate of plasma cells, lymphocytes, and some histiocytes and neutrophils are seen in the dermis. On silver staining, the causative organism can be seen between the cells of the epidermis. In the secondary stage, lesions show essentially the same histopathologic changes, and in the tertiary stage the hyperpigmented areas show atrophy of the epidermis with absence of melanin in the basal layer; the dermis presents accumulations of melanophages intermingled with a moderate number of lymphocytes. Treponema are present in considerable numbers among the cells of the epidermis, and the depigmented lesions show atrophy of the epidermis, complete absence of melanin, no inflammatory infiltrate, and no treponemata.

Diagnosis of this disorder is made by isolation of the *treponema carateum* by darkfield examination and serologic testing. In the late dyschromic stage of pinta, strongly positive serology is present in almost all patients with this disorder. The disease runs a progressive course and penicillin (a single injection of 1.2 to 2.4 million units of benzathine penicillin G) remains the treatment of choice.

PROTOZOAL DISORDERS

Leishmaniasis

The term leishmaniasis refers to three different diseases caused by the protozoan parasite of the genus *Leishmania*: (1) cutaneous leishmaniasis (oriental sore, Delhi boil, Jericho sore) caused by *Leishmania tropica*, prevalent throughout tropical and subtropical zones of the world; (2) mucocutaneous (American) leishmaniasis, a somewhat similar disease caused by *L. braziliensis*; and (3) visceral leishmaniasis (Kala-azar), caused by *L. donovani*. This terminology represents an oversimplification of the conditions but is maintained for descriptive purposes. Primarily a parasite of wild and domestic animals, for which man is only an accidental host, it is transmitted by various species of the phlebotomus sandfly that harbor the flagellated form of the parasite in their gut.[37, 38]

Cutaneous leishmaniasis. As with so many other tropical disorders, increase in travel to endemic areas of South and Central America has led to an increase in the number of cases of cutaneous leishmaniasis diagnosed in the United States. In endemic regions, visceral leishmaniasis is seen in children more frequently than adults. The disease has an average incubation period of about two months, but this may vary from two weeks to more than a year and is seen primarily on an exposed area (generally the face). There are four clinically distinct forms of cutaneous leishmaniasis: a moist or rural type, a dry urban type, a tuberculoid type, and a lepromatoid type.

The moist or rural type first appears as a maculopapule that tends to enlarge slowly over a period of a few months to form a nodule, finally becomes ulcerated and crusted, and, after a period varying from several months to a year or longer, spontaneously resolves, leaving a depressed pigmented scar. The dry, urban, or later ulcerative form appears as a small brownish nodule, develops more slowly, and forms a slowly extending plaque 1 to 2 cm in diameter over a period of approximately six months. At this stage, a shallow ulceration appears in the center. It develops a closely adherent crust. Multiple secondary nodules may occur (much less frequently than in the moist form), and after a period of 8 to 12 months, the lesion begins to regress and the ulcer heals, leaving a scar. The average time from nodule to scar is about a year (twice that of the moist form).

Chronic lupoid leishmaniasis (leishmaniasis recidivans), the result of a peculiar host reaction, is manifested by red to yellowish-brown papules that appear in or close to a scar of an old lesion of cutaneous leishmaniasis, or in distant normal skin. Lesions coalesce to form a ring or plaque and spread peripherally on a common erythematous base, often resembling lupus vulgaris with apple-jelly nodules (the lupoid type). Leishmaniasis recidivans is exceedingly chronic and frequently reaches a considerable size.

A fourth, non-ulcerating generalized form, the lepromatoid type, is characterized by papillomatous nodules over the entire body. Lesions resembling lepromatous leprosy occur chiefly on the face and ears. Patients with this form of the disorder present a public health hazard, since the skin is heavily infested and may act as a reservoir for transmission by the Phlebotomus fly.

Mucocutaneous (American) Leishmaniasis. Mucocutaneous (American) leishmaniasis, due to *Leishmania braziliensis*, is an endemic and rural disease of damp forested country of Central and South America, generally seen in young men who work as foresters or tea or cocoa plantation workers. The disorder is characterized by fungating oral and nasopharyngeal lesions that develop along with nodules and ulcers resembling those of the cutaneous form. The disease differs from the cutaneous form by its predisposition to involve mucocutaneous lesions, as the result of spread of the original cutaneous lesion (the uta form) or as a particularly mutilating form that develops several months after healing of the primary site (the espundia form). Lesions may heal without treatment in a period of 6 to 15 months. Secondary infection with regional adenitis and lymphangitis is common, and in some cases, nodular and vegetative (rather than ulcerative) lesions may occur. Secondary mucous membrane lesions occasionally attack the nasal septum and nasopharynx. In this form the disorder may be characterized by erosions and necrotic ulcers, which if untreated, may erode soft tissue and cartilage, with resulting deformities of the nose, lips, and palate.

Visceral Leishmaniasis. Visceral leishmaniasis (Kala-azar, Dum-dum fever), caused by *L. donovani*, is endemic in Asia, along the Mediterranean coast, and in Africa and South America. In India the disease is transmitted from man to man; in some endemic areas of China, the Mediterranean countries, and Brazil, dogs represent an animal reservoir, their cutaneous lesions allowing the Phlebotomus fly direct access to the infected macrophages.

The diagnosis of leishmaniasis is based upon the demonstration of non-flagellated (amastigote) intrahistiocytic forms (Leishman-Donovan bodies) in the stained smears of material scraped or aspirated from cutaneous lesions, lymph nodes, bone marrow, spleen, spinal fluid, or in stained tissue, by the Leishman skin test, or by culture of the organism on Nicolle-Novy-MacNeal (NNM) media. The leishmania organisms appear as round or oval bodies 2 to 4 microns in diameter. Although visible in routine stains, they are best seen when stained with Giemsa, Wright, or Feulgen stain. They have no capsules, but within the body, there is a relatively large, peripherally placed round nucleus with a small rod-like paranucleus (the kinetoplast) at a tangent to the nucleus.

Delayed skin test reactions (the Montenegro or leishmanin intradermal test) becomes reactive three months after infection and is positive in 95 per cent of cases of cutaneous leishmaniasis. The test is performed with a suspension of leptomonad antigen, 0.1 to 0.2 ml injected intradermally and read 48 to 72 hours later. The reaction reaches its maximum at 48 hours, appears as a papule or nodule formation with an erythematous halo, and disappears in four to five days. Although the Montenegro antigen is not available commercially in the United States, it is available from Instituto Adolfo Lutz, São Paulo, Brazil and from Burroughs Wellcome, England.[39]

Tissue may be cultured at room temperature on Nicolle-Novy-MacNeal (NNM) media. In the fluorescent antibody test the patient's serum is layered on promastigote forms of *Leishmania* obtained from cultures on NNM media and counterstained with fluorescein-labeled antihuman gamma globulin. Unfortunately this test lacks sensitivity and gives a substantial number of false-negative results. Walton and associates recently described a new fluorescent antibody for South American leishmaniasis. In this test the antigen used is the amastigote form of *L. braziliensis* obtained by osmotic lysis of cultured monkey kidney cells infected with leishmania organisms. Since the amastigote form is the only one found in infected human tissue, it provides a more specific antigenic assay in serologic tests. This new fluorescent antibody test, however, is not as yet generally available in the United States.[39, 40]

Amphotericin B is a highly effective leishmanicidal agent, but its toxicity has limited its use to cases resistant to antimony compounds. Antimony sodium stibogluconate (Solustibosan, Pentostam) (10 mg/kg, with a maximum 600 mg) administered intramuscularly into the buttocks for periods of 6 to 10 days is effective for all forms of visceral leishmaniasis, and pyrimethamine is effective in cutaneous and mucocutaneous forms of the disorder. Reactions to pentavalent antimony compounds are not severe, as a rule. They include gastrointestinal disturbances, jaundice, albuminuria, weakness, dermatitis, cough, pneumonia, and ECG changes. Because of its limited demands, Pentostam, available in the United States only from the Parasitic Disease Drug Service, Center for Disease Control, is restricted by federal law to investigational use only.[40] Pentamides, particularly stilbamidine, have been employed for cases failing to respond to antimony compounds. Pyrimethamine, a folic acid antagonist available as Daraprim (Burroughs Wellcome), although not listed as an antileishmaniasis agent in the manufacturer's instructions, is effective in a dosage of 0.5 mg/kg for a period of two weeks, repeated, if necessary, after a one week rest period. When pyrimethamine is used in the treatment of young children, it is advisable to give supplements of folinic acid.

References

1. Marples RR: Bacterial infections. Fundamental cutaneous microbiology. In Moschella SL, Pillsbury DM, Hurley HJ Jr (Eds.): Dermatology, W. B. Saunders Co., Philadelphia, 1975, 482–491.

   Principles of cutaneous microbiology and infection.

2. Stewardson-Krieger PB, Esterly NB: Pyogenic infections. In Solomon LM, Esterly, NB, Loeffel ED.: Adolescent Dermatology. W. B. Saunders Co., Philadelphia, 1978, 163–183.

   A review of cutaneous bacterial infections in childhood.

3. Kligman AM, Leyden JJ, McGinley KJ: Bacteriology. J. Invest. Dermatol. 67:161–168, 1976.

   Microflora of the skin, their ecology and role in disease.

4. Wannamaker LW: Impetigo contagiosa. Progress in Dermatology 7:11–14, 1973. (Dermatology Foundation, Philadelphia).

   Two clinical forms of staphylococcal pyoderma have been described: a bullous impetigo associated with phage group II staphylococci that later form thin varnish-like crusts, (2) a thick-crusted variety that is vesicular in its early stages and yields either streptococci alone or a mixture of streptococci and staphylococci.

5. Ross S, Rodriquez W, Controni G, et al.: Staphylococcal susceptibility to penicillin G. The changing pattern among community strains. JAMA 229:1075–1077, 1974.

   Findings in a survey of 309 children under 10 years of age reveal a trend to increasing penicillin G resistance of community strains of S. aureus similar to that already observed among hospital strains.

6. Leyden JJ, Kligman AM: The case for topical antibiotics. Progress in Dermatology 7:11–14, 1973. (Dermatology Foundation, Philadelphia)

   Topical antibiotics are helpful in the therapy of superficial staphylococcal pyodermas. Although effective in the great majority of cases of streptococcal pyoderma, systemic antibiotics produce a swifter clinical response with fewer failures.

7. Wannamaker LW: Medical progress: Differences between streptococcal infections of the throat and skin. N. Engl. J. Med. 282:23–31, 78–85, 1970.

   The prevention of nephritis by penicillin preceding respiratory infection of streptococcal etiology is only partially successful; it is even more difficult and generally is unsuccessful in patients with streptococcal impetigo.

8. Anthony FB, Kaplan EL, Wannamaker LW, et al.: Attack

rates of acute nephritis after type 49 streptococcal infection of the skin and respiratory tract. J. Clin. Invest. *48*:1697–1704, 1969.

In study among children at the Red Lake Indian Reservation in Minnesota acute nephritis or unexplained hematuria developed in 28.8 per cent of children with type 49 streptococcal skin infection.

9. Lasch EE, Frankel V, Vardy PA, et al.: Epidemic glomerulonephritis in Israel. J. Infect. Dis. *124*:141–147, 1971.

Penicillin treatment of streptococcal pyoderma, given early and adequately, succeeded in eradicating most of the streptococci, but did not prevent the appearance of glomerulonephritis nor have any effect on the course and severity of the nephritic process.

10. Green M, Fousek MD: Hemophilus influenzae type b cellulitis. Pediatrics *19*:80–83, 1957.

Six cases of cellulitis due to *Hemophilus influenzae* type b suggest a characteristic picture of tender, dusky bluish-red discoloration in individuals with this disorder.

11. Thirumoorthi MC, Asmar BJ, Dajani AS: Violaceous discoloration in pneumococcal cellulitis. Pediatrics *62*:492–493, 1978.

Bluish-red discoloration also can occur with cellulitis due to organisms other than *H. influenzae*, and *H. influenzae* cellulitis may occur in the absence of violaceous discoloration of the involved skin.

12. Feigin RD: Meningococcal disease. In Gellis SS, Kagan BM (Eds.): Current Pediatric Therapy 8. W. B. Saunders Co., Philadelphia, 1978, 560–561.

A review of the management of meningococcemia and meningococcal meningitis in childhood.

13. Melish ME, Glasgow LA: The staphylococcal scalded skin syndrome — development of an experimental model. N. Engl. J. Med. *282*:1114–1119, 1970.

Seventeen children with exfoliative dermatitis associated with phage Group II staphylococci.

14. Melish ME, Glasgow LA: Staphylococcal scalded skin syndrome: the expanded clinical syndrome. J. Pediatr. *78*:958–967, 1971.

Twenty-eight patients with dermatologic disease associated with phage Group II staphylococcus (staphylococcal scalded skin syndrome).

15. Sarai Y, Nakahara, H, Ishikawa T, et al.: Bacteriological study on children with staphylococcal toxic epidermal necrolysis in Japan. Dermatologica *154*:161–167, 1977.

Bacteriologic study of 21 infants and children with typical staphylococcal toxic epidermal necrolysis revealed that exfoliatin production is not necessarily restricted to staphylococcal phage Group II.

16. Elias PM, Fritsch P, Epstein EH Jr: Staphylococcal scalded skin syndrome. Clinical features, pathogenesis, and recent microbial and biochemical developments. Arch. Dermatol. *113*:207–219, 1977.

A review article contrasting the essential clinical features of staphylococcal scalded skin syndrome (SSSS) and other forms of toxic epidermal necrolysis (TEN).

17. Berendes H, Bridges RA, Good RA: A fatal granulomatosis of childhood. Minn. Med. *40*:309–312, 1957.

The first definitive description of chronic granulomatous disease of childhood.

18. Bridges RA, Berendes H, Good RA: A fatal granulomatous disease of childhood — the clinical, pathological, and laboratory features of a new syndrome. AMA J. Dis. Child. *97*:387–408, 1959.

A description of four male children suffering from a previous unreported syndrome consisting of chronic suppurative lymphadenitis, hepatosplenomegaly, pulmonary infiltrations, and eczematoid dermatitis of characteristic distribution.

19. Windhorst DR, Good RA: Dermatologic manifestations of fatal granulomatous disease of childhood. Arch. Dermatol. *103*:351–357, 1971.

Cutaneous lesions, the first manifestation of chronic granulomatous disease of childhood, can lead to early recognition of this disorder.

20. Quie PG, Kaplan EL, Page AR, et al.: Defective polymorphonuclear-leukocyte function and chronic granulomatous disease in two female children. N. Engl. J. Med. *278*:976–980, 1968.

Although chronic granulomatous disease in males in X-lined, studies of leukocyte function in two girls demonstrate that defective bactericidal function and metabolic abnormalities of polymorphonuclear leukocytes associated with chronic granulomatous disease are not necessarily familial and are not limited to male patients with X-linked hereditary disease.

21. Holmes B, Park BH, Malawista SE, et al.: Chronic granulomatous disease in females — a deficiency of leukocyte glutathione peroxidase. N. Engl. J.Med. *283*:217–221, 1970.

Leukocyte glutathione peroxidase, necessary for optimal killing of bacteria presumably through production of hydrogen peroxide in females, distinguishes their disease from that of male patients with X-linked chronic granulomatous disease.

22. Johnstone RB Jr, Baehner RL: Chronic granulomatous disease: correlations between pathogenesis and clinical findings. Pediatrics *48*:730–737, 1971.

Simple screening tests can readily confirm a clinical diagnosis of chronic granulomatous disease, and prolonged therapy with specific antibiotics may suppress the frequency of serious infections.

23. Bannatyne RM, Skoworn PN, Weber JL: Job's syndrome: a variant of chronic granulomatous disease. J. Pediatr. *75*:236–242, 1969.

The occurrence of Job syndrome in two sisters, the absence of the disease or defect in either parent, and the demonstration of consaguinity between the parents strongly suggests an autosomal recessive basis in this disease of young, fair-skinned girls.

24. Hill HR, Quie PG, Pabst HF, et al.: Defect in neutrophil granulocyte chemotaxis in Job's syndrome of recurrent "cold" staphylococcal abscesses. Lancet *2*:617–619, 1974.

Studies of four girls with Job syndrome suggest that chemical mediators released by interaction of leukocytes, IgE, and specific antigen are responsible for the functional leukocyte dysfunction seen in this disorder.

25. Somerville, DA: Erythrasma in normal young adults. J. Med. Microbiol. *3*:57–64, 1970.

A diphtheroid organism that fluoresced when grown in tissue culture media was demonstrated in 42 per cent of students with erythrasma of the toe webs.

26. Munro-Ashman D, Wells RS, Clayton YM: Erythrasma in adolescence. Br. J. Dermatol. *75*:401–404, 1963.

Coral-red fluorescence was detected in 17 per cent and *Corynebacterium minitussimum* was cultured from 14 per cent of individuals during an epidemic of erythrasma at a boys' boarding school.

27. Freeman RG, McBride ME, Dunkin WC, et al.: Pathogenesis of trichomycosis axillaris. South. Med. J. *62*:78–80, 1969.

Studies in seven patients with trichomycosis axillaris suggest Corynebacterial infection of the hair cuticle (with rare involvement of the cortex or medulla) as the etiology of this disorder.

28. Loria PR: Minocycline hydrochloride treatment for atypical acid-fast infection. Arch. Dermatol. *112*:517–519, 1976.

Three patients with swimming pool granulomas with an excellent response to minocycline hydrochloride within a period of two weeks.

29. Fisher I, Orkin M: Primary tuberculosis of the skin. JAMA *195*:314–316, 1966.

A review of four childhood cases of primary inoculation type tuberculous chancre.

30. Nemir RL: Tuberculosis. In Gellis SS, Kagan BM (Eds.): Current Pediatric Therapy 8 W. B. Saunders Co., Philadelphia, 1978, 597–600.

Current recommendations of tuberculosis therapy in the pediatric age group.

31. Lauer BA, Lilla JA, Golitz LE: Experience and reason: Leprosy in a Vietnamese adoptee. Pediatr, *65*:335–337, 1980.

This report of a 10-year-old Vietnamese adoptee with lepromatous leprosy serves to remind us that leprosy is a common infection among Vietnamese and, because of its long incubation period, may not become manifest for several years.

32. Stewardson-Krieger PB, Esterly NB: Actinomyces infections. In Solomon LM, Esterly NB, Loeffel ED (Eds.): Adolescent Dermatology. W. B. Saunders Co., Philadelphia, 1978, 296–299.

A review of actinomycosis and nocardiosis, uncommon gram-positive fungus-like bacterial infections primarily seen in debilitated or immunodeficient individuals.

33. Beaman BL, Burnside J, Edwards B, et al.: Nocardial infections of the United States, 1972–1974. J. Inf. Diseases *134*:286–289, 1976.

A survey of members of the Infectious Diseases Society of America indicates that nocardial infections are not rare and that probably 500 to 1000 cases are recognized in the United States each year.

34. Rudolph AH, Olansky S: Syphillis In Demis DJ, Dobson RL, McGuire J: Clinical Dermatology, Vol. 3. Harper and Row, Hagerstown, Md. 1977, 16–22, 1–37.

A comprehensive review of syphilis, its pathogenesis, clinical manifestations, and treatment.

35. Tavs LE: Syphilis. In Solomon LM, Esterly NB, Loeffel ED (Eds.): Adolescent Dermatology. W. B. Saunders Co., Philadelphia, 1978, 222–256.

A review of the classification, manifestations, diagnosis, and management of syphilis, with emphasis on childhood and adolescent forms of the disorder.

36. Litt IF: Venereal disease, Syphilis. In Gellis SS, Kagan BM (Eds.): Current Pediatric Therapy 8, W. B. Saunders Co., Philadelphia, 1978, 707–708

The management of syphilis in childhood and adolescence.

37. Price, SM, Silvers, DN: New World Leishmaniasis. Serologic aides to diagnosis, Arch Dermatol *113*:1415 1410, 1977.

A case of cutaneous leishmaniasis in a 20-year-old college student from New York who developed the disorder while studying in Peru and the importance of the fluorescent antibody test as an aid to rapid diagnosis.

38. Moschella SL: Benign reticuloendothelial lesions. Leishmaniasis. In Moschella SL, Pillsbury DM, Hurley HJ Jr (Eds.): Dermatology, W. B. Saunders Co., Philadelphia, 1975, 801–808.

A comprehensive review of the various forms of leishmaniasis.

39. Moriarty PL, Pereira C: Letters to the editor. Diagnosis and prognosis of New World leishmaniasis. Arch. Dermatol. *114*:962–963, 1978.

Tips on serologic testing and therapy of leishmaniasis.

40. Koerber WA Jr, Koehn MC, Jacobs PH, et al.: Treatment of cutaneous leishmaniasis with antimony sodium gluconate. Arch. Dermatol. *114*:1226, 1978.

Successful treatment of a 45-year-old man with antimony sodium gluconate (Pentostam).

11

VIRAL DISEASES OF THE SKIN

Viruses are ultramicroscopic organisms that grow only within living cells. The antigenic material responsible for viral immunologic reactions is present in the outer protein membrane (capsid) of the virus. The nucleoprotein core is composed of either deoxyribonucleic acid (DNA) or ribonucleic acid (RNA), but not both. Lacking ribosomes, viruses depend on the use of the host cells' enzyme systems. Here they blend with metabolic material of the host cell and frequently remain undetected until some stimulus incites the production of new viral particles.

Viral infections of the skin vary in their morphologic appearance from inflammatory changes (macules, papules, vesicles, or pustules) to localized growths or tumors composed of virus-laden cells and their products (warts, molluscum contagiosum, milkers' nodules). The following discussion will describe the common cutaneous viral disorders of childhood (warts, herpes simplex, herpes zoster, molluscum contagiosum) and viral-like disorders of the oral mucosa.

HERPES SIMPLEX

Herpes simplex, one of the most common viral infections of man, is caused by *Herpesvirus hominus*, a relatively large (175 nm) DNA virus. There are two major antigenic types of *H. hominus*. Type 1 herpes simplex virus (HSV-1) has traditionally been associated with oral herpes

(herpes labialis) and other non-genital infections, and herpes simplex virus type 2 (HSV-2), with genital infection. However, oral type 2 and genital type 1 infections have become increasingly common, probably as a result of more liberal and orogenital sexual activity and promiscuity. Both type 1 and type 2 herpes simplex viruses produce primary and recurrent infections. Although infections due to type 1 and type 2 viruses are clinically indistinguishable, differentiation of the two types can be made by differences in growth in chick embryo cells, microneutralization tests, and immunofluorescent techniques.

Infections with herpesvirus are classified as primary or recurrent. Primary infections occur in exposed individuals without circulating antibodies. They may appear as subclinical or inapparent infections, characterized only by the development of antibodies to the virus, as a localized or generalized eruption, or as a serious systemic infection with encephalitis, hepatosplenomegaly, high fever, and, at times, serious sequelae.

Recurrent herpes simplex infection occurs only in individuals who have been previously infected, either clinically or subclinically. It is characterized by repeated infections manifested by repeated eruptions of vesicles on an erythematous base at or close to one particular affected site.[1] Cultures of herpes simplex virus in spinal ganglia of mice and humans suggest that the viruses are maintained in a quiescent state from which they

238

may be reactivated, thus producing overt disease.[2,3]

do not kill the herpetic virus, but they exert their effect by interference with viral synthesis of DNA.[4]

Herpetic Gingivostomatitis

The most common clinical presentation of primary herpesvirus type 1 infection is gingivostomatitis. It may occur at any age, but its peak incidence is in children between the ages of 1 and 5 years. The clinical presentation is frequently associated with fever, restlessness, irritability, and sudden high fever. Vesicles develop in the oral cavity and soon become eroded and ulcerated, white plaques appear in the mouth and pharynx, and the gingiva swell, redden, and bleed easily. Salivation may be present, there may be a foul odor to the breath, soreness and dysphagia may interfere with intake of food or fluids, and marked cervical lymphadenopathy is common. The fever generally subsides in three to five days, but the oral manifestations usually persist for ten days to two weeks.

Gingivostomatitis is often falsely diagnosed as Vincent's infection, hand-foot-and-mouth disease, aphthous stomatitis, erythema multiforme, or Behçet's disease. The diagnosis can be confirmed by the Tzanck test and viral cultures. Therapy consists of aspirin; lidocaine (Xylocaine 2 per cent viscous solution) to decrease pain and allow intake of fluids; avoidance of citruses or spiced foods; and, on occasion, intravenous fluids for individuals (generally infants or small children) who become dehydrated as a result of poor fluid intake.

Herpetic Keratoconjunctivitis

Primary herpetic infection of the eye often causes a severe purulent conjunctivitis characterized by edema, erythema, and vesicles, with opacity and superficial erosion or ulceration of the cornea. Marked pain, photophobia, lacrimation, and discharge from the eye is common, and the eyelids may be discolored or inflamed. Although uncomfortable and alarming in appearance, most cases of primary herpetic keratoconjunctivitis generally heal within a period of two weeks, without residual corneal damage. Occasionally, however, secondary infection and ulceration may persist and, in severe cases, may cause serious impairment of sight.

Herpetic keratoconjunctivitis should be treated by an ophthalmologist. Cortisone therapy, either topical or systemic, should be avoided, since it appears to facilitate increased dissemination of virus, with subsequent scarring and, in some cases, perforation. The treatment of herpetic keratoconjunctivitis has been facilitated by the use of 5-iodo-2'-deoxyuridine (IDU), available as Herplex Liquifilm ophthalmic solution or Stoxil ophthalmic solution or ointment, and by the use of adenine arabinoside (Ara-A), available as vidarabine (VIRA-A ophthalmic ointment). These agents

Herpetic Vulvovaginitis

In contrast to herpetic gingivostomatitis, acute herpetic vulvovaginitis is a relatively uncommon disorder. In young women and adolescent girls it is usually caused by herpes simplex virus type 2 (HSV-2) and is associated with sexual contact. It should be noted, however, that it may also occur with type 1 HSV infection[5] and in young children without sexual contact.

This disorder may be accompanied by fever, malaise, and regional lymphadenopathy and is characterized by burning vaginal pain, vesicles (often with a yellowish-gray membrane), superficial ulcerations and extensive erosions on the vaginal mucosa, erythema, and edema of the mons pubis, perineum, labia majora and minora, and vagina, accompanied by intense soft tissue edema and exquisite pain. The vesicles generally measure 2 to 4 mm in diameter, but with coalescence, they frequently result in the formation of larger ulcerations on the affected mucosal and cutaneous surfaces.

The treatment of herpetic vulvovaginitis is largely symptomatic and consists of warm nonmedicated sitz baths, topical anesthetics, topical antibacterial ointment to prevent secondary infection, and oral analgesics. The fever and constitutional symptoms subside within a period of five to seven days, lesions crust over and tend to resolve within a period of 10 to 14 days, and healing is generally complete within a period of two to four weeks.

Herpes Progenitalis

Although rare in young children, genital herpes has become extremely common in adolescents and young male adults. Usually but not necessarily associated with type 2 herpes simplex virus, herpes progenitalis in the male most commonly involves the penile shaft, and less frequently the glans, urethra, or scrotum, and is manifested by single or multiple painful vesicular eruptions that are transformed to painful shallow ulcers covered with exudate (Fig. 11–1). Urethral discharge is uncommon. When it occurs, it should suggest the possibility of another etiology, such as a gonococcal or chlamydial infection.

The severity of the disorder depends upon the individual's previous history. If it is a primary infection, systemic symptoms can be severe and the duration is close to two or three weeks; in recurrent infections the disorder usually runs its course in about eight days.

Treatment consists of topical analgesics, open wet compresses with Burow's solution or tap water, and topical antibiotics to help prevent secondary infection.

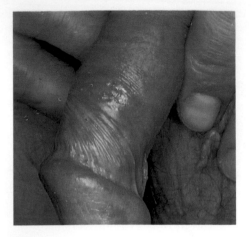

Figure 11–1 Herpes progenitalis. Multiple painful vesicles and ulcerations on the penile shaft, usually but not necessarily associated with herpes simplex type 2 infection.

Neonatal Herpes

Neonatal herpes usually develops when infants are born vaginally to mothers who have genital herpes. Like other herpetic infections this disease varies considerably in severity, with a wide spectrum of illness ranging from death or recovery with severe central nervous system involvement or ocular damage to a mild or asymptomatic infection with complete recovery (see Chapter 2, Figs. 2–13 and 2–14).

Neonatal herpes may be categorized as disseminated, local, or asymptomatic. Although the relative frequencies of the various forms are unknown, it is convenient to remember that about one-half of the infants with neonatal herpes have skin manifestations, and one-half of these, if untreated, either go on to die or suffer serious neurologic or ocular sequelae. Systemic iododeoxyuridine (IDU) and cytosine arabinoside (Ara-C), once recommended for treatment of disseminated and central nervous system herpes, are no longer recommended. Adenine arabinoside (Ara-A), however, enters the cerebrospinal fluid without toxicity and appears to be safe and beneficial if given early in the course of the disease (10 to 15 mg/kg daily) in a continuous 12 to 15 hour drip for 10 to 15 days.[6] (For further discussion of neonatal herpes, please see Chapter 2.)

Kaposi's Varicelliform Eruption

Kaposi's varicelliform eruption is generally seen as a form of herpes simplex infection in infants with atopic dermatitis but may also be seen in patients with Darier's disease. It is characterized by the sudden appearance of umbilicated vesicles distributed principally in the areas of the dermatitis (Chapter 3, Fig. 3–17). Treatment is symptomatic and requires maintenance of adequate hydration, control of fever, and prevention of bacterial superinfection. Lesions frequently resemble an extensive burn. Topical application of silver sulfadiazine is beneficial, and in patients with severe viral infection, systemic administration of adenine arabinoside (Ara-A) should be considered (see Chapter 3).

Primary Cutaneous Inoculation Herpes

Primary cutaneous inoculation herpes (herpetic whitlow) may be found anywhere on the cutaneous surface. Herpetic whitlow is a special type of cutaneous inoculation herpes. Seen primarily in physicians, dentists, dental hygienists, and nurses who work in the mouth or genital regions of patients with herpetic lesions, the virus is inoculated into the skin of one or more fingers, causing a superficial vesiculopustular or extremely painful deep vesicular eruption that forms a honey-combed, bullous, whitish-blue swelling (Fig. 11–2).[7, 8] The pain usually subsides in 10 days, but the disorder takes about three weeks to resolve.

Diagnosis is assisted by Tzanck test preparations of vesicular lesions and viral culture. Systemic antibiotics and surgical drainage are ineffective. Analgesics may be prescribed as needed. Drilling of the nail to relieve pressure followed by compresses helps reduce inflammation, and exposure to the air, topical applications of ether, Castellani's paint, and/or topical antibiotics may help prevent scarring, secondary bacterial infection, and loss of the overlying nail.

RECURRENT HERPES SIMPLEX

CLINICAL MANIFESTATIONS. Recurrent herpes simplex infection appears in previously infected individuals in whom the herpes virus remains latent. Upon reactivation, a recurrent infection ensues. Triggering mechanisms believed to be responsible for reactivation include febrile

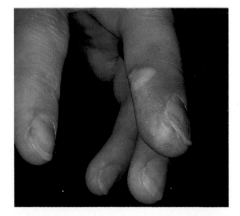

Figure 11–2 Primary cutaneous inoculation herpes (herpetic whitlow). A bullous swelling on the finger of a house staff physician acquired from a patient with herpes simplex infection.

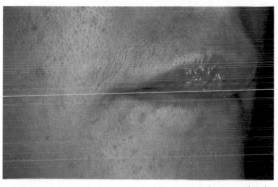

Figure 11-3 Herpes labialis. Recurrent herpes simplex infection with grouped vesicles on the upper lip. Generally caused by herpes simplex type 1 infection, this disorder usually follows an acute febrile illness or intense sun exposure.

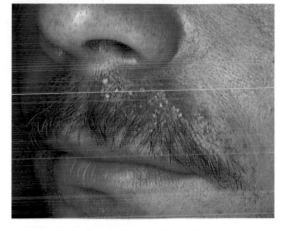

Figure 11-5 Herpes simplex. Grouped vesicles and vesicopustules on the mustache area. The period from the appearance of vesicles to complete healing generally lasts 8 to 10 days, occasionally longer.

illness, menstruation, emotional disturbances, gastrointestinal upset, sunburn, or local trauma. It is not clear where the virus resides during the latency period between attacks, but it appears to be the regional nerve ganglion. From here it is activated or triggered by any of the above factors and spreads distally to the skin.[2]

Recurrent infections differ from primary infections in the smaller size of vesicles, their close grouping, and the usual absence of constitutional symptoms. They occur most commonly on the lips, perioral region, cheeks, or chin, but may occur in any cutaneous area (Figs. 11-3 to 11-8). Grouped herpetic vesicles generally appear at or near previous areas of involvement. Following an initial period of itching, stinging, or burning (a few hours to two or three days prior to the eruption), the area becomes tender, swollen, and red, and soon thereafter several closely set thick-walled tense vesicles containing yellowish serous fluid appear.

The individual vesicles are small at their onset, do not coalesce, and overlie an erythematous base. They persist for varying short periods, ordinarily two or three days. The lesions then become purulent and form scabs that eventually fall off. Before the skin lesions appear, satellite lymph nodes may enlarge and become tender, remaining inflamed during the infection and regressing slowly after the lesions heal. An individual attack of recurrent herpes simplex may last for a period of four or five days (small lesions) or for as long as two, and sometimes three, weeks.

Recurrent Genital Herpes. The genital region is an increasingly common site for herpes simplex infection. Usually associated with herpesvirus type 2 infection, the changes in sexual mores and the concomitant increase in orogenital sexual exposures make herpes progenitalis a common venereally induced disorder, with an associated increase in the incidence of type I herpesvirus infection in this area. In males, lesions appear on the prepuce, glans, or sulcus, and occasionally on the shaft or in the urethra. Frequent sites in the

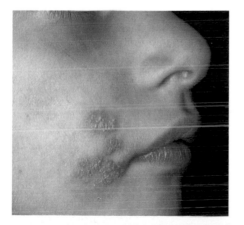

Figure 11-4 Recurrent herpes simplex infection. Grouped vesicular lesions appear on a tender red swollen area at or near previous areas of involvement.

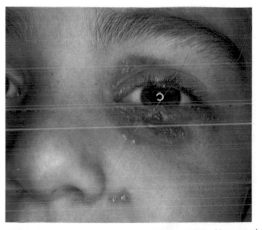

Figure 11-6 Herpes simplex of the eyelids. Herpes simplex infection around the eye requires search for the possibility of herpetic keratitis.

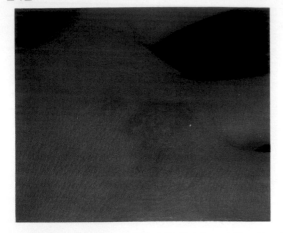

Figure 11–7 Recurrent herpes simplex on the skin of the dorsal aspect of the hand of a 2-year-old child.

female are the labia, vulva, clitoris, and cervix. The disorder is manifested by single or clustered vesicles which rupture, generally within a few days, to form erosions and ulcers. Lymphadenopathy, although uncommon, may also be present at times. Symptoms include pain, burning, and dysuria, and, occasionally, malaise, headache, and anorexia may accompany the cutaneous lesions. The infection runs its course in about eight days, and healing does not produce scarring (Fig. 11–1).

Recurrent Ocular Herpes. The most important type of recurrent herpes simplex is that which affects the eye. Presenting as a recurrent marginal keratitis or dendritic corneal ulcer, vesicles may be noted on the eyelids and palpebral conjunctivae as well as on the surrounding skin. Prevention of bacterial infection is of utmost importance, and broad-spectrum ophthalmic antibiotics are valuable in the management of this disorder. If keratitis is severe or if uveitis appears, tonometric examination is important, and mydriatic and anti-

inflammatory therapy, preferably under the management of an experienced ophthalmologist, is recommended.

Recurrent herpes simplex lesions must be differentiated from lesions of impetigo, herpes zoster, primary syphilitic chancre, and contact dermatitis. Although mixed viral and bacterial infections are not unusual, the history of itching or burning prior to the eruption and clear or straw-colored serous fluid-filled vesicles on an erythematous base is characteristic of recurrent herpetic infection.

DIAGNOSIS. When the true nature of the disorder is not apparent, rapid diagnosis can be confirmed by demonstration of multinucleated giant cells, balloon cells, and on rare occasion, intranuclear inclusions on a Giemsa-stained smear of the scraping of the base of vesicles (the Tzanck test) (see Fig. 2–15), by tissue culture of vesicular fluid or crusts, indirect fluorescent antibody studies using the fluid scraped from the base of the vesicles, and complement fixation or viral neutralization tests. It should be noted, however, that the cytological appearance of a scraping of herpes simplex cannot be differentiated from that of varicella, and that complement fixation and viral neutralizing antibody tests are not helpful in the diagnosis of recurrent herpes infections, since viral antibody titers are usually high at the time of the eruption. In order to distinguish between primary and recurrent infections, it is necessary to demonstrate a rising antibody titer in acute and convalescent sera.

The characteristic histopathologic features of a herpetic infection consist of an intradermal vesicle produced by degeneration of epidermal cells, marked acantholysis, reticular degeneration, ballooning degeneration, and, as in varicella and herpes zoster infection, inclusion bodies located within the nucleus. This is in contrast to lesions of variola in which the inclusion bodies lie predominantly in the cytoplasm.

TREATMENT. There is no single therapeutic modality that is fully effective in decreasing the duration or recurrence rate of cutaneous herpes simplex infection. The evidence that herpesvirus persists in nerve cells, specifically within the nuclei of the cells found in the sensory ganglia, should suggest the limited effectiveness of any topical approach to the treatment of herpesvirus infections of the skin.[9] Although agents that interfere with viral reproduction and the resulting damage to cells may possibly abort the infection and lead to somewhat more rapid healing, if used early in the course of recurrent cutaneous herpes infection, in controlled studies none of the currently recommended therapeutic regimens has proved to be consistently beneficial.

The key to management of recurrent herpetic infections of the skin appears to be early treatment. Once the virus has stopped spreading and no more tissue damage is occurring (usually within one or two days of the appearance of lesions), the goal is to aid the healing of damaged

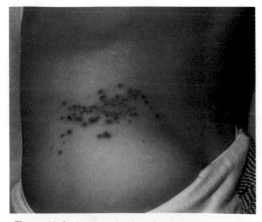

Figure 11–8 Herpes simplex simulating herpes zoster on the lateral aspect of the trunk of an immunosuppressed child with leukemia.

tissue and to prevent secondary bacterial infection.

When vesicles first appear, merely opening the lesions and treating them with any liquid preparation will result in the dilution of viral particles and help to shorten the course of infection. There is theoretical justification, therefore, for the use of 70 per cent alcohol or ether, which destroys the lipoprotein particles and renders them non-infectious.[9] Ethyl ether is a topical anesthetic agent and lipid solvent that dissolves the capsule of the herpesvirus particle. Although reports of clinical results are controversial, topical applications of ether with a cotton swab or moistened pledget until the skin blanches and local anesthesia is produced, three or four times a day to *early* recurrent lesions, has been recommended in an effort to obtain symptomatic relief and help decrease the duration of lesions.[9, 10] Possible reasons for the failure of either to change the clinical course or reduce virus titers in herpes lesions in careful double-blind placebo-controlled studies were the failure of ether to penetrate the infected cells and the fact that the ether may have penetrated the cells but had no effect on virus replication.[11, 12]

Thymol is also available as a topical anesthetic and antiviral agent that interferes with protein synthesis. Topical application of 4 per cent thymol in chloroform (also a lipid solvent capable of dissolving the herpesvirus capsule) twice daily at the earliest sign of a new lesion can also produce symptomatic relief and possibly decrease the duration of lesions. A light freeze with liquid nitrogen on a cotton applicator to a very early recurrent lesion may also help prevent further progression of the herpetic infection.

Ophthalmic preparations of 0.1 per cent 5-iodo-2'-deoxyuridine (idoxuridine, IDU) in solution or ointment base (Stoxil, Herplex, or Dendrid) and 3 per cent adenine arabinoside (VIRA-A, Ara-A), although beneficial in the treatment of herpetic keratoconjunctivitis, appear to be ineffective in recurrent disease such as herpes labialis, herpes genitalis, and herpetic whitlow. Photodynamic inactivation by exposure to a daylight-type fluorescent bulb of lesions treated with heterotricyclic dyes (proflavine, neutral red, methylene blue), appear to be effective against herpes simplex virus in vitro. Although initial trials in humans suggested that this method could enhance healing and decrease recurrence rates, recent studies also cast doubt on the efficacy of this mode of therapy.[13] Furthermore, although viral activity in vitro is destroyed, oncogenic capacity remains intact. Accordingly, until further long-term studies on the efficacy and safety of this form of therapy are completed, photodynamic inactivation is not recommended for the treatment of this disorder.[9]

Double-blind studies of repeated smallpox vaccinations for the management of recurrent herpes simplex infection indicate that repeated smallpox vaccination is not effective in the prevention or management of recurrent herpes simplex infection. Since this approach also appears to be potentially hazardous, it is not recommended in the management of this disorder.[14]

Since patients with recurrent herpes simplex infections have high circulating humoral antibody titers to herpesvirus, there is good reason to suspect that a herpesvirus vaccine might not prove effective in the therapy of recurrent diseases. Recent animal model evidence suggests that herpesvirus vaccines and circulating antiherpesvirus IgG may interact with the cell-mediated immune system and enhance resistance against herpes simplex infection. This approach, however, is controversial and remains in the investigational stage.[15]

Another recent recommendation for the management of cutaneous herpes simplex virus infections has been the oral administration of the amino acid L-lysine monohydrochloride (Lysine). A daily dose of 800 to 1000 mg during overt infection appears to be effective in the reduction of pain during acute infection, in the prevention of the development of new vesicles, and in a more rapid resolution of new lesions. Of further interest is the suggestion that a maintenance dose of 500 mg of Lysine given daily between infections may even prevent recurrences of this disorder.[16] Since arginine appears to encourage and lysine to antagonize herpesvirus replication and cytopathogenicity, nuts, seeds, and chocolate (foods high in arginine) are discouraged with this form of therapy. Although lysine treatment of cutaneous herpesvirus lesions at this time appears to have merit, carefully controlled double-blind studies are necessary before oral lysine can be accepted as an effective cure for cutaneous infection by herpes simplex virus.

Another encouraging form of therapy has been the recommendation of the use of acyclovir (9-[2-hydroxyethoxy) methyl]guanine), a new antiviral agent currently under study against a variety of herpesvirus infections. In addition to its apparent high selectivity for infected cells and low toxicity, although further studies are needed, acyclovir appears to be effective in the treatment of herpes simplex virus encephalitis and herpetic infection of the eye, skin, and mucous membranes.[17]

HERPES ZOSTER

Herpes zoster (shingles) is an acute vesiculobullous infection of the skin caused by chickenpox virus (herpesvirus varicellae), the same virus that produces chickenpox (Fig. 11-9).[18-20] The pathogenesis of herpes zoster is not well understood. It has been suggested (but not verified) that, after an initial varicella infection, the varicella-zoster (V-Z) virus remains dormant in cells of the dorsal root ganglia or cranial nerve ganglia, inapparent and non-replicating until reactivation and subsequent propagation of the virus along the nerve to the skin where infection of the dermis gives rise to the grouped vesicular erup-

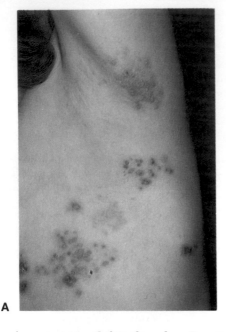

A

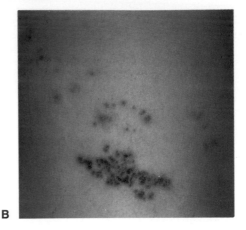

Figure 11–9   A and B. Herpes zoster. Typical segmental papulovesicular eruptions on an inflammatory base in an interrupted band with dermatomal distribution.

B

tion characteristic of this disorder. Reactivation, although not fully defined, may result from a re-exposure to varicella, physical trauma to the spinal column, x-ray therapy, immunosuppressant drugs, cancer, leukemia, or Hodgkin's disease. Acting as a trigger mechanism, any of these may release the virus from the dorsal root ganglia (a situation perhaps analogous to recurrent herpes simplex infection).

Although herpes zoster is chiefly a disease of adults, the disorder has been noted as early as the first week of life, presumably in infants born of a mother who contracted varicella during pregnancy.[20] It has been suggested that the infrequent occurrence of this disorder in infants and young children (Fig. 11–10)[18, 19, 20] might be due to the relatively low incidence of previous varicella (chickenpox) infection in this age group. Since 50 per cent of children have varicella by age five years and 80 to 90 per cent by fifteen years of age, a more likely hypothesis suggests that a long latent period is required after primary infection (a period during which various aspects of immunity pre-

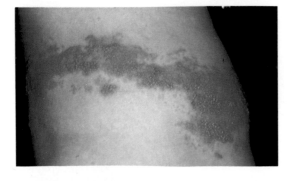

Figure 11–10   Herpes zoster on the trunk of a 7½-month-old infant following exposure to varicella (The infant's mother had chickenpox during the eighth month of pregnancy).

sumably decrease, thus allowing herpes zoster to develop on re-exposure to varicella virus).

CLINICAL MANIFESTATIONS.   Herpes zoster is characterized by a segmental papulovesicular eruption on an inflammatory base arranged in a continuous or interrupted band along the dermatomes of the skin supplied by the affected sensory nerves or extramedullary cranial nerves, usually with a degree of hyperesthesia, pain, and tenderness. The most frequently affected dermatomes are those innervated by the second dorsal to second lumbar nerves (C_2 to L_2) and the fifth and seventh cranial nerves.

Patients typically develop pain of variable severity in a dermatomal distribution four to five days (occasionally one to ten days) before the eruption appears. Herpes zoster generally tends to appear first at a point nearest the central nervous system and extends peripherally along the course of the nerve, thus producing its characteristic band-like distribution of lesions. Generally the eruption is unilateral but may cross the mid-line and, at times, may involve (to a lesser degree) the contralateral side. Successive crops continue to appear for a period of about seven days. They extend along the course of the nerve and eventually dry out and crust over in the course of another five to ten days. In 90 per cent of individuals under the age of 20 the disorder resolves in a period of 7 to 14 days. Occasionally, however, particularly in older individuals, the process may persist for a period of one to five weeks. During this time, mild constitutional symptoms, low grade fever, and/or regional lymphadenopathy may be present. It is not unusual to see a few randomly scattered vesicular lesions beyond the primary dermatomal involvement. Such scattered lesions do not constitute disseminated zoster.

Infection associated with the ophthalmic branch of the fifth (trigeminal) nerve may involve the cornea with keratitis and uveitis, and may lead to permanent damage. This disorder (zoster ophthalmicus) appears only when the nasociliary branch is involved and, accordingly, is present only in those individuals who manifest cutaneous involvement of the nose (an important clinical and prognostic sign).

Zoster of the maxillary division of the trigeminal nerve produces vesiculation of the palate, uvula, and tonsillar area (Fig. 11–11). Involvement of the mandibular division produces vesicular involvement of the anterior aspect of the tongue, floor of the mouth, lips, and buccal mucous membranes. Involvement of the geniculate ganglion produces lesions on the tongue, the ear, and the skin of the auditory canal. When accompanied by Bell's palsy and disturbances of hearing and equilibrium, it is part of the Ramsay-Hunt syndrome.

Herpes zoster in prepuberal children is usually a mild disease and it is unusual to see a prolonged course. Neuralgia, so common to adults (particularly those over 65 years of age), is unusual but occasionally may be seen in adolescents. Hematogenous dissemination of herpes with viremia and resulting spread of the eruption may occur in approximately 2 per cent of cases. Such patients initially present with the usual zosteriform eruption, which progresses, becomes generalized, and assumes a varicella-like distribution. The majority of patients with this complication have a serious underlying disease, usually a malignancy of the reticuloendothelial system. Generalized zoster is a serious disorder and occurs mainly in immunosuppressed individuals, patients with Hodgkin's disease, lymphoma, or leukemia, or those on immunosuppressive medications.[21]

DIAGNOSIS. The diagnosis of herpes zoster is based upon the presence of a painful unilateral, grouped vesicular eruption along the course of a sensory nerve. The Tzanck test may demonstrate multinuclear giant cells, and viral culture of vesicular fluid generally can confirm the clinical impression. The characteristic histologic picture is similar to that of herpes simplex and varicella.

MANAGEMENT. The management of herpes zoster is limited to symptomatic treatment and prevention of secondary infection. Uncomplicated cases may be treated with local applications of heat, open wet compresses, topical application of drying lotions such as calamine lotion (plain or with 1 per cent phenol), and ethyl chloride spray. When present, intractable pain and postherpetic neuralgia, seldom a problem in preadolescent children, can frequently be controlled with analgesics.

Patients with severe involvement or ophthalmic infection and individuals over 60 years of age (in the absence of contraindication) may be given systemic corticosteroids, preferably administered early in the course of the disorder. Administration of prednisone (or its equivalent), 40 to 60 mg daily for one week, 30 mg daily for one week, and then 15 mg daily for one week, frequently decreases the severity of the illness and, particularly in those over age 60, appears to decrease the incidence as well as the duration of postherpetic neuralgia.[22] Subcutaneous sublesional injection of 15 ml of triamcinolone acetonide and procaine has also been found to be helpful in the treatment of postherpetic neuralgia.[23]

Lesions of the tip of the nose indicate involvement of the nasociliary nerve and possible ocular involvement. In ophthalmic zoster ocular complications occur in about 50 per cent of cases. The conjunctiva is red and swollen, and superficial or deep keratitis may develop. Although fortunately relatively uncommon, uveitis, when it occurs, may be intense and prolonged and may produce keratitic precipitates, secondary glaucoma, and, in severe cases, permanent loss of vision. Patients with herpes zoster ophthalmicus, accordingly, should be referred to an ophthalmologist early in the course of the disease.

Patients with disseminated herpes zoster may be treated with adenine arabinoside (Ara-A), although this use is not listed in the manufacturer's official directive. Given early in the course of the disease, Ara-A, administered intravenously in a dosage of 10 to 20 mg/kg/day over a 12 hour period for one week, appears to be safe and effective for treatment of individuals with disseminated herpes zoster.[24] The use of hyperimmune convalescent zoster serum is of debatable value, and chemotherapy with idoxuridine is not effective. While the use of hyperimmune convalescent zoster serum or zoster immune globulin (ZIG) is probably of little use in therapy, it is effective and valuable (if given within 72 hours of exposure) for prevention or modification of varicella-zoster infections in immunocompromised individuals.[25]

VIRAL-LIKE DISORDERS OF THE ORAL MUCOSA

Aphthous Stomatitis

Recurrent aphthous stomatitis is a common disorder characterized by recurrent single or mul-

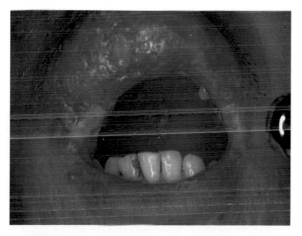

Figure 11–11 Herpes zoster with vesiculation of the lips and hard palate.

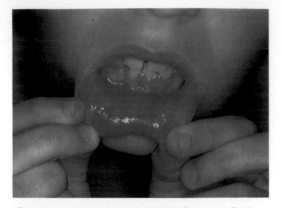

Figure 11–12 Aphthous stomatitis. Tiny superficial grayish-white erosions and ulcerations surrounded by sharp borders and narrow, slightly elevated, bright red areolae.

tiple ulcerations (canker sores) that appear on the inner cheeks, lips, gums, tongue, palate, and pharynx (Fig. 11–12). Previously believed to represent a manifestation of herpes simplex, attempts to isolate a virus have been uniformly unsuccessful, and recent investigations favor an autoimmune phenomenon as the basis of this disorder.[26] Aphthous stomatitis occurs in individuals of all ages but is relatively uncommon in children. Before puberty the sexes are affected equally; in adult life, however, the disorder appears somewhat more frequently in women, with a peak incidence during the third decade of life.

Prior to the clinical appearance of lesions the patient is frequently aware of their impending development by a tingling or stinging sensation. Twenty-four to 48 hours later a focal erythema develops, and soon thereafter tiny superficial grayish-white erosions appear. Usually one to three in number, the area of erosion increases in size and evolves into one or more sharply defined shallow ulcers covered by gray membranes and surrounded by sharp borders and narrow, slightly elevated, bright red areolae. Lesions measure 3 to 6 mm in diameter and, if left untreated, generally persist for a period of 8 to 12 days (sometimes longer) and heal without scarring.

Studies suggest that emotional stress, trauma, and hormonal changes such as menstruation appear to play an important role in the precipitation of attacks. Commonly, one to three ulcers develop at irregular intervals of weeks or months, and many patients are almost continually afflicted.

Aphthous stomatitis must be differentiated from herpetic stomatitis, Vincent's angina, candidiasis, traumatic ulcers, mucous patches of early syphilis, erythema multiforme, pemphigus, Behçet's syndrome, and Reiter's disease.

In general there is no one specific treatment for aphthous stomatitis. To date the most effective topical therapy appears to be the use of tetracycline suspension (250 mg/5cc), held in or swished around in the mouth for two minutes and then swallowed, four times a day for five to seven days, or application of a tetracycline compress of cotton soaked in a suspension of 250 mg of tetracycline in 30 ml of water placed directly on the ulcers for 20 minutes four to six times a day.[27, 28] Although the mechanism is not known, the presence of the L-form of *Streptococcus sanguis* in lesions may explain the apparent shortening of the course of aphthous stomatitis by tetracycline.

Other useful modalities include topical anesthetic agents such as lidocaine (Xylocaine 2 per cent viscous solution), and dyclonine hydrochloride (Dyclone), 0.5 per cent, swirled around the mouth for several minutes or applied directly to the lesions. Early lesions are frequently helped by topical applications of silver nitrate or by the topical use of triamcinolone acetonide (Kenalog, 0.1 per cent, in Orabase) applied four times daily to nonulcerated lesions, and large painful ulcers frequently respond dramatically to intralesional injections of 0.1 to 0.5 ml of triamcinolone acetonide (10 mg/cc) into the base of lesions.

Acute Necrotizing Gingivitis

Acute necrotizing gingivitis (trench mouth, Vincent's stomatitis, Vincent's angina) is a painful ulcerative disorder that chiefly affects adolescents and young adults. Although formerly common in schools and military establishments, the disorder, perhaps due to improved oral and dental care, is currently generally rare in the United States and western hemisphere.

The pathogenesis remains uncertain, but *Fusobacterium fusiforme* and *Borrelia vincentii* organisms usually predominate in smears from infected tissues. Clinical findings consist of painful gingivae that bleed easily and an inflamed oropharynx with eroded hemorrhagic appearance and ulcerations at both the gingival margins and interdental papillae. The ulcerations are covered by a grayish-white slough or pseudomembrane that can be removed, leaving a raw, bleeding surface. Single or multiple papillae may be involved, and the necrotizing ulceration can be very extensive. As a result of tissue necrosis and suppuration, there is bleeding of the gums, discomfort, and a characteristic fetid odor. Systemic involvement consists of varying degrees of malaise, lymphadenopathy, and fever, depending on the severity of the disease.

The clinical manifestations are characteristic, and diagnosis generally can be made on the basis of clinical evidence alone. Smears of the lesions usually reveal spirochetes, fusobacteria, cocci, vibrios, and filamentous organisms. Since these organisms can also be found in smears from normal mouths, such findings are not specific for the disease.

It must be emphasized that Vincent's stomatitis does not usually occur in healthy individuals with normal tissue resistance. The possibility of underlying systemic disease or other predisposing factors, therefore, must be considered.

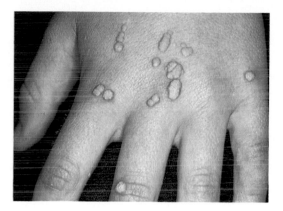

Figure 11–13 Multiple common warts (verrucae vulgaris) with Koebner phenomenon.

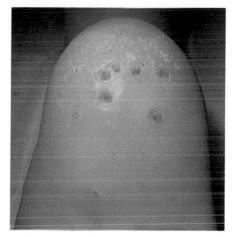

Figure 11–15 Plantar warts (verrucae plantaris) generally occur on weight-bearing areas of the heels, toes, and midtarsal areas.

The course of necrotizing gingivitis is indefinite, and the disease, if untreated, may progress into a serious and, at times, even potentially fatal complication referred to as *noma*. Extremely uncommon in the United States, this complication is seen in individuals with severe debilitating diseases such as terminal cancer, kala-azar, or kwashiorkor.

Treatment of Vincent's stomatitis consists of antibiotic therapy (penicillin, erythromycin, or tetracycline) for five to seven days, detection and relief of any underlying disorders, and the use of sodium perborate or 3 per cent hydrogen peroxide (diluted one-half to one-third with warm water) mouth washes, used every two to three hours. After the acute phase has passed, oral hygienic measures (brushing, flossing, scaling of the teeth, and removal of gingival irritants) are beneficial. Occasionally gingivectomy may be necessary to correct the deep ulcerations that may have developed between the teeth.

WARTS

Warts (verrucae) and molluscum contagiosum are common viral disorders of the skin caused by DNA viruses.

Warts are intra-epidermal tumors caused by infection with the papilloma virus of the papova group. The word "papova" is an acronym derived from the first two letters of the first three oncogenic viruses discovered, i.e.,: *pa*pilloma (wart), *po*lyoma (mouse tumors), and *va*cuolating (simian virus 40). There are four basic types of verrucae: verruca vulgaris, verruca plana, verruca plantaris, and condyloma acuminatum. Seen in 7 to 10 per cent of the population, they are among the most common skin disorders of childhood.[29] Although rarely a serious health problem, verrucae often are responsible for cosmetic problems to those who have them and therapeutic problems for those who attempt to treat them.

Seen in patients of all ages, warts generally occur during childhood and adolescence, with the highest incidence in individuals between 10 and 19 years of age. Their incubation period varies from one to six months, and although their course is totally unpredictable, the range of duration of

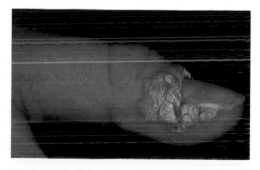

Figure 11–14 Periungual warts. Frequently seen on the fingers of cuticle pickers or nail biters.

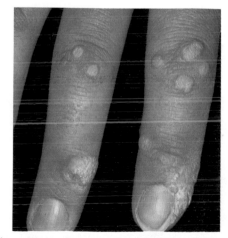

Figure 11–16 Common warts (verrucae vulgaris) on the dorsal aspect and periungual region of the fingers.

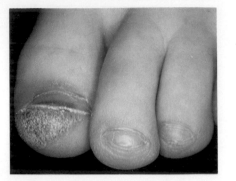

Figure 11-17 Subungual verruca with thrombosed capillaries.

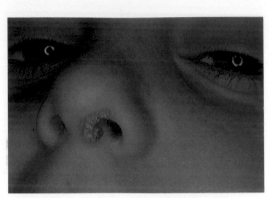

Figure 11-19 Multiple warts on the left nostril.

lesions varies from a few months to five years or more, with 25 per cent disappearing spontaneously within a period of three to six months and 65 per cent disappearing spontaneously within a period of two years.[29] Warts are inoculable from one location to another and from one person to another, through direct or indirect contact. Since local trauma promotes inoculation by the virus, most warts are seen on the fingers, hands, and elbows, along the perionychial folds (often in a linear configuration due to biting or picking of the involved areas), in areas of trauma (the Koebner phenomenon), or on the plantar surfaces of the feet (plantar warts) (Figs. 11–13, 11–14, 11–15).

Verrucae Vulgaris

Common warts (verrucae vulgaris) appear predominantly on the dorsal surface of the hands or periungual regions, but may be seen anywhere (Fig. 11–13). Occasionally they may also occur on the oral mucosa. They may vary from a solitary isolated lesion to vast numbers in any given individual. Early verrucae are usually round, discrete, flesh-colored, and pinpoint in size. With time, usually within a period of a few weeks to months, they grow to larger yellowish-tan, grayish-black or brown lesions that measure anywhere from sever-

al millimeters to a centimeter or more in diameter. Repeated irritation will often cause a wart to continue to enlarge and, with time, the surface generally takes on a roughened finely papillomatous (verruciform) surface.

Periungual warts and subungual verrucae occur around and beneath nail beds, particularly on the fingers of cuticle-pickers or nail biters (Figs. 11–14 and 11–16). These lesions, because of their location and susceptibility to trauma, frequently become irritated, infected, or tender, and are often more persistent and resistant to therapy. Satellite lesions often grow around warts, particularly those that have been irritated, manipulated, or incompletely or inadequately treated. When the diagnosis is in doubt, gentle paring with a 15-gauge scalpel blade will reveal characteristic minute black dots due to the presence of thrombosed capillaries that tend to bleed when the surface is removed (Fig. 11–17).

Digitate warts, commonly seen on the cheeks, chin, neck or scalp, are broad-based finger-like projections with a horny surface. They usually occur on the face and neck and are particularly common on the eyelids or about the ala nasi (Figs. 11–18 and 11–19). Filiform warts are seen as thread-like digitate projections with a narrow base and delicate cornified tips (Fig. 11–20). The trau-

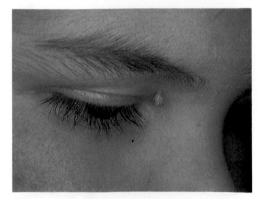

Figure 11-18 Digitate wart on medial aspect of upper eyelid.

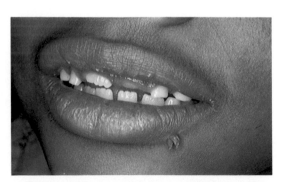

Figure 11-20 Digitate wart with bifid filiform tips.

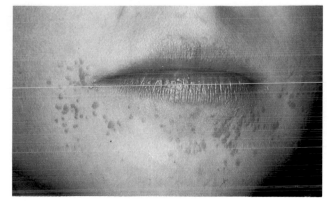

Figure 11-21 Verrucae plana (flat warts) on the chin of a 6-year-old girl.

ma of shaving plays a common role in the dissemination of filiform or digitate warts.

Verrucae Plana

Flat warts (verrucae plana) occur primarily on the face, neck, arms, and legs. They are usually seen as smooth, flesh-colored to slightly tan or brown, slightly elevated papules, 2 to 5 mm in diameter, with a round or polygonal base (Fig. 11-21). They vary from only two or three to several hundred in number in any given individual. In the bearded areas of men, and on the legs of women, irritation from shaving tends to spread flat warts in great numbers. Contiguous warts often coalesce to form firm papular plaque-like lesions. Again linear slightly elevated lesions in areas of scratch marks (the Koebner effect) are characteristic of this disorder (Fig. 11-22).

Verrucae Plantaris

Plantar warts (verrucae plantaris) occur on the plantar surface of the feet and are perhaps the most uncomfortable and therapeutically challenging form of this disorder. They generally occur on the weight-bearing areas of the heels, toes, and mid-metatarsal areas (Fig. 11-15). Pressed inward by walking, they frequently become deep, painful, and tender. Often there are several lesions on one foot. At times a cluster of small satellite warts, often pin-head in size with a grape-like vesicular appearance, may develop around a wart or group of warts. Thick keratotic plaques of closely grouped coalescent verrucae are termed mosaic warts (Fig. 11-23).

At times it may be difficult to differentiate plantar warts from corns, calluses, or scars (Fig. 11-24). Corns are localized hyperkeratoses that form over interphalangeal joints as the result of intermittent pressure and friction. Penetrating corns often appear at the base of the second or third metatarsal phalangeal joint. They can be distinguished from plantar warts by a lack of thrombosed capillaries, a characteristic hard semiopaque core, and by the fact that, in contrast to verrucae plantaris, they are more painful on direct rather than lateral pressure. *Soft corns* are macerated hyperkeratotic lesions that persist at points of friction and pressure in intertriginous areas. They are usually seen on the lateral aspect of the toes, or in the webs between the fourth and fifth toes.

Black heel ("talon noir") is a common condition frequently confused with plantar warts (Fig.

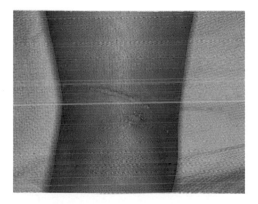

Figure 11-22 Verrucae with Koebner effect in the line of a scratch on the leg

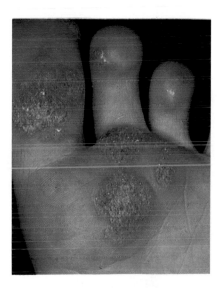

Figure 11-23 Mosaic plantar warts.

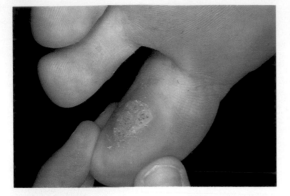

Figure 11–24   Verrucae on the medial aspect of the great toe. The presence of thrombosed capillaries helps differentiate them from soft corns.

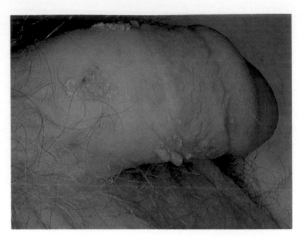

Figure 11–26   Condylomata acuminata (genital warts) on the penis shaft in a 16-year-old male.

11–25). In this disorder, papillary capillaries are ruptured by the shearing action associated with sudden stops in athletic individuals, usually tennis, handball, or basketball players.[30] Clinically this is characterized by clusters of brown or bluish-black pinpoint petechial hemorrhages in the horny layer along the back or side of the heels or lateral edges of the feet. Gentle paring of the surface of suspected lesions with a 15-gauge scalpel blade can help differentiate this condition from malignant melanoma, calluses, corns, scars, and plantar warts.

Condylomata Acuminata

Condylomata acuminata (genital warts) are fleshy verrucae that occur around mucocutaneous junctions and intertriginous areas (the glans penis, the mucosal surface of the female genitalia, and around the anus) as soft, flesh-colored, elongated, sometimes pedunculated or polypoid nodules (Figs. 11–26, 11–27, 11–28). In some patients, particularly young women, these lesions multiply and coalesce into large cauliflower-like masses (Figs. 11–29 and 11–30). Condylomata acuminata may be transmitted by sexual contact (the so-

called venereal warts) or may be associated with verrucae on other parts of the body. Condylomata acuminata must be differentiated from the moist wide-based 1 to 3 centimeter papular or nodular lesions of secondary syphilis (condylomata lata), which occur in the same regions. In rare instances, condylomata acuminata may attain considerable size, particularly on the penis of non-circumcised males. Known as giant condylomata acuminata of Buschke and Lowenstein, they frequently resemble squamous cell carcinomata (Fig. 11–31).

Common warts and plantar warts are characterized by sharply demarcated localized hyperplasia of the epidermis with marked acanthosis, papillomatosis, and hyperkeratosis with interspersed areas of parakeratosis. The rete ridges are elongated and at the periphery of individual verrucae are frequently bent inward so that they appear to point radially toward the center of the lesion. The characteristic feature that distinguishes verrucae vulgaris from other papillomas is the presence of large vacuolated cells in the upper stratum malpighii and granular layer. The dermal papillae are thin and elongated and contain blood vessels that project high into the wart itself. These vessels appear as punctate dark spots when thrombosed and bleed when the wart is pared down or traumatized. Verrucae plana show hyperkeratosis,

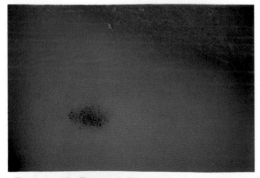

Figure 11–25   Talon noir (black heel). A common condition caused by rupture of papillary capillaries due to shearing action associated with sudden stops by tennis, handball, or basketball players.

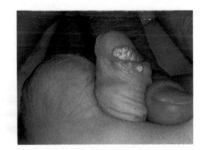

Figure 11–27   Verrucae of the glans penis and corona in an 8-month-old infant.

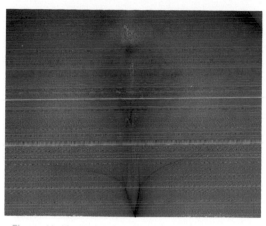

Figure 11-28 Perianal verrucae in a 9-year-old child.

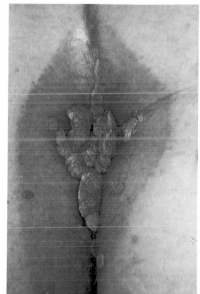

Figure 11-30 Condylomata acuminata of the perianal region.

acanthosis, and slight elongation of the rete ridges. In contrast to lesions of verrucae vulgaris, they have no papillomatosis and no areas of parakeratosis. The histologic picture of verrucae plantaris resembles that of verrucae vulgaris. The stratum corneum, however, is much thicker and frequently shows more extensive parakeratosis. In condyloma acuminatum the stratum corneum is only slightly thickened and is composed, as is usual on mucosal surfaces, of parakeratotic cells. The stratum malpighii shows papillomatosis, considerable acanthosis, and thickening and elongation of the rete ridges.[31]

TREATMENT. There is no single effective treatment for warts. They are capricious (unpredictable), occasionally highly resistant to therapy, and have a recurrence rate that varies from 5 to 10 per cent no matter what the therapeutic approach. Whether or not warts should be treated depends entirely upon the patient's and the patient's parents' desires. Only those with verrucae that are painful, spreading, enlarging, subject to trauma, or cosmetically objectionable need be treated. If treatment is to be given, the cardinal principle is

that it shall not be harmful. It should be emphasized that some modalities employed for the treatment of warts in adults are neither feasible nor desirable for the treatment of warts in children. The choice of therapy, therefore, depends upon the age and personality of the patient and the number, size, and location of the lesions. Whatever method the physician may select, he should be guided by conservatism if excessive trauma and scarring are to be avoided.[32]

To be effective, any treatment must remove the entire wart and eradicate all virus; otherwise, recurrences are common.[33] The simplest topical agents are keratolytic preparations. These include lactic acid and salicylic acid (in concentrations of 5, 10, or 16 per cent in flexible collodion). This can be applied to the surface of each wart, preferably at night (with a tooth-pick, not a cotton applicator

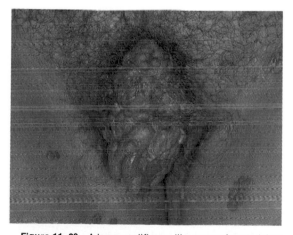

Figure 11-29 A large cauliflower-like mass of warts (giant condylomata acuminata).

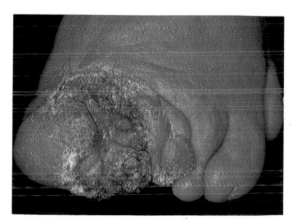

Figure 11-31 Giant verrucae (may at times resemble a squamous cell carcinoma).

or glass rod), and allowed to remain on for periods of up to 24 hours. The preparation then can be peeled off, preferably after soaking in water for a few minutes, and a fresh application is made. This procedure is usually followed for periods of three to four weeks. Care should be exercised, however, to insure that the adjacent normal tissues are not inadvertently treated, with resulting irritation. If irritation or discomfort occurs, two day intervals can be allowed between periods of application. This method can be used for flat warts (verrucae plana) if salicylic and lactic acids are kept at relatively low (5 per cent) concentrations.

Suggestion. The power of suggestion, or "charming of warts," is simple, non-traumatic, and in susceptible individuals (usually young children five to ten years of age) may cure warts within a few days, leaving no trace of the previous lesion. How this works is unknown; however, it may explain the multiple spontaneous cures attributed to various inert preparations such as cod liver oil, lime juice, bits of hamburger, potato, garlic, and so on). Although at times parents may wonder about the credibility of the physician prescribing such therapy, it is harmless, non-traumatic, and, when it works, can save many a child, parent, and physician from embarking on a long-term or more traumatic therapeutic approach. It is advisable to enlighten the parents to what the limits of the "power of suggestion" are, and to have an alternate therapeutic plan available for those patients for whom this simple, but unfortunately not always reliable, approach fails. Most of the innumerable folk remedies for warts depend upon the tendency of warts to spontaneously resolve and possibly the influence of suggestion.

An ointment containing ascorbic and pantothenic acids in a bland starch base, available as Vergo (Daywell Laboratories), is safe and reputedly effective for the treatment of some patients with verrucae vulgaris or plantaris.[34] Although I personally have not been impressed with the results of this preparation, the ease of administration and its cosmetic acceptibility make it a benign agent that can be attempted by physicians, perhaps for its "power of suggestion" if not its clinical effect.

Cantharidin. Cantharidin, a potent blistering agent, is the purified active ingredient of cantharides, the dried powdered blister beetle (Spanish fly). A 0.7 per cent solution of cantharidin in acetone and flexible collodion, available as Cantharone (Seres Laboratories), is easy to use and frequently effective, particularly in the management of periungual and plantar warts. At times it can be utilized for the treatment of other verrucae, particularly in children for whom other modalities may be painful, frightening, or traumatic. The disadvantage to the use of this agent, however, is the fact that occasionally a ring of satellite warts may develop at the periphery of the blister (Fig. 11–32).[35] Cantharidin is applied lightly with a toothpick, cotton-tipped applicator, or glass adaptor, allowed to dry, and occluded by a nonporous plastic tape and then by a strip of regular

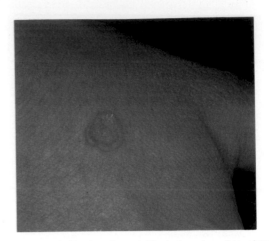

Figure 11–32 Annular satellite lesions in a "doughnut" formation following cantharidin treatment of a wart on the dorsal aspect of the hand.

adhesive tape. After a period of 24 to 48 hours, the adhesive is removed.

The cantharidin produces a blister which, in approximately ten days, dries and peels off, removing part of the wart and leaving no scar. Following gentle debridement of the remaining verrucous tissue, cantharidin may be reapplied at one to four week intervals until the wart completely disappears. Although most patients note little discomfort, some may experience tingling, itching, or burning within a few hours, and at times may become tender for several days. When there is discomfort within the first 24 to 48 hours of occlusion, relief may be obtained by removing the tape, puncturing a blister if present, and soaking the area with cool water for an hour or more.

Other methods of treatment include the topical application of formaldehyde (4 ml of 40 per cent formaldehyde in 15 gm of Aquaphor), once daily for three of four weeks or until the warts disappear, or saturated solution of trichloroacetic acid (or formalin in concentrations of 10 to 20 per cent) in combination with topical occlusion with 40 per cent salicylic acid plaster for a period of three to six weeks, or until the warts improve.[36]

Cryosurgery. Cryosurgery with liquid nitrogen (−196° C), although at times somewhat discomforting, is frequently a highly effective therapeutic approach to the treatment of individuals with multiple warts. A cotton-tipped applicator is dipped into the liquid nitrogen and applied to the lesion for periods varying from two or three to ten seconds for superficial lesions to longer periods for deeper lesions. The freezing induces blister formation just above the dermal-epidermal junction, thus removing the cells infected with the virus while leaving the basement membrane intact. Care must be employed, however, in order not to freeze the warts too vigorously, particularly on the first occasion in young children, as there is considerable variation in pain threshold and the resulting reaction. The lesion should be re-examined at two to four week intervals. Remaining warty tissue or debris can be gently pared, and liquid nitrogen can be reapplied at each visit until the wart is completely destroyed. Speed and the simplicity of this technique make this method particularly valuable, since little or no scarring occurs and local anesthesia is not required.

Cryosurgery may at times be uncomfortable, and some children will not accept this mode of therapy. Although liquid nitrogen may be used for the treatment of warts in all areas, it is particularly effective and well tolerated in the treatment of flat warts. If periungual lesions are treated, however, extreme discomfort may be produced.

One particularly undesirable complication, that of neuropathy, has been reported as the result of liquid nitrogen therapy over superficial nerves on the volar or lateral aspects of the proximal phalanges of the fingers and medial epicondyle of the humerus at the elbow, over the common peroneal nerve at the head of the fibula, and over the digital plantar nerves to the toes. In treatment of lesions on the dorsum of the hand, sliding the skin back and forth over the underlying fascia during treatment may minimize the freezing effects on nerves lying between the skin and fascia.[37]

An alternate use of cryosurgical technique is that of gentle curettage of the verrucous lesions while the area under treatment is numb and temporarily frozen to a semisolid state by topical application of liquid nitrogen. This modification of cryosurgery is easy, convenient, and frequently can be utilized without the use of local anesthetic injection.

Smallpox Vaccination. The use of smallpox vaccination has been suggested for the treatment of verrucae. Although direct inoculation of smallpox vaccine into the wart may provide a remission rate in 30 to 60 per cent of cases, the risk of a permanent scar at the site of treatment and the possible pain or severe systemic reaction or both make this method unsound. Smallpox vaccination, therefore, is *not* a recommended form of therapy in the management of verrucae.[38]

Podophyllum Resin. Podophyllum resin, often useful in the treatment of moist warts (condylomata acuminata) in concentrations of 20 to 25 per cent in tincture of benzoin, acts as a cytotoxic agent, arresting epidermal mitoses in metaphase, with cellular disruption of the hypoplastic tissue. In order to prevent excessive irritation, this preparation must be applied carefully (only to lesions, with care to avoid adjacent tissues) and must be washed off with soap and water within a period of four to six hours. Sitting in a tub bath with gentle washing of the treated area for a period of 20 to 30 minutes is a simple and effective measure for removal of the podophyllum preparation. Treatment may be repeated at weekly to monthly intervals, but failure of response after several treatments requires a change in therapy (possibly to liquid nitrogen or electrodesiccation and curettage).

When extensive verrucae are present at the perianal mucocutaneous junction, proctoscopic examination may reveal warts within the anal mucosa. These verrucae of the anal mucosae require treatment by a gastroenterologist if recurrences are to be avoided. It is important to note that podophyllum resin derivatives occasionally have been shown to produce toxic hematologic effects (leukopenia and thrombocytopenia) when administered orally. Therefore, the container must be clearly labeled, and when using large quantities on mucous membranes, the preparation should be used with extreme care and caution.[39]

X-ray. X-ray, although effective in the management of recalcitrant — particularly plantar — warts, is not recommended for use in children because of the possibility of injury to underlying epiphyseal centers and the fact that instances of annoying or serious sequelae may result from such therapy.

Surgical Excision. Since some surgical procedures may lead to scarring that can be more painful and ugly than the wart itself, the physician should be guided by conservatism in the therapeutic management of warts. Surgical excision is not recommended, since it is painful and produces a scar, with warts frequently tending to recur in the area of the scar.

Electrodesiccation and curettage, however, is highly effective and often the method of choice for individual large warts (especially in older children). Since warts are entirely epidermal, electrodesiccation should be neither extensive nor deep. The top of the lesion may be gently seared until the wart softens. It can then be curetted easily with gentle electrodesiccation of bleeders. Excessive coagulation of the base of the lesion is undesirable and may produce slow healing and undue scarring without better results or decrease in recurrence rate. This procedure should also be used with extreme caution on weight-bearing areas of the foot because of the possibility of painful and extensive scarring.

In summary, there is no single treatment for warts. All cases should be individually assessed, with the choice of therapy dependent upon the age and personality of the patient and the number, size, and location of lesions. Whatever method the physician selects, he should be guided by conservatism if excessive trauma (psychological as well as physical) is to be avoided.

MOLLUSCUM CONTAGIOSUM

Molluscum contagiosum is a viral disorder of the skin and mucous membranes characterized by discrete single or multiple flesh-colored dome-shaped umbilicated papules (Figs. 11–33 and 11–34). Seen most frequently in childhood, molluscum lesions may appear at any age. The greatest incidence of this disorder appears in children between the ages of 3 and 16; the youngest reported case is an infant with molluscum lesions noted during the first week of life.[40]

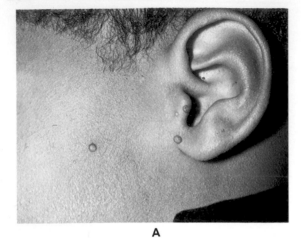

A

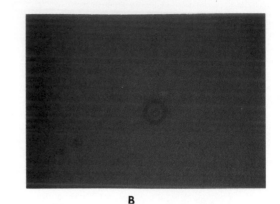

B

Figure 11–33   A and B. Molluscum contagiosum. Discrete flesh colored, semitranslucent dome-shaped papules with central umbilication.

Both contagious and auto-inoculable, in children lesions are generally located on the face, trunk, extremities (particularly in the axillae, antecubital, and crural regions), and sometimes on the mucous membranes of the lips, tongue, buccal mucosa, and conjunctiva. In adults, involvement of the pubic, genital, and perineal areas is common. The tendency for auto-inoculation is supported by the presence of linear lesions in areas that are scratched. The contagious nature is suggested by the presence of lesions in areas of direct human contact, as is seen in wrestlers and masseurs, and the predominant genital distribution noted in sexually active individuals.[41] An epidemiologic study in Alaska revealed that multiple cases in families can occur (but are unusual), that males are more susceptible than females of similar age, and that the duration of lesions may vary from two weeks to one and one-half years.[42]

The causative agent of molluscum contagiosum is a brick-shaped DNA virus of the pox virus group. Measuring 200 to 300 millimicrons in diameter, it shares, with the viruses of psittacosis and lymphogranuloma venereum, the distinction of

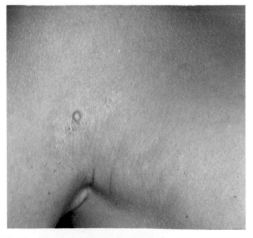

Figure 11–34   Molluscum contagiosum dermatitis. An umbilicated papule with a surrounding dermatitis. The inflammatory reaction may represent a delayed hypersensitivity reaction to the molluscum virus antigen.

being one of the largest viruses known to infect man. Although lesions are produced only rarely following experimental inoculations, most studies indicate incubation periods varying anywhere from 14 days to 6 months.[41] Recent reports of widespread lesions of molluscum contagiosum in individuals with atopic dermatitis and in patients receiving prednisone and methotrexate support a correlation between depressed cellular immunity and the use of immunosuppressive agents and increased susceptibility to viral disease.[43, 44]

CLINICAL MANIFESTATIONS.   Most lesions of molluscum contagiosum are asymptomatic. They begin as small pinpoint elevations of the skin and gradually or rapidly increase in size, generally reaching 2 to 5 mm in diameter. Larger lesions measuring 10 to 15 mm in diameter are occasionally seen, and a giant molluscum lesion may even reach a diameter of 2 or 3 cm.[41] Papules of molluscum contagiosum are initially firm, solid, and flesh-colored. With time they generally become soft and develop a waxy or pearly-gray semitranslucent quality with a centrally located dimpled umbilication and a pulpy curd-like core, which can be expressed with a comedo extractor or a small sterile needle (Fig. 11–33). In some individuals an area of dermatitis may surround the molluscum lesions (Fig. 11–34). This inflammatory reaction, seen in up to 10 per cent of affected persons, may represent a delayed hypersensitivity to molluscum virus antigen and may vary from a mild reaction extending 5 mm around a discrete lesion to 10 cm areas of active dermatitis.[45] In some patients a chronic conjunctivitis or superficial punctate keratitis may complicate lesions located on the conjunctiva or eyelid margin. In such cases the dermatitis and conjunctivitis clear spontaneously after the molluscum lesions are treated.[46]

DIAGNOSIS.   The diagnosis of molluscum contagiosum is usually easily established by the appearance of distinctive flesh-colored papules with central umbilication. When the diagnosis remains in doubt, confirmation may be achieved by direct microscopic examination of the curd-like material extracted from lesions and, when necessary, by histopathologic examination of individual papules or nodules. The histopathologic changes of molluscum contagiosum are highly characteristic and consist of lobular proliferation of epidermal cells into the dermis. Individual epithelial cells contain large intracytoplasmic inclusion bodies (the so-called molluscum bodies), which give a unique and highly diagnostic histologic appearance to the lesions.

The treatment of molluscum contagiosum depends upon the age of the patient and the size, number, and distribution of individual papules or nodules. Untreated lesions may involve spontaneously in a period of several months to years. However, because of the cosmetic appearance and occasional explosive nature of the disorder some form of treatment is generally indicated.

TREATMENT. Treatment generally depends on minor destructive techniques and should produce as little scarring or discomfort as possible. It is important to inform the parent or patient at the first visit that, no matter which method is utilized, new lesions of microscopic size may be incubating and may possibly evolve within a period of several weeks. The easiest form of therapy is a light two to three second application of liquid nitrogen to each individual papule or nodule. This method, relatively painless and non-scarring, generally results in resolution of most lesions with two or three applications at intervals of two to four weeks.

Other methods include removal of individual lesions by gentle curettage (with or without cryosurgery) or piercing of each papule or nodule with a small needle and expression of the plug under aseptic technique; by light electrodesiccation; by touching the base of each lesion with silver nitrate, 7 to 9 per cent iodine, 1 per cent phenol, or 30 to 50 per cent trichloroacetic acid; or by the application of 0.7 per cent cantharidin (Cantharone, Seres Laboratories) alone or followed by occlusion with a waterproof tape such as Blenderm for periods of up to 6 to 10 hours. The latter method, although easily and painlessly done in the office, may create a severe inflammatory reaction and, at times, a painful blister several hours later. Lesions on the eyelids and conjunctivae are probably best removed by light applications of liquid nitrogen or gentle curettage under local anesthesia. No matter which method of therapy is utilized, since the disease is transmissible by autoinoculation, care must be taken to insure that all molluscum lesions are destroyed.

References

1. Nahmias AJ, Roisman B: Infection with herpes simplex viruses 1 and 2. N. Engl. J. Med. 289:667–674, 719–725, 781–789, 1973.

   A comprehensive review of herpes simplex virus and associated infections.

2. Stevens JG, Cook ML: Latent herpes simplex in ganglia of mice. Science 173:843–845, 1971.

   Cultures of herpesvirus obtained from spinal ganglia of mice suggest that these viruses are maintained in a "quiescent" state from which they may be reactivated, thus producing overt disease.

3. Baringer JR: Recovery of herpes simplex virus from human sacral ganglions. N. Engl. J. Med. 291:828–830, 1974

   Viral cultures of S3 and S4 ganglions of 4 patients suggest that virus residing in sacral sensory ganglions may serve as a source for recurrent genital infection.

4. Leopold IH: Clinical experience with nucleosides in herpes simplex eye infections in man and animals. Ann. N.Y. Acad. Sci. 130:181–191, 1965.

   Iododeoxyuridine (IDU) is shown to be effective in the management of eye infections due to herpes simplex virus.

5. Smith IW, Peutherer JF, Robinson DHD: Characterization of genital strains of herpesvirus hominis. Br. J. Ven. Dis. 49:385–390, 1973.

   Isolates of genital strains of herpes simplex virus from 65 patients with genital herpes revealed 11 individuals with type 1 and 54 with type 2 herpes simplex virus infection.

6. Chi'en LT, Whitley RJ, Nahmias AJ, et al.: Antiviral chemotherapy and neonatal herpes simplex virus infection; a pilot study — experience with adenine arabinoside (ARA-A). Pediatrics 55:678–685, 1975.

   Studies of Ara-A in the treatment of 13 infants with neonatal herpes simplex virus infection.

7. Haburchak DR: Recurrent herpetic whitlow due to herpes simplex virus type 2. Arch. Intern. Med. 138:1418–1419, 1978.

   A case of herpetic whitlow attributed to transmission from genital herpesvirus infection.

8. Kanaar P: Primary herpes simplex infection of fingers in nurses. Dermatologica 134:346–350, 1967.

   An occupational hazard seen in individuals who work in patients' mouths.

9. Jarratt M: Herpes simplex. In Conn HF: Current Therapy 1978. W. B. Saunders Co., Philadelphia, 1978, 613–616.

   A current review on the management of herpes simplex infection.

10. Sabin AB: Misery of recurrent herpes: what to do? N. Engl. J. Med. 293:986–988, 1975.

    Topical application of ethyl ether is recommended as a mode of therapy for recurrent herpes simplex infection. (It should be noted that subsequent studies failed to substantiate the value of this approach.)

11. Corey L, Reeves WC, Chiang WT, et al.: Ineffectiveness of topical ether for treatment of genital herpes simplex virus infection. N. Engl. J. Med. 299:237–239, 1978.

    In 17 ether-treated and 18 control patients with genital infections due to herpes simplex virus, topical ether therapy did not reduce the duration of primary or recurrent genital herpes and did not prevent or delay recurrent episodes.

12. Guinan ME, MacCalman J, Kern ER, et al.: Topical ether and herpes labialis. JAMA 243:1059–1061, 1980.

    In a double-blind, placebo-controlled study of 51 patients with recurrent herpes simplex labialis there was no noteworthy difference between groups given ether or placebo in progression of lesions, healing time, duration or intensity of pain, and duration or quantity of virus excretion.

13. Myers MG, Oxman MN, Clark JE, et al.: Failure of neutral red photodynamic inactivation in recurrent herpes simplex virus infections. N. Engl. J. Med. 293:945–949, 1975.

    In a study of 170 episodes of recurrent herpes simplex virus infection, those treated with attempted photodynamic inactivation with neutral red and light did not show a significant difference in duration of discomfort, time to crusting, or healing.

14. Neff JM, Lane JM: Vaccinia necrosum following smallpox vaccination for chronic herpetic ulcers. JAMA 213:123–125, 1970.

Smallpox vaccination, a futile and potentially hazardous form of therapy for recurrent herpes simplex infection.

15. Jarisch R, Sandor I: The MIF determination for treatment control of recurrent herpes simplex: treatment with levamisole, BCG, urushiol and herpes antigen vaccine. Arch. Dermatol. Res. 258:151–159, 1977.

Studies in 30 patients with recurrent herpes simplex and six controls suggest a therapeutic effect in patients treated with levamisole and with herpes antigen.

16. Griffith RS, Norins AL, Kagan C: Multicentered study of lysine therapy in herpes simplex infection. Dermatologica 156:257–267, 1978.

In a study of 45 patients with frequently recurring herpes infection, L-lysine monohydrochloride in a daily dose of 800 to 1000 mg during overt infection appeared to relieve pain, prevent appearance of new vesicles, and hasten resolution of lesions. Of further significance was an apparent prevention of recurrences by a maintenance dose of 500 gm or more daily.

17. Gunby P: Medical News. New anti-herpes virus drug being tested. JAMA 243:1315, 1980.

Acyclovir, a new antiviral agent currently under investigation, appears to be an attractive candidate for the treatment of a variety of herpetic infections.

18. Winkelman RK, Perry HO: Herpes zoster in children. JAMA 171:876–880, 1959.

Seven cases of herpes zoster in seven children seven months to five years of age.

19. Brunnell PA, Miller LH, Lovejoy F: Zoster in children. Am. J. Dis. Child. 115:432–437, 1968.

Fifteen infants and children, ages 3 1/2 months to 14 years, with herpes zoster.

20. Feldman GV: Herpes zoster neonatorum. Arch. Dis. Child. 27:126–127, 1952.

A case of herpes zoster in one of a pair of four-day-old twins.

21. Keiden SE, Mainwaring D: Association of herpes zoster with leukemia and lymphoma in children. Clin. Pediatr. 4:13–17, 1965.

Five children, two with Hodgkin's disease and three with acute leukemia, with herpes zoster.

22. Ashton H., Beveridge CW, Stevenson CJ: Management of herpes zoster. Br. J. Derm. 81:874–876, 1976.

Systemic corticosteroids in disseminated herpes zoster and post-zoster neuralgia.

23. Epstein E: Treatment of herpes zoster and post zoster neuralgia by sublesional injection of triamcinolone and procaine. Acta Dermatovener. 50:69–73, 1970.

The subcutaneous sublesional injection of triamcinolone-procaine solution appears to help control post-herpetic pain.

24. Whitley RJ, Chi'en LT, Dolin R, et al.: Adenine arabinoside therapy of herpes zoster in the immunosuppressed. N. Engl. J. Med. 294:1193–1199, 1976.

Adenine arabinoside given intravenously in a dose of 10 mg/kg over a period of 12 hours daily is effective in the treatment of immunosuppressed patients with herpes zoster when given in the first six days of disease.

25. Groth KE, McCullough J, Marker SC, et al.: Evaluation of zoster immune plasma. Treatment of cutaneous disseminated zoster in immunocompromised patients. JAMA 239:1877–1879, 1978.

Since zoster immune plasma (ZIP) did not alter the clinical course of zoster, and because zoster patients produced high antibody titers without ZIP, it is suggested that ZIP is not useful for the treatment of cutaneous disseminated zoster and should be reserved for the prevention or modification of varicella in exposed susceptible immunocompromised patients.

26. Driscoll EJ, Ship II, Baron S, et al.: Chronic aphthous stomatitis, herpes labialis and related conditions: combined staff metting of the National Institutes of Health. Ann. Intern. Med. 50:1475–1496, 1959.

Viral and immunologic studies of recurrent aphthous stomatitis fail to demonstrate herpes virus in the etiology of this disorder.

27. Rostas A, McLean DI, Wilkinson RD: Management of recurrent aphthous stomatitis. A review. Cutis 22:183–189, 1978.

A review of various therapeutic approaches to the problem of recurrent aphthous stomatitis.

28. Shelly WB: Aphthous stomatitis. In Consultations in Dermatology II. W.B. Saunders Co, Philadelphia, 1974, 190–195.

The problem of aphthous stomatitis as manifested by a 26-year-old woman who had repeated attacks of painful ulcers in the buccal mucosa, tongue, and palataine arch and lost 25 pounds over a period of two months because of her inability to eat solid food.

29. Massing AM, Epstein WL: Natural history of warts. A two year study. Arch. Dermatol. 87:301–310, 1963.

Observations on 1000 institutionalized children revealed that two-thirds of their warts resolved spontaneously within a period of two years.

30. Crissey JT, Peachey JC: Calcaneal petechiae. Arch. Dermatol. 83:501, 1961.

The pigment in "talon noir" (black heel) appears to be hemoglobin that has extravasated from capillaries on the sides and back of the heels and edge of the foot of athletes due to the shearing effect of sudden stopping on hard surfaces.

31. Lever WF: Verruca. In Histopathology of the Skin, 4th ed. J. P. Lippincott Co., Philadelphia, 1967, 375–382.

A review of the histopathology of verrucae.

32. Perlman HH: The innocent wart. Clin. Pediatr. 2:238–246, 1963.

Whatever method the attending physician may select for the removal of warts, conservatism should be the watchword if excessive scarring is to be avoided.

33. Shelley WB: Warts. In Consultations in Dermatology with Walter B. Shelley. W. B. Saunders Co., Philadelphia, 1972, 8–13.

In the management of warts, treatment is successful only if the total virus-containing wart tumor is removed or destroyed.

34. Linn E: Conservative management of warts. Clin. Med. 74:39–42, 1967.

Since untreated warts may undergo spontaneous resolution alone or by suggestion therapy, results associated with the use of an ointment containing ascorbic and pantothenic acid are difficult to assess.

35. Epstein WL, Kligman AM: Treatment of warts with cantharidin. Arch. Dermatol. 77:508–511, 1958.

Although cantharidin appears to be beneficial in the treatment of warts, patients should be forewarned of the possibility of recurrences in the surrounding blister margin.

36. Tromovitch, TA, Kay, DM: Plantar warts: treatment with formalin and salicylic acid occlusion. Cutis 12:87–88, 1973.

A 94 per cent cure rate in 18 of 19 patients with plantar warts by formalin, salicylic acid plaster, and plastic tape occlusion.

37. Nix TE: Liquid-nitrogen neuropathy. Arch. Dermatol. 92:185–187, 1965.

In an effort to minimize the possibility of neuropathy, caution should be exercised in the use of liquid nitrogen on those sites where nerves are known to lie close to the skin surface.

38. Committee on Cutaneous Health and Cosmetics: Treatment of verrucae with smallpox vaccine. JAMA 206:117, 1968.

Even if vaccinia-induced inflammatory reactions may cause the resolution of verrucae, potential serious side effects associated with smallpox inoculation of warts makes this a medically unsound method of therapy.

39. Perez-Figaredo RA, Baden HP: The pharmacology of podophyllum. Prog. Dermatol. *10*:1–4, 1976.

Podophyllum resin, the most frequently used drug in the treatment of genital warts, is cytotoxic and when used over large areas or in children, should be used with appropriate precautions.

40. Mandel MJ, Lewis RJ: Molluscum cantagiosum of the newborn. Br. J. Derm. *84*:370–372, 1970.

Molluscum contagiosum lesions noted during the first week of life.

41. Lynch PJ, Minkin W: Molluscum contagiosum of the adult. Probably venereal transmission. Arch. Dermatol. *98*:141–143, 1969.

Lesions of molluscum contagiosum confined to the genital areas and inner thighs in fifty-five adult patients suggest a venereal transmission of the disorder in this group of military personnel.

42. Overfield TM, Brody JA: An epidemiologic study of molluscum contagiosum in Anchorage, Alaska. J. Pediatr. *69*: 640–642, 1966.

Proximity as a factor in 9 of 13 children (ages 10 months to 13 years) with molluscum contagiosum.

43. Paul CR, Artis WM, Jones HE: Atopic dermatitis, impaired cellular immunity and molluscum contagiosum. Arch. Dermatol. *114*:391–393, 1978.

Patients with atopic dermatitis may have a functional defect or defects in cell-mediated immunity that may impair host defense and predispose to increased susceptibility to molluscum contagiosum.

44. Rosenberg EW, Yusk JW: Molluscum contagiosum, eruption following treatment with prednisone and methotrexate. Arch. Dermatol. *101*:439–441, 1970

Two patients under therapy with prednisone and methotrexate developed florid eruptions with hundreds of molluscum contagiosum lesions.

45. DeOrea GA, Johnson HH Jr, Binkley GW: An eczematous reaction associated with molluscum contagiosum. Arch. Dermatol. *74*:344–348, 1956.

Patchy eczematoid eruptions around lesions of molluscum contagiosum.

46. Kipping HF: Letters to the editor. Molluscum dermatitis. Arch. Dermatol. *103*:106–107, 1971.

In 200 consecutive cases of molluscum contagiosum, 19 patients were observed to have a surrounding inflammatory dermatitis, which cleared after the molluscum lesions were treated.

12

THE EXANTHEMATOUS DISEASES OF CHILDHOOD

Varicella (Chickenpox)
Rubeola (Measles)
Scarlet Fever
Rubella (German Measles)
"Dukes' Disease"
Erythema Infectiosum
Roseola Infantum
Exanthems Due to Enteroviruses
    Coxsackie
    ECHO
    Reovirus
Exanthems Associated with *Mycoplasma pneumoniae*
Smallpox
Infectious Mononucleosis
The Rickettsial Diseases

Many viral and bacterial illnesses are accompanied by generalized erythematous eruptions called exanthems. These rashes, composed of macules, papules, vesicles, pustules, or petechiae, may be produced by many microorganisms. The classic exanthems of childhood include chickenpox, smallpox, measles, scarlet fever, rubella, erythema infectiosum, and roseola infantum. Other disorders added to this list of childhood exanthems include the exanthematous eruptions produced by echoviruses, coxsackieviruses, reoviruses, and the Epstein-Barr virus (infectious mononucleosis). Because of their exanthematous nature, the rickettsial diseases, caused by microorganisms that occupy an intermediate position between bacteria and viruses, are also included in this chapter.

Varicella (Chickenpox)

Varicella is a highly contagious disease of childhood, and occasionally adulthood, caused by a primary infection with a complex herpes group DNA virus (herpesvirus varicellae), the varicella-zoster (V-Z) virus. Transmission is by close contact and droplet infection from individuals affected with the disorder and, since varicella and herpes zoster are caused by infection with the same virus, occasionally from contact with individuals with herpes zoster.

In normal children systemic symptoms are usually mild, and serious complications are rare. In adults and children on systemic corticosteroids,

immunosuppressive drugs, or with deficiencies in cell-mediated immunity, the disorder is more likely to be characterized by an extensive eruption, severe constitutional symptoms, and, occasionally, varicella pneumonia with, at times, a potentially fatal outcome.[1]

Because of its highly contagious nature this disorder is usually seen during childhood but may occur at any age, including the newborn period. Approximately 50 per cent of the cases occur prior to the fifth year of age and 80 to 90 per cent by the age of 15 years. The disorder occurs in epidemics with a peak incidence during late winter and spring and recurring high rates of incidence at intervals of two to five years.

CLINICAL MANIFESTATIONS. Following an incubation period of 14 to 16 days (occasionally as early as 10 days or as late as 21 days) the disease begins with a low-grade fever, malaise, and the appearance of a highly characteristic vesicular exanthem manifested by delicate "tear drop" vesicles on an erythematous base (Fig. 12–1). In children the disease is characteristically a mild febrile disorder, occasionally preceded by a 24-hour prodrome of headache, malaise, and fever accompanied by successive drops of papulovesicles. Adults frequently exhibit a prodrome of one or two days, a more extensive rash, increased constitutional symptoms, and a predispostion to more severe complications.

A highly characteristic feature is the fact that all stages and sizes of lesions may be found at the same time and in the same vicinity. The eruption

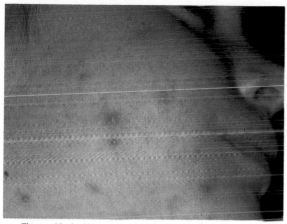

Figure 12-1 Varicella. Maculopapular lesions and "teardrop" vesicles on an erythematous base on the face of a 9-year-old girl.

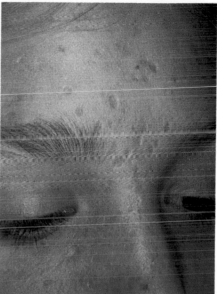

Figure 12-3 Post-varicella scars on the face of a young girl who developed chickenpox shortly after receiving systemic intramuscular corticosteroid for the treatment of poison ivy.

generally begins abruptly on the trunk, face, and scalp, with successive crops of pruritic lesions and minimal, if any, involvement of the distal aspect of the extremities. This centripetal distribution is in sharp contrast to the centrifugal distribution seen in variola (smallpox). Mucous membranes are characteristically involved, and ulcers may be present on the pharynx, palate, anterior tonsillar pillars, and occasionally on the larynx, the conjunctivae, vulva, and anal mucosa.

The average pock first appears as a small red macule, 2 or 3 mm in diameter, which, in the course of a few hours, becomes a papule. It then develops a small delicate vesicle of clear fluid (Fig. 12-1). Although many of the lesions are surrounded by an irregularly shaped red areola, this may be entirely lacking, and occasionally a vesicle may appear directly on otherwise normal-appearing skin. The vesicle of chickenpox is usually rounded or pear shaped, but may show a central depression or umbilicated appearance. Often, within a period of six to eight hours and usually within 24 hours, the rash of varicella progresses through maculopapular, vesicular, pustular, and crusted stages (Fig. 12-2). Except for secondarily infected lesions, the crusts fall off within a period of 5 to 25 days, depending on the depth of involvement. Except for immunosuppressed individuals with severe varicella, unless deep excoriation or secondary infection occurs, lesions generally tend to heal without scar formation (Fig. 12-3).

Lesions of varicella appear in successive crops over a three to five day period, with all stages of development in the same anatomic area at the same time. The lesions may be modified by pre-existing inflammation, such as may be seen in infants with diaper dermatitis, or by an increase in lesions in areas of sun-exposure or sunburn. Although little has been written about the accentuation of viral eruptions in areas of the body exposed to sunlight, this is a well-known phenomenon that bears recognition.[2, 3]

The fever in individuals with chickenpox is variable in severity and duration, and roughly parallels the extent and severity of the rash. Successive lesions usually appear over a period of three days. Crusting of lesions occurs within five days in mild cases and within 10 days in severe cases. The disorder is considered to be contagious for a period of approximately 24 hours preceding the rash and for a period of five to seven days afterward (when all vesicles have crusted). Infectivity, however, may persist much longer in patients with an altered immune response, as fresh

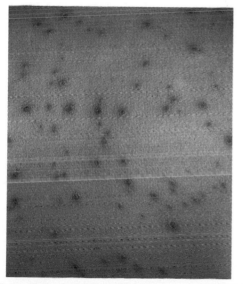

Figure 12-2 Varicella. Crusted lesions on the seventh day of illness.

moist lesions continue to appear. As in most other viral exanthems, although varicella generally confers lasting immunity, second attacks are rare but can occur.

Unusual forms of chickenpox may also occur. Varicella in an immunocompromised individual may be characterized by a hemorrhagic, progressive, and/or disseminated infection with severe viremia and a potentially fatal outcome.[4] Infants born to mothers who had varicella early in pregnancy may be born with multiple congenital anomalies (microphthalmia, cataracts, micrognathia, cutaneous scars, or atrophy of a limb), suggesting an intrauterine teratogenic potential to the varicella-zoster virus. Although transplacental IgG antibody passes from the mother to the infant in utero, the protection from this antibody is not as good as that of other viral disorders such as rubeola. Maternal varicella, accordingly, just prior to or at term may result in a severe or fatal disseminated disorder of the newborn (varicella neonatorum) characterized by hemorrhagic lesions and involvement of the lungs and liver. When an infant contracts the infection from its mother or through exposure to a sibling or other individual during the first three months of life, the disorder is usually relatively mild and uncomplicated, except for the diaper area (where the eruption may be modified by diaper dermatitis or secondary infection).

When an adult contracts the disease, it generally appears in a more severe form, constitutional symptoms are more profound, and viral pneumonia is a common sequela. Although varicella pneumonia generally runs a fairly mild course, it may at times progress and result in fatality. Most such progression has been observed in patients on systemic corticosteroids or in individuals with neoplastic disease or on immunosuppressive drug therapy. Bacterial infections of the skin due to excoriation are the most frequent complications. Other complications include appendicitis, orchitis, nephritis, cardiac and circulatory involvement, and encephalitis. Unlike other complications, encephalopathy (seen in 0.01 to 0.1 per cent of all cases of varicella) is not related to the severity of the primary disorder and the prognosis of varicella central nervous system disease is generally favorable. In 80 per cent of cases complete recovery can be anticipated, and the mortality of those afflicted is low (possibly in the order of 5 per cent).[5]

TREATMENT. The treatment of chickenpox should be directed to alleviation of itching and prevention of secondary bacterial infection. Pruritus may be decreased by starch baths or Aveeno baths, topical application of calamine lotion (to which 0.25 to 0.5 per cent menthol and 0.5 to 1.0 per cent phenol may be added), the administration of acetylsalicylic acid for fever or discomfort, and, when necessary, the use of topical or systemic antibiotics for secondary bacterial infection.

Patients on systemic corticosteroids who are exposed to varicella should have the dosage reduced to physiologic levels, and other drugs that may depress immune response should be reduced or deleted whenever possible. For immunologically depressed patients exposed to varicella, gamma-globulin prophylaxis (1.3 ml per kg of body weight) or zoster immune globulin (ZIP) may be used to attenuate the subsequent clinical disease.[6, 7, 8]

It furthermore should be noted that an attenuated strain of varicella has been used successfully in Japan in an attempt to prevent or modify varicella in sick children with no history of varicella and no detectable complement-fixing antibody. Although this vaccine has been used safely in children (with or without underlying disease, including those on steroid therapy), it is not as yet available in the United States, and further studies must be performed before this vaccine can be accepted as prophylaxis against varicella.[9, 10]

Rubeola (Measles)

Prior to 1963 measles was the most common viral exanthem of childhood. It was not unusual to see a young child with high fever, cough, coryza, conjunctivitis, Koplik's spots, and a characteristic morbilliform rash, which involved the head, face, neck, trunk, and extremities and faded after a period of three to seven days. This disorder, unfortunately, produced a variety of complications, including otitis media, bronchopneumonia, subacute sclerosing panencephalitis, and encephalitis. The latter complication occurred in 1 of 1000 affected individuals and proved fatal in 15 per cent of cases. Of those who survived, 45 per cent were left with permanent central nervous system damage — hearing loss, mental retardation, or seizure disorders.

CLINICAL MANIFESTATIONS. Transmitted by direct contact with droplets from infected persons, rubeola is caused by the measles virus (an RNA-containing paramyxovirus) with an incubation period of 10 to 14 days. The classic picture of unmodified measles begins with a prodromal period lasting 3 to 4 days, in occasional cases 1 to 6 days, manifested by systemic toxicity, with high fever (101 to 104° F. or higher), chills, malaise, headache, perspiration, prostration, oculonasal catarrh, conjunctivitis, photophobia, coryza with mucopurulent discharge, and a persistent dry hacking cough refractory to most antitussive agents.

Approximately two days before the development of the characteristic morbilliform exanthem, Koplik's spots appear on the buccal mucous membranes opposite the first molar teeth and, as they become more numerous, all over the inside of the cheeks and, at times, on the mucous membranes of the gums and lips. When marked, these spots are characterized by many pinpoint blue-white elevations resembling grains of salt sprinkled on an erythematous background. Koplik's spots are highly diagnostic of unmodified measles and usually disappear as the exanthem becomes full blown.

The exanthem of unmodified measles first makes its appearance three to four days after the

No !

onset of illness. It begins as an erythematous maculopapular eruption first on the scalp and hairline, the forehead, the area behind the ear lobes, and the upper part of the neck. It then spreads downward to involve the face, neck, upper extremities, and trunk and continues until it reaches the feet by the third day, the rash then fading in the same order as it appeared (Fig. 12–4). With the disappearance of the rash, a fine branny desquamation may be noted over the sites of the most extensive previous involvement.

The illness reaches its climax between the second and third days of the rash. At this time the temperature is at its peak, the eyes are puffy and red, the coryza is profuse, and the cough is most distressing. During this period the child feels miserable and looks "measly," but within the next 24 to 36 hours the temperature falls, the conjunctivitis and coryza clear, the cough decreases in severity, and within a few days, the child feels normal. Fever persisting beyond this point usually suggests a complication of the disorder.

Modified measles may develop in children who have been immunized with gamma globulin after exposure to the disease or in infants whose transplacental passive immunity has partially waned. The incubation period may be prolonged to 14 to 20 days, the usual prodromal period of three to four days may be absent or decreased to one or two days, there may be a low grade fever or the temperature may be normal, the cough, coryza, and conjunctivitis may be minimal or absent. Koplik's spots are absent or few in number and, if they develop, usually disappear within a day or less, and the exanthem is generally sparse or so mild that it may be missed.

The typical unmodified form of measles is usually easily recognizable. When the diagnosis is

in doubt, it can be confirmed by a variety of serologic procedures such as complement-fixation of hemagglutination inhibition studies. Lesions of the skin and oral mucosa (Koplik's spots) share the following similar histologic features: parakeratosis, acanthosis, intercellular and intracellular edema, foci of multinucleate giant cells with pale-staining cytoplasm, and a sparse lymphohistiocytic inflammatory infiltrate around the dilated blood vessels in the dermis. Electron microscopy reveals viral microtubular aggregates within nuclei and cytoplasm of the syncytial giant cells. These microtubules are indistinguishable from those seen in tissue cultures infected with measles virus. These findings indicate that the measles virus initiates a similar pathologic process in lesions of the skin and oral mucosa.[11]

MANAGEMENT. In 1954 a breakthrough in the control of this disease occurred with the isolation of measles virus by Enders and Peebles, a milestone in the control of measles. Shortly thereafter two measles vaccines were developed and, following extensive trials, licensed in 1963: a "killed" formalin-inactivated alum-precipitated vaccine and an attenuated Edmonston-B type live vaccine. Because febrile reactions caused by immunization with live Edmonston-B measles virus vaccines were common, many physicians preferred to use the killed measles virus vaccine, the live vaccine with a simultaneous injection of immune serum gamma globulin, or a combined killed and live measles virus regimen.

In 1965 an atypical form of measles following exposure to natural measles in children who had previously received killed vaccine was observed and, by 1967, it was apparent that the immunogenic and protective effects of inactivated measles virus vaccine were transient and that individuals with short-lived immunity were being seen with a bizarre new clinical syndrome termed "atypical measles."

Atypical measles is manifested by extremely high fever, cough, headache, myalgia, abdominal pain, pneumonitis, pleural effusion, peripheral edema, and an unusual macular, vesicular, or petechial rash, principally involving the hands and feet, thus frequently suggesting a diagnosis of Rocky Mountain spotted fever (Fig. 12–5).[12]

There are two theories regarding the pathogenesis of atypical measles. In one, it has been suggested that this disorder represents a generalized Arthus reaction in an individual exposed to wild measles virus — an individual who has lost his protective antibody level but has been left with a persistent cell-mediated hypersensitivity to the virus. The second is that it is due to an imbalance between T-cell function and the lack of humoral antibody. Recent evidence favors this aberrant cell-mediated response.[13]

Despite the fact that measles vaccine is easily available and highly effective (95 per cent), the control of measles is not as yet completely resolved. Current data suggest that 10 to 20 per cent of immunized children remain susceptible to

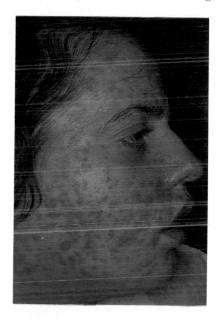

Figure 12–4 Rubeola. Purplish-red maculopapular eruption on the face.

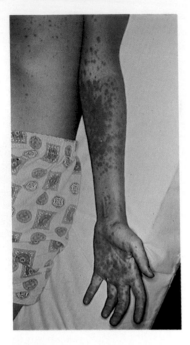

Figure 12–5 Purpuric rash on the trunk, forearm, and hand of a patient with the atypical measles syndrome (Courtesy of William E. Lattanzi, M.D.).

measles. This problem has been created primarily by the age at which vaccine was administered, the fact that many of those who apparently were properly immunized may have received vaccine that lost its potency because of exposure to heat or light, and the fact that many children still have not received measles vaccine.[14]

Current recommendations are that live measles vaccine should be administered at 15 months of age. Children who have not received vaccine during infancy may be immunized at any age; adults who have not been immunized or have not had natural measles should be immunized with live attenuated measles vaccine, and children who were initially vaccinated before 12 months of age should receive a booster immunization dose. Although there is no evidence that booster doses of measles vaccine are necessary in children who previously had primary immunization, many children were initially immunized improperly, accordingly do not have complete immunity, and therefore should be reimmunized. Although revaccination of children who previously received killed vaccine can result in mild local or severe general manifestations of hypersensitivity, most reactions are localized and the risk does not appear to be a deterrent to revaccination of such individuals.

Contraindications to live measles virus vaccine are pregnancy; leukemia, lymphoma, or other malignancy; diseases in which cell-mediated immunity is impaired; therapy that depresses resistance and immunity, such as steroids, irradiation, antimetabolites, and alkylating agents; severe febrile illness; and untreated active tuberculosis.

No adverse effect has been reported in egg-sensitive children from administration of live measles vaccine grown in chick fibroblast culture, probably because egg albumin and yolk components of the egg are essentially absent from the culture.

Scarlet Fever

Scarlet fever (scarlatina), although of bacterial origin, is commonly considered in the differential diagnosis of viral exanthems. The diffuse punctate erythematous eruption of scarlet fever results from an erythrogenic toxin produced by Group A streptococci, usually as the result of a pharyngeal infection, occasionally of a cutaneous infection (surgical scarlet). The disorder affects individuals of all ages and has its highest incidence in the late fall, winter, and early spring. The only difference between streptococcal tonsillitis or pharyngitis and scarlet fever is the fact that the latter disorder is accompanied by a cutaneous eruption.

CLINICAL MANIFESTATIONS. The clinical manifestations of streptococcal disease are governed by the portal of entry, the patient's age, and his immune status. The disease usually occurs in children, the maximal incidence being in the one-year to ten-year age group, and only rarely in adults. Although streptococcal infections are not uncommon in infants and very young children, scarlet fever is rarely seen in this age group.

The chief sources of pathogenic streptococci are discharges from the nose, throat, ears, and skin of patients or carriers. After an incubation period of two to five days (with a range of one to seven days), the disease is generally ushered in by the abrupt onset of fever, headache, vomiting, malaise, and sore throat. The enanthem includes lesions of the tonsils, pharynx, tongue, and palate. The oral mucous membranes are bright red and there may be scattered petechiae and red punctate lesions on the soft palate. During the first few days the tongue is heavily coated. By the second or third day reddened and edematous papillae project through the white coating, producing the so-called white strawberry tongue. By the fourth or fifth day the coating peels off, leaving a red, glistening tongue studded with prominent papillae, thus presenting the appearance of a red strawberry.[1]

Within 12 to 48 hours an erythematous punctate rash that blanches on pressure appears, first on the upper trunk, and then becomes generalized, rapidly within a period of a few hours or more gradually over a period of three to four days (Fig. 12–6). The face is flushed but rarely shows a punctate erythematous rash and there is a relative pallor from the triangle of the nose to the chin (circumoral pallor). The punctate lesions of scarlet fever give the skin a rough sandpaper-like texture. This is more intense in skin folds such as the axillae, antecubital, popliteal, and inguinal regions, and at sites of pressure such as the buttocks,

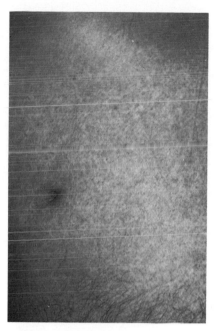

Figure 12–6 Fine punctate erythematous rash on the abdomen of a patient with scarlet fever.

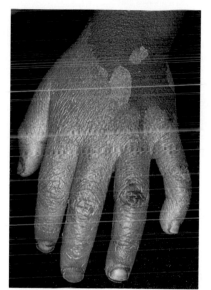

Figure 12–8 Post scarlet fever exfoliation of the skin on the hand of a black child.

the small of the back in bed patients, over the sternum, and between the scapulae. The lower legs generally are involved least and last. Capillary fragility is increased, and the eruption often exhibits transverse areas of hyperpigmentation with a petechial character in the antecubital fossae, axillary folds, and inguinal region (Pastia's lines) (Fig. 12–7). If the eruption is severe, minute vesicular lesions (sudamina) may be scattered over the abdomen, hands, and feet.

In mild cases the rash may be localized to the trunk and may be seen only as a faint erythema. In an effort to reassure anxious parents, this milder form, although actually the same disorder, is frequently referred to by physicians as scarlatina rather than scarlet fever. The eruption may become less pronounced when the circulation is poor or when the patient is cold, and generally

may be brought out more strongly by wrapping the patient warmly in blankets. In dark-skinned individuals the exanthem often is visible only where pigmentation is less pronounced (on the palms and soles); in other areas the rash is frequently difficult to recognize and may consist only of punctate papular elevations resembling cutis anserina (goose flesh).

The exanthem lasts for four or five days, but in mild cases may be transient and short lived. As the exanthem fades it leaves a scale, which is branny in most areas but which may appear as large exfoliative lamellar scales on the hands, palms, soles, fingertips, elbows, creases, and feet (Figs. 12–8, 12–9). The extent and duration of the desquamation are directly proportional to the intensity of the rash. When present, this is a most characteristic feature of scarlet fever.

The diagnosis is usually made on the basis of

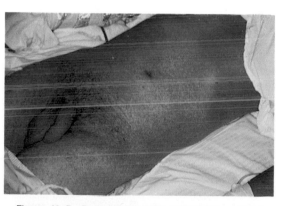

Figure 12–7 Scarlet fever with exaggeration of lesions (Pastia's sign) in the antecubital fossae and inguinal region.

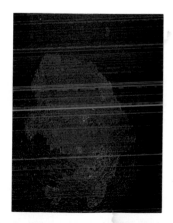

Figure 12–9 Post scarlet fever exfoliation of the skin on the knee of a black child.

clinical features of fever, pharyngotonsillitis, a characteristic enanthem, strawberry tongue, a punctate erythematous rash with circumoral pallor, postscarlatinal desquamation, isolation of Group A streptococci from the pharynx, and a rising antistreptolysin-O titer.

The cutaneous histopathology consists of perivascular collections of polymorphonuclear leukocytes and red blood cells, dilated small blood vessels, and focal accumulations of exudate. The latter are responsible for the punctate erythematous eruption characteristic of this disorder.

Staphylococcal Scarlet Fever. It should be noted that a slightly similar syndrome (staphylococcal scarlet fever) caused by an exfoliative exotoxin produced by staphylococci of bacteriophage Group II, types 3A, 3C, 55, 71, and 85, has also been documented.[15] Staphylococcal scarlatiniform disease is characterized by generalized erythema with a sandpaper-like texture and diffuse tenderness of the skin. This disorder can be differentiated from streptococcal scarlet fever by the absence of streptococcal pharyngitis or palatal enanthem, negative bacterial cultures, the absence of elevated antistreptolysin titers, and a lack of the characteristic desquamation that frequently follows streptococcal scarlet fever.

TREATMENT. The prognosis for adequately treated streptococcal infection is excellent. Early complications of inadequately treated scarlet fever include otitis media, bronchopneumonia, occasionally mastoiditis, septicemia, and osteomyelitis. Late complications include rheumatic fever and acute glomerulonephritis. Although their pathogenesis is unknown, poststreptococcal rheumatic fever and glomerulonephritis are thought to be due to a hypersensitivity to group A hemolytic streptococci or some of their byproducts.

The optimum treatment for streptococcal scarlet fever, as for other streptococcal disease, is pencillin. A single intramuscular injection of benzathine penicillin G is the most effective and secure mode of therapy (600,000 units for children under 60 pounds, and 1.2 million units for those over 60 pounds). If oral penicillin is prescribed, the patient should receive a full 10 days of therapy in order to eradicate the streptococci and help prevent rheumatic fever. Oral penicillin may be administered as 200,000 units of penicillin V three or four times a day for a period of ten days for children under 60 pounds, and 400,000 units three or four times a day for those 60 pounds or more. Although adequate treatment appears to reduce the incidence of rheumatic fever, it is unclear if early treatment of pharyngitis can regularly prevent the development of acute glomerulonephritis. Erythromycin, 40 mg/kg per day in four divided doses (not to exceed a total of 1 gm a day), is the drug of choice for patients with a history of penicillin allergy.

Followup cultures of patients are important, particularly for those individuals treated with oral therapy. Throat cultures should be obtained 7 to 10 days following a course of oral penicillin or four to five weeks after an injection of benzathine penicillin. If followup cultures are found to be positive, retreatment with intramuscular benzathine penicillin is recommended for those individuals not allergic to penicillin. For those with a history of penicillin allergy, a repeat course of therapy with erythromycin or with one of the cephalosporin group of antibiotics is advisable.

Staphylococcal scarlatiniform eruptions should be treated by a semi-synthetic beta lactamase-resistant (penicillinase-resistant) penicillin (dicloxacillin, methicillin, nafcillin, or oxacillin). If there is a history of previous allergic reaction to penicillin, antistaphylococcal cephalosporins (cephalothin, cephapirin, or cephazolin) should be utilized. However, it should be noted that in 5 to 15 per cent of patients there is a cross-reactivity with penicillin and the cephalosporins and that, because of possible renal toxicity associated with cephaloridine, this agent should not be administered to individuals in the pediatric age group.

[handwritten: MMR given 15 mos]

Rubella (German Measles)

Rubella is a common viral disease of children and young adults manifested by a generalized maculopapular rash and enlargement of the posterior occipitocervical lymph nodes. Although usually benign in its course and sequelae, rubella infection has additional significance during pregnancy owing to its potential for developmental defects in the fetus.

CLINICAL MANIFESTATIONS. The portal of entry of the rubella virus is the respiratory mucosa and the incubation period is approximately 16 to 18 days, with a range of 14 to 21 days. The exanthem, usually the first evidence of the disorder, generally begins about the hairline and face and spreads rapidly to involve the neck, trunk, and extremities, generally within a period of 24 hours. The duration and extent of the rash may be variable. Although it generally lasts for about three days, it may be evanescent and may disappear in less than a day, or it may be prolonged and last for as long as five days.

The eruption is characterized by innumerable small, discrete, rose-pink maculopapules, which are generalized and discrete on the first day, fade on the face and coalesce over the trunk on the second day, and usually disappear by the third day (Fig. 12–10). The rash tends to fade as it spreads, and the face and shoulders may be fairly clear while the eruption remains prominent elsewhere on the body. The most notable feature of the exanthem is its rapid change in appearance, frequently over a few hours. The characteristic pink-red lesions of rubella differ from the more vivid purplish-red lesions of measles and the fine punctate yellow-red lesions of scarlet fever. After severe rubella eruptions, a fine flaky desquamation may be observed in areas of maximum involvement. In contrast to measles, however, the erup-

[handwritten left margin: Not any more]

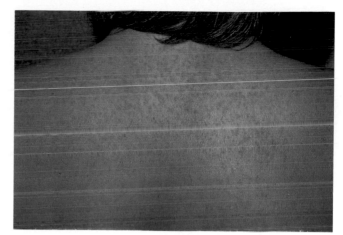

Figure 12–10   Rubella. Multiple light reddish-pink lesions on the back of a child with German Measles

tion is not followed by a temporary period of hyperpigmentation.

In children, the temperature may be normal or slightly elevated and rarely persists beyond the first day of the exanthem. In adolescents and adults, however there may be a prodromal period. Lasting one to five days it consists of headache, malaise, anorexia, mild conjunctivitis, coryza, sore throat, and cough, and at times, there is a low-grade fever during the prodromal period and first day of the rash. An enanthem termed Forchheimer's sign may be observed in up to 20 per cent of patients during the prodromal period or first day of the rash. Located on the soft palate, it is manifested by petechiae or reddish spots, pinpoint or larger in size.

Besides the eruption, the other notable feature of rubella is the involvement of the lymph nodes in the back of the neck, particularly the suboccipital and postauricular nodes. This glandular involvement may precede the appearance of the rash by one to five days, ordinarily lasts for two to seven days, and usually subsides quickly after the rash has disappeared. It is important to recognize the fact that, although highly characteristic, suboccipital, postauricular, and cervical lymphadenopathy are suggestive but not diagnostic of the disorder. They also may be associated with diseases such as measles, chickenpox, adenovirus infections, infectious mononucleosis, and others.

The clinical diagnosis is suggested by a maculopapular rash, which begins on the face, progresses rapidly downward to the trunk and extremities, and subsides, generally within a few days, accompanied by postoccipital and postauricular lymphadenopathy, which precedes the appearance of the rash, a low-grade fever or absence of fever, and absent or mild prodromal symptoms. When the diagnosis is indeterminate, rubella virus may be recovered from the pharynx as early as 7 days before and as late as 14 days after the onset of the rash. Since the introduction of the hemagglutination inhibition (HI) test in 1967, serologic studies have become increasingly important. The HI antibody test has the advantages of high sensitivity and speed with which results are obtained.[16]

A serologic diagnosis depends upon acute and convalescent serum determinations. Ideally, the first blood should be drawn as soon as possible after the rash is noted, and a second blood test should be performed two to four weeks later. Evidence of a fourfold or greater rise in rubella titer is indicative of rubella infection.

Except for possible infection of the fetus during pregnancy, rubella is one of the most benign of all infectious diseases of childhood. A pregnant woman who contracts rubella in the first trimester of pregnancy has a high probability that intrauterine transmission will give rise to the congenital rubella syndrome. In the first few weeks of pregnancy the chance of transmission is 30 to 50 per cent, at five to eight weeks it is 25 per cent, and from 9 to 12 weeks the risk is 8 per cent (for a discussion of the congenital rubella syndrome, refer to the discussion in Chapter 2.)

In older children and adults arthritis may affect about 30 per cent of females and five per cent of males. The clinical picture is variable but characteristically involves the small joints of the hands and feet, occasionally the knees, elbows, shoulders, and spine. Occasionally the arthropathy lasts up to two weeks and has been associated with mild elevations of the erythrocyte sedimentation rate and false positive latex fixation tests (the latter generally revert to normal within a period of 18 months). Other rare complications include thrombocytopenic or non-thrombocytopenic purpura, and in approximately 1 in 6000 cases encephalitis has been reported. Most patients with purpura improve and become symptom free within two weeks. The clinical manifestations of encephalitis are similar to those observed in other types of postinfectious encephalitis and, although fatalities have been reported, complete recovery generally is the rule.[1]

Present prophylactic recommendations for rubella include vaccination of all children with live attenuated rubella vaccine between the ages of 15 months and puberty. As with measles prophylaxis, rubella vaccine should not be administered to infants under 15 months of age because of possible interference from persisting maternal rubella antibody. Since infection of the fetus with attenuated virus may take place in pregnant women, routine immunization of adolescent and adult females should be undertaken with caution, and rubella vaccine should not be administered to pregnant women or to those who might become pregnant within a period of two months.

"Dukes' Disease"

Historically the exanthems of childhood have been classified on a numerical basis (Table 12–1). This classification is no longer tenable and is included only for its historical significance.

This disorder is included here only because of its historical significance. The name Dukes' disease (fourth disease) is an antiquated term used to describe a group of exanthematous disorders described by Clement Dukes in 1900. Unfortunately, Dukes' descriptions were based on clinical and morphologic examination, before modern laboratory facilities were available to allow proper evaluation and classification. The disorder, or perhaps more correctly, disorders, as originally described were characterized by a mild prodromal period manifested by headache, anorexia, drowsiness, chills, and backache, followed by a diffuse, slightly red, raised eruption and a slight edema of the skin, which disappeared on the fourth or fifth days when a branny desquamation took place. In retrospect it now appears that Dukes described variants of rubella, rubeola, scarlet fever, or perhaps viral exanthemata of the Coxsackie-ECHO group.

Erythema Infectiosum   *Fifth Disease*

Erythema infectiosum (fifth disease) is a mildly contagious disease of childhood that tends to affect children from 3 to 12 years of age. Its incubation period has an estimated range of 6 to 14 days, and it is characterized by three stages: (1) an erythematous malar blush that suddenly develops in an asymptomatic child, giving the patient a "slapped cheek" or "sunburned" appearance (Fig. 12–11); (2) a second stage that begins the next day with an erythematous maculopapular eruption on the extensor surfaces of the extremities, and less often the trunk and buttocks; and (3) a third stage that begins on or about the sixth day, when the rash fades, particularly on the proximal extremities, with areas of central clearing creating a reticulated or lacy marble-like pattern. The lesions of the second stage persist for several days to a week or more, after which they subside. The reticulated rash is the most characteristic finding of fifth disease. Its presence in a patient with little or no constitutional symptoms is highly pathognomonic.[17, 18]

The duration of the reticulated rash varies from 3 to 24 days, with an average of 9 to 11 days, and after the rash has seemed to subside, it frequently reappears, often several times, in response to friction, temperature changes, or sun

Table 12–1   THE NUMBERING OF EXANTHEMS*

First disease	Measles
Second disease	Scarlet fever
Third disease	Rubella
Fourth disease	"Dukes' disease"
Fifth disease	Erythema infectiosum
Sixth disease	Roseola infantum

*This classification is antiquated and included only because of historical significance.

exposure. There is no enanthem and rarely the disease may be accompanied by low-grade fever, malaise, fatigue, irritability, general aches and pains, and, at times, mild arthritis and arthralgia. Joint manifestations, when present, are transient, self-limiting, and more common in adults than in children.

The diagnosis of erythema infectiosum is dependent on clinical and epidemiologic grounds without any available laboratory confirmation. Although misdiagnosis often occurs, the characteristic "slapped cheek" appearance and subsequent lacy marble-like pattern on the upper arms and thighs generally helps establish the diagnosis.

Although viral etiology is suspected, attempts to isolate the agent to date have not been successful. Eosinophilia, lasting only a few weeks and occasionally accompanied by lymphocytosis, occurs in some patients. Cutaneous biopsies reveal slight perivascular lymphocytic infiltration with mild edema of the dermis. Complications seldom occur, but arthritis and arthralgia, pneumonia, hemolytic anemia, and encephalopathy have been noted.[18] Isolation is not required and, in most cases, treatment is unnecessary.

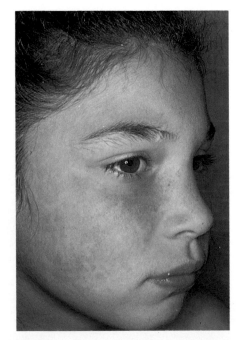

Figure 12–11   Erythema infectiosum ("fifth disease"). The "slapped-cheek" or sunburn-like malar flush.

Roseola Infantum

Roseola infantum (exanthem subitum) appears to be the most common exanthem in children under three years of age. It has been estimated that about 30 per cent of children develop this disorder, the condition appearing in a majority of instances either as an inapparent infection or as a febrile illness without a rash. Assumed to be caused by a virus, it appears that roseola infantum is not a specific one-agent disease but rather an age-related host response to several viral infections (ECHO 16, Coxsackie B5, several adenoviruses, and others).

The illness is of sporadic, non-seasonal occurrence without known contact, and the incubation period varies from 5 to 15 days. Although there are epidemics, communicability is quite low and one attack usually confers lasting immunity.[19] The disorder is characterized by constant or intermittent high fever which usually drops by crisis (occasionally by lysis). The appearance of a rash coincides with the subsidence of the fever, generally on the third or fourth day. Occasionally the rash may not be apparent until one day of normal temperature, and at times it may appear before the fever has subsided.

The eruption is characterized by discrete rose-pink macules or maculopapules, 2 to 3 mm in diameter, that fade on pressure, rarely coalesce, and are similar in appearance to those of rubella and modified measles. The rash characteristically first appears on the trunk and, at times, may spread to the neck, upper extremities, and lower extremities (Fig. 12–12). The duration of the eruption is usually one to two days; occasionally it may be evanescent, arising quickly and disappearing in a matter of hours (hence the name exanthem subi-

tum). In spite of the elevated temperature the patient is frequently alert and playful and generally does not appear to be acutely ill. Periorbital edema is common and, when present in a febrile but otherwise apparently well child, frequently is a useful clue to diagnosis during the pre-exanthematous stage.

A diagnosis of exanthem subitum is made chiefly on the basis of the striking contrast between the infant's general appearance and clinical course, periorbital edema (when present), and the appearance of the rash as the fever subsides. The white blood count is usually low (but may be slightly elevated during the first two days of the illness), and leukopenia with relative lymphocytosis as a rule does not develop until the third day of the illness.

Febrile seizures, in all probability related to the abrupt rise of temperature, as in many other febrile disorders of childhood, are a common complication. Seen in less than 6 per cent of cases in private practice, they represent a common problem in children admitted to hospitals with this disorder.

There is no specific therapy for patients with exanthem subitum other than aspirin, fluids, and phenobarbital for those with a history of febrile seizures either during the current or a previous illness.

OTHER VIRAL EXANTHEMS

Recognition of a specific virus as the etiologic agent responsible for a particular exanthematous disorder frequently is difficult. During epidemics or localized outbreaks of similar cutaneous eruptions, an etiologic association may be established by the recovery of a particular viral agent or by serologic demonstration of an acute infection in a statistically greater number of ill patients than in a similar group of well subjects from the same community. Even in situations where a specific etiologic agent cannot be identified, recognition of characteristic clinical findings or symptoms during epidemics will frequently suggest the association of specific etiologic agents with certain cutaneous eruptions.[20]

Exanthems Due to Enteroviruses

Enteroviruses, a subgroup of the picorno virus, are a common cause of exanthems. Although unknown 30 years ago, there now appear to be at least 30 types that have been associated with cutaneous eruptions. Polio viruses, Coxsackie viruses, and ECHO and Reo viruses are grouped under this classification because of their many similarities and their habitat in the human enteric tract.[1] These viruses, spread by contact from person to person, initiate infection first in the pharynx and shortly thereafter in the gastrointestinal tract.

The exanthems associated with Coxsackie and ECHO virus infections frequently are morbilli-

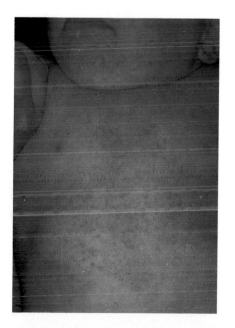

Figure 12–12　Roseola infantum (exanthem subitum).

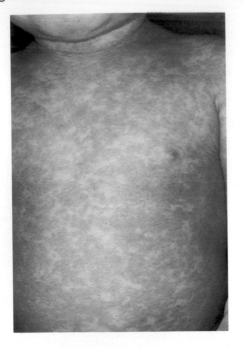

Figure 12–13 Erythematous maculopapular exanthems of the Coxsackie-ECHO group.

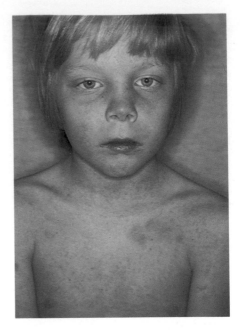

Figure 12–14 Erythematous maculopapular exanthems of the Coxsackie-ECHO group.

form in appearance (Figs. 12–13 and 12–14). Cutaneous lesions usually are generalized, nonpruritic, and maculopapular, but also have been described as scarlatiniform, vesicular, zosteriform, urticarial, petechial, or purpuric in nature (Tables 12–2 and 12–3).[20, 21, 22]

Coxsackie Virus Exanthems. Eruptions associated with Coxsackie virus vary markedly (Table 12–2). They may resemble maculopapular ECHO virus disorders, may be suggestive of roseola infantum, or may consist of urticarial lesions. In some cases lesions may resemble varicella but, unlike the latter, they heal rapidly without pustular formation, crusting, or scarring.

Hand, Foot, and Mouth Disease. The most distinctive exanthem-enanthem complex of the

"newer exanthems" is that caused by Coxsackie A16 (occasionally A5 and A10) and appropriately called the hand, foot, and mouth syndrome. First described in the mid 1950's, there have been repeated outbreaks of this disorder in the United States since 1963.[20] Infections are more common in late summer and fall. The disorder is highly contagious in a susceptible population and may occur as an isolated phenomenon or in epidemic form. During epidemics the virus is spread from child to child (horizontal spread) and then adults (vertical spread) in various family groups.

The disorder is characterized by fever and a vesicular eruption that begins after a three to six day incubation period, occasionally with a brief prodrome of low-grade fever, anorexia, a sore

Table 12–2 EXANTHEMS CAUSED BY COXSACKIE VIRUSES

Virus	Time	Distribution	Cutaneous Manifestations
Coxsackievirus A 16	During fever	Hands, feet, buttocks	Maculopapules and vesicular lesions, ulcerations on tongue, soft palate, buccal mucosa, and gums
Coxsackievirus A 9	During fever	Face, trunk, (occasionally palms and soles)	Erythematous maculopapules, vesicles, occasionally petechiae, purpura, or urticaria
Coxsackievirus A 5	During fever	Hands, feet, occasionally legs, trunk, and buttocks	Maculopapules, vesicles, ulcers on tongue, soft palate, buccal mucosa, and gums
Coxsackievirus B 5	During or after defervescence	Initially face and neck followed by spread to the trunk and extremities	Maculopapules, occasionally petechiae and urticaria

mouth, malaise, and abdominal pain, which precedes the enanthem by one to two days; the exanthem occurs shortly after the enanthem. The fever lasts for two or three days, and temperatures average 101° F. The oral lesions begin as small red macules and evolve into small vesicles 1 to 3 mm to 2 cm in diameter on an erythematous base, which then ulcerate and last for a period of one to six days. Similar lesions may also be seen on the soft palate, hard palate, buccal mucosa, gingivae, and tongue. The tongue is involved in 44 per cent of patients with this disorder, and lesions are suggestive of aphthous stomatitis. Involvement of the palate, uvula, and anterior tonsillar pillars (the classic herpangitic enanthem) is noted in about one-third of cases.[20]

One-quarter to two-thirds of affected patients also have highly characteristic vesicular lesions on the hands and feet, more commonly on the dorsal aspect, but also involving the lateral borders of the feet, the palms, soles, and buttocks, and occasionally the arms, legs, and face. The lesions on the skin are maculopapular at first, many later forming superficial gray vesicles on an erythematous base. The vesicles vary in size from 3 to 7 mm in diameter and are thin-walled, superficial, and nonloculated. They contain a clear fluid, sometimes coalesce to form bullae, and only occasionally are tender or pruritic. Vesicles are most frequently seen on the dorsal aspect of the fingers and toes as well as on the lateral borders of the feet and frequently have a characteristic elliptical football-shaped appearance (Figs. 12–15, 12–16). Although the palms and soles are not involved as frequently, when affected they may show the greatest number of lesions. The vesicles, frequently surrounded by a red areola, usually clear by absorption of the fluid within two to seven days, and on occasion, the vesicles may rupture, leaving a superficial scab.

The disorder tends to be more severe in infants and children than in adults, but is usually mild, and the temperature falls after a few days. Some patients are afflicted with high fever,

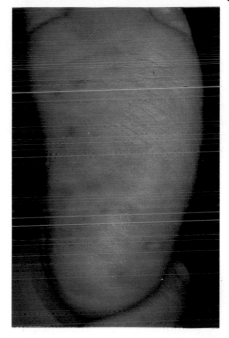

Figure 12–16 Hand, foot, and mouth disease. Linear and crescentic vesicular lesions with surrounding zone of erythema.

marked malaise, diarrhea, and occasionally joint pains. In 22 per cent of cases, marked cervical or submandibular adenopathy may be present. A few cases may recur at intervals for several months, and although the prognosis is generally excellent, rare cases of myocarditis, pneumonia, and meningoencephalitis have been reported.[23, 24, 25]

Other Exanthems Associated with Coxsackie Virus. Coxsackie A9 virus, a common cause of aseptic meningitis, is also a common cause of exanthematous eruptions. The rash, most commonly erythematous and maculopapular, starts on the face and neck and spreads to the extremities. It is usually discrete and has been described as morbilliform, but urticarial and petechial or purpuric lesions simulating meningococcemia have been reported. The duration of the rash is from one to seven days. Patients are usually febrile during the period of the rash and, except for those with aseptic meningitis, the majority of affected patients are generally not very ill.

In addition to the occasional association of hand, foot, and mouth syndrome due to Coxsackie A5 and A10 viruses, Coxsackie A5 also has been associated with scattered 4 to 5 mm yellow vesicles on the legs, which spread to the trunk; maculopapular lesions on the buttocks; and an enanthem consisting of 3 to 4 mm papules and vesicles on the soft palate. Coxsackie A10 virus has also been associated with an enanthem involving both the anterior and posterior oral cavities. Coxsackie B1 has been associated with a maculopapular rubelliform eruption with fever, headache, and aseptic meningitis and a roseola-like syndrome. Coxsackie B3 virus has been described

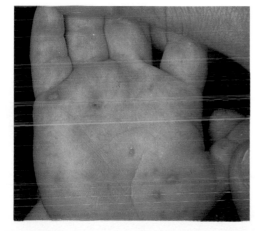

Figure 12–15 Hand, foot, and mouth disease. Linear and crescentic vesicular lesions with surrounding zone of erythema.

in individuals with a maculopapular rash, fever, headache, diarrhea, splenomegaly and hepatomegaly, lesions typical of hand, foot, and mouth syndrome, and, on occasion, petechial rashes suggesting a diagnosis of meningococcemia.[20]

Coxsackie B5 virus, a frequent cause of human illness, may occasionally be associated with aseptic meningitis, encephalitis, paralytic disease, pleurodynia, myocarditis, pericarditis, peritonitis, vesicular pharyngitis, orchitis, and hepatitis. The exanthem occasionally described in association with Coxsackie B5 infection varies considerably. Although maculopapular in the majority of instances, petechiae and urticaria have also been noted in isolated patients. The maculopapular exanthem associated with this infection appears first on the face and neck and spreads to the trunk and extremities in a period of 4 to 24 hours. The head and neck have been described as most heavily involved. The cutaneous lesions associated with Coxsackie B5 virus occur during or after defervescence and last about 36 hours.

Small outbreaks of enteroviral exanthems have also been associated with Coxsackie A4 infection. Initial symptoms in affected patients consist of anorexia, drooling, sore throat, coryza, and fever, and a typical herpangitic enanthem lasting for periods of 1 to 10 days has been described. The exanthem may begin with or after defervescence as 2 to 5 mm maculopapular lesions on the face and trunk. The lesions last one to four days and then disappear or become vesicular. The vesicular lesions have been described as occurring in crops and spreading to the extremities with exclusion of the palms and soles. Initially the vesicles tend to be yellowish, opaque, and 5 to 10 mm in size. Later they may become firm, may have a central punctum with a "bug-bite" appearance, persist for one to two weeks, and regress with brownish discoloration without crusting, pruritus, or desquamation.

Exanthemata Associated with ECHO Virus Infections. Except for the polio viruses, ECHO 9 viral infections are the best studied of all enteroviruses. Exanthems have been noted in about 35 per cent of all ECHO 9 viral illnesses, but in young children the incidence is greater than 50 per cent.[21] The rash most frequently occurs as a rubelliform eruption, but in addition, or as the sole manifestation, petechiae occasionally are noted. Lesions first appear on the face and neck and then spread rapidly to the trunk and extremities, including the palms and soles. Although the rash is usually discrete, on occasion confluence, particularly on the face, may be noted. The rash and fever usually occur simultaneously, but on occasion the rash has been noted to precede the fever by as much as two days and, in most instances, the duration of the exanthem is about three to five days. Of particular importance is the fact that disease due to enteroviruses (particularly those associated with ECHO 9 virus infection) with petechial exanthems and meningitis may closely mimic meningococcemia (Table 12–3).[26]

The "**Boston exanthem**" is an uncommon roseola-like infection caused by ECHO 16 virus. Seen in large epidemics, summer outbreaks of this disease were first observed in Massachusetts in 1951 and then in Pittsburgh in 1954. After 22 years of relative absence, the demonstration of ECHO 16 virus in ten States in 1974 suggested a general increase in the incidence of this disorder.[27]

Approximately one-third of individuals with ECHO virus infection have a rubelliform eruption consisting of discrete pinkish-red macules that are noted early in the course of the disease. Affecting first the face and neck, then the upper trunk and extremities, and only occasionally the palms and

	Table 12–3 EXANTHEMS CAUSED BY ECHOVIRUSES		
Virus	**Time**	**Distribution**	**Cutaneous Manifestations**
ECHO virus 2	With fever	Trunk, neck, and face	Pink to red papules, sometimes becoming coppery
ECHO virus 4	With fever	Trunk, neck, and face	Macules, maculopapules, occasionally petechiae, rarely vesicles
ECHO virus 5	After the onset of fever	Most marked on limbs and buttocks, also noted on trunk and face	A faint pink macular rash (a zosteriform eruption has also been noted)
ECHO virus 9	Generally with but occasionally prior to fever	Face and neck, then trunk, extremities, and occasionally palms and soles	Rubelliform macules, maculopapules, occasionally petechiae, rarely vesicles
ECHO virus 11		Trunk and extremities	Erythematous maculopapules, vesicles, urticarial lesions
ECHO virus 16	During or after defervescence	Initially head and trunk, then generalized (occasionally palms and soles)	Macules, maculopapules, punched-out ulcers on soft palate and pillars

Table 12–4   EXANTHEMS CAUSED BY REOVIRUSES

Virus	Time	Distribution	Cutaneous Manifestions
Reovirus 2	With fever	Trunk, neck, and face (then occasionally the extremities)	Maculopapules

soles, the incubation period is usually three to eight days, with fading of the lesions, usually within four or five days. Fifty per cent of cases show sparse yellow or grayish-white lesions on the oral mucous membranes with, at times, lesions resembling Koplik's spots on the membranes opposite the molars. Fever, gastrointestinal symptoms (anorexia, nausea, vomiting, and colicky abdominal pain), respiratory symptoms, sore throat, cough, and conjunctivitis may be present. Characteristically the eruption in the Boston exanthem develops during or shortly after defervescence (this roseola-like feature sets ECHO 16 and Coxsackie B5 virus infections apart from other enteroviruses). The exanthem consists of pink or salmon-colored discrete macular or maculopapular lesions measuring 0.5 to 1.5 cm in diameter, is centrifugal, and lasts for periods of from one to two days to about a week.

Other exanthemata seen with ECHO virus infection include those associated with ECHO 2 infection, a macular or rubelliform rash on the abdomen and back with spread, in some cases, to involve the chest, face, and neck. The cutaneous eruption has been noted to be coppery on the second day and persists for a period of two to seven days. Patients with this disorder have been noted to have rhinorrhea, pharyngitis, fever, cervical adenopathy, and, on occasion, aseptic meningitis and fatal paralytic infection. ECHO 4 virus has been associated with aseptic meningitis, meningoencephalitis, and, in about 15 per cent of patients during epidemics, with a macular, nonpruritic erythematous rash, which has its onset one to three days after the onset of symptoms, lasts for two days, and begins on the trunk and occasionally the face, becomes semi-confluent, and spreads to the extremities.

An unusual epidemic of ECHO 5 virus has been described in newborns with fever, malaise, vomiting, diarrhea, and a faint pink macular rash which, most marked on the limbs and buttocks, also was noted on the trunk and face. The cutaneous eruption appeared 24 to 36 hours after the onset of fever and cleared after a period of two days. In another child with ECHO 5 infection, fever, back pain, and an erythematous macular rash with a zosteriform distribution on the trunk has been noted.

ECHO 6 virus, a frequent cause of neurologic illness, has only sporadically been noted in association with an exanthem (usually a morbilliform eruption). It should be noted, however, that a zosteriform eruption has also been noted in association with this disorder.[22]

Exanthems associated with ECHO 11 infection have been described as urticarial and vesicular in nature, and in ECHO 17 and ECHO 25 virus infections, transient erythematous, macular, maculopapular, and vesicular eruptions have been noted. In the latter, the rashes had their onset following three days of fever (during the period of defervescence), were most marked on the trunk, usually lasted two to three days, and then cleared without desquamation.

Other less common exanthemata have, on occasion, been noted with other ECHO viruses. These include generalized erythematous maculopapular, morbilliform, and scarlatiniform eruptions and, as with many other enteroviral exanthems, do not appear to be particularly characteristic or diagnostic in appearance.[20] The various ECHO virus infections are self-limiting, the vast majority of patients recover completely, and there is no effective remedy for this group of disorders. Diagnosis is established on clinical grounds, on isolation of the affecting organism from the throat, rectum, or spinal fluid, and on serial antibody studies performed during the course of the illness and two weeks later.

Reoviruses. Reoviruses are common infectious agents of man and lower animals. Despite their prevalence, human disease due to reoviruses has only occasionally been recognized (Table 12–4). Reovirus 2 infections were seen in seven children under the age of 10 years in Boston during the summer of 1960. Of these, one child was asymptomatic. Of the other six, five had maculopapular eruptions and one child had a vesicular eruption.[28] The eruption was mildly pruritic, persisted for periods of three to nine days, and then began to fade, first from the face and then from other affected areas. Other associated symptoms and signs included fever, which persisted for a total of five days, anorexia, and mild pharyngitis without exudate or cervical adenopathy.

Exanthems Associated with *Mycoplasma pneumoniae* (Eaton Agent) Infection

For many years the agent (Eaton agent) of cold agglutinin-positive primary atypical pneumonia was thought to be a virus. In 1962 it was shown not to be a virus but a pleuropneumonia-like organism (PPLO). Skin rashes, often of short duration and usually described as maculopapular or urticarial, have occurred in up to 16 per cent of cases. Other cutaneous eruptions associated with *M. pneumoniae* infection include erythema multiforme (and its severe bullous form, Stevens-Johnson syndrome), erythema nodosum (see

Chapter 18), and on rare occasions, pityriasis rosea and purpura.[1, 20]

Smallpox (Variola)

Smallpox (variola) is an acute, highly contagious, frequently deadly but preventable disease caused by poxvirus variolae, a specific virus immunologically related to vaccinia virus. Due to vigorous mass immunizations, skillful management, and sound epidemiologic principles, it appears that except for possible laboratory accidents, the goal of a world free of smallpox is now at hand.[29] Although the disease currently appears to be controlled, the disorder still requires worldwide awareness for a period of several more years to assure that it is no longer smoldering in isolated pockets in Africa or Asia.

The smallpox virus (poxvirus variolae) probably first invades the upper respiratory tract where it multiplies locally in the mucosa and spreads to the regional lymph nodes from where it enters the blood stream. The incubation period of classic smallpox, variola major, is 12 days, with a range of approximately 8 to 16 days. The disease usually begins with chills, fever, headache, backache, severe malaise, delirium, and, particularly in children, seizures.

In some cases a transient eruption may develop during the prodromal period. It may be morbilliform, scarlatiniform, or petechial, with a characteristic bathing-trunk distribution. In most instances it disappears within one or two days. The duration of the prodromal period ranges between two and four days and, in most cases, it is terminated by the end of the third day.

The exanthem first appears on the face and forearms, spreads to the upper arms and trunk, particularly the back, and finally reaches the lower extremities. The eruption is characteristically more severe on the face, the distal parts of the arms and legs, and least severe over the trunk and abdomen (this centrifugal distribution is distinct from that of varicella, which tends to be centripetal).

The initial lesions are macular. First detected on the third or fourth day of illness, they rapidly become papular (within a matter of hours) and by the end of the sixth day the papules develop into vesicles that measure up to 6 mm in diameter and are usually surrounded by red areolae. Between the seventh and ninth days the vesicles become pustular and measure up to 8 mm in diameter. During this stage the temperature again begins to rise and constitutional symptoms return, now aggravated by the intensely painful lesions. On the tenth day the pustules begin to rupture and dry and finally form crusts.

Lesions do not appear in crop-like fashion (a helpful point in diagnosis), and the mature pustular lesions are thick-walled (in contrast to the thin-walled, dewdrop-like vesicles of varicella), discrete or confluent, umbilicated, and unilocular. Mucosal lesions are common and affect the mouth, nasopharynx, larynx, trachea, esophagus, and vagina as well as other areas and, among susceptible (previously unexposed or unvaccinated) populations, the fatality rate is high (up to 40 per cent).

The diagnosis is based upon clinical manifestations, tissue culture, ultramicroscopic techniques, the Tzanck test, and hemagglutination and virus neutralization tests.

Patients suspected of having smallpox should be admitted immediately to a hospital or institution where rigid isolation procedures can be enforced. There is no specific therapy for smallpox at present. Penicillin and broad-spectrum antibiotics, however, especially if started in the pustular phase (on approximately the sixth or seventh day of the disease) are highly effective in preventing secondary bacterial infection. Vaccinia immune globulin (available from Hyland Laboratories or from the Center for Disease Control, Atlanta, Georgia) helps to prevent or modify smallpox in persons known to have been exposed, if given in the incubation period or in the pre-eruptive phase of the disease.

Prophylaxis of exposed individuals requires vaccination and the administration of methisazone (Marboran, Burroughs-Wellcome), a derivative of thiosemicarbazone (1.5 to 3 gm orally, twice a day for two days) that decreases the incidence and severity of the disease in contacts even late in the incubation period. Methisazone may reduce the mortality rate in the severe types of smallpox in vaccinated patients but has little effect on severe cases in unvaccinated patients.[30]

Infectious Mononucleosis

Infectious mononucleosis is an acute infectious disease caused by the Epstein-Barr virus. Although infection with EB virus is exceedingly common in young children, illness in this age group is rare, inapparent, or so mild and atypical that the diagnosis is unrecognized. In contrast, infectious mononucleosis is common in adolescents and young adults between the ages of 15 and 25 years.

Transmitted by direct contact with a low degree of contagiousness, the incubation period of infectious mononucleosis is said to be between 33 and 49 days. The disorder begins insidiously with headache and malaise, and the early course is frequently marked by fevers of 101° to 104° F. Fever usually lasts 4 to 14 days, rarely up to three or four weeks. A sore throat commonly develops a few days after the onset of the illness, and an extensive membranous tonsillitis is characteristic. Lymphadenopathy begins early, is often generalized, and the cervical glands are usually most conspicuously affected. The spleen is moderately enlarged in one-half to two-thirds of cases, hepatomegaly is common, and icteric hepatitis is reported in 5 to 10 per cent of affected individuals.

An exanthem occurs in 10 to 15 per cent of cases, usually between the fourth and sixth days, and appears as a macular or maculopapular mor-

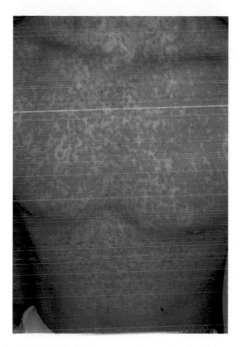

Figure 12–17 Infectious mononucleosis. Erythematous maculopapular eruption (seen in 10 to 15 per cent of patients with this disorder).

billiform eruption of the trunk or upper arms, and occasionally the face, forearms, thighs, and legs (Fig. 12–17). The eruption may last for only a few days and may be followed by an urticarial or erythema multiforme–like eruption. Upper eyelid edema occurs in 50 per cent of cases, frequently with narrowing of the eyelid aperture. An enanthem appears in 25 per cent of cases on the palate between the fifth and seventeenth days of the illness. Manifested by discrete bright red petechiae 0.5 to 1.0 mm in diameter, these lesions, seen at the junction of the hard and soft palates, are considered to be highly characteristic of the disorder and fade to a brownish hue in two days.

In most cases spontaneous recovery occurs in 10 to 20 days, and virtually all patients return to their normal state of health and activity within four to six weeks after the onset of the illness. Deaths are extremely rare and, when reported, generally are associated with splenic rupture.

Diagnosis is established on the basis of the clinical picture, a white blood count of 10,000 to 40,000, with lymphocytosis and abnormally large lymphocytes that are basophilic and contain foamy cytoplasm. Heterophile antibody studies (agglutination of sheep erythrocytes by the Paul-Bunnell test) resulting in titers of 1:112 or higher are diagnostic, and the Mono test, a slide test utilizing formalized horse cells (available from Wampole Laboratories), is a valuable presumptive test for rapid diagnosis.[31]

The treatment of infectious mononucleosis is symptomatic. During the acute phase, rest is the most important aspect of treatment. In severe forms of the disorder corticosteroids have been shown to reduce the duration and severity of the illness, and 20 to 25 per cent of patients are reputed to have a concurrent beta-hemolytic streptococcal infection. Penicillin or erythromycin is beneficial for those individuals with streptococcal disease, but ampicillin should be avoided, since 80 to 90 per cent of individuals with infectious mononucleosis have an unusual sensitivity to this drug characterized by copper-colored maculopapular lesions that occur five to eight days after the initiation of therapy.[32, 33] The reason for this unusual sensitivity is unknown. It appears that the skin reaction to ampicillin is part of a transient serologic abnormality involving a number of antigens during infection with this disease.[34]

Rickettsial Diseases

Rickettsial infections are arthropod-borne diseases caused by microorganisms that occupy an intermediate position between bacteria and viruses. Spread by blood-sucking insects such as the body louse, the flea, tick, and mite, the various rickettsial diseases that occur in the United States include endemic or murine typhus, rickettsialpox, Rocky Mountain spotted fever, and Q fever.

Epidemic Typhus Fever. Epidemic typhus fever (louse-borne typhus) is an acute, severe, potentially fatal infectious disease caused by *Rickettsia prowazekii* and characterized clinically by high fever, headaches, general aches and pains, and a centripetal maculopapular eruption that, in severe cases, becomes hemorrhagic. The diagnosis can be established by the clinical picture, isolation of *R. prowazekii* from the blood, and the Weil-Felix agglutination reaction with *Proteus* OX-19.

Endemic Typhus Fever. Endemic typhus fever (flea-borne or murine typhus) is an acute, relatively mild infection caused by *Rickettsia mooseri* and characterized chiefly by headache, fever, malaise, and a centripetal maculopapular eruption. Essentially a modified version of epidemic typhus, it is spread to man by the rat flea *Xenopsylla cheopis* and is diagnosed on the basis of the clinical picture, isolation of the organism by inoculation of the patient's blood into guinea pigs and adult white mice, and a positive Weil-Felix agglutination reaction with *Proteus* OX-19.

Rickettsialpox. Rickettsialpox is an acute benign infectious disease caused by *Rickettsia akari*, spread by the rodent mite *Allodermanyssus sanguineus* and ectoparasites of the mouse, *Mus musculus* (the reservoir of the infection). The disorder is characterized by an initial papule at the site of the bite, a grippe-like syndrome, and a papulovesicular eruption (papules surmounted by vesicles) with an irregular distribution. Diagnosis can be made on the basis of the clinical picture, isolation of the causative agent from the blood during the acute stage of the disease, negative Weil-Felix agglutinations, and a complement fixation test that shows a fourfold or greater rise in antibody titer in paired sera obtained early and late in the disease. It should be noted that because of cross-reactions, the Rocky Mountain spotted fever complement fixation test is positive and accordingly should not be misdiagnosed in patients with this disorder.

Q Fever. Q fever, caused by *Rickettsia burnetti*, is manifested by an acute pneumonitis and hepatitis. In contrast to the other rickettsial diseases it is not characterized by a cutaneous eruption.

Rocky Mountain Spotted Fever. Rocky Mountain spotted fever is an acute febrile exanthematous illness caused by *Rickettsia rickettsii* and transmitted by the bite of a wood tick. Although for years a disorder primarily confined to the Rocky Mountain states, the disorder is also endemic in the South Atlantic states, and cases are now reported from all parts of the United States.[35] In the western United States, *Dermacentor andersonii*, the wood tick, is the most important vector and the disease usually occurs in men who acquire a wood tick bite in wooded areas; in the eastern United States, *Dermacentor variabilis*, the dog tick, is the usual vector, and most patients are women and children.[36]

The incubation period usually is five to seven days. Most often the rash begins on the third or fourth day of illness as a maculopapular eruption on the extremities (the flexors of the wrists and ankles), spreads centrally to involve the back, chest, and abdomen, and within two days becomes generalized. At first the macules are erythematous, later become purpuric, and the palms and soles usually are involved. Occasionally the face is also affected. The lesions are at first discrete, macular, and maculopapular, blanching on pressure. Within one or two days the rash becomes hemorrhagic, and the severity and extent of the eruption are directly proportional to the severity of the disease (Fig. 12–18).

The history of a tick exposure in a child with fever, headache, a peripherally distributed hemorrhagic eruption, conjunctivitis, and peripheral and periorbital edema suggests the possibility of Rocky Mountain spotted fever.[36] Diagnosis can usually be confirmed by Weil-Felix agglutinations positive with OX-19 and OX-2 strains by the second or third week of the infection and by complement fixation tests. Since the pathogenic organism cannot routinely be cultured and the Weil-Felix or complement fixation tests may be negative during the acute stages of the disorder, a high index of suspicion and careful epidemiologic history are important.[37] When diagnosis is in doubt, a rapid diagnosis can be obtained by direct immunofluorescence of a cutaneous punch biopsy.

Rocky Mountain spotted fever (RMSF) is a curable but potentially fatal disease with a confirmed death rate of about 20 per cent, with a range of 13 to 40 per cent without treatment.[1] Fatalities are more common in individuals over age 40 and less common in children and young adults. With effective rapid therapy, however, mortality can be lowered to 5 per cent. The primary factor in patient survival is early diagnosis and therapy. Reduction of deaths from RMSF, accordingly, requires that a presumptive diagnosis be made early enough for appropriate antibiotic therapy to be effective.[37]

Tetracyclines and chloramphenicol have replaced para-aminobenzoic acid in the treatment of Rocky Mountain spotted fever. The preferred drug, tetracycline, may be administered orally in a dosage of 40 mg/kg per day (in four equally divided doses) with a maximum of 2 gm daily for seven to ten days. When administered intravenously, the dosage of tetracycline is 20 mg/kg/day. In the more severely ill, intravenous chloramphenicol (50 to 100 mg/kg per day, with a maximum of 2 to 4 grams per day) may be utilized. When chloramphenicol is given, patients and their families should be advised of the potential toxicity of this preparation, complete blood counts should be done every two days (or daily if the white blood count is below 7000/cu/mm), and chloramphenicol should be replaced with tetracycline if the white blood count decreases to below 5000/cu/mm or the polymorphonuclear cell count becomes less than 30 per cent.

All patients with Rocky Mountain spotted fever have vasculitis to a varying degree. The more severely ill patients may have edema involving the periorbital area, face, and extremities. Disseminated intravascular coagulopathy or purpura fulminans (Fig. 9–29), myocarditis, and heart failure are common complications of patients severely ill with this disorder. Though rarely necessary, the platelet deficit may be lessened temporarily by platelet or whole blood transfusion and intravenous heparin (50 to 100 units/kg intravenously every four to six hours appears to decrease or stop the progression of the coagulopathy). Central nervous system vasculitis, when present, is manifested by delirium, confusion, stupor, and

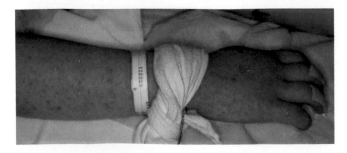

Figure 12–18 Maculopapular and hemorrhagic eruption on the forearm and hand (Rocky Mountain spotted fever).

seizures. Phenobarbital sodium, intravenously, in a dose of 4 mg/kg will usually control the seizures. Widespread increase in capillary permeability and hyponatremia may be prominent abnormalities in patients with Rocky Moutain spotted fever. Accordingly, intravenous therapy with plasma and whole blood infusions followed by appropriate fluid and electrolyte replacement is frequently necessary.[38]

References

1. Krugman S, Ward R, Katz SL: Infectious Diseases of Children. The C. V. Mosby Company, St. Louis, 1977.

   An up-to-date practical reference on the infectious diseases of childhood.

2. Cupoli JM: Photodistribution of viral exanthems (letter). Pediatrics 59:484, 1977.

   A profound photodistribution of viral exanthems as manifested in a brother and sister with varicella.

3. Gilchrest B, Baden H: Photodistribution of viral exanthems. Pediatrics 54:136–138, 1974.

   Two children with viral exanthems (echovirus 9 and varicella) with the eruption almost exclusively in sun-exposed areas.

4. Feldman S, Hughes WT, Daniel CB: Varicella in children with cancer: seventy-seven cases. Pediatrics 56:388–397, 1975.

   Of 77 children with cancer who contracted varicella, no complications were noted in the children not treated with corticosteroids or chemotherapeutic agents at the time of infection. In contrast, 32 per cent of 60 children receiving anticancer therapy had evidence of visceral dissemination and 7 per cent died of varicella pneumonia or encephalitis.

5. Jenkins RB: Severe chickenpox encephalopathy. Treatment with intravenous urea, hypothermia, and dexamethasone. Amer. J. Dis. Child. 110:137–139, 1965.

   A six-year-old girl with chickenpox complicated by severe varicella encephalopathy.

6. Roth KE, McCullough J, Marker SC, et al.: Evaluation of zoster immune plasma. Treatment of cutaneous disseminated zoster in immunocompromised patients. JAMA 239:1877–1879, 1978.

   A study of 20 immunocompromised patients with cutaneous disseminated zoster in which zoster immune plasma (ZIP) did not alter the course of their disorder suggests that ZIP be reserved for prevention or modification of varicella in exposed, susceptible immunocompromised patients.

7. Balfour HH, Groth KE, McCullough J, et al.: Prevention and modification of varicella using zoster immune plasma. Am. J. Dis. Child. 131:693–696, 1977.

   Zoster immune globulin (ZIP) administered to 31 susceptible immunocompromised children one to seven days following exposure to varicella suggests that ZIP is effective in preventing or modifying varicella in immunocompromised patients if given shortly after exposure is recognized.

8. Brunnell PA, Gershon AA, Hughes WT, et al.: Prevention of varicella in high risk children: a collaborative study. Pediatrics 50:718–722, 1972.

   Zoster immune globulin (ZIG) in adequate dosage, administered within 48 hours of exposure, may be expected to prevent or modify varicella in high risk children.

9. Takahashi M, Otsuka T, Okuno Y, et al.: Live vaccine used to prevent spread of varicella in children in hospital. Lancet 2:1288–1290, 1974.

   Twenty-three hospitalized children were apparently successfully vaccinated with an attenuated varicella virus vaccine.

10. Asano Y, Takahashi M: Clinical and serologic testing of live varicella vaccine and two year follow-up of immunity of the vaccinated children. Pediatrics 60:810–814, 1977.

    On the basis of two-year clinical and serologic follow-up studies of 181 susceptible children who received live varicella vaccine, it appears that live varicella vaccine may be used safely in children and produces an immunity that lasts for at least two years.

11. Suringa DWR, Bank LJ, Ackerman AB: Role of measles virus in skin lesions and Koplik's spots. N. Engl. J. Med. 283:1139–1142, 1970.

    On the basis of histopathologic and electron microscopic features, measles virus appears to initiate a similar pathologic process in lesions of the skin and oral mucosa.

12. Cherry JD, Feigin RD, Lobes LA Jr, et al.: Atypical measles in children previously immunized with attenuated measles virus vaccines. Pediatrics 50:712–721, 1972.

    Twelve children with clinical illnesses suggesting "atypical measles" during an epidemic of measles during the winter and spring of 1970 to 1971.

13. Krause PJ, Cherry JD, Naiditch MJ, et al.: Revaccination of previous recipients of killed measles vaccine: clinical and immunologic studies. J. Pediatr. 93:565–571, 1978.

    Clinical and immunologic studies suggest low serum antibody and increased measles specific lymphocyte reactivity as the cause of the atypical measles syndrome and severe local reactions following reimmunization with live measles vaccine.

14. Yeager AS, Davis JH, Ross LA, et al.: Measles immunization. Successes and failures. JAMA 237:347–351, 1977.

    Measles hemagglutination (HI) titers measured in 465 immunized children suggest that vaccine failure, not waning antibody, accounts for the majority of inadequate titers in immunized children.

15. McCloskey RV: Scarlet fever and necrotizing fasciitis caused by coagulase-positive hemolytic staphylococcus aureus, phage type 85. Ann. Int. Med. 78:85–87, 1973.

    The syndrome of scarlet fever and necrotizing fasciitis typically associated with group A hemolytic streptococci due to an exfoliative toxin caused by Staphylococcus aureus phage type 85.

16. Stewart GL, Parkman PD, Hopps HE, et al.: Rubella-virus hemagglutination inhibition test. N. Engl. J. Med. 276:554–557, 1967.

    The hemagglutination-inhibition (HI) test is simple, rapid, economical, and reliable for the detection of rubella infection.

17. Balfour HH Jr: Fifth disease: full fathom five (marginal comments). Am. J. Dis. Child. 130:239–240, 1976.

    Erythema infectiosum, a mild evanescent disorder of childhood is presumed to be a viral disorder, although the etiologic agent has not yet been established.

18. Hall CB, Horner FA: Encephalopathy with erythema infectiosum. Am. J. Dis. Child. 131:65–67, 1977.

    The second reported case of encephalitis following erythema infectiosum and apparently the first with permanent sequelae.

19. Berenberg W, Wright S, Janeway CA: Roseola infantum (exanthem subitum). N. Engl. J. Med. 241:253–259, 1949.

    A review of the clinical and laboratory features of roseola infantum (exanthem subitum).

20. Cherry JD: Newer viral exanthems. In Schulman I, Bongiovanni AM, Kempe CH, et al.: Advances in Pediatrics, Vol. 16. Year Book Medical Publishers, Inc., Chicago. 1969, 233–286.

    An extensive review of the newer viral exanthems and their cutaneous lesions

21. Lerner AM, Klein JP, Cherry JD, et al.: Medical progress, new viral exanthems. N. Engl. J. Med. 269:678–685, 736–740, 1963.

A review of the various enteroviruses and the cutaneous manifestations seen in association with these agents.

22. Meade III RH, Chang T: Zoster-like eruption due to Echovirus 6. Am. J. Dis. Child. *133*:283–284, 1979.

A 7-year-old boy with a unilateral vesiculobullous eruption, which on the basis of viral culture of fluid from several bullae and the development of high titers of serum neutralizing antibody appeared to be associated with echovirus type 6 infection.

23. Tindall JP, Miller GD: Hand, foot and mouth disease. Cutis *9*:457–463, 1972.

A review of hand, foot, and mouth disease, its clinical and laboratory aspects.

24. Goldberg MF, McAdams AJ: Myocarditis possibly due to Coxsackie group A, type 16, virus. J. Pediatr. *62*:762–765, 1963.

A 10½-month-old girl with interstitial myocarditis, cardiac failure, and death presumably due to an infection with Coxsackie Group A type 16 infection.

25. Wright HT Jr, Landing BH, Lennette EH, et al.: Fatal infection in an infant associated with Coxsackie virus Group A, type 16. N. Engl. J. Med. *268*:1041–1044, 1963.

A fatal case of hand, foot, and mouth disease in a seven-week-old male infant with enteritis, interstitial myocarditis, lymphohistiocytic arachnoiditis, and what was interpreted as a non-specific interstitial pneumonia.

26. Frothingham TE: ECHO virus type 9 associated with three cases simulating meningococcemia. N. Engl. J. Med. *259*:484–485, 1958.

Three patients with ECHO virus type 9 infection, aseptic meningitis, and a petechial rash.

27. Hale CB, Cherry JE, Hutch MH, et al.: The return of the Boston exanthem. Echovirus infections in 1974. Am. J. Dis. Child. *131*:323–328, 1977.

Ten children aged one week to seven years with the Boston exanthem in Rochester and Los Angeles.

28. Lerner AM, Cherry JD, Klein JO, et al.: Infections with reoviruses. N. Engl. J. Med. *267*:947–952, 1962.

Seven children under age 10 years with reovirus 2 infection.

29. Wehrle PF: Smallpox eradication. A global appraisal. JAMA *240*:1977–1979, 1978.

Barring unforeseen problems, it appears that a world free from smallpox is now at hand.

30. Kempe CH: Smallpox. In Gellis SS, Kagan BM: Current Pediatric Therapy 8. WB Saunders Co., Philadelphia, 1978, 619–620.
An outline of the management of smallpox by a leader in the fight to eradicate this disorder.

31. Hoff G, Bauer S: A new rapid slide test for infectious mononucleosis. JAMA *194*:119–121, 1965.

Of 426 cases suspected of infectious mononucleosis, the the correct diagnosis was reached in 98.5 per cent by rapid slide test.

32. Patel BM: Skin rash with infectious mononucleosis. Pediatrics *40*:910–911, 1967.

A 100 per cent incidence of a copper-colored maculopapular rash in 13 patients with infectious mononucleosis treated with ampicillin.

33. Levene G, Baker H: Ampicillin and infectious mononucleosis. Br. J. Dermatol. *80*:417–418, 1978.

Infectious mononucleosis appears to have a tendency to render patients sensitive to ampicillin.

34. Lund A, Bergan T: Temporary skin reactions to penicillins during acute stage of infectious mononucleosis. Scand. J. Dis. *7*:21–28, 1975.

Studies in 19 patients with infectious mononucleosis allergic to penicillin and ampicillin during the acute stages of their illness with reversal of the reactivity after recovery from the disease.

35. Cawley EP, Wheeler CE: Rocky Mountain spotted fever. JAMA *163*:1003–1007, 1957.

Seventy-four cases of Rocky Mountain spotted fever encountered at the University of Virginia Hospital from 1945 through 1954.

36. Haynes RE, Sanders DY, Cramblett HG: Rocky Mountain spotted fever in children. J. Pediatr. *76*:685–693, 1970.

A review of 78 children with Rocky Mountain spotted fever.

37. Bradford WD, Hawkins HK: Rocky Mountain spotted fever in childhood. Am. J. Dis. Child. *131*:1228–1232, 1977.

Review of 138 cases of Rocky Mountain spotted fever indicates that the characteristic rash in combination with fever, tick bite, low serum sodium concentration, and thrombocytopenia is helpful in recognition of this serious and potentially lethal infectious disease.

38. Hattwick MAW, Retailliau H, O'Brien RJ, et al.: Fatal Rocky Mountain spotted fever. JAMA *240*:1499–1503, 1978.

Comparison of 44 fatal and 50 non-fatal cases of Rocky Mountain spotted fever emphasizes the need for early diagnosis and therapy of this disorder.

SKIN DISORDERS DUE TO FUNGI

Fungi are a group of simple plants that lack flowers, leaves, and chlorophyll and get their nourishment from dead or living organic matter, thus depending on plants, animals, and man for their existence. Fungal infections that affect man may be superficial, deep, or systemic, and sometimes fatal. Often regarded as trivial, diseases caused by fungi are no longer unimportant and remote problems in medicine and public health. Although they do not rank as pathogens with the bacteria or viruses, a number of species once thought to be ubiquitous and harmless have been implicated in various diseases, and with increasing use of broad-spectrum antibiotics, steroids, and potent cytotoxic agents, fatal deep mycoses have become increasingly frequent and significant.

The pathogenic fungal diseases are divided into superficial and deep infections. The superficial infections are those that are limited to the epidermis, hair, nails, and mucous membranes. The deep fungal infections are those in which the organisms affect other organs of the body or invade the skin through direct extension or hematogenous spread.

SUPERFICIAL FUNGAL INFECTIONS

There are three common types of superficial fungus infection, the dermatophytoses, tinea versicolor, and candidiasis (moniliasis). Those caused by dermatophytes are termed tinea, dermatophy-

277

tosis, or, because of the annular appearance of the lesions, ringworm.

The dermatophytes are a group of related fungi that live in soil, on animals, or humans, digest keratin, and invade the skin, hair, and nails, producing a diversity of clinical lesions. Depending upon the involved site, the infection may be termed tinea capitis, tinea barbae, tinea corporis, tinea manuum, tinea pedis, tinea cruris, or onychomycosis (tinea of the nails). The diagnosis and management of fungal diseases of childhood have become easier in the past decade owing to the development of more effective diagnostic techniques and therapeutic agents.

DIAGNOSIS OF FUNGAL INFECTIONS

Tests for fungal infection are rewarding procedures readily available to all physicians, not merely to those trained in dermatology.[1, 2] Diagnosis of ringworm of the scalp can frequently be aided by the presence of fluorescence under a Wood's light, by direct microscopic examination of cutaneous scrapings or infected hairs, or by fungal culture. These tests can be performed simply, inexpensively, and rapidly, as an office procedure. With the ready availability of these tests, I feel that it is best not to treat a possible fungal disorder without fungal culture, just as it is best not to treat a possible streptococcal throat infection without bacterial culture.

WOOD'S LIGHT EXAMINATION. The discovery in 1925 that hair infected by certain dermatophytoses would fluoresce when exposed to ultraviolet light filtered by a Wood's filter led to a helpful but occasionally improperly utilized diagnostic tool. When Wood's light examination is performed, it must be remembered that infected hairs, not the skin, fluoresce when exposed to light rays emitted in the 3560 Ångstrom (356 nanometer) range by this lamp. Although the nature and the source of the fluorescent substance in infected hairs are not fully understood, this phenomenon is believed to be the result of a substance, perhaps a pteridine, emitted when the fungus invades the hair (Fig. 13–1).

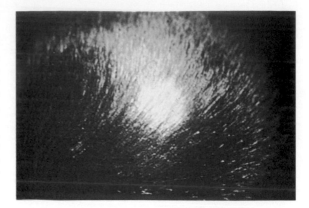

Figure 13–1 Tinea capitis. Fluorescence with Wood's light (Courtesy of Alfred S. Kopf, M.D., New York University Medical Center).

Optimally, a powerful Wood's lamp should be used in a completely darkened room. Under these conditions the majority of cases of tinea capitis will show fluorescence. Hairs infected by the *Microsporum* organisms *audouini* and *canis* produce a brilliant green fluorescence, and those infected by *Trichophyton schonleini* produce a pale green fluorescence. It must be remembered, however, that infections due to *Trichophyton tonsurans* and *violaceum* do not fluoresce. Sources of error include Wood's light examination in an insufficiently darkened room; the bluish or purplish fluorescence produced by lint, scales, serum exudate, or ointments containing petrolatum; and failure to remember that it is the infected hair and not the skin that fluoresces.

POTASSIUM HYDROXIDE WET-MOUNT PREPARATIONS. Microscopic examination of scrapings of cutaneous fungal infection is an important but frequently overlooked aid in the diagnosis of suspected fungal infection of the skin or hair. This examination will yield rapid results but requires considerable experience, as a consequence of which, unfortunately, it has achieved wide use only by those trained in the dermatologic disciplines (Fig. 13–2).

Material for mycological study should be

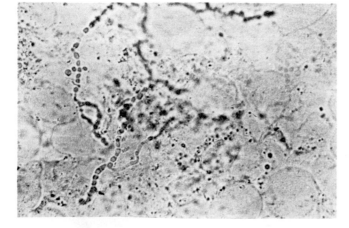

Figure 13–2 Fungal elements (hyphae) as seen on microscopic examination of a potassium hydroxide preparation (Courtesy of Alfred W. Kopf, M.D., New York University Medical Center).

taken by gently scraping outward from the active border of a suspected lesion with a dull scalpel blade. Cut hairs, nail scrapings, subungual debris, and material from the edge of the affected nail may also be utilized for wet-mount examination. Suspected material should be placed on a glass microscope slide with care and spread out flat and evenly in a single layer. A coverslip is applied, and one or two drops of 10 to 20 per cent potassium hydroxide are added at the side of the coverslip until the entire space between coverslip and slide is filled. This preparation should be heated slowly and gently (with care to prevent boiling of the potassium hydroxide, since this will cause crystallization) until the horny cells and debris are rendered translucent. If the potassium hydroxide solution contains dimethylsulfoxide (DMSO), the slide should not be heated, since heating a DMSO potassium hydroxide preparation will dissolve fungi as well as epidermal cells.[1]

After preparation of the specimen, gentle pressure is applied to the coverslip. When the material has been softened, this will improve the preparation by forcing out trapped air and thinning the specimen, thus allowing better visualization of fungi. It is further recommended that the light of the microscope condenser be dimmed, to enhance contrast between branched hyphae and epidermal elements.

FUNGAL CULTURE. Although direct microscopic examination of skin scrapings will often confirm the suspicion of a fungal disorder, definitive identification of the responsible agent requires isolation of the fungus by culture. There are several types of fungal culture media, but those with Sabouraud's maltose peptone agar, selective for fungi because of an acid pH, are most popular. However, since non-pathogenic fungi grow as well and more rapidly than most pathogenic organisms, a simple modification includes chloramphenicol to inhibit bacterial growth and cycloheximide to discourage non-pathogenic fungi.

The formulation and introduction of Dermatophyte Test Medium (DTM) in 1969 brought a new dimension to the gross screening of pathogenic dermatophytes.[2, 3] Dermatophyte Test Medium has antibiotics (cycloheximide, gentamycin, and chlortetracycline), which inhibit saprophytic fungi and bacteria. Of particular significance is the fact that the medium also contains phenol red as a color indicator. Non-pathogenic fungi ferment the glucose in culture media with an acidic byproduct. Thus, when not inoculated by a pathogenic dermatophyte, the medium maintains its original yellow color. Dermatophytes, conversely, do not cause fermentation of glucose but utilize nitrogenous ingredients, resulting in the production of alkaline byproducts and a color change from yellow to red. Although not quite as reliable as standard Sabouraud's media, DTM (available from Chester A. Baker Laboratories) is 95 to 97 per cent accurate, thus making it particularly useful for physicians who lack detailed knowledge of fungus colony morphology.[2, 3, 4]

Tinea Capitis

Tinea capitis, the most common dermatophytosis of childhood, is a fungal infection of the scalp characterized by scaling and patchy alopecia. Generally a disease of prepuberal children, chiefly those between two and ten years of age, it only rarely affects infants. Boys are afflicted five times more frequently than girls, and infection beyond the age of puberty may occur but is uncommon. The cause of resistance to tinea capitis infection after puberty is unknown but has been attributed to a higher content of fungistatic fatty acids in the sebum of postpuberal individuals. Although this hypothesis has not been proved, it has widespread acceptance and support.[5]

CLINICAL MANIFESTATIONS. Primary lesions of tinea capitis are characterized by the presence of broken-off hairs, 1 to 3 mm above the scalp, and partial alopecia. The infected areas are round or oval, sometimes irregular, and there may be coalescence of lesions, with formation of gyrate patterns. Individual patches generally measure 1 to 6 cm in diameter, and multiple patches are common (Figs. 13-3, 13-4).

Tinea capitis is produced only by species of *Microsporum* and *Trichophyton*. Lesions can be classified clinically as inflammatory or non-inflammatory. The latter type is exemplified by lesions of *Microsporum audouini*. The designation non-inflammatory is actually a misnomer. On histologic examination tinea capitis displays an inflammatory response and, with careful clinical examination, the presence of erythema and slight scaliness can be detected in most cases. However, the term "inflammatory" has gained wide acceptance and is useful in the description of lesions of tinea capitis associated with widespread pustulation, suppuration, or kerion formation. Tinea capitis due to *M. audouini* is characteristically non-inflammatory at the outset, and most

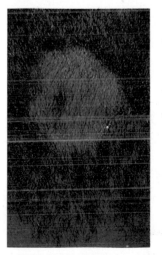

Figure 13-3 Tinea capitis. Broken hairs in a sharply circumscribed area of alopecia.

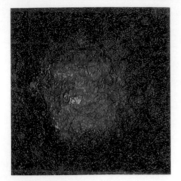

Figure 13-4   Inflammatory tinea capitis.

cases remain so throughout the course of the disease. In the early phases the features of the lesions are similar to those of tinea infection of glabrous skin. The central areas show scaling, and the borders are active and slightly elevated. The disorder is characterized by sharply delineated, usually rounded areas of alopecia on the scalp, which is not devoid of hair but covered with short lusterless stubs of hair broken off at 1 to 3 mm of length. The term "gray patch ringworm" has been applied to this disorder. Although *Microsporum audouini* heretofore has been the most common cause of tinea capitis in the United States, it is apparent that currently it is being replaced in many areas of the United States by *Trichophyton tonsurans*, the major cause of tinea capitis in Europe.[6]

Any dermatophyte causing tinea capitis may at times produce a sharply demarcated inflammatory indurated boggy granulomatous tumefaction called a kerion (Figs. 13–5 and 13–6). The onset of this condition is acute, lesions usually remain localized to one spot, and the area of involvement

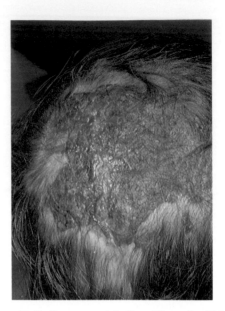

Figure 13-6   *T. tonsurans* infection of the scalp with kerion and alopecia.

is boggy, indurated, and studded with vesicles and pustules. Elicited most often by *Microsporum canis* and *Trichophyton tonsurans*, and in rural areas by *Trichophyton verrucosum*, an inflammatory kerion is believed to be associated with an intense allergic sensitization to the fungi.[6]

"Black dot" ringworm is a form of tinea capitis caused by *Trichophyton tonsurans* and *violaceum* and characterized by multiple small circular patches of alopecia, with only a few involved hairs, which are broken off very close to the cutaneous surface, resulting in a polka dot–like appearance. This type of involvement tends to produce a chronic diffuse alopecia. It should be noted that the "black dot" sign is probably overemphasized and, although present, is frequently relatively inconspicuous.[7]

Favus, a severe chronic form of tinea capitis rarely seen in the United States, is caused by the fungus *Trichophyton schonleini*. This disorder is characterized by scaly erythematous patches with honeycomb-yellow cup-like crusts that are termed scutula. It begins as a yellowish or red papule surrounded by a circle of vesicles, which progress to form friable nummular crusts that are yellowish brown to greenish brown; they coalesce to form plaques and exudate with a characteristic mouse-like odor. Such infections frequently result in considerable scarring and permanent alopecia.

DIAGNOSIS.   Tinea capitis may occasionally mimic other scalp conditions and may be confused with seborrheic dermatitis, psoriasis, alopecia areata, trichotillomania, folliculitis, impetigo, lupus erythematosus, folliculitis decalvans, and pseudopelade. When the diagnosis remains uncertain, Wood's light examination, demonstration of the fungus by potassium hydroxide wet-mount preparations of loose hairs removed from suspected areas, and fungal culture will help confirm the

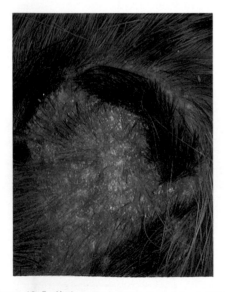

Figure 13-5   Kerion. An inflammatory boggy mass with pustules. This represents an exaggerated host response to a fungal infection.

diagnosis. It must be re-emphasized, however, that hairs infected with *Trichophyton tonsurans* and *violaceum* do not fluoresce.

Microscopic examination of a potassium hydroxide preparation of an infected hair will reveal tiny arthrospores surrounding the hair shaft in *Microsporum* infection (ectothrix involvement) and chains of arthrospores within the hair shaft (endothrix type) in *Trichophyton tonsurans* and *violaceum* infections (Fig. 13–7). Final definitive diagnosis may be obtained by planting several of the infected hairs or epidermal scales on appropriate culture media (Sabouraud's glucose agar or Dermatophyte Test Medium). A distinctive growth appears within 5 to 14 days on Sabouraud's agar. With DTM medium, a color change from yellow to red in the medium surrounding the fungus colony suggests the presence of a dermatophyte.

The color change in DTM may begin within a period of 24 to 48 hours for fast-growing dermatophytes and appears as a pinkish or red zone around the developing colony. The color will intensify as growth proceeds, with full color development for most cultures in three to seven days. When DTM medium is used, however, the culture should not be evaluated for color after 10 days, since contaminant fungal growth may cause color change by this time, thus leading to false positive results. It must be remembered that fungi grow best at room temperature and require oxygen. Accordingly, the culture media should be left at room temperature, and the tops of the culture tubes or bottles should be left slightly unscrewed

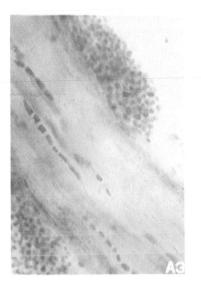

Figure 13–7 Tinea capitis: microscopic examination of a potassium hydroxide preparation. Endothrix infections (e.g.: *T. tonsurans* and *T. violaceum*) show spores within the hair shaft; in ectothrix involvement (e.g.: *Microsporum* infection) the arthrospores surround the hair shaft (Courtesy of Alfred W. Kopf, M.D., New York University Medical Center).

(or the tubes may be covered only with a cotton plug) to allow aeration of the preparation.

TREATMENT. Currently available topical antifungal agents do not appear to reach the hair bulb and therefore are ineffective in the treatment of tinea capitis. The introduction of griseofulvin (a metabolic product of several species of Penicillium) in 1958 marked the first effective systemic antidermatophytic agent, one that was curative for tinea capitis. The effect of griseofulvin appears to be related to its capacity to attach to newly formed keratin in skin, hair, and nails, where it exerts a fungistatic effect. Administered for periods of six to eight weeks or more, it is effective against all forms of tinea. The oral dose of microcrystalline griseofulvin is 10 to 20 mg/kg per day (generally 125 to 250 mg per day for children weighing 30 to 50 pounds, and 250 to 500 mg per day for those weighing over 50 pounds). For children unable to swallow tablets, Grifulvin-V suspension, 125 mg per teaspoon (Ortho) may be recommended, or Grisactin capsules, 125 mg (Ayerst), can be pulled apart and the powder dispensed in milk or other suitable vehicles.

A new form of ultramicrocrystalline griseofulvin dispersed in polyethylene glycol is available as Gris-Peg (Dorsey). This ultramicronized form has allowed the dosage to be cut to one half of the recommended dose of the microcrystalline forms. The manufacturer's recommended dosage of griseofulvin ultramicrosize (Gris-Peg) is not yet established for children two years of age or younger. Children over two who weigh 30 to 50 pounds should receive 62.5 to 125 mg per day; those weighing over 50 pounds should receive 125 to 250 mg of Gris-Peg daily. It should be recognized, however, that except for enhanced bioavailability and lower dosage schedules, the ultramicrocrystalline preparation does not appear to offer any significant increase in efficacy or safety over other available microsized formulations.

Griseofulvin appears to be absorbed more rapidly after a fatty meal and therefore is probably best given after ingestion of a meal containing fats (milk or ice cream may be recommended for this purpose). Medication should be continued for periods of four to eight weeks (two weeks after all clinical and laboratory examinations confirm absence of the fungus). Although a single 3 to 4 gm dose of microcrystalline griseofulvin will result in cure of most children with tinea capitis (particularly those cases due to *Microsporum* species that fluoresce under Wood's light examination), the six to eight week dosage regimen appears to have a higher curative rate with fewer recurrences.

Reported reactions to griseofulvin consist of hypersensitivity (morbilliform eruptions, urticaria, and angioneurotic edema), photosensitivity, gastrointestinal disturbances, mental confusion, dizziness, headaches (particularly in adults), insomnia, paresthesias of the hands and feet, albuminuria, leukopenia, and aplastic anemia. Although administration of griseofulvin should be discontinued if granulocytopenia occurs, most reported side effects are minor and probably have been exaggerated.

Griseofulvin also has some effect on porphyrin metabolism, and there have been reports of precipitation of acute porphyria in patients receiving this antibiotic. It also induces microsomal enzymes in the liver, thus decreasing the activity of warfarin-type anticoagulants; it is embryotoxic and teratogenic in rats; and evidence suggests hepatic carcinogenicity in male mice when given in amounts and duration comparable to dosages used in humans. More than 20 years of use, however, have revealed no evidence of hepatic carcinoma in humans. Griseofulvin, accordingly, should be avoided in patients with porphyria or hepatocellular failure and in pregnant women. Griseofulvin should be reserved for ringworm infections of the scalp, severe tinea infection of the nails, or for severe proven ringworm infections in other sites that have not responded to topical agents.

Although griseofulvin appears to be beneficial in the treatment of tinea capitis, concomitant topical therapy often is beneficial. Twice daily application of a topical antifungal agent may decrease dissemination of spores and infected particles and appears to hasten involution. Available topical antifungal agents include clotrimazole (Lotrimin and Mycelex), haloprogin (Halotex), miconazole (MicaTin), and tolnaftate (Tinactin). Of these, clotrimazole and miconazole appear to be more effective and also have an additional antimonilial effect (of particular value in fungal disorders in which monilia may be involved).

If a kerion is present, remember that this deep boggy inflammation is caused by an allergic reaction to the fungus. In resistant cases, a combination of prednisone and griseofulvin generally will ensure rapid clearing and help keep atrophy and permanent hair loss to a minimum.[6, 8] The oral administration of saturated solution of potassium iodide has also been recommended for the treatment of patients with kerion. Although I have had no personal experience with this modality for the treatment of tinea infection, Dr. Richard L. Dobson reports good results with this agent and feels that this form of therapy can eliminate the need for systemic steroid therapy for patients with resistant kerion formation.[9] The dosage of potassium iodide solution is discussed under the treatment of sporotrichosis in this chapter.

Tinea Barbae

Tinea barbae is an uncommon fungal infection of the bearded area and surrounding skin of adolescent and adult males. Since the most common etiologic agents are zoophilic species of *Trichophyton mentagrophytes* and *Trichophyton verrucosum* (occasionally *T. violaceum* and *T. rubrum*), it occurs primarily among individuals from rural areas in close contact with cattle or other domestic animals.

The infection generally is solitary or confluent and confined to one side of the face. Its clinical appearance is dependent upon the species of organism producing the infection. The majority of infections are characterized by highly inflammatory lesions with purulent follicles, inflammatory papules, pustules, exudate, crusts, and boggy nodules. The hairs in infected areas are loose or absent, and pus may be expressed through the follicular openings. Spontaneous resolution may occur, or the lesions may persist for months with resultant alopecia and scar formation.

Occasionally, a less inflammatory superficial variety may appear. This variant is characterized by mild pustular folliculitis, erythematous patches with or without broken-off hairs, and a raised vesiculopustular border and central clearing similar to that seen in lesions of tinea corporis.

Tinea barbae must be differentiated from bacterial folliculitis of the bearded area (sycosis barbae), contact dermatitis, herpes zoster, or severe herpes simplex. Sycosis barbae may be differentiated by the presence of papular and pustular lesions pierced in the center by a hair that is loose and easily extracted; herpes simplex or zoster frequently can be diagnosed by the presence of characteristic balloon cells on Tzanck smear preparations. When the diagnosis remains indeterminate, microscopic examination of a potassium hydroxide wet-mount for fungal elements and fungal culture generally will establish the correct diagnosis.

Although superficial inflammatory cases of tinea barbae frequently resolve spontaneously, generally after a period of months, both forms of tinea barbae may result in scar formation and alopecia. Warm saline compresses frequently aid in the removal of crusts, and topical antibacterial agents may help to control secondary bacterial infection. As in patients with tinea capitis, oral microcrystalline griseofulvin is generally required and will produce clearing, frequently within a period of four to six weeks.

Tinea Corporis

Superficial tinea infections of the non-hairy (glabrous) skin are termed tinea corporis. Sites of predilection include the non-hairy areas of the face (particularly in children), the trunk, and limbs, with exclusion of ringworm of the scalp (tinea capitis), bearded areas (tinea barbae), groin (tinea cruris), hands (tinea manuum), feet (tinea pedis), and nails (onychomycosis).

Tinea corporis tends to be asymmetrically distributed and is characterized by one or more annular, sharply circumscribed scaly patches with a clear center and scaly vesicular, papular, or pustular border (hence the term "ringworm") (Figs. 13–8 and 13–9). When multiple lesions are present, they may join together, thus giving rise to bizarre polycyclic configurations. Although the infection may involve people of all ages, the

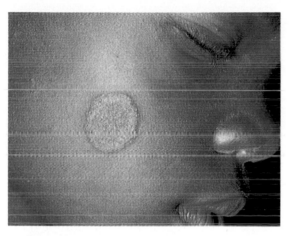

Figure 13–8 Tinea corporis. Ringworm with a clear center and a circinate papulovesicular border.

disorder is most commonly seen in children, in individuals in warm, humid climates, or in those with systemic diseases, such as diabetes mellitus, leukemia, or other debilitating illnesses. Although dermatophyte infections are rare in infancy, they may be seen during the first few weeks of life and have even been described (but not proved by culture) in an infant within six hours of birth.[10] Contact with domestic animals, particularly young kittens and puppies, is a common cause of the affliction in children. The causative organism frequently is *M. canis*, occasionally *M. audouini* or *T. mentagrophytes*. In adults, *T. rubrum*, *T. verrucosum*, *T. mentagrophytes*, or *T. tonsurans* is more likely to be found. In children with infection caused by *T. rubrum* or *Epidermophyton floccosum*, parents with tinea infection are commonly noted to be the source of infection.

CLINICAL MANIFESTATIONS. Tinea corporis is frequently manifested as a classic ringworm with annular, oval, or circinate lesions. At times, however, the pattern can vary and may mimic a wide variety of other dermatoses. Lesions may be eczematous, vesicular, pustular, and, less often, granulomatous in nature. Lesions may resemble the herald patch of pityriasis rosea, nummular eczema, psoriasis, contact dermatitis, seborrheic dermatitis, tinea versicolor, vitiligo, erythema chronicum migrans, various granulomatous lesions (particularly granuloma annulare), fixed drug eruptions, and lupus erythematosus. The use of topical corticosteroids may further mask the diagnosis by amelioration of signs and symptoms while the infection persists (Fig. 13–10). The term "tinea incognito" has been suggested for this phenomenon.[11] Of further significance is the fact that individuals with certain immunologic abnormalities such as atopic dermatitis, presumably due to a decreased cell-mediated delayed sensitivity and an increase in humoral (IgE) response, are particularly prone to chronic and recurrent dermatophyte infections.[12]

Although granulomatous lesions are uncommon in children, a perifollicular granulomatous disorder (Majocchi's granuloma) may appear, especially on the limbs of young women who shave their legs closely. This distinctive variant of ringworm is essentially a granulomatous folliculitis and perifolliculitis caused by *Trichophyton rubrum*, the primary focus frequently being a diffuse *T. rubrum* infection of the feet. The nodular lesions in this disorder usually involve only one leg, rarely exceed a centimeter in diameter, and are flat or only slightly elevated. If observed early, a hair may be noted in the center of the lesion. It is this infected ingrown hair (secondary to close shaving) that presumably incites the surrounding granulomatous skin infection.

The classic erythematous scaling with a sharply defined papulovesicular border is by no means the most common expression of this disorder, and any red scaly rash should be suspect for fungus until proved otherwise. Accordingly, a potassium hydroxide wet-mount examination and fungal cultures of appropriately collected cutaneous scrapings should be performed on any sus-

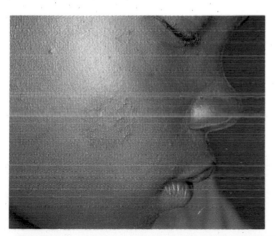

Figure 13–9 Resolving tinea corporis following two weeks of treatment with a topical antifungal preparation.

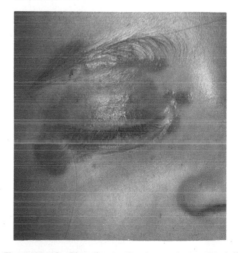

Figure 13–10 Tinea incognito. An atypical presentation of tinea corporis (the characteristic clinical features are masked owing to the use of topical corticosteroids).

pected lesions. As previously described, fluorescence under a Wood's light is not helpful in diagnosis of suspected lesions on glabrous (hairless) skin unless the lanugo hairs are infected. In this case, if the infection is associated with the *Microsporum* species, a light green fluorescence similar to that of *Microsporum*-induced tinea capitis may be observed. Infection of lanugo hairs, however, is extremely unusual. Accordingly, Wood's light examination of suspected tinea corporis generally is fruitless and unnecessary.

MANAGEMENT. Unfortunately there currently is considerable confusion among nondermatologists regarding the classification and management of cutaneous infection due to fungus. By definition, the term fungus infection incorporates disorders due to both tinea and monilia infection. It must be recognized, however, that dermatophytes and monilia are not synonymous, and that although nystatin is effective against monilial infection, it is inappropriate and ineffective in the treatment of tinea (dermatophyte) infection. Tolnaftate and undecylenic acid, although beneficial in the management of dermatophytoses such as tinea pedis, cruris, and corporis, also are ineffective against disorders due to monilial (candidal) infection. Topical antimonilial agents include nystatin, fungizone, and iodochlorhydroxyquin. Clotrimazole, haloprogin, and miconazole are effective in the topical therapy of both dermatophytes and monilia.

Most patients with tinea corporis, therefore, will respond to clotrimazole (Lotrimin and Mycelex), haloprogin (Halotex), micronazole (Mica-Tin), or tolnaftate (Tinactin) gently rubbed into the affected area and surrounding skin morning and evening. Even though clinical clearing and relief of pruritus is frequently seen within the first seven to ten days after initiation of therapy, treatment should be continued for a minimum period of two to three weeks after the affected area is clinically clear and fungal cultures are no longer positive. If a patient shows no clinical improvement after four weeks of therapy, the diagnosis should be reevaluated, and in unusually severe or extensive disease, a course of therapy with griseofulvin (as described for the treatment of tinea capitis) may be required.

Tinea Cruris

Tinea cruris ("jock itch") is an extremely common superficial fungus disorder of the groin and upper thighs. Seen primarily in adolescent and adult males, it may occur but is less common in females. It is more symptomatic in hot, humid weather and is most frequently noted in obese individuals or persons subject to vigorous physical activity, chafing, and tight-fitting clothing such as athletic supporters, jockey shorts, wet bathing suits, panty hose, or tight-fitting slacks. *Epidermophyton floccosum* traditionally has been associated with this infection, but both *Trichophyton*

rubrum and *Trichophyton mentagrophytes* frequently are responsible for this disorder, and it is commonly seen in association with tinea pedis.

The eruption is sharply marginated, is usually but not invariably bilaterally symmetrical and involves the intertriginous folds near the scrotum, the upper inner thighs, and occasionally the perianal regions, buttocks, and abdomen. The scrotum and labia are usually spared or only mildly involved, unless the eruption is caused by *Candida albicans*, overtreatment, or an associated neurodermatitis (Fig. 13–11). The margins are abrupt, frequently half-moon shaped, and the skin in the involved area is erythematous and scaly. The color may vary from red to brown, central clearing may be present, and an active vesiculo-pustular border, although uncommon, may be noted. In chronic infection the redness and scaling may be slight, the active margin may be subtle or ill defined, and lichenification may be present.

Tinea cruris must be differentiated from intertrigo, seborrheic dermatitis, psoriasis, primary irritant dermatitis or allergic contact dermatitis (generally due to therapy), or erythrasma (a fairly common chronic superficial dermatosis of the crural area caused by the diphtheroid *Corynebacterium minutissimum*. A characteristic coral-red fluorescence under Wood's light is helpful in diagnosis of the erythrasma (see Chapter 10). The presence of tinea cruris can be confirmed by potassium hydroxide microscopic examination of cutaneous scrapings and by fungal culture on appropriate media.

The treatment of tinea cruris consists of topical therapy with clotrimazole, haloprogin, micronazole, or tolnaftate preparations gently rubbed into the affected region and surrounding skin twice daily for a period of three to four weeks, reduction of excessive chafing and irritation by loose-fitting cotton underclothing, reduction of friction and perspiration by the use of a bland absorbent powder such as ZeaSorb Medicated Powder (Steifel), and for dermatophyte-induced lesions that are resistant or recur frequently, oral

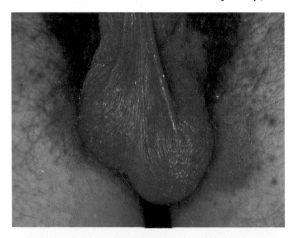

Figure 13–11   Scrotal infection caused by *Candida albicans*.

griseofulvin for a period of four or five weeks. For candida-induced infections, iodochlorhydroxy-quin (Vioform or Vioform HC, Ciba; Vytone Cream, Dermik) or clotrimazole (Lotrimin or Mycelex), haloprogin (Halotex), or micronazole (MicaTin) may be utilized. The last three preparations are effective in the management of both tinea- and monilia-induced disorders.

Tinea Pedis

Tinea pedis, or athlete's foot, is an extremely unusual dermatophyte infection in young children. More common in adolescents and adults, it represents the most prevalent ringworm infection seen in adults. Although children are not completely immune, most instances of "athlete's foot" in individuals below the age of puberty actually represent misdiagnosed examples of foot eczema, shoe dermatitis, or some other dermatosis[13] (Fig. 13–12).

The etiologic agents usually responsible for tinea pedis are *Trichophyton rubrum* and *Trichophyton mentagrophytes*, and less often *Epidermophyton floccosum*. The disorder may present clinically as an intertriginous inflammation, as a vesiculopustular eruption, or as a chronic scaling disorder with or without hyperkeratosis. Of these, interdigital lesions are the most common expression of the disorder and appear as fissuring, maceration, and interdigital scaling, generally in the web between the fourth and fifth toes, accompanied by maceration and peeling of the surrounding skin. In many instances the disorder remains localized to the interdigital webs and sides of the toes. In others, it may spread to affect the soles and, less often, other parts of the feet (Fig. 13–13). Contrary to the eruption seen in foot eczema, the dorsal aspect of the toes and feet generally remain clear.

The inflammatory vesiculopustular lesions generally result from *T. mentagrophytes* infection. Lesions may involve all areas of the foot, including the dorsal surface, but usually are patchy in

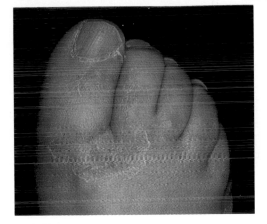

Figure 13–13 Tinea pedis with extension to the dorsal aspect of the foot.

distribution, with a predisposition to the midanterior plantar surface or instep (Fig. 13–14). Lesions occur most often in summer, and allergy to fungal elements may be reflected by a vesicular eruption on the palms and sides of the fingers, and occasionally by an erythematous vesicular eruption on the extremities and trunk, the so-called dermatophytid ("id") response. Although the mechanism of this frequently described but relatively uncommon eruption is not completely understood, it appears to result from absorption of the fungus or fungal products and an associated reaction between circulating antigen originating from the primary infection site and skin-sensitizing antibodies.

While vesicular dermatophytid reactions of the fingers and palms may appear as "id" reactions to tinea pedis, other causes of eczematous dermatitis or dyshydrotic eczema frequently are misinterpreted as true dermatophytid reactions in individuals with tinea pedis. The diagnosis of an "id" reaction accordingly is dependent upon absence of fungus in the area of the id reaction, a demonstrable focus of pathogenic fungus (generally on the feet), and spontaneous disappearance of the rash when the focus of infection has been eradicated.

The scaly hyperkeratotic variety of tinea pedis

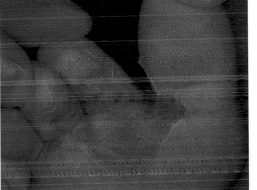

Figure 13–12 Tinea pedis in a 21-month-old child. This disorder (uncommon in prepuberal children) is characterized by fissuring, maceration, and scaling of the interdigital webs.

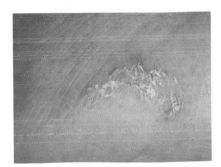

Figure 13–14 Tinea pedis. Scaly vesicular eruption on the instep of the foot.

is extremely chronic and resistant to treatment and may affect the soles, heels, and sides of the feet. In this form of tinea pedis, seen in adults more frequently than children, the disorder is generally bilateral (occasionally unilateral) and is characterized by a dull red or skin-colored, diffuse, often bran-like scaling, relative lack of inflammation, and extreme chronicity. When the process becomes diffuse over the entire plantar surface, the term "moccasin foot" is applied to this disorder.

The diagnosis of tinea pedis is dependent upon the clinical picture, with corroboration by potassium hydroxide examination of cutaneous scrapings and fungal culture. Tinea pedis frequently is difficult to control because of the moist and warm environment of the feet. Efforts to keep the feet dry are helpful. These include thorough drying of the feet after bathing, avoidance of occlusive footwear, frequent airing of the affected areas, avoidance of nylon socks or other fabrics that interfere with dissipation of moisture, and the wearing of sandals or perforated shoes to permit drying of the affected areas. Absorbent powders such as ZeaSorb or those containing undecylenic acid (Desenex powder) or tolnaftate (Tinactin Powder) may be used liberally once or twice a day, and 3 to 6 per cent salicylic acid in rubbing alcohol, aluminum chloride 20 per cent in anhydrous ethyl alcohol (available as Drysol, Person and Covey), or aluminum chloride in a 30 per cent concentration is an aid in the management of the hyperhidrosis commonly associated with persistent or recurrent lesions.[14]

Acute vesicular lesions should be treated with open wet compresses (Burow's solution 1:80) applied for 10 to 15 minutes three to four times a day for three to five days (see Chapter 3), bed rest if the disorder is severe, and topical antifungal preparations such as clotrimazole, haloprogin, miconazole, or tolnaftate. Severe, chronic, and recalcitrant forms of tinea pedis that are uncontrollable by topical therapy may require treatment with systemic microsize griseofulvin (10 to 20 mg per kg of body weight per day) for periods up to 6 to 12 months. "Id" reactions, when present, are best treated by open wet compresses, topical corticosteroids, and eradication of the primary source of infection.

Tinea Manuum

Ringworm infections of the hand (tinea manus, tinea manuum) are uncommon in childhood and, when present, generally are seen on the palms in postpubertal individuals. The disorder is usually unilateral and has morphologic changes similar to those seen in individuals with chronic scaly dermatophytosis of the feet. Usually it is caused by the same fungi responsible for tinea pedis, *Trichophyton rubrum*, *Trichophyton mentagrophytes*, and *Epidermophyton floccosum*, and may be seen in association with ringworm infection of the feet.

Clinical manifestations range from diffuse hy-perkeratosis of the fingers and palm, accompanied by a fine branny adherent scale that is especially prominent in the flexural creases, to a less common patchy inflammatory vesicular reaction. Other clinical variants include discrete erythematous papular and follicular scaly patches or severe scaling and exfoliation (Fig. 13–15). Involvement of the fingernails frequently occurs in association with this disorder. When present, it is seldom that all the nails of the involved hand are infected. Total nail involvement, when seen, should make one suspect psoriasis and, less commonly, lichen planus.

Ringworm infections of the hand frequently masquerade as psoriasis, allergic contact or primary irritant dermatitis, dyshidrosis, and, less commonly, as a dermatophytid reaction. The fact that the infection frequently is unilateral is a clue to the diagnosis, which then can be corroborated by potassium hydroxide microscopic examination and fungal culture of cutaneous scrapings.

The management of tinea manuum is essentially the same as that recommended for tinea pedis, with the exception of the environmental measures outlined for the treatment of dermatophytosis of the feet. It must be remembered, however, that ringworm of the hand often is accompanied by tinea pedis, and that when both sites are affected they generally should be treated simultaneously.

Tinea Unguium (Onychomycosis)

Tinea unguium (onychomycosis) is a chronic fungal infection of the fingernails or toenails caused by *Trichophyton rubrum*, *Trichophyton mentagrophytes*, and *Epidermophyton floccosum* (the dermatophytes that usually affect the hands and feet), and, at times, *Candida albicans*. Rarely seen in children, the disorder generally occurs in association with tinea pedis or tinea manuum, but may occur as a primary infection or in association

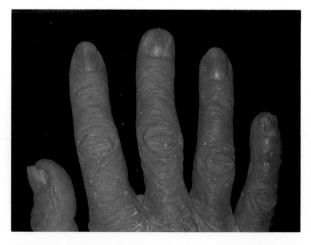

Figure 13–15 Onychomycosis. Tinea of the hand (tinea manuum) with nail involvement.

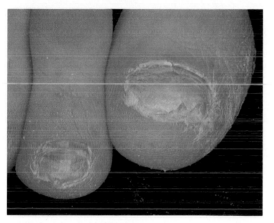

Figure 13–16 Onychomycosis. Thickening, discoloration, and crumbling of the nail plate in a 16-year-old boy.

with other dermatophytoses (Figs. 13–15 and 13–16).

The disorder usually has its origin at the distal edge of the nail and first becomes evident at the lateral border of the distal tip of the nail. The onset is slow and insidious, and toenails are affected more frequently than fingernails. The disorder first begins as an opaque white or silvery, then yellow and later brown, patch at the sides and distal tip of the nail plate. Subungual debris collects and actual invasion of the nail plate then occurs, and the nail slowly becomes discolored, thickened, deformed, and friable, and because of accumulation of subungual keratin, loosened from the nail plate.

In onychomycosis due to *Candida albicans* there often is an associated paronychia (Fig. 13–17). The adjacent cuticle is pink, swollen, and tender, and on pressure, occasionally a small amount of pus may be expressed from the lateral border. In other instances the nail plate may show brown or gray discoloration at the lateral nail edge or white or gray spots without development of further dystrophy. In contrast to onychomycosis

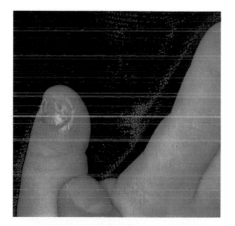

Figure 13–17 Onychomycosis due to *Candida albicans*. Candidal onychomycosis, in contrast to onychomycosis due to tinea infection, almost exclusively affects fingernails rather than toenails.

due to tinea infection, candidal onychomycosis almost exclusively affects the fingernails rather than toenails and is seen more commonly in individuals who frequently have their hands in water.

Onychomycosis must be differentiated from psoriasis, dystrophy secondary to eczema or chronic paronychia, trauma, tetracycline-induced photo-onycholysis, pachyonychia congenita, lichen planus, nail-patella syndrome, and other nail dystrophies (see Chapter 17). It must be remembered that onychomycosis is seldom symmetrical and that it is common to find involvement of only one, two, or three nails of only one hand. In all suspected cases the feet should be examined with care, since infection is frequently found there, and if all ten fingernails are abnormal, some cause other than ringworm should be sought.

Accurate diagnosis depends upon direct microscopic examination of potassium hydroxide preparations and identification of the organism by fungus culture. When collecting specimens it is essential to obtain samples from the ventral nail plate and subungual keratinous material rather than from the nail surface, and since the responsible organism in onychomycosis is difficult to demonstrate, repeated scrapings and cultures frequently may be necessary.

Despite recent advances in antifungal therapy, topical agents are rarely effective, and oral administration of griseofulvin (for periods of 6 months for fingernails, 12 to 18 months for toenails) for the treatment of dermatophyte-induced tinea unguium is frequently disappointing. Since the treatment of onychomycosis is a long-term process, patients should be advised that even prolonged therapy may not lead to cure, and that recurrences are all too frequent.[15]

If the disorder proves to be associated with *Candida albicans*, topical application of clotrimazole, haloprogin, miconazole, nystatin, or Mycolog to the periungual region generally is beneficial. With this organism, however, therapy will not be effective unless the affected digits (usually the fingers) are kept dry. Exposure to water should be kept to a minimum, and inexpensive cotton gloves should be worn under protective rubber or latex gloves when immersion in water cannot be avoided. Cotton-lined rubber gloves are of relatively little value, since the lining frequently becomes saturated with perspiration. A solution of 4 per cent thymol in chloroform applied under the nail folds two or three times daily and immediately following immersion in water frequently will help keep the area dry and may prove helpful in the management of persistent monilial-induced nail disorders.

TINEA VERSICOLOR

Tinea versicolor (pityriasis versicolor) is an extremely common superficial fungal disorder of the skin characterized by multiple scaling, oval macular and patchy lesions, usually distributed over the upper portions of the trunk, proximal

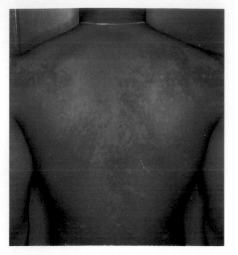

Figure 13–18 Tinea versicolor. Multiple oval hypopigmented macules with fine, almost imperceptible scales.

arms, and occasionally the face or other areas (Fig. 13–18). The lesions may be hypopigmented or hyperpigmented (fawn-colored or brown), depending upon the patient's complexion and exposure to sunlight. This disorder is caused by the dimorphic fungus *Pityrosporum orbiculare* (originally called *Malassezia furfur)*, which exists predominantly in the yeast phase on normal skin and causes clinical lesions only when substantial numbers of filamentous forms develop. The reason for proliferation of hyphal forms in lesions is unknown, but findings of glycogen granules in unusual amounts in the normal skin of patients with tinea versicolor suggests the presence of some underlying disorder such as malnutrition, poor general health, treatment with steroids, or a genetic predisposition to the disorder.[16]

Usually seen as a disorder of adolescents and young adults 15 to 30 years of age, it has been found in senior citizens, prepubertal children, and, at times, even in infants.[17, 18] Generally asymptomatic and extremely chronic, the lesions become more prominent during the summer months when the patient is exposed to sunlight and the involved areas fail to tan following sun exposure. Lesions accordingly become lighter than the surrounding skin in summer and relatively darker during winter, hence the term tinea versicolor. In the past, the hypopigmentation was attributed to a sun-screening effect. However, closer observations do not support this hypothesis but suggest that the organism may suppress the formation of melanin or that an abnormal transfer of pigment from melanocytes to keratinocytes may be the cause of the pigmentary disturbance seen in this disorder.[19]

DIAGNOSIS. The eruption in tinea versicolor usually is distinctive and the diagnosis frequently can be made on clinical grounds and confirmed by potassium hydroxide wet-mounts of cutaneous scrapings. Conditions most commonly confused with this disorder include pityriasis alba, postinflammatory hypopigmentation, vitiligo, me-

lasma, seborrheic dermatitis, pityriasis rosea, and secondary syphilis. When the diagnosis is uncertain, demonstration of a coppery orange, bronze, or blue-white fluorescence under the Wood's light (in a darkened room) or demonstration of highly characteristic fungal hyphae and spores in grape-like clusters (in a "spaghetti-and-meatballs" appearance) on microscopic examination of a potassium hydroxide slide preparation of scrapings from lesions generally will help confirm the diagnosis. Fungal cultures, however, are unsatisfactory, owing to the fact that the organisms are difficult to grow on culture media.

TREATMENT. Tinea versicolor generally responds readily to a variety of topical preparations. However, since the course of the disorder generally is chronic and the primary etiologic agent *(P. orbiculare)* is a normal saprophytic inhabitant of the skin, treatment generally must be thorough and recurrences are common. Wood's light fluorescence of lesions of tinea versicolor is valuable in the management of this disorder, since it helps to delineate distal areas of involvement not seen in ordinary light. Selenium sulfide shampoo (Exsel, Iosel, or Selsun) in a 2.5 per cent concentration is a convenient, rapid, and highly effective mode of therapy for this disorder.[20] This is accomplished by application of a thin layer of the preparation to the affected area overnight, with care to see that the entire cutaneous surface is covered, once a week for a period of three to four weeks, followed by monthly applications for three months (in an effort to help prevent recurrences of this disorder). The preparation is washed off in the morning by bath or shower, at which time the patient should be instructed to change all night clothes, bedding, and undergarments.

Response to therapy should be assessed by potassium hydroxide wet-mount microscopic examination of cutaneous scrapings. The patient should be advised that this is a benign, occasionally pruritic, but otherwise primarily cosmetic disorder, that the hypopigmentation will not return to normal until sun exposure allows remelanization of the affected areas, and that recurrences, especially during the hot and humid months, are common. Recurrences, when noted, should be treated early in an effort to prevent extensive cutaneous involvement. Alternate remedies include a 15 to 25 per cent solution of sodium hyposulfite or thiosulfate. Twenty-five per cent sodium thiosulfate with 1 per cent salicylic acid is readily available as Tinver lotion (Barnes-Hind) and should be applied twice daily for a period of two to four weeks. Antifungal agents such as clotrimazole, haloprogin, miconazole, and tolnaftate, although effective, are relatively more expensive and, except perhaps in cases resistant to other modes of therapy, do not appear to offer any substantial advantage.

CANDIDIASIS (MONILIASIS)

Candidiasis (moniliasis) is an acute or chronic infection of the skin, mucous membranes, and occasionally the internal organs, caused by yeast-like fungi of the *Candida* genus. Although other candidal species can be responsible for human infection, *Candida albicans* is the most frequent cause of this disorder.

Candida albicans is not a saprophyte of normal skin. It exists in the microflora of the oral cavity, gastrointestinal tract, and vagina and becomes a cutaneous pathogen when an alteration in the host defenses, either localized or generalized, allows the organism to become invasive.

Factors that predispose to candidiasis include endocrinologic disorders (diabetes mellitus, hypoparathyroidism, and Addison's disease), genetic disorders (Down's syndrome, acrodermatitis enteropathica, chronic mucocutaneous candidiasis, granulomatous disease of childhood), debilitating disorders such as leukemia or lymphoma, and the administration of systemic antibiotics, corticosteroids, anovulatory drugs, or immunosuppressive agents.

Newborns are physiologically susceptible to candidal infection, which may be manifested as oral moniliasis (thrush) or, less commonly, as a localized or generalized dermatitis. Candidiasis in the infant is traceable almost invariably to an infected mother who may be a vaginal or intestinal carrier of the organism. These infants invariably harbor *Candida albicans* in the mouth or intestinal canal (see Figs. 2–20 and 2–21) and the infected saliva or stools constitute a focus for cutaneous infection.[21] See Chapter 2 for a more in depth discussion of monilial diaper dermatitis.

Oral Candidiasis (Thrush)

Oral candidiasis (thrush) is a painful inflammation of the tongue, soft and hard palates, and buccal and gingival mucosae characterized by whitish-gray, often confluent, friable, cheesy pseudomembranous patches or plaques on a markedly reddened mucosa (Fig. 2–21). Often not clinically apparent until eight or nine days of life, the disorder is acquired at the time of delivery during passage through the vaginal canal. The overall incidence of maternal vaginitis has been estimated to be 20 to 25 per cent. In a study of 1442 mothers, 18 per cent had positive vaginal cultures of *Candida albicans* in early labor. Oral cultures were positive in 20 per cent of infants of mothers who had positive vaginal cultures and, of these, one-half (55 per cent) had clinical thrush.[22]

Occurrences of oral thrush in adults, infants, and children are clinically similar and can be diagnosed by gentle removal of the curd-like plaques, which, unlike milk particles, adhere to the underlying oral mucosa, by gently rubbing the area with a cotton applicator or tongue blade with a resulting underlying inflammatory mucosal erosion. The organism may be identified by potassium hydroxide wet-mount preparation or a Gram's stain of material removed from a plaque, or by fungal culture. Lesions usually respond promptly to careful removal of the curd-like lesions after each feeding by a cotton applicator dipped into a mixture of one-quarter teaspoon of baking soda and one or two drops of liquid detergent mixed in a glass of warm water or to careful removal of lesions by a cotton applicator dipped into a nystatin suspension (Mycostatin Oral Suspension or Nilstat Oral Suspension). Persistent or recurrent lesions in infants and young children may be treated by oral administration of nystatin (100,000 units per ml of Mycostatin Oral Suspension or Nilstat Oral Suspension) 2 ml four times a day until 48 hours after the lesions have disappeared and cultures have been normal for 48 hours (generally a period of 7 to 14 days). Oral candidiasis in older individuals can be treated by Mycostatin Oral Tablets, one to three tablets (500,000 to 1,000,000 units) three times daily, or by the use of antimonilial vaginal tablets (although not FDA-approved for this purpose), available as Mycostatin Vaginal Tablets or as Gyne-Lotrimin or Mycelex-G Vaginal Tablets, held in the mouth and allowed to dissolve, two or three times a day, for a period of one to two weeks).

Cutaneous Candidiasis

Candidiasis may present a variety of cutaneous manifestations. The moist warm conditions found in intertriginous areas favors its development. Accordingly the disorder frequently affects the folds of the body (the groin, perineum, intergluteal, and, particularly in obese individuals, the inframammary folds). It also affects the interdigital spaces, particularly those of the third and fourth fingers; see *erosio interdigitalis blastomycetica* below.

Two types of candidiasis have been reported in the newborn period, a congenital form in which the skin lesions are present at birth or shortly thereafter and a neonatal form commonly seen after the first week of life.[23] In the congenital form the skin lesions involve the head, face, neck, trunk, and extremities. The diaper area is spared, but the intertriginous areas, posterior aspect of the trunk, and extensor surfaces of the extremities may be severely affected. Occasionally, the nails, palms, and soles may be involved. The rash begins with an intense erythema and small white papules that gradually increase in number and become pustular.[24]

The syndrome of congenital cutaneous candidiasis differs from the classical form of candidal dermatitis of the newborn infant. Whereas congenital cutaneous candidiasis represents an intrauterine infection, candidal dermatitis of the newborn is acquired by passage through an infected vagina, with onset of cutaneous lesions at a later date. The clinical period of congenital cutaneous candidiasis may resemble erythema toxicum, bacterial folliculitis, bullous impetigo, congenital herpes, varicella, or syphilis.[24] It is distinguished by a progressive but relatively benign course, absence of constitutional signs, and the recovery of *Candida* organisms by direct smear and fungal culture from the cutaneous lesions. The prognosis is good. Lesions progress from erythema and pustules to a drying exfoliative stage and clear spontaneously after a period of several weeks. With systemic and topical nystatin therapy, however, the disorder generally resolves within a period of three to ten days.

In late-onset neonatal candidiasis, in contrast to congenital cutaneous candidiasis, early lesions radiate from the perianal area into the gluteal folds with satellite lesions and spread to the perineum, genitalia, suprapubic areas, buttocks, and inner thighs. The infection may be restricted in extent or may go on to involve the entire area. The typical vivid-red hue, glistening skin, and characteristic pustulo-vesicular border, when present, are the hallmarks of this disorder (Fig. 2–20). It is highly significant that a majority of older infants with cutaneous candidiasis harbor *C. albicans* in the intestine, suggesting infected stools as the primary focus of candidiasis in the diaper area.[21]

Occasionally a widespread cutaneous dermatitis may occur, either as a result of progression from an untreated localized area or by contamination of the skin from an infected maternal vagina during the process of delivery. In this variant, superficial vesiculopustules rupture, leaving a denuded surface. Lesions spread peripherally and form confluent plaques of dermatitis with generalized scaling. When the etiology of the dermatosis is not readily apparent, direct microscpic examination of cutaneous scrapings (particularly the white scale and the edge of lesions) and fungal culture will help establish the correct diagnosis (Figs. 2–22 and 2–23).

The treatment of superficial infections of the skin caused by *Candida albicans* consists of the use of topical antimonilial agents such as 1 per cent topical clotrimazole cream or lotion (Lotrimin or Mycelex), 2 per cent miconazole cream or lotion (MicaTin), 1 per cent haloprogin cream or solution (Halotex), or nystatin, 100,000 units per gram (available as Candex Creme or Lotion or Nilstat Topical Cream or Ointment). Although Mycolog cream or ointment (a formulation of nystatin, neomycin, gramicidin, and triamcinolone acetonide) is also effective, many authorities avoid these preparations because of the presence of a topical corticosteroid (triamcinolone) and possible hypersensitivity to the neomycin, gramicidin, paraben, or ethylenediamine contained in them. It should be noted that ethylenediamine and parabens are contained in the cream, but not in the ointment formulations.

Candidal Vulvovaginitis

Candida albicans is a common inhabitant of the vaginal tract, but its incidence increases in diabetes and pregnancy, and in females taking antibiotics or oral anovulatory preparations. When vulvovaginitis occurs, the labia become edematous and red, white patches appear on an erythematous mucosal surface, and leukorrhea develops, with painful itching, burning, and an associated discomfort on micturition. The infection may spread to the perineum, perianal region, gluteal folds, and upper inner aspects of the thigh.

Diagnosis is established by the clinical signs and symptoms and by demonstration of the fungus by potassium hydroxide microscopic examination and fungal culture. Treatment consists of nystatin vaginal tablets, available as Mycostatin Vaginal Tablets (Squibb), 100,000 units, deposited high in the vagina by means of an applicator twice daily for 7 to 14 days, or clotrimazole vaginal tablets, available as Gyne-Lotrimin Vaginal Tablets or Mycelex-G Vaginal Tablets, 100 mg per tablet inserted intravaginally at bedtime for seven consecutive days.

Perlèche

Perlèche, angular cheilitis, is a common disorder characterized by fissuring and inflammation of the corners of the mouth, with associated maceration and softening of the adjacent cutaneous surface (Fig. 13–19). This condition is not due to vitamin B deficiency. It is associated with moisture collecting in the corners of the mouth. In adults it is generally due to ill-fitting dentures; in children it is seen in conjunction with overbite, overlapping, the wearing of braces, and poor closure of the mouth. This disorder is best managed by the use of petrolatum or steroid ointments applied two or three times a day to the corners of the mouth, avoidance of the habit of lip-licking, and, when monilia or secondary bacterial infection is present, the application of topical antibiotics and topical antimonilial agents, alone or in combination.

Erosio Interdigitalis Blastomycetica

Erosio interdigitalis blastomycetica (derived from the Latin, meaning an erosion between digits caused by a budding fungus) is a red, itchy, and occasionally slightly painful, well-defined oval-shaped eruption of the webs between and extending to the sides of fingers (Fig. 13–20). Usually, but not necessarily, involving the area between the third and fourth fingers (occasionally the second and third or fourth and fifth fingers, and rarely a

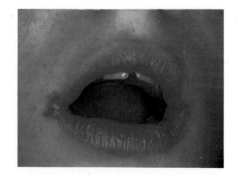

Figure 13–19   Perléche. Maceration, erythema, and fissuring of the corners of the mouth associated with *Candida albicans*.

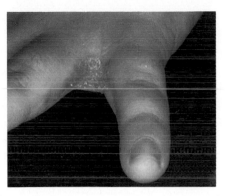

Figure 13-20 Erosio interdigitalis blastomycetica. Cutaneous candidiasis of the interdigital web.

corresponding surface of the toes), the disorder is manifested by fissuring, maceration, and exfoliation of the affected region, with a characteristic scaly and occasionally vesicular or papulovesicular border. It appears to be associated with infection due to *Candida albicans* and an associated, possibly syngergistic gram-negative infection, particularly in individuals who tend to perspire a great deal or who frequently have their hands immersed in water.[25] Treatment of erosio interdigitalis blastomycetica consists of avoidance of moisture to the intertriginous webs and the use of topical antibacterial as well as topical antimonilial preparations.

Black Hairy Tongue

Black hairy tongue is a term used to describe a disorder of adults and occasionally adolescents characterized by hypertrophic elongated filiform papillae, which form a dense black, bluish-black, or brown mat-like surface on the mid portion of the dorsum of the tongue (Fig. 13–21). The etiology of this disorder is unknown, but it frequently is attributed to the prevalence of *Candida albicans*, aspergillosis, or the filamentous mycelia of fungi that grow on the tongue's dorsal surface, and is

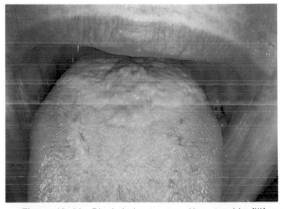

Figure 13-21 Black hairy tongue. Hypertrophic filiform papillae on the dorsal aspect of the tongue due to *Candida albicans* (a complication of long-term systemic tetracycline therapy for acne vulgaris).

often associated with prolonged use of antibiotics.

The most effective treatment consists of discontinuation of possible offending systemic antibiotics and gentle brushing of the dorsum of the tongue with a soft tooth-brush, alone or with a papain paste made up of a solution of four parts water and one part Adolph's Meat Tenderizer. This helps remove retained debris and generally results in clinical improvement of the disorder.

Systemic Candidiasis

While superficial skin and mucosal infections are common in the neonatal period, serious *Candida* infections are encountered much less frequently. Systemic candidiasis presents a major challenge to the clinician, since neither diagnostic nor therapeutic measures are entirely satisfactory. The disorder may affect the lungs, bronchial tree, meninges, kidneys, bladder, joints, and, less commonly, the liver, myocardium, endocardium, and eyes. Drug addiction and in-dwelling intravenous catheters, as well as direct trauma during intracardiac surgery, have been implicated in this disorder.[26]

Although almost indistinguishable from corresponding bacterial, viral, or other fungal diseases, the disorder may be suspected in patients with intermittent, spiking, therapy-resistant fever, with cutaneous or unusual candidal lesions or cellulitis at the site of an intravenous catheter. The diagnosis is confirmed by isolation of *Candida* from blood, abscesses, urine, or other body fluids, by demonstration of the organism in cutaneous biopsy or other surgical specimens, and by the presence of hypergammaglobulinemia and precipitating antibodies to cytoplasmic antigens of *C. albicans*.

Treatment is directed toward removal of iatrogenic factors, treatment of the underlying illness, and specific antifungal therapy. Nystatin, 1 to 1.5 million units per day in infants or 3 to 6 million units per day in older children, may be administered as the oral suspension (for infants) or in tablet form (for older individuals). Amphotericin may be administered in dosages of 0.25 mg/kg to 1 mg/kg intravenously daily, or 1.5 mg/kg every other day. The toxicity of amphotericin B (anemia, thrombocytopenia, and nephrotoxicity), however, requires caution with the use of this preparation. In such cases, oral clotrimazole (60 to 150 mg/kg per day) in three divided doses, flucytosine (100 mg/kg/day) divided into four doses, or intravenous miconazole (30 to 60 mg/kg daily), given at eight-hour intervals, may be administered.[27, 28] Although flucytosine may be given orally and is relatively safe, resistant strains of *Candida* often develop during therapy.[29]

Chronic Mucocutaneous Candidiasis

Chronic mucocutaneous candidiasis is a progressive candidal infection that usually is associated with endocrinopathy or immunologic deficiency, with severe defects in the thymus-controlled lymphocyte defense system. Although the disorder may have its onset in the neonatal period, it usually manifests itself later in infancy or early childhood.

It may begin as an oral candidiasis (thrush), candidal diaper dermatitis, candidal intertrigo, or paronychia that is persistent and resistant to the usual modes of therapy. The disorder persists and spreads to involve the scalp, eyelids, nose, hands, and feet, and may be characterized by intertrigo, pathognomonic satellite pustules, erythematous lesions covered with dry scaly patches, or thick macerated crusts (Fig. 10–12). Coalescence of individual lesions often leads to the formation of crusted granulomatous areas with verrucous surfaces and horn-like projections. Dystrophy of the nails, scarring, and loss of hair are common sequelae.

Although the disorder to date has been refractory to therapy, systemic candidiasis is uncommon. Death, when it occurs, is usually seen in individuals with immunodeficiency syndromes and associated severe and recurrent infections of various types.[30] Although there are patients with chronic mucocutaneous candidiasis who also have extensive and persistent dermatophytosis, this is usually not seen in association with this disorder.

Nystatin and amphotericin B in the past have been the treatments of choice for this disorder. Unfortunately, neither of these antifungal antibiotics are absorbed from the gastrointestinal tract sufficiently to be of value in the oral treatment of systemic infection. Although the intravenous or prolonged administration of amphotericin B may result in clearing of chronic mucocutaneous candidiasis, recurrence invariably occurs when treatment is discontinued, and nephrotoxicity precludes its continued use.

In recent years, there have been reports of successful treatment of chronic mucocutaneous candidiasis with the newer antifungal agents. Clotrimazole (60 to 150 mg/kg per day taken in three divided doses) or intravenous miconazole (30 to 60 mg/kg daily, given at eight-hour intervals) may be administered. Clotrimazole can be given orally, and side effects are limited to gastrointestinal intolerance, leukopenia, and elevated liver enzymes, all of which are reversible. Because the drug induces hepatic microsomal enzymes that affect its metabolism, the manufacturer (Delbay Pharmaceuticals) recommends that it be given for two-week courses, followed by a two-week rest period.[31]

DEEP FUNGAL DISORDERS

In contrast to the superficial dermatophytes, which are confined to dead keratinous tissue, certain mycotic infections have the capacity for deep invasion of the skin or produce skin lesions secondary to systemic visceral infection, usually of the lungs and reticuloendothelial system.

SUBCUTANEOUS MYCOSES

The subcutaneous mycoses are a group of disorders caused by a number of fungi that exist as soil saprophytes and are normally of low virulence. Although these infections (sporotrichosis, chromoblastomycosis, histoplasmosis, blastomycosis, coccidiomycosis, and cryptococcosis) are found most often in adults with occupational exposure to soil and plants, all age groups are potentially susceptible.[32]

Sporotrichosis

Sporotrichosis is a granulomatous fungal infection of the skin and subcutaneous tissues caused by *Sporotrichum schenkii*, a dimorphous fungus of worldwide distribution commonly isolated from soil and plants. It occurs in patients of all ages and is observed most commonly in adult males who, because of their occupation or leisure-time activities, are likely to be exposed to contaminated soil or vegetation (farmers, florists, gardeners, forestry workers, miners, individuals who work with contaminated packing material, or children at play). It appears that children are just as susceptible to this disease as adults; the relatively infrequent reports of childhood forms of this disorder probably reflect a lesser degree of exposure to contaminated material among individuals in this age group.[33, 34, 35]

Lymphocutaneous sporotrichosis is the most common manifestation of the disease. Seen in 75 per cent of all reported cases, it follows a wound inflicted by an object, such as a splinter, thorn, straw, grain, rock, or glass, contaminated with the organism. The initial lesion is characterized by a small, firm, painless dusky papule that develops at the site of trauma, slowly enlarges and eventually ulcerates, and is followed by a series of subcutaneous nodules with overlying erythema and occasional ulceration along the course of lymphatic drainage (Fig. 13–22). The disorder is almost always unilateral. A well-developed lesion appears as a 2 to 4 cm violaceous nodule with central ulceration, undermined edges, and considerable crusting. In adult cases most lesions occur on exposed surfaces of the arms and legs; in childhood cases, lesions on the face and trunk are fairly common as well.[33]

The second most common form of sporotrichosis is a fixed cutaneous form, which appears in endemic areas, in which infection in a previously sensitized person does not spread along lymphatic channels but remains localized at the site of entrance of the organism. Localized forms of this disorder range from scaly maculopapular lesions to verrucous and weeping ulcerations with or without satellite lesions. In other instances there may be primary chancriform lesions, with enlarge-

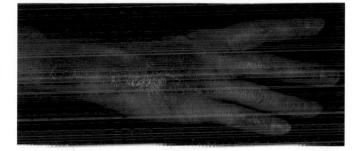

Figure 13-22 Sporotrichosis. Subcutaneous nodules, ulceration, and erythema along the course of lymphatic drainage.

ment of the regional lymph nodes without intervening nodules along the lymphatic channels, and in some cases, mucous membrane involvement may give rise to suppurative ulcerating, vegetative, or granulomatous lesions.

Disseminated sporotrichosis is an uncommon manifestation of this disorder seen in individuals with compromised immunologic capacity, such as those with sarcoidosis, malignant neoplasms, diabetes mellitus, or chronic alcoholism. In such cases, the cutaneous lesions may be widespread and may be located on the extremities in a pattern suggestive of embolic spread.[34, 36]

Atypical mycobacterium infections, localized granulomatous lesions, bacterial infections, primary syphilis, cat-scratch disease, leishmaniasis, tuberculosis, anthrax, blastomycosis, tularemia, and occasionally nocardial infections can all cause lesions that mimic cutaneous sporotrichosis. When the diagnosis is uncertain, demonstration of the organism on fungal culture, preferably from ulcerative lesions or aspiration of unopened nodules, is confirmatory. Direct examination of smears or biopsy material is usually unrewarding, but a fluorescent antibody-staining technique may aid in rapid diagnosis of this disorder.[32]

The treatment of choice for cutaneous sporotrichosis is orally administered saturated solution of potassium iodide, five drops three times a day, increased by one drop each day until a maximum of 25 to 40 drops per day is reached, or until signs of intolerance (salivation, burning mouth, headache, or gastric intolerance) appear. This is administered after meals and if necessary may be supplemented by intravenous sodium iodide. Treatment is continued for four to six weeks after resolution of lesions. The therapeutic effect of iodides is not due to a fungistatic activity, but to some unknown influence on tissue reaction which increases the resistance of the host.

Amphotericin B, given by slow intravenous infusion (0.25 mg/kg to a maximum of 1.0 mg/kg) with appropriate precautions is the method of choice for extracutaneous (disseminated) sporotrichosis, especially in the presence of a rising titer with agglutination or complement fixation tests.

Chromoblastomycosis

Chromoblastomycosis (chromomycosis) is an uncommon chronic cutaneous and subcutaneous fungal infection of the skin caused by several

species of *Phialophora* or *Cladisporium*, all of which are common inhabitants of soil and decaying vegetation. Confined most frequently to one of the lower extremities, the disorder usually results from a puncture or splinter of wood and occurs most frequently among barefoot farm laborers in rural tropical or subtropical countries, but it has also been seen in North America, Northern Europe, and Australia, and has occurred in children as young as three years of age.

Chromoblastomycosis is characterized by the formation of small papular, verrucous nodules, plaques, and tumor masses, usually on the distal portion of one of the extremities (most frequently the foot, occasionally an upper extremity, rarely the face, neck, or trunk). Lesions have a dull reddish-gray color, may be slightly scaly, and are usually painless unless secondary infection is present. In early stages of this disorder the appearance is not very distinctive and may resemble other granulomatous disorders. The occurrence of verrucous lesions is an outstanding feature of all cases of chromoblastomycosis, thus accounting for the name dermatitis verrucosa, once given to this disorder. Eventually, after a period of months or years, the extremity may become edematous and swollen, enlarged masses may form with exudate, debris, and crusts, and lesions may become papillomatous, with masses of elevated, hard, brownish or reddish nodules surmounting the plaques, with a resultant cauliflower-like appearance.

Chromoblastomycosis can be diagnosed by recognition of the causative fungus in microscopic examination of potassium hydroxide preparations, in biopsy specimens from clinical lesions, or in fungal culture. When the foci of infection are localized and limited in number, the treatment of choice is surgical removal of the infected tissue by excision, electrodesiccation, or cryosurgery. In cases of long duration and extensive involvement, although the organism may be sensitive to amphotericin B, the required local concentration generally is too high for intravenous infusion to be effective. In such instances, the use of intralesional amphotericin B given in a concentration of 5 mg per ml in dextrose and water or in 2 per cent lidocaine may be curative.[37]

Mycetoma

Mycetoma, also termed Madura foot or maduromycosis, is a chronic localized granulomatous disorder of the subcutaneous tissues followed by marked invasion of the fascia, muscles, and bone, and, when an extremity is involved, enlargement of the affected area. Although the majority of lesions are seen on the foot or hand, lesions also may occur on the shoulder, buttocks, or knees; thus the term Madura foot actually is inappropriate for this disorder.

The infection may be caused by various species of true fungi, *Allescheria boydii*, *Madurella mycetomi*, *M. grisea*, *Phialophora jeanselmi*, *Cephalosporium recifei*, and aerobic fungus-like bacteria, actinomycetes (usually species of *Nocardia* and *Streptomyces*), which occur as saprophytes in soil or on vegetable matter. Uncommon in childhood and relatively rare in the United States, mycetoma occurs most commonly in young adults and workers in rural tropical and subtropical areas who walk barefoot and accordingly are more readily exposed to the fungi.

The infection begins as one or more small nondescript firm painless papules that gradually evolve into subcutaneous nodules with sinus tracts, draining abscesses, edema, and, when an extremity is affected, enlargement of the area of involvement. The diagnostic features of mycetoma are distortion and enlargement of the involved area, draining sinus tracts, and bloody or purulent drainage with characteristic pinpoint-sized granules seen on microscopic examination of the suppurative fluid. Definitive diagnosis can be made by microscopic identification of the granules and their actinomycete or fungal nature, with confirmation by culture of the etiologic organism.

The treatment of mycetoma is dependent upon early diagnosis and the nature of the infection. Disease due to actinomycetes frequently responds to sulfonamides, penicillin, tetracycline, or chloramphenicol (alone or in combination), or in some instances to amphotericin B, and that due to *N. brasiliensis*, diaminodiphenylsulfone (Dapsone). Unfortunately, there is no single drug that can give consistently good results, and long-standing cases with extensive tissue destruction and fibrosis frequently are resistant to all forms of drug therapy. Surgery may be effective during the early stages. In more advanced cases, however, particularly when there is extensive sinus tract formation, except for amputation procedures, surgical treatment rarely is curative.

SYSTEMIC MYCOSES

The systemic mycoses comprise a group of fungal disorders that arise from internal foci, usually the lungs or upper respiratory tract. When the skin lesions result from dissemination of the disease from one or more internal foci, the prognosis is generally poor. Disorders in this group include blastomycosis, coccidioidomycosis, cryptococcosus, histoplasmosis, rhinosporidiosis, and those due to opportunistic infection, aspergillosis, and mucormycosis. Actinomycosis and nocardiosis, although frequently included under the group of disorders due to true fungi, are actually caused by fungus-like gram-positive bacteria. Accordingly,

they are described in the chapter on bacterial infections (see Chapter 10).

Blastomycosis

Blastomycosis is seen in two forms, North American and South American. North American blastomycosis is caused by *Blastomyces dermatitidis*. It occurs in three forms, primary cutaneous inoculation blastomycosis, pulmonary blastomycosis, and disseminated (systemic) blastomycosis. South American blastomycosis is a chronic granulomatous disease caused by *Blastomyces brasiliensis*. It characteristically begins on the skin or mucosa about the mouth or nasal cavity, occasionally the lungs, with dissemination by hematogenous spread to various internal organs, namely the central nervous system, brain, bones, adrenal glands, spleen, and skin.

An infrequent disorder of childhood, North American blastomycosis is almost exclusively restricted to individuals on the North American Continent from Canada to Mexico and Central America (usually males over fifty years of age), with most cases occurring in the Central Eastern and Midwestern United States. Except for rare cases of primary cutaneous inoculation blastomycosis, which appears in physicians or laboratory workers who have accidentally inoculated themselves with *Blastomyces dermatitidis* organisms, most cases of North American blastomycosis are pulmonary in origin. Those caused by inoculation show an indurated ulcerated chancriform lesion with lymphangitis and lymphadenitis of the affected limb. The primary lesion and affected nodes heal spontaneously, generally within a period of eight months, and, except for a resultant scar, the prognosis is excellent.

Pulmonary blastomyocosis may be asymptomatic or may produce mild to moderately severe acute pulmonary involvement characterized by low-grade fever, pleuritic chest pain, cough, and hemoptysis. The disorder may heal spontaneously, may cause chronic pulmonary disease with or without cavitation, or may disseminate, primarily to the skin, subcutaneous tissues, bones, and joints, and less frequently to the gastrointestinal tract, liver, spleen, and central nervous system. If untreated, pulmonary blastomycosis often progresses, with the patient's eventual demise.

Cutaneous lesions disseminated from a primary pulmonary focus are usually symmetrical and generally appear on the exposed areas of the body (the face, wrists, hands, and feet). They appear as papules or nodules, which subsequently ulcerate and discharge purulent material; as elevated verrucous crusted lesions, with active arciform or serpiginous borders and violaceous margins, and a tendency toward central healing with a thin depigmented atrophic scar; or as a raised firm subcutaneous nodule with multiple small pustules over its surface.

South American blastomycosis (paracoccidiomycosis) occurs almost exclusively in all sections of South and Central America with the exception of Chile and British French Guiana. The disorder is most frequently noted in Brazil and, as in North American blastomycosis is found more often in males than in females (in a proportion of 10 to 12 to one), with the highest incidence in inhabitants of rural areas, especially farmhands. The highest incidence occurs in individuals between 20 and 50 years of age and it is uncommon in childhood. It is thought that the organism lives as a saprophyte on vegetation or in soil, and that the infection is acquired by direct implantation into the skin or mucous membranes, possibly through the practice of cleaning the teeth with small pieces of infected vegetation or, in pulmonary lesions, by direct inhalation of the organism.

The primary lesions usually appear on the lips or in the mouth, pharynx (extending to the larynx) or nasal cavity as infiltrated ulcerated lesions. The ulcers extend and ultimately progress to destroy the nose, lips, and facies. Hematogenous or lymphatic spread results in subcutaneous abscesses, and the lymph nodes draining the affected areas are palpable, painful, adherent to the overlying skin, and occasionally go on to form chronic sinuses and suppurate.

The diagnosis of cutaneous blastomycosis is dependent upon the demonstration of characteristic round budding organisms in potassium hydroxide mounts or stained smears of material from skin, ulcers, or purulent discharge, or by culture of the organisms on Sabouraud's agar. Amphotericin B is the drug of choice for both North American and South American forms of blastomycosis. This is administered by slow intravenous infusion, with precautions to reduce the potential risk of nephrotoxicity, hepatotoxicity, hypokalemia, and anemia. The initial dose is 0.25 mg per kg of body weight, with gradual increase to a maximum daily dose of 1 mg per kg. Toxicity may be reduced by alternate day dosage after clinical regression has been accomplished. Clinical and serologic followup is indispensable, and retreatment with amphotericin B must be considered if relapses occur. If amphotericin B is not tolerated, stilbamidine or its derivative 2-hydroxystilbamidine can be given. Neurotoxicity, however, particularly trigeminal neuralgia, may prove to be a frequent and distressing side effect.

Coccidioidomycosis

Coccidioidomycosis is an acute, subacute, or chronic infectious disease caused by the fungus *Coccidioides immitis*, a soil saprophyte endemic in the hot, arrid, desert areas of the southwestern United States (especially the San Joaquin Valley in California), Mexico, and parts of South America. Seen in infants as early as the first few months of life and in children as well as adults, it affects individuals of all ages, particularly adult males engaged in agricultural occupations, with a peak incidence of the acute infection among field workers during the hot months of autumn. The disease is not believed to be transmitted via the placenta, but cases of disseminated coccidioidomycosis have been reported beginning as early as two to three weeks of age.[38]

As in blastomycosis, coccidioidomycosis may also occur as a primary cutaneous inoculation, pulmonary, or systemic disorder. Primarily an airborne disease, the common pulmonary form is acquired by the inhalation of dust that contains arthrospores, and it varies in severity from a mild inapparent upper respiratory tract infection to an acute, disseminated fatal disease. The primary pulmonary disorder is the most common form of coccidiomycosis. Following an incubation period of ten days to several weeks, 60 per cent of cases are asymptomatic, and 40 per cent of affected individuals develop a respiratory infection consisting of a "flu-like" syndrome, with fever, malaise, cough, chest pain, chills, dyspnea, nodular densities, localized infiltrations in the lung, and hilar adenopathy. Ninety-five per cent of patients with clinically manifest coccidioidomycosis recover completely; 5 per cent develop pulmonary residua and complications consisting of persistent pulmonary granulomas or thin-walled cavities, pleural effusion, bronchiectasis, and pneumothorax; and 0.1 per cent progress to a disseminated disorder, with involvement of the skin, subcutaneous tissue, bone, lymph nodes, or central nervous system.

Cutaneous signs of primary pulmonary coccidiomycosis include a generalized erythematous macular exanthem that appears within the first day or two of illness (seen in up to 10 per cent of patients) or erythema multiforme or erythema nodosum (seen in up to 20 per cent of individuals with acute pulmonary form, particularly females). Supraclavicular lymphadenopathy frequently is an early sign of dissemination, and the disseminated form consists of nondescript papules or pustules, granulomas or erosions, plaques, nodules, or abscesses with thick mucoid pus or chronic ulcers with, at times, superimposed verrucous or vegetative surfaces.

Primary cutaneous inoculation is relatively rare and occurs through injury by contaminated splinters, thorns, or accidental inoculation in laboratory or autopsy rooms. This form of coccidiomycosis is characterized by a painless, indurated ulcerated lesion with lymphangitis and lymphadenopathy (similar to that seen in sporotrichosis or blastomycosis). Although healing usually takes place within a period of a few months, at least one patient with primary cutaneous inoculation went on to develop an associated coccidiodal meningitis.[39]

Diagnosis of coccidioidomycosis can be established by demonstration of the characteristic large (up to 60 micra) thick-walled globular spherules in potassium hydroxide mounts of sputum, purulent discharge, biopsy specimens, or cerebrospinal fluid or by isolation of the fungus by culture. Since *C. immitis* is highly infectious, special precautions are necessary to prevent laboratory accidents due to airborne spread of arthrospores. Serologic tests also are of value in the diagnosis and prognosis of this disorder. The coccidiodin skin test usually becomes positive in three to four weeks, but may revert to negative or never become positive in overwhelming disease. A negative test, therefore, may be misinterpreted or may indicate a poor prognosis. Complement fixation antibodies develop more slowly, increase with the severity of the disease, and diminish with clinical improvement. A high titer or complement fixation denotes severe extensive disease and poor prognosis; complement fixation antibodies in spinal fluid indicate the presence of central nervous system infection.

The majority of infections with coccidioidomycosis are self-limiting and do not require specific therapy. The illness of non-disseminated primary coccidiomycosis commonly lasts one to two months, but the disseminated course may be fulminant or may persist for several years, and until the advent of amphotericin B therapy, disseminated forms were fatal in more than 50 per cent of cases. Medical therapy today, accordingly, is dependent upon the use of amphotericin B with appropriate precautions to avoid toxicity.[39] An alternative mode of therapy includes intravenous miconazole and transfer factor, although the latter drug remains investigational at this time.

Cryptococcosis (Torulosis)

Infection due to the encapsulated yeast *Cryptococcus neoformans* affects all age groups in a worldwide distribution and usually occurs as a systemic disease with the respiratory tract as the portal of entry. The organism has been found in various fruits, in soil, pigeon excreta, and cow's milk, and, when it affects man, there is marked predilection for the brain and meninges, although the lungs and occasionally the skin and other parts of the body may be involved. The disease usually occurs in individuals between 30 and 60 years of age and, although uncommon, does occur in children and has been seen in newborn infants. In some cases of neonatal cryptococcosis, symptoms begin so promptly after birth that the question of transplacental transmission must be considered. However, since cryptococcus is an occasional inhabitant of the female genital tract, it is believed that the infant acquires infection during passage through the birth canal.[40]

Clinically apparent cryptococcosis infection may remain localized to the lungs, producing focal pneumonia, patchy infiltrates, solitary nodules, and, infrequently, abscesses and pleural effusion. Pulmonary symptoms may be absent or minimal and, although pulmonary involvement may progress and produce death, in most instances central nervous system manifestations almost always predominate, and infection is detected only after dissemination to the central nervous system has occurred.

Central nervous system manifestations consist of occipital or frontal headaches, behavioral abnormalities, confusion, dizziness, vomiting, stiff neck, and, with progression, cranial nerve palsy, seizure disorders, delirium, coma, and death. Although most patients have isolated meningeal involvement occasionally accompanied by pulmonary infiltrates, other organs, including the liver, spleen, kidney, bones, and lymph nodes, may be involved. Skin lesions, when present, may be related to trauma or extension from bony involvement, but are usually due to hematogenous spread from a pulmonary focus. Approximately 30 per cent of cases of disseminated cryptococcosis are associated with some form of reticuloendothelial system malignancy (usually Hodgkin's disease). The presence of cutaneous involvement, therefore, suggests a search for a possible underlying malignant disorder.

Cutaneous lesions, seen in 10 to 15 per cent of cases, are located most commonly on the head and neck (including the scalp); less commonly they are found on the extremities or thorax. Lesions usually begin as painless, well-demarcated firm pink, red, or bluish-purple papular, pustular, acneiform eruptions without surrounding inflammation. These lesions are especially characteristic of widespread infection and often occur around the nose and mouth. As the lesions enlarge they form infiltrated plaques and develop firm rubbery indolent tumors, subcutaneous abscesses, or ulcers, often with raised papillomatous borders.

The diagnosis of cryptococcosis is dependent upon demonstration of the organism by examination of spinal fluid, pus from skin lesions, sputum, or tissue sections, by indirect immunofluorescence, or by culture on Sabouraud's dextrose agar. The organisms are oval or rounded thick-walled spherules 5 to 20 micra in diameter. The organism is surrounded by a polysaccharide capsule, often with characteristic budding. This is best demonstrated by the addition of one drop of India ink to potassium hydroxide wet-mounts and spinal fluid preparations, or by special staining with methylene blue, alcian blue, or mucicarmine.

Untreated cryptococcosis is fatal in 90 per cent of cases; intravenous and intrathecal amphotericin B, however, will result in cure in about 80 per cent of cases of disseminated forms of this disorder. Intravenous amphotericin B is administered in increasing increments, beginning with 0.1 to 0.3 mg/kg/day (never exceeding a total daily dose of 1.5 mg/kg). Sterilization of foci of cryptococci is accomplished in 10 to 14 days, and treatment should be given daily, generally for a period of two months, with a total intravenous dose of 30 mg per kg. For patients with central nervous system involvement, intrathecal therapy in addition to intravenous therapy often produces a cure.

Oral 5-fluorocytosine (5-FC), an antifungal fluorinated pyrimidine chemically related to fluorouracil and available as flucytosine (Ancoban, Roche), 150 to 200 mg/kg of body weight administered daily in four divided doses, is effective. Since emergence of fluorocytosine-resistant strains has been a major cause of treatment failure, the combination of 5-FC with intravenous amphotericin B is now recommended in order to avert development of resistant strains and to avoid the potential toxic effects associated with high doses of amphotericin B.[40]

Histoplasmosis

Histoplasmosis is a common, highly infectious disorder affecting primarily the lungs caused by the fungus *Histoplasma capsulatum*. The disease is widely distributed throughout the world, is endemic in the Mississippi and Ohio valleys of the United States, and affects infants and children as well as adults. *H. capsulatum* exists as a saprophyte in the soil in endemic areas, most often in soil contaminated by chicken feathers or droppings. Infection is usually acquired by inhalation and is contracted more frequently in rural rather than urban areas. In children, who are more likely to have generalized histoplasmosis, the frequency of extensive ulcers along the gastrointestinal mucosa that give rise to diarrhea and other gastrointestinal disturbances suggests that organisms of histoplasmosis may be ingested rather than inhaled in these individuals. Approximately three-quarters of infected individuals have asymptomatic benign, self-limiting pulmonary infections, which may leave calcified residua in the lungs. Twenty-five per cent develop a "flu-like" pulmonary infection, and less than 1 per cent progress to the disseminated form of the disease.

Many classifications of histoplasmosis have been recommended. The most recognized include an acute pulmonary form, a febrile disorder of varying severity in which there may be malaise, cough, chest pain, chills, dyspnea, and nodular densities or localized infiltration in the lung; chronic pulmonary forms often resembling tuberculosis clinically and roentgenographically; disseminated forms with fever, hepatosplenomegaly, anemia, and weight loss (more commonly seen in young children and individuals over 50 years of age); and an extremely rare traumatic primary form (seen in laboratory or autopsy room workers) characterized by chancriform lesions at the site of inoculation accompanied by regional lymphadenopathy.

Cutaneous lesions are uncommon but may be seen in the disseminated form of histoplasmosis. Quite variable in nature, they include lesions of erythema multiforme and erythema nodosum, purpura, papules, pustules, plaques, chronic abscesses, patches of impetiginized or exfoliative dermatitis, vegetative lesions, characteristic ulcerations of the nose, mouth, pharynx, genitalia, and perianal regions, and punched-out or circumscribed granulomatous ulcers.

The diagnosis of histoplasmosis consists of identification of the small intracellular yeast-like organisms in sputum, peripheral blood, smears from open or ulcerated tissue, biopsies of cutaneous lesions, lymph nodes, liver, or bone marrow, and fungal culture on Sabouraud's dextrose agar. Since in endemic areas as many as 90 per cent of the population react positively, the skin test is not diagnostic. In infants a positive reaction probably indicates active infection, but in older children and adults it may signify past or present infection and accordingly is reliable only as a screening procedure. It must be remembered, however, that the histoplasmin skin test does not become positive for two or three weeks after infection and that it may be negative in extensive debilitating disease.

Serologic tests may be of value, but blood for serologic studies must be collected prior to skin testing, since the skin test itself may produce a rise in serologic titer. Serologic tests (agar gel precipitin test, yeast phase complement fixation, and collodion or latex particle agglutination) usually are positive except in chronically ill patients with severe disseminated lesions. Since low titers frequently are present in healthy persons living in endemic areas, titers less than 1:16 should be viewed with suspicion, and titers exceeding 1:32, although not conclusively diagnostic, are highly suggestive of histoplasmosis infection.

In more than 99 per cent of infections histoplasmosis has a benign self-limiting course. The disseminated forms, however, particularly in the very young and very old, have a high mortality. Amphotericin B, as in blastomycosis and coccidiomycosis, is the treatment of choice for this disorder. Lesser infections may be treated with triple sulfa, but since there is considerable tendency to spontaneous resolution, controlled studies are lacking.

Rhinosporidiosis

Rhinosporidiosis is a rare chronic disorder caused by the fungus *Rhinosporidium seeberi*. Endemic in India and Sri Lanka (Ceylon), it occurs in other parts of the world, including the southern part of the United States. Males are infected most commonly (11 to 1) and the disease occurs at any age, but it is more common in children and young adults.

The disorder is characterized by papules, nodules, and pedunculated vascular polypoid growths on the mucous membranes of the nose, nasopharynx, and soft palate (in 75 per cent of cases) and in upper respiratory passages, the conjunctivae, lacrimal sacs, the skin, larynx, genitalia, or rectum. The surface of the growth has a raspberry-like appearance and is studded with tiny white or yellowish nodules containing the fungal spores.

The lesions become hyperplastic and may reach enormous size, and symptoms are associated with obstruction of the respiratory passages or esophagus. Typical lesions are recognizable by their pink to purple color, friable consistency, and the presence of the white sporangia within the lesion itself. Diagnosis is confirmed by microscopic demonstration of typical sporangia on the surface of the polyps or in tissue section, and treatment consists of electrosurgical destruction and surgical removal of lesions when feasible.

OPPORTUNISTIC MYCOTIC INFECTIONS

With the frequent use of broad-spectrum antibiotics and potent cytotoxic agents, fatal deep mycoses have become increasingly frequent. Opportunistic mycoses (e.g., aspergillosis, mucormycosis) are those that are very low in pathogenic potential but capable of causing infection when alteration or breakdown of host defenses occurs, thus permitting them to invade the host.

Aspergillosis

Aspergillosis is an uncommon opportunistic fungal disease of the respiratory tract and other sites caused by a variety of *Aspergillus* species. Although *A. fumigatus* is the most commonly identified pathogen, *A. niger* and an increasing number of species have been reported in recent years. There is no predilection for sex or race, and although a state of altered susceptibility is more common in adults, it also occurs in susceptible infants and children.

The fungi are ubiquitous, normally nonpathogenic, and primarily affect debilitated individuals in the respiratory tract, although the skin, cornea, external auditory canal, gastrointestinal tract, nasopharynx, vagina, and urethra may also be affected. There are no features pathognomonic of aspergillosis, the clinical picture being related to the organs of involvement.

One of the most common characteristic manifestations of aspergillosis is the pulmonary intracavitary fungus ball. This is composed of colonies of *Aspergillus*, inflammatory exudate, cells, and fibrin in the form of a sphere, which may measure from 1 to 5 cm in diameter. Although it occasionally causes hemoptysis, most patients with fungus balls are asymptomatic.

In some patients, especially those with lymphoma or malignancy and those who are receiving systemic corticosteroids or other immunosuppressive therapy, the fungus may invade the tissues directly and spread hematogenously to other organs, characteristically the central nervous system, kidney, liver, spleen, gall bladder, heart, aorta, thyroid, bones, lymph nodes, uterus, and skin. Less commonly, an opportunistic infection of the paranasal sinuses may result in mucopurulent or blood-tinged nasal discharge, headache, periorbital neuralgia, rhinitis, and, with extension, the face may become erythematous, swollen, warm, and tender, suggesting a diagnosis of cellulitis or erysipelas. Cutaneous lesions are rare, but various species of *Aspergillus* have been recovered from the external auditory canal. Whether the fungus is a causative factor of otomycosis, however, remains controversial.

Although aspergillus organisms may be identified on culture, clinical findings must be carefully evaluated before a diagnosis of aspergillosis is established. Clinical material should be examined carefully for the presence of hyphae, and although culture of the organism is ideal, this is not always possible. Treatment consists of amphotericin B or oral fluocytosine (5-FC) and surgical removal of pulmonary fungus balls, when present. As with cryptococcosis, amphotericin B and fluocytosine in combination are recommended, to avoid toxicity and development of resistant strains.[40]

Phycomycosis (Mucormycosis)

Phycomycosis (mucormycosis) is an opportunistic infection that occurs in patients with a variety of debilitating diseases, such as diabetes, anemia, heart or liver disease, burns, leukemia or other lymphomas, and in individuals receiving corticosteroids, cytotoxic agents, or immunosuppressive therapy. It may involve any organ of the body but most commonly affects the skin, lungs, meninges, gastrointestinal tract, and structures in the head and neck.

The causative fungi of mucormyocosis belong to the class *Phycomycetes* and include species of *Mucor*, *Rhizopus*, *Absidia*, *Mortierella*, and *Cunninghamella*, the portal of entry varying with the site of the disease. The term phycomycosis refers to the subcutaneous form of the disorder. Caused by *Basidiobolus* and *Entomophthura* species, this form is characterized by inflammatory subcutaneous swellings that spread over the upper part of the chest, neck, or arms; involve the fat, muscle, and fascia; and heal spontaneously.

Cutaneous or subcutaneous infections are rare and occur most frequently in diabetics with recurrent acidosis or in patients with severe burns. They are characterized by papular lesions, chronic indolent ulcers, and slowly enlarging painless subcutaneous nodules. The initial lesion is usually a small area of macular discoloration or dusky erythema, which gradually enlarges and ulcerates. Necrosis may be marked and there is usually a profuse foul-smelling purulent exudate, and, in some cases, cutaneous infarction resembling ecthyma gangrenosum.[41, 42] Subcutaneous phycomycosis is seen most frequently in children and adolescents. It is characterized by localized subcutaneous nodular eosinophilic granulomas, usually with an intact but inflamed epidermis, multiple purulent ulcerations, and paronychia.

The cerebral form may be recognized by a suppurative necrotizing infection of the paranasal sinuses, orbital pain, swelling, edema, proptosis, ptosis, pupil fixation, and loss of vision. Acute inflammation, infarction, or necrosis in the lungs, gastrointestinal tract, orbits, and the central nervous system in a patient debilitated by disease or immunosuppressant therapy should suggest the possibility of mucormycosis.

Diagnosis depends upon microscopic examination of the organism in clinical lesions and definitive fungal culture. Therapy requires treatment of the underlying disease process, discontinuation of predisposing therapeutic agents whenever possible, and, when necessary, the use of intravenous amphotericin B.

References

1. Zaias N, Taplin DM: Improved preparation for the diagnosis of mycologic diseases. Arch. Dermatol. 93:608–609, 1966.

Microscopic demonstration of fungi in skin, nail, and hair scrapings can be facilitated by the use of 20 per cent potassium hydroxide in a solution of 60 per cent water and 40 per cent dimethyl sulfoxide (DMSO).

2. Rockoff AS: Fungus cultures in a pediatric outpatient clinic. Pediatrics 63:276–278, 1979.

In a total of 76 fungal cultures, of which 24 yielded dermatophytes, results on dermatophyte test medium (DTM), read by non-mycologists (pediatric house officers), compared favorably with those on standard media processed in a laboratory.

3. Taplin D, Zaias N, Rebell G, et al.: Isolation and recognition of dermatophytes on a new medium (DTM). Arch. Dermatol. 99:203–209, 1969.

Dermatophyte Test Medium (DTM) contains a phenol red indicator, enabling the non-myocologist to determine the presence of dermatophytic fungi by a change in the color of the agar from yellow to red.

4. Rosenthal SA, Furnari D: Efficacy of "Dermatophyte Test Media." Arch Dermatol. 104:486–489, 1971.

Although not quite as reliable as Sabouraud's media, the distinctive color change in DTM is helpful in the evaluation of fungal cultures for those not proficient in dermatophyte colony morphology.

5. Kligman AM: Tinea capitis due to M. audouini and M. canis. II. Dynamics of host-parasite relationship. Arch. Dermatol. 71:313–337, 1955.

Clarification of the pathogenesis of tinea capitis through sectioned biopsy specimens taken from the scalps of experimental subjects inoculated with M. audouini and M. canis.

6. Zaias N, Taplin D, Rebell G: Evaluation of microcrystalline griseofulvin therapy in tinea capitis. JAMA 198:805–807, 1966.

A study of 324 children with scalp ringworm infection demonstrates an increasing incidence of non-fluorescent T. tonsurans as a cause of tinea capitis in the United States.

7. Friedman L, Derbes VJ: Tinea capitis. In Demis DJ, Dobson RL, McGuire JS: Clinical Dermatology, Vol. 3. Harper and Row Publishers, Hagerstown, Md., 1979, 17–6, 1–23.

A current review of tinea capitis, its epidemiology, clinical features, diagnosis, and management.

8. Kahn G: Letters to the Editor. Kerion treatment. Pediatrics 61:501, 1978.

Prednisone with griseofulvin appears to be the most effective form of therapy for kerion.

9. Dobson RL: Editorial comment. In 1979 Year Book of Dermatology. Year Book Medical Publishers, Chicago, 1979, p. 124.

In a discussion of an article on children with tinea capitis, the editor suggests the use of oral saturated solution of potassium iodide for the treatment of kerion.

10. Yesudian P, Kamalam A: Epidermophyton floccosum infection in a three-week-old infant. Trans. St. John's Hosp. Dermatol. Soc. 59:1, 66–67, 1973.

A three-week-old infant with ringworm infection (E. floccosum) infection on the skin overlying the left hip.

11. Ive FA, Marks R: Tinea incognito. Br. Med. J. 3:149–152, 1968.

Fourteen patients with "tinea incognito," an unusual presentation of tinea corporis due to topical application of corticosteroids.

12. Jones HE, Reinhardt JH, Rinaldi MG: A clinical, mycological, and immunological survey for dermatophytosis. Arch. Dermatol. 108:61–65, 1973.

Data in a study of 180 subjects suggest that susceptibility to chronic tinea infection in atopic individuals appears to be related to a lack of delayed cell-mediated immunity coexistent with increase in antibody (presumably IgE).

13. Marples MJ, Chapman EN: Tinea pedis in a group of school children. Br. J. Dermatol. 71:413–421, 1959.

A study of 387 school children confirms the rarity of tinea pedis in prepubertal individuals.

14. Leyden JJ, Kligman AM: Aluminum chloride in the treatment of symptomatic athlete's foot. Arch. Dermatol. 111:1004–1010, 1975.

Thirty per cent aluminum chloride produces a beneficial drying effect in the soggy macerated interdigital webs and, although it does not cure athlete's foot, appears to render the interspaces less hospitable to bacteria and fungi.

15. Davies RR, Everall JD, Hamilton E: Mycological and clinical evaluation of griseofulvin for chronic onychomycosis. Br. Med. J. 3:464–468, 1967.

Griseofulvin, even when given over a two-year period, rarely cures dermatophyte infections of the toenails.

16. McGinley KJ, Lantis LR, Marples RR: Microbiology of tinea versicolor. Arch. Dermatol. 102:168–171, 1970.

Studies of normal and affected skin of patients with tinea versicolor support the dimorphous concept that Pityrosporum orbiculare becomes pathogenic when it changes from a yeast to a filamentous form.

17. Smith EB, Gellerman GL: Tinea versicolor in infancy. Arch. Dermatol. 93:362–363, 1966.

Report of an eight-week-old infant with tinea versicolor and review of the subject of tinea versicolor in infancy.

18. Michalowski R, Rodziewicz H: Pityriasis versicolor in children. Br. J. Dermatol. 75:397–400, 1963.

A study of 305 children between the ages of four months and ten years with tinea versicolor.

19. Charles RC, Sire, DJ, Johnson BL, et al.: Hypopigmentation in tinea versicolor. A histochemical and electronmicroscopic study. Int. J. Dermatol. 12:48–58, 1973.

Electron microscopic studies suggest an abnormal pigment transfer from melanocyte to keratinocyte as the cause of the pigmentary disturbance seen in lesions of tinea versicolor.

20. Albright, SD, Hitch JM: Rapid treatment of tinea versicolor with selenium sulfide. Arch. Dermatol. 93:460–462, 1966.

Selenium sulfide shampoo, applied to the skin of patients with tinea versicolor (dried and left on overnight) offers a convenient and effective therapeutic approach to the management of this disorder.

21. Kozinn PJ, Taschdjian CL, Dragutsky D, et al.: Cutaneous candidiasis in early infancy and childhood. Pediatrics 20:827–834, 1957.

In a study of 2175 infants, 100 per cent of neonates and 80 per cent of older infants and young children with candidal diaper rashes harbored C. albicans in the intestines.

22. Harris LJ, Pritzker HG, Laski B, et al.: Effect of nystatin (Mycostatin) on neonatal candidiasis (thrush). Method of eradicating thrush from hospital nurseries. Canad. Med. Ass. J. 79:891–896, 1958.

Although the prophylactic treatment of newborn infants with oral nystatin can reduce the incidence of thrush tenfold (from 4.0 to 0.4 per cent), the rarity of serious pathology due to candida does not warrant oral nystatin prophylaxis in neonates.

23. Kam LA, Giacoia GP: Congenital cutaneous candidiasis. Am. J. Dis. Child. 129:1215–1218, 1978.

Two cases of congenital cutaneous candidiasis and a summary of the clinical characteristics of this disorder and its differentiation from neonatal cutaneous candidiasis.

24. Rudolph N, Taria AA, Reale MR, et al.: Congenital cutaneous candidiasis. Arch. Dermatol. 113:1101–1103, 1977.

Macular, papular, vesiculopustular, and bullous lesions followed by desquamation are the cutaneous manifestations in three newborn infants with congenital cutaneous candidiasis.

25. Rebora A, Marples RR, Kligman AM: Erosio interdigitalis blastomycetica. Arch. Dermatol. 108:66–68, 1973.

Studies in 53 volunteer subjects suggest that *Candida albicans* evokes a dermatitis and that gram-negative rods play an important role in the chronicity of erosio interdigitalis blastomycetica.

26. Keller MA, Sellers BB Jr, Melish ME, et al.: Systemic candidiasis in infants. A case presentation and literature review. Am. J. Dis. Child. 131:1260–1263, 1977.

A 4½-month-old infant with systemic candidiasis following exchange transfusion for hyperbilirubinemia and subsequent surgical repair of a patent ductus arteriosus at 20 days of age.

27. Rockoff AS: Chronic mucocutaneous candidiasis. Successful treatment with intermittent oral doses of clotrimazole. Arch. Dermatol. 115:322–323, 1979.

Report of a 9-year-old girl with chronic mucocutaneous candidiasis who achieved a prolonged remission following treatment with the imidazole antibiotic clotrimazole.

28. Fisher TJ, Klein RB, Kershnar HE, et al.: Miconazole in treatment of chronic mucocutaneous candidiasis: Preliminary report. J. Pediatr. 91:815–819, 1977.

Evaluation of intravenous miconazole in the treatment of five children with chronic mucocutaneous candidiasis.

29. Logan RI, Goldberg MJ: *C. albicans* resistance to 5-fluorocytosine. Br. Med. J. 3:531, 1972.

A 53-year-old man who developed a 5-fluorocytosine resistant *Candida albicans* infection of the throat and blood stream while on treatment for endocarditis.

30. Higgs JM, Wells RS: Chronic mucocutaneous candidiasis: new approaches to treatment. Br. J. Dermatol. 89:179–190, 1973.

A discussion of chronic mucocutaneous candidiasis and a review of new approaches to therapy.

31. Leikin S, Parrott R, Randolph J: Clotrimazole treatment of chronic mucocutaneous candidiasis. J. Pediatr. 88:864–866, 1976.

Report of a beneficial response to oral clotrimazole in an 11-year-old girl with multiple immunologic defects and chronic mucocutaneous candidiasis.

32. Stewardson-Krieger PB, Esterly NB: Fungal infections. *In* Solomon LM, Esterly NB, Loeffel ED: Adolescent Dermatology. W. B. Saunders Company, Philadelphia, 1978, 293–325.

Review of mycotic infections as seen in children and adolescents.

33. Lynch PJ, Botero F: Sporotrichosis in children. Am. J. Dis. Child. 122:325–327, 1971.

Nine of 11 childhood cases of sporotrichosis developed their initial lesion on an exposed area of the face, arms, or legs.

34. Orr ER, Riley HD Jr: Sporotrichosis in childhood. J. Pediatr. 78:951–957, 1971.

Ten children ages 3 to 16 with sporotrichosis.

35. Dahl BA, Silberfarb DM, Sgrosi GA, et al.: Sporotrichosis in children. Report of an epidemic. JAMA 215:1980–1982, 1971.

A report of sporotrichosis in nine children who had been playing among contaminated bales of prairie hay.

36. Satterwhite TK, Kageler WV, Conklin RH, et al.: Disseminated sporotrichosis. JAMA 248:771–772, 1978.

Disseminated sporotrichosis in a 60-year-old alcoholic male who expired as the result of cardiopulmonary arrest and S. schenkii meningoencephalitis.

37. DeFeo CP, Harber LC: Chromoblastomycosis treated with local infiltration of amphotericin B solution. Report of a second case. JAMA 171:1961–1963, 1959.

Chromoblastomycosis of 22 years' duration caused by *Hormodendrum pedrosoi*, the second case of favorable response to amphotericin B injected locally in a two per cent procaine solution.

38. Townsend TE, McKey RW: Coccidiomycosis in infants. Am. J. Dis. Child. 86:51–53, 1953.

Although human transmission of coccidiomycosis is extremely rare, a 3-week-old female infant who did not live in an endemic area but was exposed to a father who lived in southwestern United States where coccidiomycosis is endemic, had pneumonitis, meningoencephalitis and positive cerebrospinal fluid cultures of *C. immitis*.

39. Winn WA: The treatment of coccidioidal meningitis. The use of amphotericin B in a group of 25 patients. Calif. Med. 101:78–79, 1964.

Intracisternal amphotericin B as an adjunct to intravenous and intraspinal therapy in the treatment of coccidioidal meningitis.

40. Smith A: Fungus infections. *In* Schaffer AJ, Avery ME: Diseases of the Newborn, 4th edition. W. B. Saunders Co., Philadelphia, 1977, 819–826.

A review of systemic fungal diseases in the neonate.

41. Kramer BS, Hernandez AD, Reddick RL, et al.: Cutaneous infarction, manifestation of disseminated mucormycosis. Arch. Dermatol. 113:1075–1076, 1978.

Cutaneous infarction resembling ecthyma gangrenosum as a manifestation of mucormycosis.

42. Meyer RA, Kaplan MH, Ong M, et al.: Cutaneous lesions in disseminated mucormycosis. JAMA 225:737–738, 1973.

An 8-year-old male with leukemia, widespread systemic mucormycosis and cutaneous vasculitis as an unusual cutaneous manifestation.

INSECT BITES AND PARASITIC INFESTATIONS

Parasites are a fascinating and important cause of skin disease in children, for pediatricians, general physicians, and dermatologists alike. They produce their effects in various ways: mechanical trauma of bites or stings, injection of pharmacologically active substances which induce local or systemic effects, allergic reactions in a previously sensitized host, persistent granulomatous reactions to retained mouth parts, direct invasion of the epidermis, or transmission of infectious disease by blood sucking insects.[1]

ARTHROPODS

Arthropods are elongated invertebrate animals with segmented bodies, true appendages, and a chitinous exoskeleton. Those of dermatologic significance are the eight-legged arachnids (mites, ticks, spiders, and scorpions) and the six-legged insects (lice, flies, mosquitoes, fleas, bugs, bees, wasps, ants, beetles), caterpillars, moths, and their larvae.

THE ARACHNIDS

The term **mite** refers to a large number of tiny arachnids, many of which live at least part of their lives as parasites upon animals or plants, or in prepared foods. Of greatest medical significance are itch mites (*Sarcoptes scabiei*), grain mites, and harvest mites (chiggers). They attack man by burrowing under or attaching themselves to the skin where they inflict trivial bites and associated dermatitides.

Scabies

Scabies is a contagious disorder caused by an itch mite, *Sarcoptes scabiei,* which attacks infants and children as well as adults. Although clinical descriptions of scabies date back to civilization's earliest records, it was not until 1687 that Bonomo first teased the mite out of a scabietic lesion and, with the aid of a light microscope, described the responsible organism and its etiologic role in scabies.[2] Unfortunately, either through ignorance or prejudice, two centuries passed before the parasite was officially acknowledged as the true cause of this disorder.

Over forty years ago John Stokes commented that scabies was both the easiest and yet the most difficult diagnosis in dermatology. This is just as true today as it was in 1936.[3] Epidemics of scabies seem to occur in 30 year cycles, each one lasting about 15 years, with a 15-year gap between the end of each cycle and the beginning of the next. It appears that we are presently in the midst of a world-wide pandemic, one which began in 1964

301

and, if estimates are correct, should last at least until 1979 or into the 1980's.[4, 5, 6] Although the current epidemic is widespread, it does not appear to be of sufficient intensity to limit the cycle to the usual 15 years and accordingly may persist longer than originally anticipated. Because of a rarity of scabies, particularly in this country until recent years, there has been a decrease in the index of suspicion, which often has led to misdiagnosis and mismanagement of this disorder.

Infestation begins with a newly fertilized female mite. Pinpoint in size and barely visible to the unaided eye, the oviporous parasite is oval, eight-legged, translucent, and pearly gray, measuring less than half a millimeter in length (Fig. 14–1). She tunnels into the stratum corneum and lives in cutaneous burrows, which may measure several millimeters to a few centimeters in length.[2] What determines the area of her burrow is unknown; apparently the parasite favors areas with a low concentration of pilosebaceous follicles and a thin stratum corneum.[7] This seems to account for a difference in the distribution of lesions in infants and young children as compared to that seen in older children and adults.

During the years from 1970 to 1976 I had the opportunity to see over 400 infants and children with scabies, ranging in age from 2 months to 18 years of age.[8, 9] The first of these was a 3-month-old white female infant who started with a pruritic, scaly, erythematous papular eruption on the trunk, the postauricular areas, and extremities at two months of age (Fig. 14–2). Microscopic examination of skin scrapings and fungal cultures were done, and the eruption was treated as a seborrheic

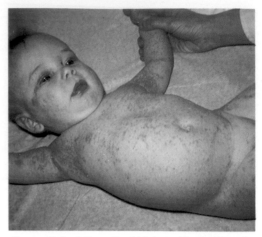

Figure 14–2 A 3-month-old infant with a scaly erythematous papular eczematoid eruption due to scabies (Hurwitz, S.: Am. J. Dis. Child. *126*:226, 1973).

dermatitis with frequent shampoos and topical fluocinolone acetonide cream.

Two weeks later the rash had spread to the back of the head and neck, the entire trunk, and all extremities, including the palms and soles. A 3 mm cutaneous punch biopsy revealed a nonspecific dermatitis with focal parakeratosis and a mild dermal mononuclear infiltrate. A second skin biopsy several days later revealed a more severe dermal mononuclear infiltrate, hyperkeratosis and parakeratosis of the stratum corneum, and a burrow within the hyperkeratotic stratum corneum, which suggested the presence of *Sarcoptes scabiei* (Fig. 14–3). Microscopic examination of skin scrapings subsequently confirmed the diagnosis of scabies.

The infant's parents and two babysitters were examined and found to have excoriated papules and nodules of the trunk, axillae, wrists, and interdigital spaces of the fingers, with involvement of the areolae of the mother, both babysitters, and the genital area of the father. Subsequently a total of 32 cases were detected through direct or indirect exposure to this infant, including my wife and myself. The initial source of exposure to the scabies mite was never determined, but the disease must have been contracted either in the hospital during the newborn period or shortly thereafter by other personal contacts, possibly babysitters.[8, 9]

CLINICAL MANIFESTATIONS. The eruption in scabies presents as a distinctive clinical syndrome of pruritic papules, vesicles, pustules, and linear burrows. Unfortunately most patients do not present this pure a picture, but rather a mixture of primary lesions, intermingled with or obliterated by excoriation, eczematization, crusting, or secondary infection (Table 14–1). Primary lesions of scabies consist of burrows, papules, and vesicular lesions (Fig. 14–4). Burrows represent the home of the invading female parasite (Fig. 14–5), the papules appear to represent temporary

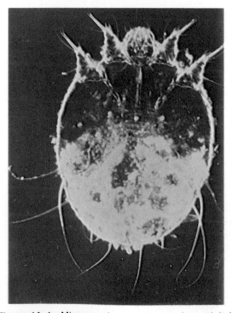

Figure 14–1 Microscopic appearance of an adult female mite of *Sarcoptes scabiei* (Courtesy of Reed & Carnrick). Pinpoint in size (less than 0.5 mm in length) and barely visible to the unaided eye, the parasite is oval, eight-legged, translucent, and pearly gray in color.

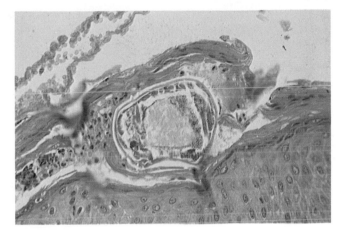

Figure 14–3 Scabies. Microscopic examination of a cutaneous biopsy reveals a burrow containing an adult female mite *(S. scabioi)* within the stratum corneum.

invasion by the larval stages of the parasite, and the vesiculation is believed to be the result of sensitization of the host. The severe itching that accompanies this disorder takes approximately four to six weeks to develop and also is thought to be related to sensitization. Until this sensitization occurs, the disorder is usually unrecognized and almost never diagnosed.[9]

In adults and older childen lesions tend to involve the webs of the fingers (Table 14–2, Fig. 14–6), the axillae, the flexures of the arms and wrists, the belt-line, and the areas around the nipples, genitals, and lower buttocks. In infants and young children the distribution is altered and includes the palms (Fig. 14–7), soles (Fig. 14–8), head, neck, and face (Figs. 14–9, 14–10). Although bullous lesions are uncommon, vesicles are often found in infants and young children, owing to the predisposition for blister formation seen in this age group.

The burrow, long considered a pathognomonic sign of scabies, unfortunately is demonstrable in a mere 7 to 13 per cent of adult patients.[10, 11] In infants and children this is even less convenient a clue, owing to frequent obliteration by vigorous hygiene, excoriation, and secondary eczematization, crusting or infection.[8, 9]

Nodular Scabies. A high percentage of children who develop scabies have been found to develop persistent reddish-brown infiltrated nodules, particularly on the covered parts of the body (the axillae, shoulders, groin, buttocks, and genital area) (Fig. 14–11). These lesions often persist for months despite therapy, and when present may be diagnosed, both clinically and on histopathologic examination, as forms of histiocytosis or lymphoma.[12]

An increased frequency of scabies, varying between 5 and 10 per cent, possibly even higher, has been noted in foreign-born children, principally from Korea and South Vietnam, who have been brought to this country for adoption. It has been noted that high numbers of these children seem to develop the granulomatous nodular lesions.[6]

Crusted (Norwegian) Scabies. This distinctive form of scabies is characterized by extensive heavily crusted skin lesions, with thick hyperkeratotic areas on the scalp, ears, elbows, knees, palms, soles, and buttocks. Crusted scabies is highly contagious, even on casual contact, because of the vast number of mites in the exfoliating scales and the lengthy period of time until the diagnosis is usually established. The predilection of this disease for the physically debilitated, mentally retarded (particularly those with Down syndrome), and immunologic deficient remains unexplained.[13]

Canine Scabies. Children can be infected by sarcoptes from domestic animals. This infesta-

Table 14–1 CLINICAL APPEARANCE OF SCABIES

A. *Primary Lesions*
 1. Pruritic papules
 2. Vesicles
 3. Pustules
 4. Burrows

B. *Secondary Lesions*
 1. Excoriations
 2. Eczematization
 3. Crusts
 4. Secondary infection

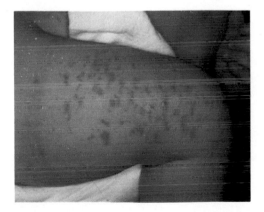

Figure 14–4 Papulovesicular lesions of scabies in a 2½-year-old child.

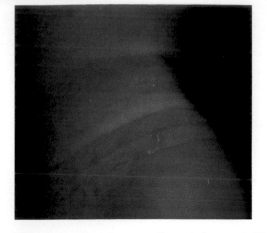

Figure 14-5   A linear burrow on the posterior aspect of the heel of an infant with scabies.

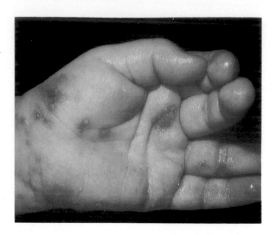

Figure 14-7   Infected scabies on the hand of an 18-month-old child (Hurwitz, S: Am. J. Dis. Child. *126*:226, 1973).

Table 14-2   DISTRIBUTION OF LESIONS IN SCABIES

A. *Older Children and Adults*
   1. Interdigital webs
   2. Flexures of wrists and arms
   3. Axillae
   4. Belt-line
   5. Areolae
   6. Genitalia
   7. Buttocks

B. *Infants and Small Children*
   1. Trunk and extremities
   2. Head, neck, palms and soles

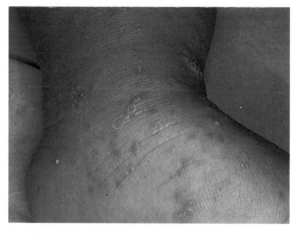

Figure 14-8   Scabies on the foot and ankle of a 10-month-old infant.

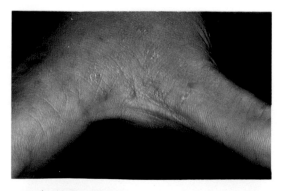

Figure 14-6   Scabietic lesions in the web between the thumb and index finger of an 11-year-old child.

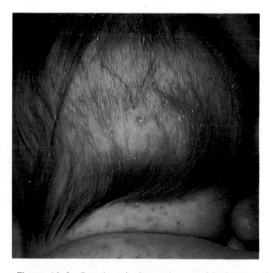

Figure 14-9   Papulovesicular and crusted lesions on the scalp and nape of the neck of an infant with scabies.

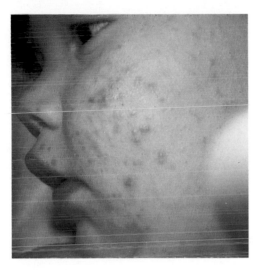

Figure 14–10 Papulovesicular lesions on the face of an 18-month-old child with scabies (Hurwitz, S: Am. J. Dis. Child. *126*:226, 1973).

tion is not permanent and dies out in a few weeks. Although persons may be susceptible to mites from a variety of domestic animals, man's close relationship to the dog makes the canine form of animal scabies the most common type transmitted to humans.[14, 15] Canine scabies, or sarcoptic mange, causes patchy loss of hair with scaling in the dog. It is seen most commonly in undernourished, heavily parasitized puppies. A presumptive diagnosis of canine scabies can be made on the basis of exposure to a pet with a pruritic papular eruption, alopecia involving mainly the head, ears, and intertriginous folds, and the characteristic mouse like odor of animals with extensive sarcoptic infestation.

In children with canine scabies the eruption is most common on the forearms, lower region of the chest, abdomen, and thighs. The distribution usually differs from that of human scabies in that it spares the interdigital webs and the genitalia. Absence of burrows and rare reports of finding the mite on microscopic examination of skin scrapings appear to be related to the fact that the mite of canine scabies does not reproduce on human skin. The infestation, therefore, is usually self-limiting and generally clears spontaneously within four to six weeks if the patient is not re-exposed to the canine source.

Secondary Complications. Eczematous changes due to scratching and rubbing of involved areas or to topical therapeutic agents are common complications of scabies in infants and children. They are frequently aggravated by excessive bathing, overzealous attempts at hygiene, and associated dryness and pruritus. In infants, young children, and atopic individuals, such complications may be particularly severe and widespread.[8, 16]

Corticosteroid administration (topical or systemic) may further mask the diagnosis of scabies by amelioration of signs and symptoms while the infestation and its transmissability persist. This frequently results in unusual clinical presentations, atypical distributions, and unusual extents of involvement, in some conditions closely simulating a variety of other entities (Fig. 14–12). It has been suggested that unusual features of scabies associated with the use of topical steroids may be related to a suppression of hypersensitivity cell-mediated immunity.[17, 18] The term "scabies incognito" has been suggested for this phenomenon.[6]

Secondary infection, seen as pustulation, bullous impetigo, severe crusting, or ecthyma, is frequently seen as a complication of scabies in young children (Fig. 14–7). Recent epidemics of nephritis suggest that scabietic lesions are particularly favorable for the growth of virulent M-strains of nephritogenic streptococci. These are distinctive from the streptococcus found in the throat and are associated with a high incidence of nephritis, reportedly in the neighborhood of 12 per cent.[19] This nephritogenic strain of streptococcus is not as

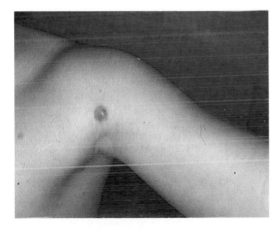

Figure 14–11 Postscabietic nodules (nodular scabies). The result of a hypersensitivity to the mite, these pruritic reddish-brown infiltrated nodules generally appear on covered parts of the body (the axillae, shoulders, groin, buttocks, and genital area) and often persist for months.

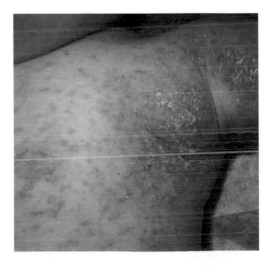

Figure 14–12 Eczematoid scabies (scabies incognito) following long-term topical corticosteroid therapy.

common in the northern part of the United States as it is in the south, the Island of Trinidad in the West Indies, and parts of Africa.[20]

DIAGNOSIS. The diagnosis of scabies is best made by the history of itching, a characteristic distribution of lesions, the recognition of primary lesions, particularly the pathognomonic burrow when present, and the presence of disease among the patient's family or associates (Table 14–3). In infants and children, however, the diagnosis of scabies is often overlooked because of a lower index of suspicion, an atypical distribution that includes the head, neck, palms, and soles, and obliteration of demonstrable primary lesions as a result of vigorous hygienic measures, excoriation, crusting, eczematization, and secondary infection.

Rapid and definitive confirmation can be made by microscopic examination of scrapings of suspicious lesions, with demonstration of the adult mite, ova, larva, or fecal matter (Fig. 14–13). The best lesions for microscopic examination are fresh papules or identifiable burrows, ideally those where potential organisms and ova have not been scratched or excoriated. Potassium hydroxide, time-honored for microscopic examination of skin scrapings, dissolves the organisms, their ova, and excreta, thus making the diagnosis even more difficult and less reliable. In practical application, a drop of mineral oil on the suspected lesion will allow easier scraping of the lesion and more definitive identification of the pathogenic organism.[21]

Although positive microscopic identification of the parasite is dramatic, convincing, and helpful to the physician, I find the yield of such examinations in infants and small children to be particularly low, frustrating, and frequently unrewarding. When lesions are atypical or obliterated, therefore, diagnosis must be made by the history of intractable, particularly nocturnal pruritus, the character and distribution of the eruption, and the presence of associated contact cases. Despite the low yield and the time required for careful microscopic examination, I firmly believe that all suspected lesions should be scraped and minutely examined.

In patients in whom the true nature of the dermatosis remains undiagnosed, a cutaneous punch biopsy, although not always diagnostic, may rule out other diagnoses and assist in establishing the final correct diagnosis (Fig. 14–3). Most skin biopsies of scabies demonstrate intra and intercellular edema, with or without vesicle formation, and a non-specific lymphocytic infiltrate in the dermis.[22] The histopathologic demonstration of a sarcoptic burrow within the stratum

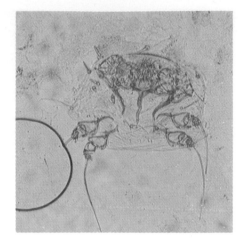

Figure 14–13 A gravid female of *S. scabiei* as seen on microscopic examination of a skin scraping of a patient with scabies (Hurwitz, S: Am. J. Dis. Child. *126*:226, 1973).

corneum is uncommon and frequently fortuitous. Except in overwhelming infestations such as crusted scabies, it is often found only after multiple sectionings and repeated biopsies.

In the differential diagnosis of scabies in infants and young children, atopic, contact, and irritant dermatitides are the most frequently confused and misdiagnosed. Other common misdiagnoses include Letterer-Siwe disease (histiocytosis X), seborrheic dermatitis, dermatitis herpetiformis, and papular urticaria. An awareness of scabies, the morphology and distribution of lesions, a history of itching or lesions in other members of the family, microscopic examination of skin scrapings, and histopathologic examination of lesions usually will help differentiate scabies from these cutaneous disorders.

TREATMENT. Present-day therapy of scabies consists of topical application of 1.0 per cent gamma benzene hexachloride (lindane, available as Kwell), 10 per cent crotamiton (Eurax), 6 to 10 per cent precipitate of sulfur in petrolatum, or a suspension of benzyl benzoate in a 12.5 to 25 per cent concentration (Table 14–4). Other preparations suggested for the management of scabietic infestation include phenylbutazone and thiabendazole. Until further studies are available, however, these two preparations should be reserved only for those patients unresponsive to other presently available therapeutic agents.[9, 23]

Gamma Benzene Hexachloride (Lindane). Lindane is currently the most extensively used

Table 14–3 DIAGNOSIS OF SCABIES

1. History of intractable itching
2. History of exposure to other cases
3. Character and distribution of lesions
4. Burrows (when present)
5. Microscopic examination of skin scrapings
6. Cutaneous biopsy

Table 14–4 TREATMENT OF SCABIES

1. 1.0% lindane
   (gamma benzene hexachloride, Kwell)
2. 10% Crotamiton (Eurax)
3. 6 to 10% sulfur in petrolatum
4. 12.5 to 25% benzyl benzoate
5. Antipruritics (systemic and topical)
6. Appropriate antibiotics when necessary

scabicide in the United States. Because of its widespread use and anecdotal communications suggesting possible toxicity associated with its use, this preparation has come under close scrutiny during the past several years. In 1974, Felman and Maibach demonstrated transcutaneous absorption of gamma benzene hexachloride and suggested that prolonged or repetitive application might lead to elevated blood levels of this potentially toxic agent.[24] In view of this potential toxicity, 1976 the Academy of Pediatric and the Federal Drug Administration warned of possible toxicity due to misuse of this preparation.[25]

The problem of possible toxic effects becomes more acute in infants and small children, owing to a relatively greater skin surface and possibly higher blood level accumulations in this age group. Since this alert, systemic reactions associated with accidental ingestion or excessive topical application of this preparation have been documented. These include eczema, urticaria, aplastic anemia, possible alopecia, and central nervous system toxicity, manifested by irritability, nausea, vomiting, amblyopia, headache, dizziness, and convulsions.[26-29] It should be emphasized that these reactions were almost invariably associated with ingestion or excessive use of medication. It is apparent, therefore, that careful guidelines be established for this agent, particularly for use in the therapy of infants and small children.

Current recommendations for the use of gamma benzene hexachloride (lindane) suggest a 12-hour period of application of this preparation, in a 1 per cent cream or lotion. Following the prescribed time of application the preparation should be washed off thoroughly. Allergic contact dermatitis from this agent has not been documented; irritant contact dermatitis, however, from excessive use is not uncommon.[16] Current studies on file at Reed & Carnrick Research Institute suggest that 1 per cent lindane may be ovicidal against ectoparasitic mites. A second application may be required one week later to destroy recently hatched larvae not eliminated by the initial treatment if there is evidence of failure of compliance, reinfestation, or apparent resistance. There is no justification, however, for repeated treatment at more frequent intervals. This practice, unfortunately all too common, may result in toxicity due to abnormally high blood levels of this potentially toxic agent.[28, 29, 30]

Recent studies in scabies have demonstrated that a 6-hour application of lindane appears to be effective as previously recommended 12 and 24-hour treatment regimens (personal communication, David Taplin). One 4-hour application is curative in 85 per cent of cases, and one 12 hour application cures 96 per cent of cases. Further studies on the efficacy of concentrations less than the recommended 1 per cent, blood level determinations to demonstrate the degree of cutaneous absorption in various age groups, and a comparison study on the relative efficacy of the available scabicidal agents are necessary. Present recom-

mendations also suggest a hot bath prior to the application of lindane. If a bath is indeed deemed necessary, it seems reasonable that the skin be allowed to dry and cool in order to limit transcutaneous permeability and possible excessive levels of absorption.

Twenty-four hours after effective treatment, the patient is no longer capable of transmitting the disease, and resistance to scabicides has not been proved. However, symptoms and signs may not clear for weeks, since the hypersensitivity state does not cease immediately after eradication of the infection. The patient and his family should be alerted to this possibility so that they will know what to expect and will not be tempted to continue excessive, unnecessary, and potentially hazardous therapy.

Studies have shown that the scabies mite is unable to live for more than five minutes in temperatures above 120° Fahrenheit (50° Centigrade), or when away from its human host for periods of two days or more. Thus, if personal bedclothing of treated individuals is changed, stored, or laundered in a washing machine or dryer, reinfection can usually be prevented.

Crotamiton. Of the other available therapeutic agents, crotamiton (Eurax) has no reported systemic effect and may be used as a safe alternate in the treatment of pregnant women, infants, and small children. Whether it is more or less efficacious than lindane is not known.[16] Crotamiton however, can be irritating on raw or denuded skin and reportedly has caused sensitization after prolonged use in patients with eczema. This agent, therefore, may be used in infants and small children, but should be used with caution in patients with acutely inflamed, weeping cutaneous surfaces or atopic dermatitis.

Benzyl Benzoate. Used extensively for the management of scabies in the United Kingdom and Canada, although not readily available in the United States, benzyl benzoate can be compounded and used in concentrations of 12.5 to 25 per cent. This preparation is effective and cosmetically acceptable, but can result in an increase in pruritus or irritation. In such cases, topical or systemic antipruritic agents can be beneficial. Particular care should be exerted in the use of benzyl benzoate so as to avoid conjunctivitis or irritation to the eyes.

Sulfur. Although I personally have treated over 40 infants with gamma benzene hexachloride without apparent adverse reaction, until further studies are completed I recommend a 6 per cent sulfur precipitate in petrolatum for the management of scabies in infants and small children. When in contact with living tissue, this preparation readily forms hydrogen sulfide and pentathionic acid ($CH_2S_5O_6$), both of which appear to have germicidal and fungicidal activity. Though perhaps somewhat messy, odoriferous, and staining to clothing, I find this preparation to be safe, effective, and well tolerated in this age group. The preparation can be applied nightly for three nights, and if evidence of infestation persists, this regimen may be repeated in one week.

Coal Tar Preparations. A high percentage of children with scabies have been found to develop persistent reddish-brown infiltrated nodules, particularly on the covered parts of the body (the axillae, groin, buttocks, and genital areas). These lesions, termed nodular scabies, are associated with a hypersensitivity and may persist for months despite adequate antiscabietic therapy. If treatment is desired, scabietic nodules respond to coal tar preparations (Estar gel or Psorigel), intralesional steroids, and/or corticosteroids under occlusion.

Precautions. Once a diagnosis of scabies has been made, many patients or their parents will embark on a regimen of frequent bathing and overzealous attempts at hygiene. This frequently leads to excessive dryness of the skin, secondary eczematization, and persistent pruritus. Often the generalized itch will persist long after the parasite has been eliminated by antiscabietic therapy. This itching, perhaps due to an acquired sensitivity to the mite or its products, should not be confused with resistance of the mite to therapy. Repeated examinations and skin scrapings, therefore, should also be performed in these cases to insure that infestation is no longer present. As an added precaution, in order to limit overtreatment on the part of patients and their families, only required amounts of the therapeutic agent should be prescribed, and prescription refills should be strictly limited.

Recent reports of infants with extensive scabietic infestation and unusual clinical presentation (scabies incognito), apparently promoted by extended topical use of potent corticosteroids, suggest avoidance of such preparations in the routine treatment of scabies. Systemic antipruritic agents, topical antipruritic lotions, and only low-potency hydrocortisone preparations accordingly appear to be appropriate for the management of persistent pruritus and secondary eczematization associated with scabietic infestation.

Although current evidence suggests that adequate treatment may fail to reduce the incidence of nephritis following streptococcal disease, it seems reasonable to treat all scabies infestations complicated by cutaneous streptococcal infection with appropriate systemic antibiotics.[31] Simple and effective in promptly eradicating the infecting organism, antibiotics clear the clinical infection and limit the spread of this organism to others. Because of the risk of nephritis, it is further recommended that urinalyses be done for a period of two or three weeks in all patients suspected of harboring nephritogenic strains of this organism.

Other Mites

Harvest Mites (Chiggers). The chigger, *Trombicula alfreddugesi*, or red bug, a member of the American harvest mite family, is commonly seen in the southern United States. The chigger is distinct from other mites in that only the larva is parasitic to man and animals. The eight-legged adult and nymphal stages are spent in a nonparasitic existence. They live in grain stems, in grasses, or in areas overgrown with briars or blackberry bushes, where they exist and feed upon vegetable matter, minute arthropods, and insect eggs. The six-legged larvae are responsible for the characteristic eruption seen in this disorder. They attach themselves to the skin of a passing human or animal host, inject an irritating secretion that causes itching, and then drop to the ground or are scratched off within a day or two after the itching begins.[32]

Areas affected by chiggers depend to a certain extent on the type of clothing worn, for they tend to attach themselves to areas where they meet an obstacle in the clothing, such as a belt, brassiere, garter, or boot or shoe top. A few hours after exposure itching, which may be intense, occurs. The itching reaches its peak of intensity on the second day and gradually decreases over the next five or six days. The eruption, chiefly seen on the legs and at the belt-line, is characterized by pruritic discrete bright-red papules, 1 to 2 mm in diameter, often with hemorrhagic puncta. At times there may be scratch marks, urticarial lesions, and diffuse erythema. In children the eruption is often widespread, the pruritus may persist for months, purpuric lesions or bullae may develop, and secondary excoriation and impetiginization are common. In sensitized individuals wheals, followed by papules, papulovesicles, or nodules may be noted. In severe cases, fever may be present, and an eczematous reaction may complicate the picture.

Treatment of chigger bites consists of antihistamines, cool baths or compresses, and topical corticosteroids or antihistamines. Clear nail polish applied to the individual chigger bites appears to be a simple yet highly effective measure for immediate relief.[32] Bullous lesions readily become infected, particularly in children, and may be treated with appropriate antibiotics as well as antihistamines. Materials used for protection against chiggers function more as toxicants than true repellents.[33] The good mosquito repellents — diethyltoluamide (Deet), ethylhexanediol dimethyl phthallate, and dimethyl carbate are good chigger toxicants. They provide the best protection when applied to the clothing, but if inadequate clothing is worn, it may be necessary to apply the protective material to the skin as well. Benzyl benzoate is an excellent chigger toxicant and is the only one that remains effective after rinsing, washing, or submersion in water.[33]

Grain Mites. Of medical interest is the grain itch mite (*Pyemotes ventricosus*), which feeds on the larvae of insects, infesting seeds, grains, and plant stems. Persons coming into contact with infested straw and grain are particularly susceptible to this form of dermatitis. The eruption is seen as seasonal, severely pruritic, pale-pink to bright-red, macular, papulovesicular, or pustular lesions

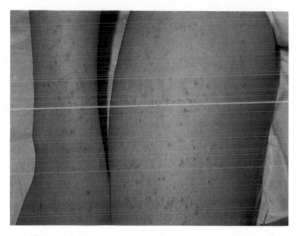

Figure 14-14 "Pigeon-mite" dermatitis. Urticarial wheals, papules, and vesicles in the areas of bites by *Dermonyssus gallinae* (a common parasite of chickens, swallows, canaries, and pigeons).

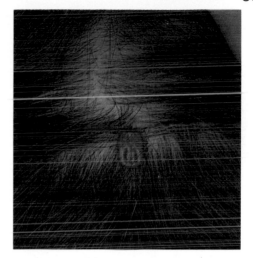

Figure 14-15 A tick embedded in the scalp of an 11-year-old child. In the removal of ticks, care must be exercised to insure that fragments of mouth parts are not left within the skin.

followed by urticarial wheals, and, at times, a purpuric eruption. In severe cases involving the entire body, constitutional reactions with fever can be confused with the eruption of varicella (chickenpox). The eruption is self-limiting and generally managed by antihistamines and topical antipruritic preparations (calamine lotion or topical corticosteroids).

Fowl Mites ("Pigeon-Mite" Dermatitis). *Dermonyssus gallinae*, a common ectoparasite of chickens and wild or domesticated birds (swallows, canaries, pigeons) may temporarily infest human beings and produce troublesome skin lesions at the site of skin puncture. The eruption is characterized by urticarial wheals, papules, or vesicles that develop at areas of bites (Fig. 14-14).

Ticks

Ticks are large, globular arachnids with short legs and hard leathery skin and are adapted for sucking blood from mammals, birds, and reptiles. They are important vectors of diseases, such as relapsing fever and a variety of rickettsial and virus infections, including Rocky Mountain Spotted Fever and possibly erythema chronicum migrans (see Chapter 18). Many species inflict troublesome bites, and some cause severe constitutional symptoms.[1]

Classified into two family groups, hard ticks (Ixodidae) and soft ticks (Argasidae), they are found in grass, shrubs, vines and bushes, from which they attach themselves to dogs, cattle, and human beings. The female tick attaches herself to the intended victim by sticking her proboscis into the skin to suck blood from the superficial vessels (Fig. 14-15). The local bite is painless and innocuous, and thus the tick is frequently undetected or noted only after several days of attachment. The local bite often results in an infiltrated lesion with

a distinct surrounding erythematous halo, which may persist for one or two weeks or more (Fig. 14-16). The bites are often followed by small, often pruritic nodules (a local foreign body reaction if the mouth parts are carelessly left in the skin or improperly removed). The resulting pruritic granulomatous nodule may persist for months or even years. In some individuals an annular erythema characterized by a raised red ring with an advancing indurated border and central clearing (erythema chronicum migrans) may result (see Fig. 18-4).[34] Whether this is induced by a rickettsia, spirochete, mycoplasma, virus, or toxic or allergic disorder is unknown, but penicillin and tetracycline are helpful in treating erythema chronicum migrans and may prevent or attenuate arthritis in patients with Lyme disease (Lyme arthritis).[35, 35a]

Tick bite pyrexia, manifested by fever, chills, headache, vomiting and abdominal pain, is presumably caused by a toxin secreted by the female tick. Removal of the engorged tick results in improvement of symptoms, usually within a period of 12 to 36 hours.

Tick paralysis, a reversible disease of the nervous system, manifested by incoordination, weakness, and flaccid paralysis, is due to a neuro-

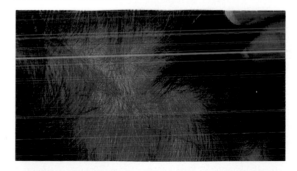

Figure 14-16 Infiltration with surrounding erythema (cutaneous reaction to a tick bite on the scalp of a 4-year-old child).

toxin that is injected into the victim while the tick is engorging. In this disorder it appears that the tick must feed for several days before paralysis occurs. Although there is wide variation in individual susceptibility, paralysis generally occurs about six days after attachment of the tick. The paralysis usually starts in the legs and gradually ascends upward over the body. Bulbar paralysis, dysarthria, dysphagia, and death from respiratory failure may occur unless the tick is found and removed. Most cases of tick paralysis occur in children, especially girls. The tick is usually attached to the scalp, where it is hidden by the hair, but it may attach to any part of the skin, especially the ear, axilla, back, groin, or vulva (Fig. 14–15). Prompt recovery from tick paralysis generally occurs, often within 24 hours, after the tick is removed.[36]

Various methods of tick removal have been advocated. Recommended methods include heat from a previously lighted match; covering the area with nail polish, mineral oil, or petrolatum; a few drops of chloroform or ether; ethyl chloride spray; and cryotherapy with liquid nitrogen. It is important that ticks not merely be plucked off, but that care be exercised to insure that no fragments of the mouth parts or proboscis be left behind within the skin. Should a portion be retained, a cutaneous punch biopsy generally will effectively remove it. In infested areas protection for tick bites is best accomplished by the use of repellents in clothing — diethyltoluamide (N,N-diethyl-m-toluamide, Deet), Indalone (butyl-3,4-dihydro-2,2-dimethyl-4-oxo-1,2,H-pyran-6-carboxylate), dimethyl carbate, dimethyl phthalate, and benzyl benzoate.[33]

Spiders

Spiders, because of their menacing appearance, are unjustifiably blamed for more damage than they actually create. Virtually all the spider bites on the North American continent are caused by *Lactrodectus mactans* (the black widow spider) and *Loxosceles reclusa* (the brown recluse spider).

The Black Widow Spider (Lactrodectus mactans).   The female black widow spider, the dangerous spider of southern Canada, the United States, Cuba, and Mexico, is recognized by its coal-black color and globular body (1 cm across) with a red or orange hour-glass marking on the underside of its abdomen. A web-spinner (in contrast to burrowing spiders) she lives in cool dark places in out-buildings and little used structures and often spins her web across outdoor privy seats. Therefore, a large number of bites in the southern United States are received around the genitalia and buttocks.

The black widow spider bites humans only in self-defense. Two red punctate marks and local swelling may be seen, and burning or stinging develops at the site of the bite. This is followed, within ten minutes to an hour, by severe cramp-like pain, which increases to a maximum in about three hours. Although the bite may be fatal in approximately 5 per cent of children, most patients recover spontaneously in two or three days.

Treatment consists of specific antivenin (Lyovac, Merck Sharp & Dohme) and intravenous calcium gluconate. Methocarbamol (Robaxin, A. H. Robins) is thought to be of more benefit than 10 per cent calcium gluconate and produces more prolonged relief of symptoms. Although safety and effectiveness of methocarbamol in children below the age of 12 years have been established only in tetanus, the injectable form can be administered intravenously (10 ml over a 5-minute period, with a second 10 ml ampule in 250 ml of a glucose or saline drip solution intravenously at 20 drops per minute).[37] Neostigmine methylsulfate may help relieve muscle spasm, and in severe cases ACTH or systemic corticosteroids may be helpful.

The Brown Recluse Spider (Loxosceles reclusa).   The recluse spider *(Loxosceles reclusa)* is slightly smaller than the black widow spider and has an overall diameter of 3 to 4 cm. It has an oval light-fawn to dark chocolate-brown body (about 1 cm in length and 4 mm in width). A dark violin-shaped band (extending from the eyes back to the end of the cephalothorax) and three pairs of eyes, rather than the four seen in other spiders, differentiate *Loxosceles reclusa* from other brown spiders. The spider has been found and bite reactions have been reported from Colorado to the eastern coast of the United States, from southern Illinois to the Gulf coast, and more recently in the western states of California and Arizona.[38] When in the house, the brown recluse spider is found in storage closets (among clothing); when outdoors, it generally resides in grasses, rocky bluffs, and barns. Because of its normal shyness and predilection for dark recesses, it bites only in self-defense when molested.[39]

The venom of the *Loxosceles* spider is hemolytic and necrotizing and contains a spreading factor. Two types of reaction, a localizing cutaneous response and a severe, potentially grave systemic reaction, may occur. These reactions are not mutally exclusive and individual patients may exhibit either or both reactions. In localized reactions the initial symptom may be a mild itching or

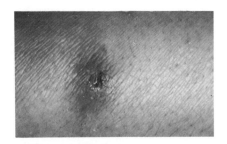

Figure 14–17   Cutaneous reaction eight days after a spider bite on the arm of a young woman.

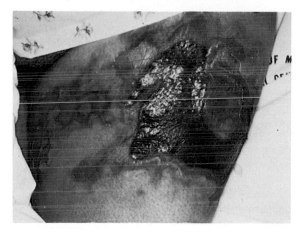

Figure 14-18 Eschar due to the bite of a Brown Recluse Spider (Courtesy of Larry E. Millikan, M.D. and Richard Berger, M.D.).

stinging at the time of the bite. Mild to severe pain begins after a period of two to eight hours, followed by swelling and tenderness, a hemorrhagic vesicle or blister, and finally a gangrenous eschar with surrounding zones of edema, erythema, and ischemia (Figs. 14–17, 14–18). Lymphangitis, manifested by a linear erythema along the course of the lymphatics, is not uncommon when the bite occurs on an extremity. In about a week the central portion becomes dark, demarcated, and gangrenous and may produce a large necrotic ulceration that can extend many centimeters in width and may last for months before healing occurs.

In 25 per cent of patients, the bite evokes a systemic reaction in addition to the cutaneous reaction. This reaction may include nausea, vomiting, chills, fever, malaise, muscle aches and pains, a generalized erythematous, often purpuric macular eruption, thrombocytopenia, hemolytic anemia, hemoglobinuria, shock, coma, and eventual renal failure. Severe systemic reactions are noted more often in children than adults and have been responsible for the deaths of at least two children and one adult.[40]

Treatment of brown recluse spider bites is difficult. Some patients, particularly those with progressive ischemia, cyanosis, and bulla formation at the site of the bite, appear to benefit from early intralesional steroids at the site of the bite, systemic corticosteroids, oral antihistamines, and systemic antibiotics for secondary infection. Some authors suggest excision when necrosis appears inevitable (usually within two to five days) in an effort to reduce spread of the toxin and reduction of secondary infection. In patients in whom necrosis has occurred, the entire area should be excised with subsequent split-thickness skin grafts.[37]

Scorpions

Scorpions are tropical photophobic arachnids that hide by day and hunt by night. They differ from other arachnids in that they have an elongated abdomen ending in a stinger. Found all over the world, particularly in the tropics, in North America they are generally seen in the southern United States and Mexico.

The venom apparatus is carried in the curved sting at the tip of the tail, which is swung over the scorpion's head to penetrate the victim's skin. During the day scorpions hide in shoes, closets, clothing, and crevices. Some species of ground scorpions, however, may burrow and hide in gravel or children's sandboxes. They rarely attack man but will sting humans when accidentally disturbed, brushed against, or stepped upon.

The sting of the scorpion is extremely dangerous, since it releases two principle noxious agents: a localized hemolytic toxin and a dangerous neurotoxic venom. The hemolytic toxin may cause a painful burning sensation, with pronounced redness, swelling, discoloration, lymphangitis, severe necrosis, and, in some patients, disseminated intravascular coagulopathy or renal failure. The purpuric area around the bite is a sign that distinguishes spider bites from the bites of other insects. The degree of damage at the site of the sting varies; the variations are most likely due to polypeptide variations in the different venoms and the amount of venom injected.[41] The neurotoxic venom may produce local numbness and a severe generalized reaction consisting of sweating, salivation, tightness in the throat, abdominal cramps, cyanosis, convulsions, and, particularly in small children, respiratory paralysis and death. In a tabulation of deaths according to age, 75 per cent are in infants and children less than three years of age.

Treatment of scorpion stings consists of immediate application of a tourniquet above the area whenever possible, applications of ice or cold water, and, in severe reactions, the administration of epinephrine, specific antitoxin serum, and/or systemic steroids. The site of the sting should not be incised, and neither opiates nor paraldehyde should be given. Shock, when present, is treated with parenteral fluids, and barbiturates should be administered to patients with extreme irritability or convulsions, or both.

INSECTA

Insects are the class of arthropods characterized by division into three parts (a head, thorax, and abdomen). Noxious insects are ubiquitous, affecting all human beings in some manner at one time or another. The insects of medical significance include lice, bugs, bees, wasps, ants, fleas, moths and their larvae, flies, and mosquitoes.

Pediculosis — Disorders Due to Lice (Anoplura)

Lice have plagued man since ancient times. Although infection is most common during times

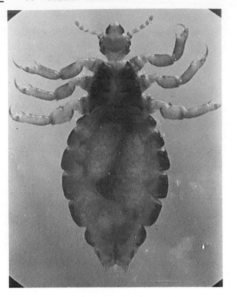

Figure 14–19   The head louse *(Pediculus humanus capitis).* A six-legged wingless insect (1 to 4 mm in size) with a translucent grayish-white body that becomes red when engorged with blood (Courtesy of Reed & Carnrick). Body lice are lighter in color and 10 to 20 per cent larger than head lice.

Barely visible to the naked eye, they measure 1 to 4 mm in size. The head contains a pair of eyes and a pair of short segmented antennae. The mouth parts consist of stylets modified for piercing and sucking (retractable when not in use) and six pairs of hooks by which they attach to the skin while feeding (Fig. 14–19). In general body lice are 10 to 20 per cent longer than head lice and are often lighter in color.[42]

Three varieties of pediculi attack man. These include *Pthirus pubis* (the crab louse), *Pediculus humanus capitis* (the head louse), and *Pediculus humanus corporis* (the body louse). Although the crab louse is a distinct genus and species, some doubt exists as to the status of the two forms of *Pediculus humanus.* Most authorities feel that the head louse represents the ancestral type and that the body louse evolved when man began wearing clothes. Each variety has a predilection for certain parts of the body and rarely migrates to other regions. In piercing the skin they exude a poisonous salivary secretion, which, together with the mechanical puncture, produces a pruritic dermatitis. In addition, the body louse is the carrier of certain rickettsial diseases (louse-born typhus and trench fever) and a spirochetal disorder (relapsing fever).

Head and body lice may be acquired by personal contact or by putting on infested clothing. Head lice may also be acquired by contact with upholstered chairs and the use of infested combs or brushes.

Crab lice are spread chiefly by sexual contact and perhaps occasionally by close personal contact or the proverbial toilet seat. The crab louse has a shorter abdomen, bearing hairy lateral tufts, and large second and third legs, which give it its crab-like appearance (Fig. 14–20). Small children may become infected with crab lice on their eyebrows or eyelashes from their mothers or by close contact with infested adults. For some unknown reason blacks are relatively resistant to louse infestation.

The ova or nits are oval, grayish or yellowish-white in color, and are seen as tiny pin-head specks measuring 0.3 to 0.8 mm. They may be

of stress, such as war, crowded situations in schools, camps, or institutions, following widespread use of DDT after the end of World War II there were relatively few reports of pediculosis in the United States. Subsequent to restrictions in the use of DDT in this country since January, 1973, however, the number of cases has recently increased, particularly pediculosis capitis and, with our present climate of sexual permissiveness, pediculosis pubis.

Human lice occur wherever there are people. They spend their entire life as ectoparasites, living on man, depending on the blood they extract from their victims for sustenance. Their existence, therefore, independent of humans is impossible. They are small, six-legged, wingless insects with translucent, almost gray or grayish-white bodies, which become red when engorged with blood.

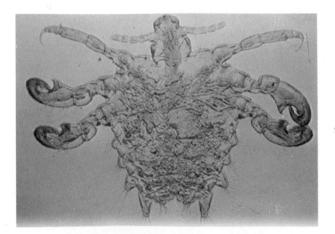

Figure 14–20   *Pthirus pubis* (the crab louse) (Courtesy of Reed & Carnrick).

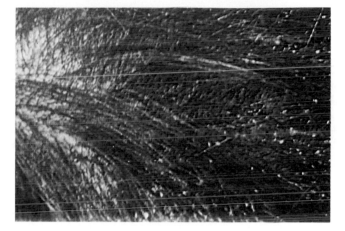

Figure 14–21 Pediculosis capitis. Oval grayish to yellowish-white nits in the hair of the scalp (Courtesy of Reed & Carnrick). Nits measure about 0.5 mm in length, fluoresce under Wood's light, and are not easily flicked off or moved along the hair shaft

found in the scalp in pediculosis capitis, the pubic and anal regions in pediculosis pubis, and on the seams of clothing in pediculosis corporis (Figs. 14–21, 14–22). They are laid within 24 to 48 hours after mating and, incubated by the heat of the body, hatch in about eight days. It takes another eight days for the emerging larvae to reach maturity. The ova can be identified by fluorescence under Wood's light and by examination under the microscope. They have a chitinous ring at the base by which they are fastened securely to the hair. The egg may have an embryo visible inside and a cap at the free end (operculum) for breathing purposes (Fig. 14–23).

Pediculosis Corporis. The body louse is slightly larger (10 to 20 per cent) than the head louse, generally lives in clothing or bedding, lays eggs along the seams of clothing, and only visits the human host long enough to feed. Its nits attach firmly to the fibers of clothing (where they may remain viable for several weeks) and hatch out, owing to body warmth when the clothing is worn by the human host. The parasite is rarely observed on the skin; it obtains its nourishment by clinging to the patient's clothing and piercing the skin by its proboscis. The primary lesion is a small pinpoint red macule, papule, or urticarial wheal, with a characteristic hemorrhagic central punctum. Due to the intense generalized pruritus associated with this disorder, primary lesions are frequently obliterated by scratching and, therefore, are seldom seen. Diagnosis is established by a generalized pruritus, parallel scratch marks (particularly in the interscapular region), fleeting wheals, secondary eczematization, bacterial infection, bloody crusts, and in cases of prolonged duration, postinflammatory hyperpigmentation. The diagnosis can be confirmed by the finding of lice or nits in the seams of clothing (Fig. 14–22).

Pediculosis Capitis. Pediculosis capitis, except during situations that cause crowding and insanitary conditions, is the most common form of louse infestation. Children, particularly girls, are more susceptible to infestation than adults. Presumably the higher incidence in females is due to their usually longer hair styles. For some unknown reason, blacks are relatively resistant to this disorder. Itching is the principal symptom of pediculosis capitis. Infestation is frequently complicated by bacterial infection and should not be overlooked when overshadowed by impetigo of the scalp, furunculosis, or postoccipital lymphadenopathy.

Nits are chiefly found in the hairs above the

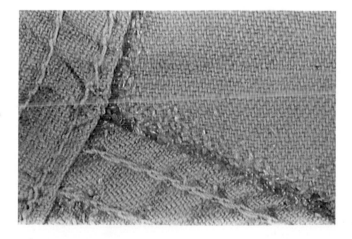

Figure 14–22 Nits in the seams of clothing. Diagnostic of *Pediculus humanus corporis* (Courtesy of Reed & Carnrick).

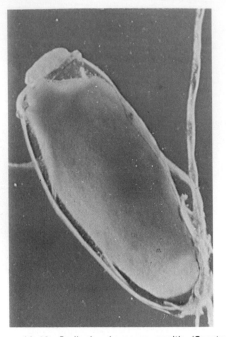

Figure 14–23 *Pediculus humanus capitis* (Courtesy of Reed & Carnrick). Note chitinous attachment to the hair shaft, an embryo in situ, and the intact operculum. Microscopic examination of nits readily establishes the proper diagnosis.

ears and in the occipital region, usually one-quarter inch or so from the scalp (Fig. 14–21). The nits are small, oval, whitish in color, and measure about 0.5 mm in length. They are laid close to the scalp near the bottom of the hair shaft and, as hairs grow out, are carried outward. Nits present away from the scalp and along the shafts or tips of long hairs signify long-standing infection or residual nits from previously treated infestation. It is important not to mistake epidermal scales or hair casts as pediculosis capitis or nits. Such errors may have severe psychological consequences for the patients, their families, and, at times, even school authorities.[43] Of diagnostic importance is the fact that nits fluoresce under Wood's light examination and are not easily flicked off or moved along the shaft with the fingers. If the differentiation is doubtful, snipping of the hair and low power

microscopic examination of suspected nits will usually clarify the diagnosis (Fig. 14–23).

Pediculosis capitis may be transmitted by shared hats, clothing, towels, combs, or hair brushes. Traditionally confined to the scalp, the head louse, on occasion, also has been known to be responsible for pediculosis of the eyelids, particularly in children.

Pediculosis Pubis. Pediculosis pubis is caused by the crab louse (*Pthirus pubis*) (Fig. 14–20). It should be noted that the scientific name of the insect is often misspelled as *Phthirus pubis*. This parasite normally inhabits the hairs of the pubic region, but may also involve the eyelashes, beard, mustache, axillary, and other body hairs. Infestation of the pubic region is most frequently seen in adolescents and young adults as the result of transmission by sexual intercourse, although it may also be transmitted by clothing, bedding, or towels. The crab louse is shorter and broader than the head and body louse. Itching may be the initial symptom, but in persistent cases eczematization or secondary infection may occur (Fig. 14–24). A heavy infestation is occasionally accompanied by asymptomatic bluish or slate-colored macules, 0.5 to 1.0 cm in diameter (maculae ceruleae), that do not blanch upon pressure with a glass slide. They may be seen on the trunk, thighs, or upper arms, and often last for months. Although frequently described in clinical descriptions of pediculosis pubis, they are not commonly seen in mild infestations and therefore should not be relied upon as a clinical feature in the differential diagnosis of this disorder.

Pediculosis Palpebrarum. In children *Pthirus pubis* (occasionally *Pediculus humanus capitis* or *corporis*) may locate in the eyelashes or eyebrows (pediculosis palpebrarum). When the eyelids are involved it usually is related to infestation in an adult, often the mother. In this disorder the nits must be differentiated from the scaling seen in blepharitis associated with seborrheic dermatitis.

TREATMENT OF PEDICULOSIS. 1.0 per cent gamma benzene hexachloride (lindane), available as Kwell lotion or shampoo, is highly effective in the treatment of pediculosis capitis and pediculosis pubis. Since in pediculosis cor-

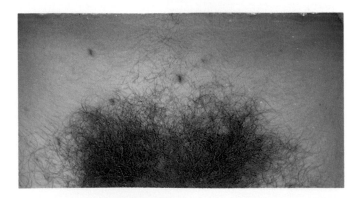

Figure 14–24 *Pediculosis pubis.* Excoriated cutaneous lesions and nits.

poris the body louse ordinarily does not inhabit the body, therapy mainly consists of proper hygiene and frequent showering or bathing, with change of underclothes and bedding. Underclothing and bedding should be laundered with hot water or boiled. Dry cleaning destroys lice in articles that cannot be laundered. Pressing woolens with a hot iron is also satisfactory, but special attention should be given to the seams of the clothing. All likely contacts (members of the household and close contacts in institutions) should be examined and treated if there is evidence of infestation.

Pediculosis capitis is treated by 1 per cent lindane (Kwell) as a shampoo or lotion. When lindane shampoo is used, the patient's scalp should be thoroughly shampooed for four minutes with one tablespoon or less of the preparation. If the lotion is used, it may be applied to the scalp, left on overnight, and then washed out carefully. A second treatment may be repeated after one week if viable eggs persist. Other children in the family should be examined, and those with evidence of infestation should be treated.

Live nits can be differentiated from dead ones by use of a Wood's lamp in a completely darkened room (live nits glow with a pearly fluorescence while dead nits do not), or by microscopic examination of nits (the absence of an embryo or operculum in ova that have hatched). Since nits are firmly attached to the hair shaft, removal (although not necessary) may be facilitated by the use of a fine-tooth comb, or tweezers, or by soaking the hair with white vinegar or a 3 to 5 per cent acetic acid solution, followed by wrapping with a damp towel soaked in the same solution. The towel may be removed after about an hour, and removal of the nits can be facilitated by a shampooing and the use of a fine-tooth comb (the acetic acid dissolves the chitin, which binds the nits to the hair shafts).[44]

In pediculosis pubis, a thin layer of lindane lotion is applied to the infested and adjacent hairy areas, with particular attention to the pubic mons and perianal region. The lotion is left on for 12 hours, then washed off thoroughly, with reapplication in one week if viable eggs persist. Sexual contacts should be treated simultaneously, but other household members need not be treated. At the conclusion of therapy, treated individuals should change their underclothing, pajamas, sheets, and pillow cases. These articles should be washed by machine, automatically dried or laundered, ironed, or boiled in order to destroy remaining ova or parasites.[30]

Pediculosis of the eyelashes may be treated by petrolatum or yellow mercuric oxide applied thickly to the eyelashes twice daily for eight days, followed by mechanical removal of remaining nits. Although petrolatum applied to the eyelashes is the treatment of choice, physostigmine ophthalmic preparations (Eserine) are also effective if applied topically to the eyelid margin (twice daily for 24 to 48 hours). Because of the parasympathetic effect of physostigmine, miosis should be watched for as a possible side effect.

Mosquitoes and Flies

Flies and mosquitoes belong to the order Diptera. One of the largest orders of insects, it includes the two-winged biting flies, gnats, and mosquitoes. Of these, mosquitoes, worldwide in distribution, are the most important from the standpoint of human health. They are vectors of many important diseases (encephalitis, malaria, yellow fever, and filariasis). In the United States the most common insect bites of infants and children are those of mosquitoes.

Mosquitoes are attracted to bright clothing, heat, humidity, and human odors, particularly those of young children. In unsensitized individuals, the ordinary mosquito bite only produces a local irritation. Following the initial bite there may be a slight stinging sensation and a small pruritic erythematous papule with some transient discomfort. In sensitized individuals, however, bites may produce itching; urticarial wheals, which may last for several hours to several days; or firm papules or nodules, which may persist for longer periods of time. Occasionally, particularly in the young, mosquito bites may produce blisters or hemorrhagic lesions, and, owing to pruritus and excoriation, may result in secondary eczematization and impetiginization. Although the diagnosis of insect bites is often obvious, differentiation from other papular, vesicular, and pruritic eruptions can be assisted by a characteristic grouping of lesions, a central punctum when present, and the seasonal incidence of the disorder.

Treatment of mosquito bites consists of oral antihistamines, cool compresses, calamine lotion, and topical corticosteroids. Insect repellents are recommended for individuals who are sensitive to mosquito bites. When out of doors, children prone to insect bite reactions should wear a head covering, shoes, trousers, clothing with long sleeves, and garments of smooth-finished fabrics of neutral colors (white, green, tan, and khaki do not, as a rule, attract insects). Scented hair sprays, tonics or pomades, soaps, lotions, powders, colognes, and perfumes may attract all forms of stinging insects. Although results are not definite, in some individuals thiamine hydrochloride taken orally in dosages of 75 to 150 mg a day appear to help repel insects. This innocuous vitamin apparently combines with human perspiration and produces an odor, imperceptible to the human host, but theoretically disagreeable and repelling to insects.[45, 46]

Various species of biting flies (sandflies, gnats, black flies, deerflies, horseflies) are known to attack the exposed areas of the face, neck, arms, and legs, with the production of painful, irritating, or pruritic papules or nodules, often with vesiculation. Although lesions often disappear in a few hours, they may persist for several days and can be very annoying, particularly in small children. Treatment consists of the prophylactic use of insect repellent (6-12, Deet, or Off) and symptomatic relief by aspirin, antihistamines, calamine lotion, or topical corticosteroids.

Non-biting flies, including common house-flies, tend to feed at open wounds, exudates, and cutaneous ulcers, and may produce myiasis, a far less common, but severe cutaneous disorder. Uncommon in areas where high standards of hygiene prevail, fly larvae may burrow into normal or injured skin (wounds or ulcers), invade the epidermis, and wander in the cutaneous tissues with a resulting migratory inflammatory pattern (migratory myiasis). Therapy consists of injection of a local anesthetic, surgical removal of the larvae, and antibiotics when necessary to control secondary infection.

Fleas

Fleas (Siphonaptera) exist universally among animals and human beings. Those that most commonly attack man in the United States are the human flea (*Pulex irritans*), the cat flea (*Ctenacephalides felis*), and the dog flea (*Ctenacephalides canis*). The eruption produced by a flea bite in a sensitized individual is an urticarial wheal or papule, often, but not invariably, centered by a hemorrhagic punctum (Fig. 14–25). In highly susceptible individuals, particularly young children, wheals may progress and develop into bullae. Bites are usually multiple and grouped together in linear or irregular clusters on the arms, forearms, or legs or on areas where clothing fits snugly (the thighs, buttocks, waist, and lower abdomen). Treatment consists of antihistamines, calamine lotion, or topical corticosteroids and elimination of fleas by treatment of suspected animal carriers and spraying of carpets, floors, crevices, and other potentially infested areas (such as stuffing of furni-

ture and bedding), with 5 per cent malathion powder, 1 per cent lindane dust, or, if available, 5 per cent DDT powder.

Bedbugs

Bedbugs, *Cimex lectularius* (Hemiptera), are reddish-brown blood-sucking insects, about 3 to 5 mm in size, wingless, with flattened oval bodies and three pairs of legs. They secrete themselves in crevices of floors and walls and in bedding or furniture, and normally emerge to feed only in darkness. Under normal conditions feeding takes place about once a week; in cold weather it is less frequent. The time required for feeding varies from five to twelve minutes, after which the insect leaves its victim as quickly as possible. The bedbug is capable of traveling long distances in search of food, often from one house to another, and has been known to survive without food for periods of up to six months to a year.

The bites are commonly seen on exposed areas of the face, neck, arms, or hands, often two or three in a line. Usually the host does not feel the bite. In individuals not sensitized by previous exposure the only manifestation is a symptomless purpuric macule at the site of the bite. In previously sensitized individuals, intensely pruritic papules, or wheals, often with central hemorrhagic puncta, are characteristic. A vesicle may surmount the papule or wheal. Frequently the initial lesion may evolve into a nodule that may last up to 14 days or more. Bullae are frequently seen in children, and excoriated lesions, associated eczematization, or secondary infection may alter the clinical picture.

Treatment is directed at elimination of the bug from the environment by DDT, chlordane, or lindane. Although individual lesions require no direct therapy, oral antihistamines and topical corticosteroids or calamine lotion may give subjective relief.

Papular Urticaria

Papular urticaria (lichen urticatus) is a common disease of childhood manifested by a chronic or recurrent papular eruption caused by a sensitivity reaction to the bites of mosquitoes, fleas, bedbugs, and other insects. Although cases have been described in infants as young as two weeks of age, it is seen primarily in children between two and seven years of age, particularly in those with an atopic background. The disorder appears in summer and late spring; lesions may occur on any part of the body, but tend to be grouped in clusters on exposed areas, particularly the extensor surfaces of the extremities. Although they may occur to a lesser extent on the face and neck, trunk, thighs and buttocks, they generally spare the genital, perianal, and axillary regions.[47]

Individual lesions are seen as 3 to 10 mm firm urticated papules with wheals, or wheals surmounted by papules, often with a central punc-

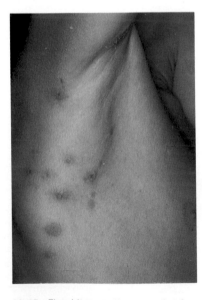

Figure 14–25 Flea bites on the upper trunk, axilla, and shoulder of a young child. Note the characteristic clustering, central hemorrhagic puncta, and urticarial wheals.

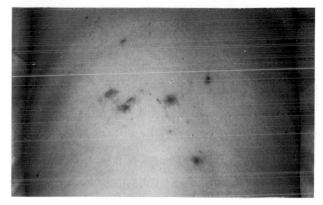

Figure 14-26 Papular urticaria. Recurrent crops of grouped papules with central puncta and urticarial wheals.

tum. (Fig. 14-26). Lesions may be rubbed or irritated, excoriated, lichenified, or secondarily infected with impetiginized crusts or inflammatory ulcerations.[48] The lesions recur in crops, and all stages of development and regression may be noted. Most lesions persist for two to ten days and, after resolution, may result in temporary postinflammatory erythema or pigmentation. If exposure to the parasite is allowed to continue, the attacks may persist for an average of three to four years, perennially or recurring seasonally; occasionally they may persist into adolescence or later.

On histopathologic examination the lesions of papular urticaria are identical to those of insect bites.[49] Affected persons give a delayed papular reaction when injected intradermally with flea, bedbug, or mosquito antigens and run a course that parallels that of papular urticaria. There is no feature of the disease, clinically, histopathological, immunologic, or epidemiologic, that is not consistent with the theory that parasite bites in specifically sensitized subjects is the cause of this disorder.[47]

The differentiation of papular urticaria from true urticaria and arthropod infestations is seldom difficult, but when indeterminate, microscopic examination of skin scrapings, examination of other household members, and skin biopsy may be indicated. In some cases the early lesions of granuloma annulare resemble nodular lesions of papular urticaria; this, too, can be differentiated by histopathologic examination of a cutaneous biopsy. The histopathologic changes in papular urticaria consist of intercellular and intracellular edema, spongiotic vesicles in the epidermis, and moderate to heavy infiltration of lymphocytes, with many eosinophils around vesicles and epidermal appendages in the middle and lower dermis.[49]

Therapy of papular urticaria consists of insect control in the household, with particular attention to baseboards, basements, bed frames, and upholstered furniture and treatment of affected dogs and cats. Antihistamines appear to be of limited value; in most cases disinfestation, simple sedation, and topical calamine lotion or corticosteroids are adequate for relief of symptoms. In patients with bullous lesions or secondary impetiginization, bacterial culture and appropriate antibiotics are indicated.

Bees, Wasps, and Ants

Bees, wasps, and ants belong to the order Hymenoptera, a large order of insects that contains about 100,000 species, of which about half are parasitic on insects or other invertebrates.[1] Like most other insects they have three pairs of legs and four wings and are recognized by the narrow isthmus separating the abdomen from the thorax.

Bees, the only insects that produce food eaten by man, live in almost every part of the world except the North and South Poles. Honey bees live and work together in large groups and do not sting unless frightened or hurt. Wasps, among the most interesting and intelligent of insects, may live together and cooperate with one another, as the so-called social wasps (hornets and yellow jackets), or may live as solitary wasps (those that build separate nests and do not live in communities). Most wasps are helpful to man. Although they sometimes damage fruit, they also destroy large numbers of flies, caterpillars, and other insects harmful to man. Wasps, just as bees, ordinarily do not sting man unless they are bothered or frightened.

Symptoms of bee or wasp stings vary from mild local pruritis, pain, and edema, to general anaphylactic reactions with associated difficulty in breathing and swallowing, hoarseness, thickened speech, gastrointestinal disturbances, abdominal pain, dizziness, weakness, confusion, generalized edema, collapse, unconsciousness, and at times, even sudden death.

Ants, like bees and wasps, have large glands at the tip of the abdomen from which they introduce venom into wounds produced by their bites. The fire ant (*Solenopsis saevissima*), imported from South America in the 1920's, has spread rapidly in the southern part of the United States and produces a venom more potent than that of other hymenoptera. Fire ants are particularly ferocious and, when molested, produce many burning and painful stings within seconds. Pivoting about the grasping jaws, which produce two hemorrhagic sites of puncture, the fire ant inserts its sting into multiple areas producing intense pain, followed by an almost immediate flare, which generally measures from 2.5 to 5.0 cm in diameter. This is rapidly followed by a wheal, which may measure from 2.0 mm to 1 cm in diameter. Eight to ten hours later cloudy and then purulent fluid develops at the puncture site. The bites generally occur in clusters and frequently result in systemic reactions (fever, gastrointestinal distress, urticaria, angioedema, and asthma).[50]

The treatment of ordinary bee, wasp, or ant stings consists of local application of antipruritic shake lotions (calamine lotion), cool compresses or cool baths, and oral antihistamines. A papain solution made up of 1 part meat tenderizer to four parts of water will frequently help relieve local symptoms of pain or discomfort. Epinephrine, oxygen, antihistamines, and systemic corticosteroids should be administered to patients with severe allergic reactions. Patients known to suffer systemic reactions to the sting of a bee, wasp, hornet, or yellow jacket should be desensitized and should have an insect sting kit readily available as a prophylatic measure. An effective insect sting kit should contain a tourniquet (to be applied above the sting when possible), a 15 mg sublingual tablet of isoproterenol for immediate use, an oral antihistamine, and a hypodermic syringe (preferably preloaded with epinephrine) for intramuscular or subcutaneous injection.[51]

If a child has responded with a generalized reaction to a hymenoptera sting, whether mild or severe, desensitization is mandatory. A history of repeated stings with progressively larger local reactions invites a program of hypersensitization. Severe local reactions, delayed reactions, particularly with angioedema and generalized urticaria, place the patient in the same category.[46]

Blister Beetles

Blister beetles (Coleoptera) contain cantharidin, a volatile substance mostly concentrated in the beetles' genitalia. The lesions produced accidentally by crushing blister beetles, by discharge of their body fluid on the skin, or by external therapeutic use of cantharidin (as in the treatment of verrucae), consist of slowly forming blisters that involve the outer layers of the skin. Treatment depends on the extent and location of lesions. Simple aseptic drainage of large bullae and cool compresses generally give adequate relief of symptoms. If vesicles are not traumatized, they usually resolve in three or four days, and the overlying epidermis usually flakes off within a period of six or seven days, requiring no further therapy.

Caterpillars and Moths

Caterpillars represent the larval stage of butterflies and moths of the order Lepidoptera. The hairs of certain moths and caterpillars are known to produce a dermatitis, often severe and incapacitating to both children and adults. In the United States, the most frequently seen and most irritating of these are those due to the hairs of the brown-tail moth (usually seen in the northeastern part of this country) and the hairs of the puss caterpillar (the larva of the "flannel" moth (*Megalopyge opercularis*), seen from Virginia southward to the states bordering the Gulf of Mexico.[52, 53, 54]

Reactions produced by contact with the hairs and spines of these moths and caterpillars appear to be due to a toxin that produces varying degrees of irritation. This may range in severity from a local dermatitis characterized by discrete pruritic, burning, or stinging maculopapular lesions, to urticarial wheals with vesicular or shallow necrotic centers.[55] Systemic reactions may consist of severe local pain, nausea, fever, swelling of the affected area, numbness, severe muscle cramps, intense headache, shock, and convulsions. Not only do the hairs themselves penetrate the skin, but slender delicate hairs are often detached and transported through air or clothing, thus resulting in widespread dermatitis or painful nodular conjunctivitis.

The diagnosis of moth or caterpillar dermatitis can be confirmed by microscopic examination of skin scrapings of involved areas, with demonstration of offending hairs. Treatment is non-specific and primarily supportive. Antihistamines and mild analgesics appear to be of little value. Immediate application of Scotch tape or adhesive over the sting may be helpful in the removal of broken-off spines. Ice packs to the involved areas may help to relieve discomfort in some patients; in others narcotics may be required to control severe pain, and intravenous calcium gluconate and systemic corticosteroids may be of distinct benefit in patients with severe generalized reactions.[52]

OTHER CUTANEOUS PARASITES

Creeping Eruption (Cutaneous Larva Migrans)

Creeping eruption (cutaneous larva migrans) is a distinctive skin disorder that results from invasion of the epidermis and subsequent migration within the superficial layers of the skin by larval parasites. This produces a tortuous linear eruption characterized by bizarre serpentine pink or skin-colored tracts, 2 to 3 mm in diameter (Fig. 14–27). Although the majority of cases are caused by larvae of the dog or cat hookworm (*Ancylostoma braziliense*), other species of parasitic nematodes have been described in this disorder. Infections are most common in warm, humid, and sandy coastal areas of tropical and subtropical regions, and in travelers to and from these areas. In the United States it occurs in states bordering the Gulf of Mexico and the Atlantic Ocean from Texas to Rhode Island. Infections are most common in children and adolescents, although infestations have been noted in adults strolling

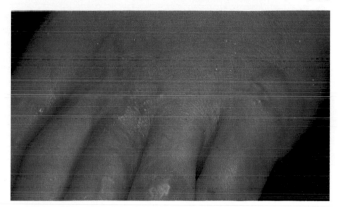

Figure 14–27 Creeping eruption (cutaneous larva migrans) with characteristic serpiginous tracts.

barefoot or walking in these areas. Infections are also frequently acquired by workmen such as plumbers ("plumbers' itch"), electricians, carpenters, pest exterminators exposed to the larvae in warm, moist sandy areas such as the crawl spaces of houses, and gardeners and fisherman working in infected areas.

Adult nematodes live in the intestines of their unnatural host (dogs or cats). Ova are deposited in the animal feces and, under favorable conditions of humidity and temperature, hatch into infective larvae. The larvae, perhaps with the aid of a collagenase or other enzyme, may then penetrate human skin that has been in contact with contaminated sandy areas. Unable to proceed through the bloodstream to the lungs and ultimately the intestines of the unnatural host, the larva remain in the skin, wander aimlessly along the dermal-epidermal junction, and produce the characteristic serpentine tracts seen in this disorder.

The onset of creeping eruption is characterized by pruritus at the site of larval penetration (usually the feet, lower legs, buttocks, or hands). The larvae may lie quietly for weeks or months, or may begin a tortuous serpentine migration along the dermal-epidermal junction. Their migration may vary from 1 mm to 1 or 2 cm a day, with resultant slightly elevated pink or flesh-colored tortuous or serpentine tracts (Fig. 14–27). The number of tracts is variable (in one study the number ranged from 1 to 50, with an average of 10.9 tracts per patient). The disease is self-limiting. In most patients the parasites may wander aimlessly for periods of a few days to several weeks. In some patients they may persist for six months or longer. In one study it was noted that 81 per cent of lesions disappeared spontaneously within a period of four weeks.[56]

For years the management of creeping eruption was inadequate and ineffective. It consisted of an attempt at larval destruction by caustic agents (trichloroacetic acid), by cryotherapy (ethyl chloride spray, carbon dioxide, or liquid nitrogen), or by electrodesiccation. These methods are effective only if the skin is damaged sufficiently to cause sloughing of the ensheathed parasite. This requires therapy aimed at a site just ahead of the advancing burrow. Unfortunately, advance of the parasite beyond the site of inflammation frequently complicates attempts at localization and destruction.

Since 1963 the broad-spectrum antihelminthic thiabendazole has been used successfully in the management of creeping eruption. Until recently the treatment of choice consisted of oral thiabendazole (Mintezol) in a dosage of 25 mg per kg of body weight, given twice a day for two to four days, with a maximum dosage of 2 grams a day.[56, 57, 58] Unfortunately, 30 to 40 per cent of patients treated in this manner develop side effects consisting of dizziness, nausea, cramps, and vomiting. These side affects, therefore, dictated the desirability of an effective topical preparation. A 2 per cent solution of thiabendazole in dimethyl sulfoxide (DMSO) was effective, but difficulties with this combination limited its use to research purposes. The use of topical thiabendazole suspension (Mintezol) under an occlusive plastic film has been shown to be effective, but produced pruritus and stinging in a substantial number of patients. Addition of a topical steroid cream to topical thiabendazole (under occlusion with Saran Wrap for 24 to 48 hours) has been shown to be a most effective method of therapy at this time.[59]

Jellyfish

Jellyfish (the common name of a type of invertebrate sea animal) are classified as Coelenterata, a phylum that includes corals, sea anemones, and hydras. The Portuguese man-of-war is a jellyfish that floats on the surface of tropical seas and the Gulf Stream. All coelenterates possess tentacles that bear numerous stinging structures (nematocysts). Upon contact each nematocyst discharges a small barb and a neurotoxin that seems to paralyze fish on contact. In man this toxin produces erythematous or urticarial ulcerations, burning pain, vesiculation, necrotic cutaneous ulcerations, and systemic reactions characterized by fever, vomiting, collapse, shock, and, at times, death.[60]

Treatment of jellyfish or Portuguese man-of-war stings consists of immediate bathing of affected areas to wash away the barbs, analgesics, application of topical corticosteroids or meat tenderizer (one part in four parts of water) to affected areas in order to relieve local discomfort. In patients with systemic reactions, antihistamines, intravenous calcium gluconate, and systemic steroids are often beneficial.

Cercarial Dermatitis (Swimmers' Itch)

Cercarial dermatitis, swimmers' itch, or schistosome dermatitis is an acute allergic cutaneous response that follows penetration of the skin by parasitic cercariae of the Schistosome family. Although global in its distribution, in North America this disorder has been noted most frequently in bathers of fresh water lakes in the north central part of the United States, with man as the accidental host of schistosomes of birds, ducks, or cattle, which utilize snails as their intermediate host.[61]

Affected individuals have no difficulty after initial exposure. Subsequent exposures, however, stimulate an allergic response to a protein residue deposited by the invading cercariae. A pricking or itching sensation may be noted at the time of cercarial penetration. This itching, which may last for periods of five minutes to an hour, is generally associated with 1 or 2 mm macules at each penetration site. The initial macules often persist or may disappear after a few hours, only to be followed, 10 to 15 hours later, by a more severe, intensely pruritic eruption characterized by 3 to 5 mm papules surrounded by variable zones of erythema. These papular lesions may or may not progress, with a resulting erythematous reaction consisting of edema, vesicles and/or urticarial wheals. In most individuals this stage of the eruption reaches its peak in two or three days, resolves within a week, and leaves a residual brown hyperpigmentation, which may persist for periods of several months or more.

The treatment of swimmers' itch is directed toward relief of symptoms and prevention of secondary infection. Administration of antihistaminic preparations and the use of shake lotions (calamine lotion) and topical corticosteroids help relieve the symptoms associated with this disorder. Systemic corticosteroids, although seldom necessary, are at times helpful for those patients with severe involvement. Prophylaxis of swimmers' itch consists of avoidance of prolonged immersion in polluted water and treatment of polluted waters with a mixture of copper sulfate and carbonate, or sodium pentochlorphenate.

Seabather's Eruption

Seabather's eruption is a term used to describe an acute dermatitis that occurs after bathing in salt water, particularly in the Caribbean area and along the Florida beaches, during the late spring and summer months (March to September). Although the cause of this disorder has not been established with certainty, it appears to be related to a species of marine cercaria of schistosomal origin.

The eruption consists of pruritic erythematous wheals or perifollicular papules that develop several hours after bathing in salt water and persist for periods of a few days to one or two weeks. A characteristic feature is localization of the eruption to areas covered by the bathing suit. Children are particularly prone to a more extensive eruption than that generally seen in adults and associated systemic reactions characterized by headache, malaise, nausea, vomiting, and fever occur. [62] Since seabather's eruption is a self-limiting disorder, therapy generally is palliative and consists of topical corticosteroids, antipruritic lotions, and the administration of antihistamines.

References

1. Rook A: Skin Diseases Caused by Arthropods and Other Venomous or Noxious Animals. In Rook A, Wilkinson DS, Ebling FJG: Textbook of Dermatology, 2nd ed. Blackwell Scientific Publications, Oxford, 1972, 845–884.

    In depth review of cutaneous disorders associated with arthropods and other invertebrates.

2. Mellanby K: Scabies, 2nd ed. E. W. Classey, Ltd., Hampton, England, 1972.

    Reissue of a classic review of scabies originally published in 1943 as one of a series of "Oxford War Manuals."

3. Stokes JH: Scabies among the well-to-do. JAMA 106:674–678, 1936.

    Scabies affects individuals from all walks of life.

4. Mellanby K: The development of symptoms, parasitic infection and immunity in human scabies. Parasitology 35:197–206, 1944.

    Studies on human volunteers suggest hypersensitivity as an explanation of some features of the clinical picture and cyclic epidemic nature of scabies.

5. Orkin M: Resurgence of scabies. JAMA 217:593–597, 1971.

    A forecast of global resurgence of scabies in epidemic proportions.

6. Orkin M: Today's scabies. JAMA 233:882–885, 1975.

    A review of scabies, with emphasis on diagnosis and management.

7. Madsen A: Why Acarus scabiei avoid the face. Acta Dermatovener 45:167–168, 1965.

    The author suggests that female mites avoid the head and face because of a greater density of hair follicles in this region (16 times that of the extremities and trunk).

8. Hurwitz S: Scabies in babies. Am. J. Dis. Child. 126:226–228, 1973.

    Scabies in infants and young children may be misdiagnosed because of a low index of suspicion, the frequent lack of burrows, secondary eczematization suggesting other conditions, and an atypical distribution in this age group.

9. Hurwitz S: Scabies in Infants and Children. In Orkin M, Maibach HI, Parish LC, et al.(Eds.): Scabies and Pediculosis. J. B. Lippincott Company, Philadelphia, 1977, 31–38.

    Scabies as it affects infants and children, with emphasis on diagnosis and management in this age group.

10. Sehgal VN, Rao TL, Rege VL, Vadiraj SN: Scabies: A study of incidence and treatment method. Int. J. Dermatol. 11:106–111, 1972.

    Analysis of 1015 cases of scabies revealed the most common lesions (in order of frequency) to be papules, vesicles, crusted lesions, pustules, burrows and wheals; burrows were seen in a mere 7 per cent of patients.

11. Friedman R: Atypical Scabies. Diagnosis by the Scrape and Smear Method. Penn. Med. J. 47:39–41, 1943.

The burrow, the so-called pathognomonic clinical sign of scabies, is demonstrated in only 13 per cent of patients.

12. Berge T, Krook G: Persistent nodules in scabies. Acta Dermatovener. 47:20–24, 1967.

Histologic study of five cases of nodules that persisted after apparent successful treatment of scabies suggest a possible allergic origin to these lesions.

13. Hubler, WR Jr, Clabaugh W: Epidemic Norwegian scabies. Arch. Dermatol. 112:179–181, 1976.

An epidemic of Norwegian scabies in a 25-patient ward of physically handicapped (mostly mongoloid) individuals.

14. Smith EB, Claypoole TF: Canine scabies in dogs and humans. JAMA 199:95–100, 1967.

A review of 22 patients with canine scabies.

15. Norins AL: Canine scabies in children. "Puppy dog" dermatitis. Am. J. Dis. Child. 117:239–242, 1969.

Canine scabies in humans is characterized by small red papular and papulovesicular lesions with predilection for the chest, abdomen, and forearms.

16. Orkin M, Maibach HI: Scabies, a current pandemic. Postgraduate Medicine. 66:52–65, 1979.

A review of the current status of scabies, its diagnosis, and therapy.

17. MacMillan AL: Unusual features of scabies associated with topical fluorinated steroids. Br. J. Dermatol. 87:496–497, 1972.

An infant with scabies treated topically with potent fluorinated steroids for four months manifested extensive scabietic infestation attributable to an adverse effect of topical steroids.

18. Burgess I: Unusual features of scabies associated with topical fluorinated steroids. Br. J. Dermatol. 88:519–520, 1973.

The prolonged application of potent topical steroids appears to suppress cell-mediated immunity, thus upsetting the normal pattern of response to scabietic infestation.

19. Wannamaker LW: Differences between streptococcal infections of the throat and skin. N. Engl. J. Med. 282:23–31, 78–85, 1970.

Streptococcal infection of the skin does not lead to rheumatic fever.

20. Svartman M, Potter EV, Finklea JF, et al.: Epidemic scabies and acute glomerulonephritis in Trinidad. Lancet 1:249–251, 1972.

Cutaneous infection due to nephritogenic strains of streptococci are responsible for epidemics of acute glomerulonephritis following scabies.

21. Muller GH, Jacobs PH, Moore NE: Scraping for human scabies. Arch. Dermatol. 107:70, 1973.

A drop of mineral oil on suspected lesions allows easier scraping and more definitive identification of scabies.

22. Ackerman AB: Histopathology of human scabies. In Orkin M, Maibach HI, Parish LC, et al. (Eds.): Scabies and Pediculosis. J. B. Lippincott Co., Philadelphia, 1977, 88–95.

The papular type of scabies, the most common manifestation in human skin, typically shows a superficial and deep perivascular mixed inflammatory cell infiltrate of lymphocytes, histiocytes, and numerous eosinophils.

23. Hernandez-Perez E: Topically applied thiabendazole in the treatment of scabies. Arch. Dermatol. 112:1400–1401, 1976.

Satisfactory response to topical thiabendazole warrants further evaluation of this drug in the treatment of scabies.

24. Feldman RJ, Maibach HI: Percutaneous penetration of some pesticides and herbicides in man. Toxicol. Appl. Pharmacol. 28:126–132, 1974.

Studies reveal that 9.3 per cent of gamma benzene hexachloride applied to adult skin can be recovered in the urine.

25. FDA Drug Bulletin: Gamma benzene hexachloride alert. 6:28, 1976.

Poorly documented reports of adverse reaction following use of gamma benzene hexachloride suggest caution in its use and the report of cases of possible toxicity to the Division of Drug Experience, FDA (HFD-210), Rockville, Maryland, 208502.

26. Lee B, Groth P, Turner W: Suspected reactions to gamma benzene hexachloride. JAMA 236:2846, 1976.

Reports of adverse reactions following imprudent use of gamma benzene hexachloride.

27. Lee B, Groth P: Letters to the editor. Scabies: Transcutaneous poisoning during treatment. Pediatrics 59:643, 1977.

Case reports of suspected CNS toxicity to excessive or inappropriate use of gamma benzene hexachloride (lindane).

28. Ginsburg CM, Lowry W, Reisch JS: Absorption of lindane (gamma benzene hexachloride) in infants and young children. J. Pediatr. 91:998–1000, 1977.

Concentrations of lindane in the blood of 20 children who received treatment with 1 per cent lindane lotion were inversely related to the body weight and surface area of the treated patients.

29. Pramanik A, Hansen RC: Transcutaneous gamma benzene hexachloride absorption and toxicity in infants and children. Arch. Dermatol. 115:1224–1225, 1979.

CNS toxicity in an infant following one topical application of gamma benzene hexachloride (lindane) to a premature malnourished infant; the level of gamma benzene hexachloride was 17 times greater than mean levels reported in children 48 hours after topical application of this agent.

30. Orkin M, Epstein E Sr, Maibach HI: Treatment of today's scabies and pediculosis. JAMA 236:1136–1140, 1976.

A review of the current approach to therapy of scabies and pediculosis.

31. Lasch EE, Frankel V, Pardy PA, et al.: Epidemic glomerulonephritis in Israel. J. Infect. Dis. 124:141–147, 1971.

Early treatment of streptococcal infection did not appear to prevent the development of acute glomerulonephritis.

32. Selfon PM: The red mite among our field personnel. Milit. Med. 127:479–484, 1962.

Clear nail polish appears to be effective for relief of chigger bites.

33. Gouck HK: Protection from ticks, fleas, chiggers, and leeches. Arch. Dermatol. 93:112–113, 1966.

Mosquito repellents are good chigger toxicants; benzyl benzoate is also effective and withstands washing and submersion in water.

34. Mast WE, Burrows WM: Erythema chronicum migrans in the United States. JAMA 236:859–860, 1976.

Although until recently only one case of erythema chronicum migrans had been reported in the United States, this disorder recently has been seen in Connecticut and Cape Cod.

35. Hollström E: Successful penicillin treatment of erythema migrans Afzelus. Acta Dermatovener. 31:235–243, 1951.

Some cases of erythema chronicum migrans appear to respond to systemic antibiotics.

35a. Steere AC, Malawista SE, et al.: Antibiotic therapy in Lyme disease. Ann. Int. Med. 93:1–8, 1980.

Studies demonstrated that antibiotic therapy shortens the duration of erythema chronicum migrans.

36. Jellison WL, Gregson JD: Tick paralysis in northwestern United States and British Columbia. Rocky Mountain Med. J. 47:28–53, 1950.

An undertaker who picked ticks off a cadaver subsequently died of tick paralysis.

37. Derbes VJ: Treatment of arthropod bites and stings. In Gellis SS, Kagan BM (Eds.): Current Pediatric Therapy, 7. W. B. Saunders Co., Philadelphia, 1976, 480–481.

A review of the treatment of arthropod bites and infestation in children.

38. Villaveces JW: Gangrenous spider bite in Los Angeles County (apparently by *Loxosceles reclusa*). California Med. *108*:305–308, 1968.

The brown recluse spider, not formerly seen in western United States, appears in Los Angeles County.

39. Medical News: Thirteen states report dangerous spider: "The Brown Recluse." JAMA *200*:19, 24, 1967.

The brown recluse spider tends to avoid humans and seeks refuge in dark recesses of buildings.

40. Dillaha CJ, Jansen GT, Honeycutt WM: North American loxoscelism. *In* Demis DJ, Dobson RL, McGuire J: Clinical Dermatology. Vol. 4. Harper and Row, Hagerstown, Md., 1977, 18–25:1–8.

The brown recluse spider: clinical manifestations and therapeutic approach.

41. Chadha JS, Leviav A: Hemolysis, renal failure, and local necrosis following scorpion sting. JAMA *241*:1038, 1979.

Renal failure associated with severe hemolysis following a scorpion sting.

42. Pratt HD, Littig KS: Lice of Public Health Importance and their Control, Publication (CDC) 76–8265. U.S. Dept. of Health, Education, and Welfare: 1976, 1–22.

Biological aspects of lice, with emphasis on diagnosis and treatment of human infestation.

43. Kohn SR: Hair casts or pseudonits. JAMA *238*:2058–2059, 1977.

Hair casts, or pseudonits, are 2 to 7 mm long, discrete, firm, shiny, white, freely movable accretions that encircle the hair shafts of the scalp and may be responsible for pseudoepidemics of pediculosis capitis.

44. Robinson HM Jr: Live nits versus dead ones, continuation. The Schoch letter. Vol. 27, 5:9, 1977.

Practical advice on the management of nits in pediculosis capitis.

45. Shannon WR: Thiamine chloride — an aid in the solution of the mosquito problem. Minn. Med. *26*:799, 1943.

Although studies on oral thiamine give conflicting results, this vitamin may offer value as a mosquito repellent.

46. Marks MB: Stinging Insects: Allergy implications. Ped. Clin. North Amer. *16*:177–191, 1969.

Fifty to seventy per cent of children with histories of severe local response to insect bites appear to improve with thiamine hydrochloride (25 mg three times a day).

47. Rook A: Papular urticaria. Ped. Clin. of North Amer. 8:817–833, 1961.

Evidence appears to support the conclusion that papular urticaria represents a cutaneous hypersensitivity to the bites of certain insects.

48. Blank, H, Shaffer B, Spencer MC, et al.: Papular Urticaria — a study of the role of insects in its etiology and the use of DDT in its treatment. Pediatrics. 5:408–412, 1950.

Seventy-seven per cent of 30 patients with papular urticaria, in contrast to 2 of 124 in a control series, proved to be sensitive to flea and bedbug antigens, thus supporting the theory of hypersensitivity as the cause of papular urticaria.

49. Shaffer B, Jacobson C, Beerman H: Histopathologic correlation of lesions of papular urticaria and positive skin test reactions to insect antigens. Arch. Dermatol. Syph. *70*:437–442, 1954.

Histologic examination of lesions of papular urticaria display similarity to ordinary insect bites and urticarial and delayed skin reactions to insect antigens.

50. Caro MR, Derbes VJ: Skin responses to the study of the imported fire ant (Solenopsis saevissima). Arch. Dermatol. *75*:475–488, 1957.

The fire ant imported from South America, a particularly destructive insect, has spread rapidly in the southern part of the United States.

51. Frazier CA: Insect Stings — a medical emergency. JAMA *235*:2410–2411, 1976.

Systemic reactions to insect stings are medical emergencies and require vigorous therapy.

52. McMillan CS, Purcell W: Hazards to health — the puss caterpillar, alias wooly slug. N. Engl. J. Med. *271*:147–149, 1964.

More than 50 species of caterpillars possess irritative hairs. Depending on the species, their effects range from a local dermatitis to a dangerous disorder with systemic signs and symptoms.

53. Daly JJ, Derrick BL: Puss caterpillar sting in Arkansas. South Med. J. *68*:893–894, 1975.

Toxin from the hairs of the puss caterpillar can produce numbness and swelling of the affected areas, severe radiating pain, regional lymphadenopathy, nausea, and fever.

54. Zaias, N, Ioannides G, Taplin D: Dermatitis from contact with moths (genus Hylesia). JAMA *207*:525–527, 1969.

Histopathologic examination of dermatitis from exposure to *Hylesia* moths suggests toxic injury as the principal cause of caterpillar dermatitis.

55. McGovern JP, Barkin GD, McElhenney TR, et al.: Megalopyge opercularis — observations of its life history, natural history of its sting in man, and report of an epidemic. JAMA *175*:1155–1158, 1961.

The symptoms of exposure to the puss caterpillar include marked local pain and swelling, lymphadenopathy, headache, shock-like symptoms, and convulsions.

56. Kata R, Ziegler J, Blank H: The natural course of creeping eruption and treatment with thiabendazole. Arch. Dermatol. *91*:420–424, 1965.

Systemic thiabendazole effective in the treatment of creeping eruption.

57. Stone OJ, Mullins JF: Thiabendazole effectiveness in creeping eruption. Arch. Dermatol. *91*:427–429, 1965.

Oral thiabendazole (in doses of 50 mg/kg daily for two days) permanently halted the activity of 99 per cent of larvae in patients with creeping eruption.

58. Jacksonville Dermatology Society: Creeping eruption treated with thiabendazole. Arch. Dermatol. *91*:425–426, 1965.

Oral thiabendazole therapy of 51 patients with extensive cutaneous larva migrans infestion gave encouraging results for a disease that previously had no satisfactory treatment.

59. Davis CM, Israel RM: Treatment of creeping eruption with thiabendazole. Arch. Dermatol. *97*:325–326, 1968.

In fifteen patients with creeping eruption, 160 of 164 tracts cleared in one week on topical treatment with 10 per cent thiabendazole suspension; symptomatic relief of pruritus was noted within three days.

60. Moschella SL: Parasitology and Tropical Dermatology. *In* Moschella SL, Pillsbury DM, Hurley HJ Jr: Dermatolgy. W. B. Saunders Co., Philadelphia, 1975, 1487–1552.

A comprehensive review of cutaneous disorders associated with parasites and tropical diseases.

62. Hoeffler DF: "Swimmers' Itch (cercarial dermatitis). Cutis *19*:461–467, 1977.

Description of an epidemic of swimmers' itch in 31 students.

62. Strauss JS: Seabather's eruption. Arch. Dermatol. *74*:293–295, 1956.

Seabather's eruption can be differentiated from swimmers' itch by the fact that seabather's eruption is limited to the bathing suit area and is associated with salt-water rather than fresh water.

BULLOUS DISORDERS OF CHILDHOOD

Blisters or bullae are rounded or irregularly shaped lesions of the skin or mucous membranes and result from the accumulation of fluid between the cells of the epidermis or between the epidermis and underlying corium. The term bullae refers to blistering lesions 0.5 cm to 1 cm or more in diameter; those less than 0.5 cm in diameter are termed vesicles. Owing to our limited knowledge, the classification of bullous or vesiculobullous disorders, until recently, was based purely upon clinical morphology and light microscopic examination, and differed according to the national background and training of individual authors, and implied neither an etiologic nor pathogenic basis to the disease process.

Although our knowledge as to pathogenetic mechanisms remains limited, current classification is based upon clinical features, electron microscopic examination, and, whenever possible, immunopathologic mechanisms. It is well recognized that the skin of infants and children is more susceptible to blister formation than that of adults. With the exception of epidermolysis bullosa, however, the blistering group of diseases in general are a relatively uncommon group of disorders in childhood.

EPIDERMOLYSIS BULLOSA

The term epidermolysis bullosa refers to a group of inherited disorders characterized by bullous lesions that develop spontaneously or as a result of varying degrees of friction or trauma.

Although categorization of types of epidermolysis bullosa in the past has been controversial and often confusing, the absence or presence of permanent scarring allows this disorder to be divided into two major groups: those that may result in complete healing without scarring and those that inevitably produce scars. As a matter of convenience, these two major divisions can be further subdivided into smaller groups based upon inheritance, clincial patterns, and theories of pathogenesis derived from histologic studies at the light and electron microscopic levels (Tables 15–1 and 15–2).[1, 2]

Epidermolysis simplex, recurrent bullous eruptions of the hands and feet, and epidermolysis bullosa letalis are characterized histologically by cleavage above the periodic acid-Schiff (PAS)–positive basement membrane. The scarring dystrophic forms are characterized by a split in the upper dermis, below the basement membrane. Although the pathogenesis of blister formation in epidermolysis is unknown, current data suggest an abnormal cytolytic enzyme within the epidermal cells in the simplex variety and an increase in dermal collagenase in the dystrophic forms of this condition.[1]

NON-SCARRING FORMS OF EPIDERMOLYSIS BULLOSA

Epidermolysis Bullosa Simplex

Epidermolysis bullosa simplex (EBS) is an autosomal dominant disease characterized by blis-

Table 15–1 NON-SCARRING EPIDERMOLYSIS BULLOSA

Type	Inheritance	Clinical Features	Electron Microscopic Features
Epidermolysis bullosa simplex	Autosomal dominant	Bullae present at birth or early infancy; in areas of trauma; generally improves in adolescence; little to no mucous membrane involvement; nail involvement in 20 per cent	Cleavage through basal cell layer above the basement membrane with formation of vacuoles in the basal cells
Recurrent bullous eruption of hands and feet (Weber-Cockayne disease)	Autosomal dominant	May present in first two years of life, but usually not before adolescence or early adulthood; bullae confined to hands and feet	Epidermal cleavage, usually in the mid-squamous area, but may be anywhere from the suprabasal to lower granular cell layer
Junctional epidermolysis bullosa (Herlitz disease)	Autosomal recessive	Usually at birth or shortly thereafter; spontaneous bullae and large areas of erosion with generalized distribution (except for palms and soles); perioral involvement and scalp lesions characteristic; if survival through first two years of life it resembles epidermolysis bullosa simplex	Cleavage at junction of dermis and epidermis (above the basement membrane)
Localized absence of the skin with blistering and nail dystrophy (Bart syndrome)	Autosomal dominant(?)	Mouth erosions; deformed nails; extensive erosions on extensor aspects of extremities, intertriginous areas, neck, and buttocks; spontaneous improvement	Intact dermis with basement membrane on dermal side of cleavage

ters that develop in areas of trauma and heal without subsequent scar formation (Fig. 15–1). The disorder usually begins at birth or shortly thereafter. In the neonatal period, blisters or large erosions tend to involve areas of friction, namely the hands, feet, neck, and lower aspect of the legs. As the infant begins to crawl and walk, the knees, ankles, feet, buttocks, elbows, and hands are the principal areas of involvement; blisters, however, may also occur in other locations, owing to rubbing or irritation from clothing. After the third year of life, usually only the hands and feet are affected. Although EBS at times may persist throughout life, the condition generally improves in adolescence.

There is considerable variation in the severity of the simplex form of epidermolysis bullosa. As in all forms of epidermolysis bullosa, heat and frictional trauma appear to be important precipitating factors in blister formation. Temporary hyperpigmentation may occur, but secondary infection is usually not a problem. EBS is characterized by blisters that generally heal without residual scarring or milia formation.

Electron microscopic examination shows cleavage through the basal layer (above the PAS-positive basement membrane of the epidermis), formation of vacuoles in the basal cells adjacent to areas of separation, and displacement of nuclei to the epidermal end of the involved cells. Although no specific histochemical abnormality has been delineated, the defect in epidermolysis bullosa simplex appears to be related to mechanical trauma and associated activation of a cytolytic enzyme or enzymes within the involved basal cells. Whether this is due to increased production of normal enzymes or abnormal enzymes or to a defect in control mechanisms, however, requires, further study.[2]

There is little to no mucous membrane involvement in EBS, and the nails are affected in only 20 per cent of cases. Nail dystrophy, when it

Table 15–2 SCARRING EPIDERMOLYSIS BULLOSA

Type	Inheritance	Clinical Features	Electron Microscopic Features
Dominant dystrophic epidermolysis bullosa (dominant dermolytic bullous dermatosis)	Autosomal dominant	Early infancy and later; of intermittent severity (between that of epidermolysis bullosa simplex and recessive dystrophic epidermolysis bullosa); little or no involvement of hair and teeth; 20 per cent have mucous membrane lesions. 80 per cent have nail dystrophy. Albopapuloid form later.	Dermal-epidermal separation beneath basement membrane
Recessive dystrophic epidermolysis bullosa (recessive dermolytic bullous dermatosis)	Autosomal recessive	Present at birth; widespread dystrophy, scarring, and deformity; severe involvement of mucous membranes and nails; retardation of growth and development, anemia, and mottled carious teeth are common	Separation at dermal-epidermal junction (beneath the basal lamina)
Acquired epidermolysis bullosa	Non-hereditary	A disease of adolescence and adulthood; affects pressure areas of ears, elbows, knees, hands, and feet; mucous membrane erosions and nail dystrophy common	Subepidermal blister beneath basement membrane

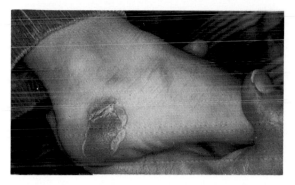

Figure 15-1 Epidermolysis bullosa simplex. Blisters develop in areas of trauma and heal without subsequent scar formation.

appears, generally occurs in those patients who manifest involvement of the fingers and toes during the first year of life. Except for occasional linear striations in the nail plate and the fact that the nails may be a bit more brittle than usual, there generally is normal regrowth of nails without evidence of residual deformity.[3]

Recurrent Bullous Eruptions of the Hands and Feet

Recurrent bullous eruptions of the hands and feet (Weber-Cockayne disease) is an autosomal dominant disorder. It is a clinical variant of epidermolysis bullosa simplex that requires a higher threshold of frictional trauma to induce blister formation. Although the pathophysiology of Weber-Cockayne disease is unknown, it appears to represent an exaggeration of the normal mechanism for production of friction blisters, possibly related to activation of a cytolytic enzyme (or enzymes) and an associated dyskeratosis of squamous cells in the epidermis.[2]

In this disorder the bullae are usually confined to the hands and feet and are associated with hyperhidrosis of the palms and soles. Although blisters can occur in the first year or two of life, they are frequently not manifested until adolescence or early adulthood. In young children, blisters develop on the knees from the frictional trauma of crawling. In adolescents and young adults, blisters may occur on the feet after long hikes or on the hands following a game of golf. In many patients, lesions only occur in hot weather. Blisters generally heal rapidly without scarring; nail involvement rarely occurs, the teeth are normal, and mucous membranes are not involved.

As in epidermolysis bullosa simplex, cytolysis of epidermal cells is the essential histologic feature of Weber-Cockayne disease. In contrast to epidermolysis bullosa simplex, the basal cells are spared. In Weber-Cockayne disease epidermal cleavage usually appears in the mid-squamous area but may occur anywhere, from the suprabasal to the lower granular cell layers of the epidermis.

Junctional Epidermolysis Bullosa

Junctional epidermolysis bullosa (previously termed Herlitz disease or epidermolysis bullosa letalis) is a severe autosomal recessive disorder. Characterized by spontaneous bullae and large areas of erosion, it usually occurs on the legs at birth or shortly thereafter, and about 50 per cent of cases result in death within the first year or two of life. Although this disease is grouped under the non-scarring disorders, it may represent a variant of the recessive form of dystrophic epidermolysis bullosa or perhaps a separate entity distinct from and unrelated to other forms of epidermolysis bullosa. When large areas of the body are involved, the patient dies in infancy because of severe fluid loss or overwhelming sepsis. If the infant survives the first two years of life, the disease tends to improve and resembles epidermolysis bullosa simplex.

Light and electron microscopy reveal blisters at the junction of the dermis and epidermis, with cleavage above the PAS-staining basement membrane. Separation occurs in the intermembranous space between the plasma membrane of the basal cell and the basal lamina. Although the cause of this abnormality is unknown, it may be the result of an enzymatic change at the dermal-epidermal junction, a structural defect of the hemidesmosomes or the hypothetical glue substance at the plane of separation, or an abnormality of the basement membrane or plasma membrane of the basal cells.[2]

In this disorder most lesions heal slowly without milia or significant scarring. Scalp lesions are common, and although perianal and esophageal lesions may occur, they do not form significant strictures and they usually are not as severe or troublesome as those seen in the recessive dystrophic form of epidermolysis bullosa. The hands and feet usually are spared. Involvement of the nail beds, with moderate thickening, dystrophy, or complete loss of nails, however, is not uncommon. The teeth are dysplastic, with an altered enamel pattern (the dental enamel breaks down easily, and a cobblestone appearance to the teeth is characteristic). Perioral involvement, with sparing of the lips, is common and is said to be pathognomic of this disorder. Although patients who survive to adulthood do so without scars, they often exhibit severe growth retardation and recalcitrant anemia.

Bart Syndrome

In 1966, Bart and associates recognized a new mechanobullous syndrome consisting of skin defects that affect the lower extremities, with blistering of the skin and mucous membranes and deformity of the nails.[4] Although the disorder appears to be autosomal dominant, isolated cases suggest the possibility of variable penetrance or spontaneous mutation.[5]

Some patients have only mouth erosion;

others have deformed nails, recurrent blistering, or the complete syndrome, with characteristic localized, sharply marginated skin defects on the legs. Other skin defects, apparently due to mechanobullous phenomena induced by local shearing trauma, may appear as extensive erosions on the extensor aspects of the extremities, intertriginous areas, neck, and buttocks. Although skin and mucous membrane erosions heal without scarring, milia and occasional residual hypopigmentation may be noted.

Histologically, skin lesions show loss of the epidermis, an intact dermis with the basement membrane on the dermal side of the split, and normal adnexa and subcutaneous tissue. A tendency toward progressive spontaneous improvement without residual defects emphasizes the importance of early recognition and conservative management of individuals with this disorder.[5]

SCARRING FORMS OF EPIDERMOLYSIS BULLOSA

The scarring (dysplastic or dystrophic) types of epidermolysis bullosa are divided into dominant and recessive forms. Although the term epidermolysis bullosa is retained, since bullae are subepidermal rather than epidermal, the term dermolytic bullous dermatosis has been suggested as a more accurate term for these disorders.[2] The dominant disease is less severe. Affected individuals are generally healthy, of normal stature, and have little or no involvement of hair and teeth. The recessive form, conversely, is severe and incapacitating. Growth and development are retarded, the teeth are abnormal, and hypotrichosis or alopecia is common (Fig. 15–2).

Histopathologic examination of involved skin in dystrophic forms of epidermolysis bullosa reveals separation at the dermal-epidermal junction, fragmentation of collagen bundles in the floor of blisters, and a lymphohistiocytic infiltrate with extravasation of erythrocytes.[6] Electron microscopy shows separation beneath the basal lamina (on the dermal side of the dermal-epidermal junction) and absence of anchoring fibrils in normal as well

as blistered skin. The abnormality resides in the dermis.

The absence of anchoring fibrils (the apparent primary structural defect in recessive forms of dystrophic epidermolysis bullosa) allows disruption of the structural integrity of the epidermal-dermal junction and subsequent blister formation.[7] Although anchoring fibrils are lacking in damaged skin of patients with dominant forms of dystrophic epidermolysis bullosa, studies of a large kindred revealed normal fibrils in the noninvolved skin of three individuals with this disorder. This suggests a possible means of differentiating dominant from recessive forms of this disorder, but it requires confirmation.

The most likely defect that would account for the pathologic alterations seen in dystrophic forms of epidermolysis bullosa therefore appears to be a structural abnormality of the dermal connective tissue, most probably the collagen, with an associated impaired function of anchoring fibrils.[7] The role of collagenase in the pathophysiology of dystrophic epidermolysis bullosa has been suggested by observations of elevated collagenase levels in friction bullae of patients with the recessive form of this disorder.[8, 9, 10] Lazarus, however, found elevated collagenase levels only in active lesions, and none of his patients had increased urinary hydroxyproline, suggesting an ongoing degradation of tissue collagen. He concludes that the increased collagenase activity in lesions of dystrophic forms of epidermolysis bullosa may be secondary to tissue injury rather than a primary abnormality in individuals with this disorder.[11]

Dominant Dystrophic Epidermolysis Bullosa

The dominant form of this scarring disorder (also termed dominant dermolytic bullous dermatosis) is of intermediate severity. It is more severe than epidermolysis bullosa simplex and considerably milder than the recessive dystrophic disease. Although the onset of bullae in mild cases may occur later in life, blisters generally appear at birth or shortly thereafter. About 20 per cent of patients

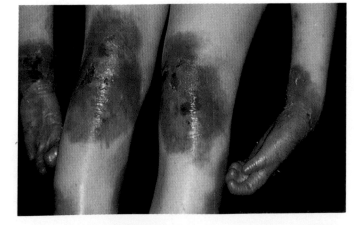

Figure 15–2 Epidermolysis bullosa, recessive dystrophic form (recessive dermolytic bullous dermatosis). Note hemorrhagic bullae, dystrophic scars, pseudosyndactyly and claw-like deformities of the hands (Department of Dermatology, Yale University School of Medicine).

show changes before the age of one year. Improvement seems to occur with age and only rarely is there deformed scarring of the hands and feet approaching that seen in the recessive disease.[2]

In the dominant form of epidermolysis bullosa dystrophica, most lesions are clearly related to mechanical trauma. Bullae may be present at birth, but often do not appear until the child begins to crawl or walk.[12] Blisters appear primarily over the bony prominences of the knuckles, wrists, and feet. Early blisters are often tense and sometimes hemorrhagic; erosions without blister formation may occur; hyperhidrosis of the palms and soles may be noted, and palmar and plantar keratoses occasionally are present.

Milia characteristically are seen as 1 to 2 mm firm white globoid lesions at the sites of healed bullae (Fig. 15-3). They are not specific for this disorder and often are present in chronically traumatized skin. Also seen in porphyria and following dermabrasion, they appear to represent retention cysts caused by occlusion of pilosebaceous units.[3] Although mutilating scars are rarely seen, soft superficial atrophic scars with wrinkled surfaces may develop as bullae heal. Erythematous plaques, due to trauma insufficient to cause blistering, are frequently seen. Hyperpigmentation or depigmentation may be found at healed blister sites, and hypertrophic and keloidal lesions occasionally occur.[2]

Mucous membrane lesions appear in 20 per cent of cases but do not present the severe problems seen in the recessive form of this disorder. The teeth generally are not affected, but oral milia resulting from detached islands of epithelium in areas of earlier bulla formation may be noted.[3] The hair is not affected; physical and mental development is normal; and, in contrast to the recessive dystrophic disorder, the conjunctiva and cornea are never involved. The nails, however, in 80 per

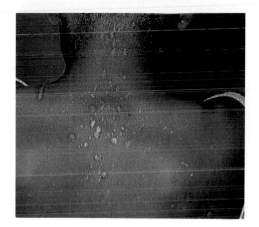

Figure 15-4 Albopapuloid form of epidermolysis bullosa. Small firm ivory-white perifollicular papules on the trunk of a patient with dominant dystrophic epidermolysis bullosa (dominant dermolytic bullous dermatosis). (Courtesy of Robert A. Briggaman, M.D.)

cent of cases are thickened, dystrophic, and, at times, completely destroyed.

The Albopapuloid Form of Epidermolysis Bullosa. A unique variant of epidermolysis bullosa, the albopapuloid form is occasionally seen as a variant of dominant dystrophic disease (Fig. 15-4). Although it may be present in infancy, this disorder usually begins in later childhood, early adolescence, or adult life. It is characterized by small firm raised ivory-white perifollicular papules that vary in size from several millimeters to a centimeter or more in diameter. They appear independent of bullae and are generally seen on the trunk, particularly the lower back. Although generally associated with dominant dystrophic epidermolysis bullosa, similar lesions occasionally may be found in the recessive form of this disorder.

Recessive Dystrophic Epidermolysis Bullosa

Autosomal recessive dystrophic epidermolysis bullosa (recessive dermolytic bullous dermatosis) is a severe distressing bullous disease characterized by widespread dystrophic scarring and deformity and by severe involvement of mucous membranes.[12] In this disorder, erosions and blisters are usually manifested at or shortly after birth (Fig. 15-5). Although some blisters may appear to occur spontaneously, most seem to arise at sites of pressure or trauma. Although any area of the skin may be involved in infants the most commonly affected areas are the hands, feet, buttocks, scapulae, face, occiput, elbows, and knees. In older children the hands, feet, knees, and elbows are most commonly involved. Bullae may be hemorrhagic, and large areas, especially on the lower extremities, may be completely devoid of skin (similar to that seen in epidermolysis bullosa letalis) (Fig. 15-6). When a blister ruptures or its roof peels off, a raw painful surface is evident. The

Figure 15-3 Recessive dystrophic epidermolysis bullosa (recessive dermolytic bullous dermatosis). Milia (1 to 2 mm firm white globoid lesions) at the sites of healed bullae.

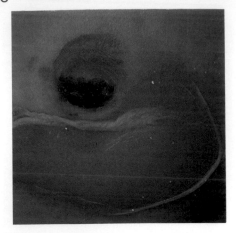

Figure 15–5 Recessive dystrophic epidermolysis bullosa (recessive dermolytic bullous dermatosis). A large blister on the lower aspect of the abdomen of a newborn.

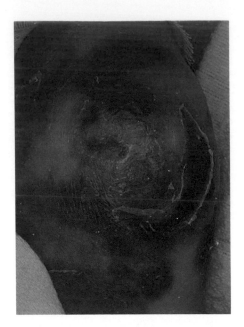

Figure 15–7 Recessive dystrophic epidermolysis bullosa (recessive dermolytic bullous dermatosis). Hemorrhagic blister, erosions, and superficial crinkled tissue paper-like appearance on the knee of a newborn.

Nikolsky sign (production or enlargement of a blister by slight pressure or the production of a moist abrasion by slight pressure on the skin) is often positive. Fluid contained in bullae, though at first sterile, may become secondarily infected, which can lead to sepsis; and in older children, nephritis has been seen as a sequela to streptococcal infection.

Bullae are often followed by atrophic scars or varying degrees of hyperpigmentation or hypopigmentation, or both. Milia frequently are seen (Fig. 15–3), and in severely affected individuals large areas of the skin surface may show a fine superficial crinkled tissue-paper appearance (Fig. 15–7). Repeated cycles of blistering, secondary infection, and healing leave wide areas of superficial scars and at times deep or hypertrophic cicatrices.[2] The hands and lower aspects of the legs are particularly susceptible to severe involvement. With repeat-

ed scarring the fingers and toes may become fused, with resultant pseudosyndactyly. As the fingers become immobile (usually over prolonged periods of time), the hands and arms may become fixed in a flexed position, with resulting contractures (Fig. 15–2). During fusion and with recurrent scarring, the digits may be bound together by a glove-like epidermal sac, with resulting claw-like clubbing or mitten-like deformities.

In recessive forms of dystrophic epidermolysis bullosa the nails may show extreme involvement, with severe dystrophy or complete absence of nails due to degeneration of the nail bed (Fig. 15–8). The eyes may develop a number of characteristic changes: blepharitis, symblepharon, conjunctivitis or keratitis or both, with associated

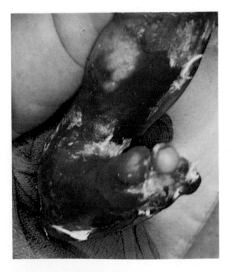

Figure 15–6 Recessive dystrophic epidermolysis bullosa (recessive dermolytic bullous dermatosis). Erosive lesions on the foot and lower aspect of the leg of a newborn.

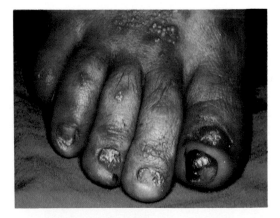

Figure 15–8 Recessive dystrophic epidermolysis bullosa (recessive dermolytic bullous dermatosis). Hemorrhagic bullae, milia, and nail dystrophy.

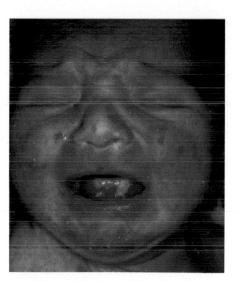

Figure 15–9 Involvement of the oral mucosa in an infant with recessive dystrophic epidermolysis bullosa (recessive dermolytic bullous dermatosis).

vesicle formation and corneal opacity.[3] Hoarseness, aphonia, or dysphagia, or all three may occur as a result of blistering of the larynx or pharynx. Laryngeal stenosis, although rare, may occur in varying degrees as the result of blistering and subsequent scarring of the larynx. Oral mucosal involvement occurs soon after birth and erosions of the esophagus may at times result in segmental stenosis (most often in the upper half) with consequent difficulty in swallowing (Fig. 15–9). Scarring in such cases is common and may resemble that seen after corrosive poisoning. Such children are reluctant to eat and, as a result, often fail to thrive. As the individual grows older there is a tendency for the disease to become less severe, but the affected individual soon learns to avoid hot drinks, rough foods, large particles, and anything that might produce blistering of the mouth, pharynx, or esophagus.[13]

The teeth in the recessive dysplastic disorder are frequently delayed in eruption, are malformed, and are particularly susceptible to early and frequently severe caries. Even routine dental care may cause the eruption of bullae on the lips, gums, and oral mucosa, and the children soon come to recognize the sequelae associated with even slight abrasions from normal toothbrushing procedures. The face often has a "puckered" appearance about the mouth due to intraoral scarring. The ears may be mildly scarred or bound down to the scalp. Scalp and body hair may be sparse, and there may be patches of cicatricial alopecia.

In some cases the dystrophy may be minimal, and differentiation from milder forms of epidermolysis may be difficult. In more severely affected individuals, death may occur during infancy or childhood as a result of septicemia, pneumonia, fluid loss from extensive areas of denuded skin, amyloidosis due to chronic and recurrent infec-

tion, renal failure (possibly due to chronic pyelonephritis), or malnutrition secondary to esophageal strictures. Other complications associated with this disorder include refractory anemia, hyperglobulinemic purpura, and clotting abnormalities. Those who have had epidermolysis for years may show a predisposition to carcinomata (both basal and squamous cell types) of the skin. The cause of this complication appears to be related to abnormal collagen in heavily scarred areas with continuing blister activity.[14] The pathogenesis is probably similar to that seen in neoplastic disorders that arise in thermal burns and other chronic scars.[15]

Acquired Epidermolysis Bullosa

Acquired epidermolysis bullosa (epidermolysis bullosa acquisita) is a non-hereditary late-onset bullous disorder that is first manifested in adolescence or adulthood and characterized by blister formation below the basement membrane. Ultrastructural findings are similar to those seen in the hereditary forms of dystrophic epidermolysis and most closely resemble those of the dominantly inherited disease. Patients with epidermolysis bullosa acquisita generally appear with a peculiar susceptibility to blister formation following trauma or pressure. The disorder is manifested by vesicles, bullae, and erosions over the pressure areas of the ears, elbows, knees, and particularly hands and feet. Scarring, milia, and nail dystrophy occur. Although the teeth are normal and mucous membrane erosions are frequently seen, the conjunctival, esophageal, and genitoanal mucous membranes are not involved.[12]

Epidermolysis bullosa acquisita has been associated with poison oak dermatitis, dermatitis herpetiformis, inflammatory bowel disorders (Crohn's disease), impetigo, scarlet fever, tuberculosis, porphyria, cutaneous amyloidosis, Ehlers-Danlos syndrome, and ingestion of sulfonamides, arsenic, and penicillamine.[6]

TREATMENT. As in any inherited disorder, it is the responsibility of the physician to inform parents of the risks associated with transmitting genetic abnormalities. When the condition is determined by a dominant gene (as in dominant dystrophic epidermolysis bullosa), if one parent is affected, there is a 50 per cent risk that each child will be so afflicted. In a family in which a child manifests abnormalities due to a recessive gene (as in recessive dystrophic epidermolysis bullosa), parents must be prepared to risk a 25 per cent possibility of this severe disorder occurring in future offspring.

The treatment of epidermolysis bullosa is palliative, with avoidance of trauma and control of secondary infection. Since blisters result from mechanical injury, measures should be taken to relieve pressure and prevent unnecessary trauma. A cool environment, avoidance of overheating, and lubrication of the skin to decrease the surface coefficient of friction are helpful in the reduction of blister formation. When blisters occur, extension may be prevented by aseptic aspiration of blister fluid. The roofs of blisters should be trimmed with a sterile scissors whenever feasible, and no ragged edges should be left under which organisms may flourish and lead to secondary infection.[15]

A water mattress and a soft fleece covering will help to limit friction and trauma. Daily baths, topical protective antibiotic dressings, or sterile Vaseline-impregnated gauze applied with sterile precautions may help reduce topical bacterial infection and assist spontaneous healing of involved areas. Large denuded areas should be treated, whenever possible, by the open method (as in treatment of burns) with intravenous fluids, appropriate systemic antibiotics when indicated, and protection of injured areas by protective dressings and Vaseline-impregnated gauze is helpful.

Although it has been stated that high concentration topical corticosteroid preparations may facilitate healing of chronically blistered areas, this has not been verified. If sepsis is to be prevented or controlled, especially in the newborn and young infant, careful monitoring of the skin and mucosal florae is essential.[16] In severe dystrophic forms of epidermolysis bullosa, prophylactic antibiotics such as penicillin and erythromycin are valuable. They lessen the tendency to local infection, sepsis, and severe scarring, and help prevent the risk of glomerulonephritis secondary to cutaneous streptococcal infection.

Oral vitamin E (DL-alpha tocopherol) has been suggested for the treatment of patients with epidermolysis.[12, 17] Vitamin E is an antioxidant that enhances the activity of some enzymes and perhaps induces the synthesis of others.[11] Although there are reports of favorable responses to oral vitamin E is dosages of up to 2000 units per day, most studies do not seem to confirm its value in the prevention of blistering and scarring.[18] Until the value or lack of effect is determined, since there appear to be no adverse side effects associated with the use of this preparation, it may be worthy of trial in severe dystrophic disease unresponsive to other forms of therapy.

Dysphagia is the major symptom of esophageal involvement in recessive dystrophic epidermolysis bullosa. It may result from a reversible inflammatory reaction or from a permanent stricture. Barium studies demonstrate esophageal lesions; endoscopy, however, is not recommended. Softening of the diet for several weeks may result in modest to marked improvement of symptoms. If conservative management fails to result in proper nourishment, bougienage, surgery, or both should be considered.[19, 20] Once bougienage has been initiated, however, some patients may require the procedure at frequent intervals. In those instances where surgery must be considered, colon transplant procedures have been successful.[21] With repeated blistering, ulceration, and scar formation, carcinomata may sometimes develop on the involved skin or mucous membrane. Although the cause of carcinoma is unknown, abnormal collagen formation in heavily scarred areas with continuous blistering activity appears to predispose to this complication.[15]

Systemic steroids have been tried in all forms of epidermolysis bullosa. Although they appear to have value in the management of junctional bullous dermatosis (epidermolysis bullosa letalis, Herlitz disease), present studies do not seem to substantiate reports that high dose systemic steroids prevent the scarring and mutilation in severe dystrophic forms of this disorder.[14, 16, 19] Moynahan, however, feels that systemic steroids in high doses (140 to 160 mg of prednisone or its equivalent per day) may be life-saving in some cases of severe dystrophic forms during the neonatal period.[16] Since high doses may be required for several weeks or months, if this form of therapy is initiated, it should be utilized only with recognition of the potential risks of associated complications, particularly sepsis. The value of systemic steroids in the long-term management of severe forms of epidermolysis bullosa remains controversial.

Oral diphenylhydantoin (Dilantin) recently has been suggested for the treatment of dystrophic forms of epidermolysis bullosa.[22] This form of therapy is based on the fact that diphenylhydantoin in pharmacological doses has been shown to cause significant inhibition of collagenolytic activity both in vivo and in vitro. Although large clinical trials are required before this can be accepted as an effective form of therapy, diphenylhydantoin (Dilantin) in dosages of 2.5 to 5.0 mg/kg of body weight per day, to a maximum dose of 300 mg per day (a dosage high enough to obtain serum levels of 5 to 12 mcg per milliliter), may prove to be helpful in the treatment of this disorder.

The nursing care of the infant or child with severe epidermolysis bullosa is time-consuming and difficult. Restoration of function in severe fusion and flexion deformities of the hands and feet often can be helped by physiotherapy and appropriate plastic surgery. Mild cases of the dystrophic and non-dystrophic types may be compatible with a nearly normal life. The severe dystrophic forms remain a challenge and require cooperation by patient, parents, and physician.

CHRONIC NON-HEREDITARY BLISTERING DISEASES OF CHILDHOOD

The chronic non-hereditary bullous diseases of childhood have given rise to nosological confusion owing to their varying responses to sulfapyridines and sulfone preparations, usually negative results from immunofluorescent studies, and histologic patterns no more characteristic than subepidermal bulla formation.[23] In 1971 Bean et al. emphasized the usefulness of immunofluorescent techniques as a diagnostic aid and suggested a classification based on the clinical, histologic, and immunologic features of each disorder.[24] In 1974,

Table 15–3 CHRONIC NON-HEREDITARY BULLOUS DERMATOSES OF CHILDHOOD

Type	Characteristics	Histology	Immunofluorescence	Treatment
Dermatitis herpetiformis Usually in children over 8 years of age.	Extremely pruritic, grouped vesicles symmetrically distributed over the lower back, buttocks, sacrum, elbows, knees, and shoulders, sparing the mucous membranes	Subepidermal micro-abscesses with accumulation of neutrophils and eosinophils	IgA and complement at tips of dermal papillae without circulating antibodies	Sulfapyridine or dapsone
Juvenile bullous pemphigoid Usually in children below 8–10 years of age.	Large, tense, sometimes hemorrhagic, bullae in a generalized distribution; generally involves the lower abdomen, anogenital region, posterior aspect of the thighs, and sometimes the face; mild to moderate erosions of the mucous membranes	Subepidermal bullae, generally without microabscesses	Smooth pattern of IgG and C_3 along basement membrane with circulating IgG basement membrane zone antibodies	Sulfapyridine, dapsone, or corticosteroids
Bullous disease of childhood Usually in preschool children.	Large, tense, clear or hemorrhagic bullae on the face, scalp, lower trunk (including the genitalia and pubis), inner thighs, legs, and dorsal aspect of the feet, with sparing of the mucous membranes	Subepidermal bullae with edema of adjacent papillae and an underlying inflammatory infiltrate	Most cases are immunofluorescence negative; in some cases granular IgA and C_3 may be present along the basement membrane	Sulfapyridine or dapsone

on the basis of additional information regarding the clinical course, immunologic characteristics, and appropriate therapy of these diseases in children, dermatitis herpetiformis, bullous pemphigoid, benign chronic bullous dermatitis of childhood, pemphigus vulgaris, and pemphigus foliaceus were grouped under the inclusive term "chronic non-hereditary blistering disease of children."[25] Each of these diseases has an adult counterpart, with the exception of benign chronic bullous dermatosis of childhood (frequently shortened to chronic bullous dermatosis of childhood). Although previously regarded as a form of bullous pemphigoid or dermatitis herpetiformis, or a combination of the two, chronic bullous dermatosis of childhood (CBDC) may be emerging as a distinct and separate entity (Table 15–3).[26]

Childhood Dermatitis Herpetiformis

Dermatitis herpetiformis (Duhring's disease) is a chronic recurrent cutaneous disease of unknown cause characterized by an intensely pruritic papulovesicular and, at times, bullous eruption that responds dramatically to orally administered doses of sulfones or sulfapyridine. Although the disorder may affect individuals of all ages, dermatitis herpetiformis generally occurs during the second to fifth decades of life. It is relatively unusual in infancy and childhood and affects males more frequently than females. Blacks are rarely afflicted.

Dermatitis herpetiformis in childhood usually occurs in children over eight years of age, persists into adulthood, and is fundamentally the same disease as that seen in adults. Diagnosis of this disorder, just as in adults, should not be based solely on the morphologic aspects and distribution of lesions, but upon the constellation of clinical appearance, histopathologic characteristics, immunofluorescent findings, and response to therapy.[27-32]

Dermatitis herpetiformis is characterized by an extremely pruritic, symmetrically grouped papulovesicular eruption that affects the extensor surfaces: the elbows, knees, sacrum, buttocks, and shoulders. In association with the onset of intense pruritus or burning, erythematous and, at times, urticarial lesions may develop. Characteristic of this disorder are minute clear, relatively tense vesicles that measure from 0.3 to 4.0 mm in diameter. These vesicles rupture easily, either spontaneously or when scratched, and frequently erythematous lesions, small grouped papules and vesicles, superficial hyperpigmented macules, and hypopigmented scars exist at the same time. The general course of this disorder is chronic (often lasting 5 to 10 years or more) with frequent exacerbations and remissions.

The most useful diagnostic histologic changes in dermatitis herpetiformis are seen in the vicinity of new blisters. Whenever possible, cutaneous biopsy should include the newest vesicle and a piece of the surrounding erythematous portion of the lesion. The initial changes are first noted in the tips of the dermal papillae and consist of subepidermal microabscesses with accumulations of neutrophils and eosinophils. Immunofluorescent studies suggest the best criteria for diagnosis of dermatitis herpetiformis to be the finding of IgA and complement deposits at the tips of the dermal papillae in a speckled distribution (or, less frequently, in a linear pattern) along the basement membrane at the dermal-epidermal junction of normal appearing skin, without detectable circulating antibody to the basement membrane.[30, 31] Although dermatitis herpetiformis and bullous pemphigoid are distinct in most instances, on the basis of clinical and immunofluorescent features it appears that mixed and overlapping cases of both disorders can occur.[32]

Dermatitis herpetiformis is generally manifested as a purely cutaneous disorder. Recent studies, however, have demonstrated that 60 to 70 per cent of patients with this disorder also have small bowel abnormalities indistinguishable from those seen in celiac-type gluten-sensitivity enteropathy.[33, 34] Although the cutaneous abnormality may not be caused by the same agent as that of gluten-sensitive enteropathy, it appears that there are strong genetic links with an unusually high frequency of leukocyte antigen HL-A1 and HL-B8 in patients with both disorders.[35, 36]

Although the cause of dermatitis herpetiformis remains unknown, there is increasing evidence that, in some individuals at least, immunologic processes may be involved in the pathogenesis of dermatitis herpetiformis and adult celiac disease. Since the immunoglobulin in the skin of patients with adult-type dermatitis herpetiformis has been shown to be IgA, it has been suggested that immunoglobulins formed in the gut lodge in the skin and produce the characteristic cutaneous lesions seen in this disorder.

TREATMENT.   Clinical experience has shown that sulfapyridine and the sulfones are effective in relieving the symptoms and suppressing the eruption of dermatitis herpetiformis in children as well as adults. Dramatic relief from the use of these agents, therefore, frequently as early as 24 to 48 hours, is often helpful in the diagnosis of this disorder.

Sulfapyridine is generally considered to be the drug of choice. The initial dose of sulfapyridine is usually 100 to 200 mg/kg/per day for children, in four divided doses (with a maximum total of 2 to 4 grams a day). Once existing lesions have been suppressed, the dosage may be tapered at weekly intervals, with a maintenance level of 0.5 gm or less as the daily required dose for most patients. Nausea and vomiting usually are the first signs of sulfapyridine toxicity. Other side effects include anorexia, headache, fever, leukopenia, agranulocytosis, hemolytic anemia, serum-sickness–type reactions, hepatitis, exfoliative dermatitis, and renal crystalluria.[37] A screening test for glucose-6-phosphate dehydrogenase (G6PD) deficiency should be performed prior to the initiation of therapy, and close observation of the patient with pretreatment and follow-up blood counts at monthly intervals is recommended. Patients should be encouraged to drink large quantities of fluid in order to avoid renal complication, and since the disease may remit spontaneously, gradual attempts at reduction of treatment should be attempted at intervals of three to six months.

Various sulfone derivatives of 4,4′-diaminodiphenyl sulfone (dapsone, DDS) are better tolerated and more economical than sulfapyridine. Their side effects, however, are more severe, and because of an increased tendency to hemolytic anemia in patients with glucose-6-phosphate dehydrogenase deficiency (G6PD), a screening test should be done prior to initiation of therapy. Available in 25 and 100 mg tablets as Avlosulfon (Ayerst), dapsone treatment may be initiated with 2 mg/kg/day, with an increase or decrease in dosage depending on the clinical response and the side effects associated with therapy. If side effects do not occur, a maximum of 400 mg a day may be reached, (the required dosage, however, is usually in the range of 50 mg three times daily).

Once a favorable response is achieved (usually within a week) the dose is decreased gradually to a minimum level (generally 25 to 50 mg daily). In addition to hemolysis, side effects include methemoboglobinemia (manifested by bluish discoloration of the face, mucous membranes, and nails), nausea, vomiting, headache, giddiness, tachycardia, psychoses, anemia, fever, exfoliative dermatitis, liver necrosis, lymphadenitis, and peripheral neuropathy. Although leukopenia rarely occurs, complete blood counts and urinalyses should be checked at monthly intervals during the first year of therapy (after that about three-month intervals appear to be adequate). Since the disease has a tendency to remission after a period of years, periodic gradual decrease in dosage levels should be attemped, as with sulfapyridine therapy.

A high percentage of patients with dermatitis herpetiformis have an associated gluten-sensitive enteropathy. Accordingly, it has been recommended that patients should have small-intestine studies for the possibility of this association. Although gluten-free diets (avoidance of foods containing wheat, rye, and barley flour) have been suggested in an attempt to reduce the symptoms of malabsorption, the conclusions of studies vary as to the efficacy of such diets on cutaneous lesions. Whereas Shuster found that treatment with a gluten-free diet did not affect the severity of the cutaneous eruption and did not permit a decrease in the dosage of sulfone required to control the disease, other investigators have reported an improvement in cutaneous lesions while on gluten-free diets.[38]

Local applications of steroid creams or shake lotions such as Calamine lotion with menthol or phenol may diminish pruritus and permit control of the disorder with lower doses of systemic preparations. For patients who can tolerate neither sulfapyridine nor sulfone therapy, systemic corticosteroids (although not very effective) may be the only available form of treatment.

Juvenile Bullous Pemphigoid

Juvenile bullous pemphigoid, the large blister variety of chronic bullous dermatosis of childhood, is an acquired chronic bullous eruption that on rare occasions affects young children below eight to ten years of age.[39–41] The youngest patient reported to date was a 3 1/2-month-old infant.[40] The course of the disease is marked by periodic remissions and eruptions and spontaneous resolution generally within a period of two or three years.

The disorder resembles the adult type of bullous pemphigoid except that the incidence of

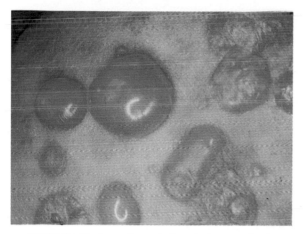

Figure 15–10 Large tense bullous lesions on the lower aspect of the abdomen of a 3 1/2-year-old boy with juvenile bullous pemphigoid.

oral lesions is higher in children. The clinical features of bullous pemphigoid are dominated by large bullae, more tense and inflamed, but otherwise similar to those of pemphigus vulgaris (Fig. 15–10). The course of bullous pemphigoid, however, is more indolent than that of pemphigus vulgaris and the Nikolsky sign usually is absent. Denuded areas tend toward spontaneous healing and do not extend or increase in size as they do in patients with pemphigus vulgaris. The disorder is characterized by mild pruritus and by large tense, sometimes hemorrhagic bullae that measure 0.25 to 2.0 cm in diameter and generally involve the lower abdomen, anogenital region, posterior aspect of the thighs, and sometimes the face. Lesions may appear on normal skin or on an erythematous base, and they frequently occur at the periphery of annular or polycyclic erythematous plaques.

Biopsy of cutaneous lesions shows subepidermal blister formation, generally without papillary microabscesses (an important diagnostic feature of dermatitis herpetiformis). Direct and indirect immunofluorescent techniques show deposition of gamma globulins and complement at the dermal-epidermal junction of lesions. The demonstration of circulating IgG antibodies to the basement membrane zone suggests that some of these children represent a juvenile counterpart to adult bullous pemphigoid. Although the etiology of bullous pemphigoid is unknown, at times it appears that this cutaneous reaction may represent an antigen-antibody complex precipitated by administration of certain drugs or antibiotics. Basal cell antibodies, however, are not specific, and their role in pathogenesis remains unclear.[23, 39]

The response to treatment of bullous pemphigoid of childhood is variable. Systemic corticosteroids may suppress the eruption. In severe and resistant cases, a combination of sulfones or sulfapyridine in conjunction with corticosteroids may be helpful. Topical corticosteroids, cool baths with colloidal oatmeal, and systemic antipruritics can also be beneficial in the management of this disorder.

Bullous Disease of Childhood

Chronic bullous dermatosis of childhood, also referred to as benign chronic bullous dermatosis of childhood (CBDC) or bullous disease of childhood (BDC), is a subepidermal blistering disease that frequently is indistinguishable both clinically and histologically from bullous pemphigoid and dermatitis herpetiformis. Whether this disorder represents a distinct entity or an aberrant form of dermatitis herpetiformis, bullous pemphigoid, or a combination of both remains to be clarified. Although it originally was proposed that bullous disease of childhood could be distinguished from bullous pemphigoid and dermatitis herpetiformis by the lack of fixed or circulating epithelial antibodies,[25] cases of BDC have shown linear deposition of IgA, IgG, or complement at the dermal-epidermal junction.[26, 40] The immunofluorescent findings in BDC are not uniform, and the majority of reported cases are negative for immunofluorescence.[12]

Bullous disease of childhood, probably the most common but least well studied chronic bullous dermatosis of childhood, is usually a disease of the first decade of life, with onset occurring most frequently during the preschool years and spontaneous remission after several months to three years of activity.[26, 42] The eruption is characterized by large, tense, clear or hemorrhagic bullae measuring 1.0 to 2.0 cm in diameter on a normal or erythematous base. The eruption is widespread, and areas of predilection include the face, scalp, lower part of the trunk (including the genitalia and pubis), buttocks, inner thighs, legs, and dorsal aspect of the feet. The bullae may form annular or rosette-like lesions composed of sausage-shaped blisters surrounding a central crust. Many patients also have erythematous plaques with polycyclic margins bordered by intact bullae. Pruritus is a variable feature. It is usually mild to moderate but may be intense and distressing or completely absent.[25, 26, 42]

Histologically BDC is characterized by a subepidermal bulla, edema of adjacent dermal papillae, and an underlying inflammatory infiltrate consisting of neutrophilic polymorphonuclear leukocytes, eosinophils, and mononuclear cells.[43] Although most cases reported are immunofluorescent negative, in some cases direct immunofluorescence demonstrates a linear band of IgA and C_3 at the basement membranes.[44, 45]

This disorder appears to differ from both pemphigoid and dermatitis herpetiformis in several ways. Bullous pemphigoid is characterized by large tense bullae on the trunk and flexor surfaces of the extremities, with mild to moderate involvement of the mucous membranes in children. It causes a subepidermal bulla with deposition of IgG and C_3 at the basement membrane. Indirect immunofluorescence shows circulating basement

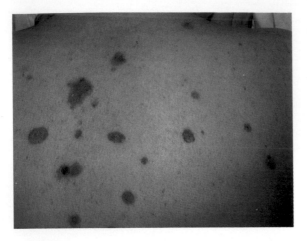

Figure 15–11 Pemphigus vulgaris. Seldom seen in childhood, this dermatosis is characterized by flaccid bullae that develop on normal appearing skin and mucous membranes.

membrane zone antibodies. Although bullous pemphigoid is usually treated with corticosteroids, some patients are reported to respond to sulfapyridine or dapsone.

Dermatitis herpetiformis is an intensely pruritic, chronic, recurrent eruption of grouped vesicles or bullae. It involves the back, buttocks, scalp, and extensor surfaces of the extremities in a symmetrical mirror-image–like distribution. Histologically it is characterized by subepidermal bullae, at the periphery of which are suprapapillary polymorphonuclear leukocytic microabscesses. Direct immunofluorescence shows granular deposition of IgA at the tips of dermal papillae. In those cases of BDC with positive immunofluorescence, the IgA is deposited in a linear pattern along the basement membrane.

Response to therapy for BDC is generally favorable. Sulfapyridine, as in dermatitis herpetiformis, is the drug of choice. If response to sulfapyridine is inadequate, sulfapyridine is discontinued and dapsone is begun. Although BDC may respond to systemic administration of steroids, because of the side effects of prolonged

corticosteroid therapy in children, this form of therapy should be avoided whenever possible.[42]

Pemphigus in Childhood

Pemphigus is a term applied to a group of severe, chronic, sometimes fatal blistering disorders characterized by flaccid bullae that develop on normal-appearing skin and mucous membranes. Although four types of pemphigus have been described (vulgaris, vegetans, foliaceus, and erythematous), on the basis of histologic criteria it now appears that this disease can be simplified into two basic disorders, pemphigus vulgaris and pemphigus foliaceus and their variants. It has been suggested that pemphigus vegetans may merely represent a variant of pemphigus vulgaris and that pemphigus erythematosus may be manifested as an early or abortive form of pemphigus foliaceus.[46]

Pemphigus Vulgaris (and Pemphigus Vegetans). Pemphigus vulgaris is a chronic vesiculobullous disease characterized by flaccid bullae and persistent erosions, with a predilection for middle-aged individuals (Fig. 15–11). Although the etiology is unknown, the finding of intercellular antibodies in the serum of patients suggests an autoimmune basis to pemphigus and its variants (Fig. 15–12).

An extremely uncommon disorder of childhood, it was reported in five children during the fifteen years from 1955 to 1969;[47, 48] in two children in 1972;[49, 50] in a 3 1/2-year-old boy in 1973,[51] and in a ninth case in 1978.[52] The apparent rarity of pemphigus in childhood may be related to difficulty in diagnosis and a low index of suspicion in this age group. With higher levels of suspicion and present histologic and immunofluorescent techniques these disorders may prove to be less rare in childhood than previously suspected.

Clinical Manifestations. The cutaneous lesions of pemphigus vulgaris favor the seborrheic areas (the face, scalp, neck, sternum, axillae, groin, and periumbilical regions) and pressure areas of the feet and back, and mucous membranes are affected in 95 per cent of patients. In more than half the patients the disorder starts with erosions

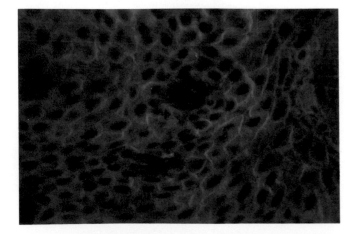

Figure 15–12 Pemphigus vulgaris. Immunofluorescent stains with IgG and complement bound to intercellular areas of the epidermis. (Courtesy of Irwin M. Braverman, M.D.)

of the oral mucosa, which are frequently present for several months before the appearance of skin lesions. Intact blisters are rarely seen on the oral mucosa, since they rupture soon after formation, leaving raw denuded painful erosions that heal slowly. Other mucosal surfaces, the anogenital areas, conjunctivae, vermilion borders of the lips, pharynx, and larynx may also be similarly involved. Since a majority of patients with proven pemphigus vulgaris present with painful oral erosions for weeks to months before they develop the characteristic bullous eruption, children with severe recurrent mucocutaneous lesions or chronic erosive mucous membrane disease should be examined carefully, and mucosal biopsy should be performed to rule out the possibility of this severe debilitating disorder.

The primary cutaneous lesions of pemphigus vulgaris appear as vesicles or bullae that arise on erythematous plaques or normal appearing skin (Fig. 15–11). The initial lesions may remain localized to one area of the skin or mucous membrane for weeks or months before other areas of the skin are involved. With the onset of new lesions, the patient may experience some pruritus, burning, or local discomfort. Blisters generally measure 1 centimeter or less at onset but may increase in size by peripheral extension to several centimeters in diameter. Vertical pressure may produce peripheral extension of lesions. The blisters rupture easily, and the resultant erosions are painful, bleed easily, and heal slowly. Scaling and crusting are common, and patients frequently are misdiagnosed as having impetigo or infected seborrheic dermatitis.

The diagnosis of pemphigus vulgaris depends upon awareness that the disorder can occur in children and upon the clinical picture, histologic examination of lesions, and immunofluorescent studies. Dislodgement of the outermost layer from the basal layer of the epidermis by gentle sliding pressure of involved as well as uninvolved skin (the Nikolsky sign) is invariably demonstrable in patients with pemphigus vulgaris. This phenomenon, a manifestation of defective epidermal cohesion, however, is not pathognomonic of this disorder, since it may also be seen in patients with epidermolysis bullosa, bullous pemphigoid, severe erythema multiforme (Stevens-Johnson disease), and toxic epidermal necrolysis. An ancillary sign of pemphigus vulgaris, however, is the peripheral enlargement of blisters by peripheral extravasation of fluid into the layers of the epidermis.

The Tzanck test is useful for the rapid demonstration of acantholytic epidermal cells in vesicles or bullae of pemphigus. After careful removal of the roof of a blister, smears from the base of the lesions stained with Giemsa or Hematoxylin and Eosin stain show typical detached acantholytic cells. Since acantholytic epidermal cells may also be seen in other disorders, this examination is a preliminary test and requires histopathologic confirmation.

For diagnostic purposes it is essential that a new bulla be examined histologically, preferably a small one that can be totally excised together with some surrounding skin. Light freezing of the bulla with an aerosol refrigerant prior to biopsy permits removal without damage to its architecture. The earliest histologic change is intercellular edema, with loss of cohesion between epidermal cells. In pemphigus vulgaris this results in the formation of clefts and bullae in a suprabasal location. The basal cells, although separated from one another, remain attached to the dermis, with a resultant "row of tombstones" appearance and frequently the base of the bulla may be irregular in contour when layers of epidermal cells (villi) project into the bullous cavity.[16]

Although the etiology of pemphigus is unknown, the demonstration of intercellular antibodies in the serum of patients with all forms of pemphigus suggests an autoimmune phenomenon as the basis of pemphigus vulgaris and its variants. Direct immunofluorescent tests show IgG and complement bound to intercellular areas of the epidermis (Fig. 15–12). Indirect immunofluorescent studies of the serum of patients with pemphigus vulgaris containing antibodies against an intercellular substance of the stratified squamous epithelial cells help confirm the diagnosis. The level of serum antibodies against the intercellular substance reflects the severity or extent of the disease; it is particularly helpful in diagnosis of very early cases and appears to be a good index of response to therapy.[53]

Pemphigus vegetans. Pemphigus vegetans is a variant of pemphigus vulgaris in patients who have an increased resistance to their disease. Some authorities recognize two types of pemphigus vegetans: one is the *Neumann* and the other the *Hallopeau* type (pyodermite vegetante). Pemphigus vegetans differs from pemphigus vulgaris in that it starts at an earlier age and is characterized by flaccid bullae, particularly on the face and genitals and in intertriginous areas, that become eroded and heal with papillomatous proliferation (the so-called vegetations). The Hallopeau type has a prolonged course, and pustules rather than bullae represent the usual primary lesions. The pustules are followed rapidly by verrucous vegetations, which have a tendency to peripheral extension, and older vegetations no longer show the pustules seen in earlier stages, but appear more papillomatous and hyperkeratotic.

Prior to the use of corticosteroids, the course of pemphigus vegetans was more protracted than that of pemphigus vulgaris. It tends to pursue a chronic course, and although spontaneous remission and even permanent healing may occur in some patients, it nearly always ends in fatality if not treated with corticosteriods.

Pemphigus Foliaceus (and Pemphigus Erythematosus).
Pemphigus foliaceus is a more superficial and less severe form of pemphigus. The disease most commonly affects middle-aged persons and, although rare in children, is more com-

mon than pemphigus vulgaris of childhood and follows a more benign and less aggressive course.[53, 54] The youngest child with this disorder to date was an 18-month-old, reported on in 1971.[55]

Histologic findings in pemphigus foliaceus are similar to those of pemphigus vulgaris and demonstrate epidermal bullae and intercellular acantholysis of the epidermis. The acantholysis seen in pemphigus foliaceus, however, is more superficial and occurs in the upper epidermis, usually in the granular layer or just beneath it, with resultant formation of clefts in a superficial, often subcorneal. location.

Oral lesions are rarely seen in pemphigus foliaceus and, when present, usually consist of small, superficial, often inconspicuous erosions. Bullae, when seen, are usually small and flaccid. They break easily, and because of their superficial location, leave shallow erosions. Patients generally are not severely ill, but complain of pruritus, pain, and burning. At times, however, the clinical picture may progress to resemble that of a severe generalized exfoliative dermatitis.

Pemphigus erythematosus. The first lesions of pemphigus foliaceus often localize to the center of the face. When the butterfly area of the face, the scalp, upper chest, and back are involved, the disorder has been termed pemphigus erythematosus. In 1926, Senear and Usher described this as an unusual form of lupus erythematosus (the Senear-Usher syndrome). Clinical course and histopathologic patterns, however, confirm pemphigus erythematosus and the Senear-Usher syndrome as variants of pemphigus foliaceus.[56]

Fogo selvagem. Fogo selvagem (Brazilian pemphigus) is a variant of pemphigus foliaceus found in tropical regions. Endemic in Brazil, it occurs in children and young adults, particularly women. It affects native Brazilians and immigrants alike and commonly affects more than one member of a family. Approximately 15 per cent of patients are children, and young women under 30 comprise 65 per cent of all patients with this variant of pemphigus. Although it is indistinguishable from non-endemic pemphigus, its localization to small foci point to an infectious agent, possibly borne by an arthropod, in the etiology of this disorder.[57, 58]

The onset of Brazilian pemphigus is similar to that of pemphigus foliaceus. In chronic cases hyperpigmentation, hyperkeratosis, and loss of hair over the scalp and body are prominent features of this disorder. In younger patients the natural course of pemphigus foliaceus is to recede gradually and subside completely. The prognosis prior to the availability of corticosteroids was dependent upon the age of the patient and whether the disease took an acute or chronic course. Once the disease has cleared, pemphigus foliaceus has less tendency to recurrence than pemphigus vulgaris.[53]

Treatment. Systemic corticosteroids at present are the treatment of choice for patients with pemphigus vulgaris and pemphigus foliaceus. Childhood pemphigus, although rare, can be just as virulent as its adult counterpart. Without appropriate treatment the disease almost invariably terminates fatally in several months to years. Prompt diagnosis, therefore, is particularly important so that therapy can be instituted early in the course of the disease.

In recent years successful treatment of pemphigus vulgaris in adults has consisted of daily high-dose prednisone (100 to 200 mg or more) or its equivalent. In children the recommended dose is 3 to 6 mg/kg/day (up to 60 to 120 mg of prednisone or its equivalent), depending upon the severity of the disorder. This dose is continued until healing occurs (often two to five months after the onset of therapy in severe cases). Treatment of pemphigus foliaceus is similar to that of pemphigus vulgaris except that patients with pemphigus foliaceus and its variants generally respond to lower steroid dosages. Although patients with Brazilian pemphigus (fogo selvagem) may respond to antimalarial therapy (quinine or quinacrine), systemic corticosteroids continue to be the treatment of choice.

Adverse reactions associated with prolonged high-dose corticosteroid therapy are a major hazard in long-term management of patients with pemphigus vulgaris. Once a maintenance dosage is attained, therefore, treatment should be reduced (by about 20 per cent every two weeks), and alternate day therapy is preferred once the disease is controlled.[55] Immunosuppressive drugs (methotrexate, azathioprine, or cyclophosphamide) have been used as ancillary therapeutic agents for patients with severe disease who cannot be controlled by steroids alone, or when prolonged high-dose steroids are undesirable.[46] Because of potential adverse effects, however, cytotoxic drugs should be used with caution in children.

Patients with pemphigus foliaceus or its variant pemphigus erythematosus may, at times, respond to topical corticosteroids. Topical corticosteroids are advisable, therefore, in an attempt to limit long-term use of systemic corticosteroid therapy in mild cases of pemphigus foliaceus and its variants.

SUBCORNEAL PUSTULAR DERMATOSIS

Subcorneal pustular dermatosis (Sneddon-Wilkinson disease) is a chronic vesiculopustular disorder of undetermined etiology first described in 1956.[59] It is characterized by pustules in an annular and serpiginous arrangement and generally involves the abdomen, axillae, and groin. This relatively rare disease occurs most frequently in middle-aged women, but can also appear in childhood.[60] Although some authorities consider this disorder to be an atypical form of dermatitis herpetiformis, lack of changes in the jejunal mucosa and absence of IgA in the tips of dermal papillae suggest that it is distinct from and unrelated to dermatitis herpetiformis.

Comparison of the disease in children and adults indicates no difference in clinical appearance, course, and histologic findings except that children frequently have a more severe toxic reaction with high fever and leukocytosis, during the acute stage of the disorder.[60] The disease generally begins with small pustules or vesicles on an erythematous base. Occasionally only vesicles may be present, but these soon change into sterile pustules. The pustules tend to appear in crops and spread to large parts of the body, forming large circinate or gyrate patterns that coalesce to form serpiginous patterns. The eruption favors the groin, abdomen, axillae, and flexural aspects of the proximal extremities. The hands, feet, face, and mucous membranes are rarely affected. Although most patients experience a mild degree of pruritus, severe itching with excoriation is uncommon. Individual lesions tend to last for periods of five days, with new lesions appearing as others disappear. As the pustules resolve they are replaced by a superficial leafy scale or crust. After the eruption resolves, a faint blotchy brown hyperpigmentation, without atrophy or scarring, remains. The condition is benign and is characterized by remissions and exacerbations that may last for periods of five to eight years.

Histopathologic examination of an intact lesion reveals a subcorneal blister filled almost entirely with neutrophilic polymorphonuclear leukocytes. The more intense itching and the subepidermal location of blisters in dermatitis herpetiformis help differentiate these two conditions. Subcorneal pustular dermatosis may be differentiated from impetigo, which has a similar histologic picture, by history, absence of pathogenic bacteria on culture, and failure to respond to antibiotics. Differentiation from pemphigus foliaceus can be made by immunofluorescent studies.

Diaminodiphenylsulfone (dapsone) and sulfapyridine are the treatments of choice. Although the response is slower than that seen in dermatitis herpetiformis, the majority of patients obtain partial, if not complete, relief. Dosage in children and precautions with dapsone or sulfapyridine therapy are similar to those utilized in the management of dermatitis herpetiformis.

FAMILIAL BENIGN PEMPHIGUS

Familial benign pemphigus (benign familial chronic pemphigus, Hailey-Hailey disease) is an autosomal dominant genodermatosis characterized by recurrent vesicles and bullae, which most commonly appear on the sides and back of the neck, in the axillae, in the groin, and perianal regions. It appears equally in males and females, occurs most frequently in Caucasians, and is relatively uncommon in Negroes and Orientals. First described by two brothers, Howard and Hugh Hailey in 1939, the disorder is not seen before puberty and usually has its onset in the late teens or early twenties.[61]

Most cases of familial benign pemphigus have a fairly constant course. The primary lesions are small vesicles that occur in groups on normal or erythematous skin. The vesicles may enlarge to form bullae and rupture easily, leaving an eroded base, exude serum, and develop crusts resembling impetigo or pyoderma. The Nikolsky sign may or may not be present. Lesions tend to spread peripherally, with an active, often serpiginous border and central resolution with peripheral extension often results in circinate lesions. In the intertriginous areas lesions tend to form erythematous plaques with dry crusting and soft, flat, and moist granular vegetations. Burning or pruritus are common, and particularly in the intertriginous areas, lesions tend to become irritating, painful, and exceedingly uncomfortable.

Although lesions of the mucous membranes rarely occur, keratoconjunctivitis and papular lesions of the vulva and oral mucosa have been described, and esophageal involvement has been demonstrated by esophagoscopy and histopathologic changes.[62] Although some patients may have spontaneous improvement, the disease generally does not clear completely. It tends to run a chronic course characterized by exacerbations and remissions and by age 50 tends to become less severe in nature.[63]

The basic disturbance in familial benign pemphigus is a defect in the desmosome-filament complex similar to that seen in patients with Darier's disease.[64] The cutaneous lesions of familial benign pemphigus are induced by numerous external stimuli, namely heat, humidity, friction, exposure to ultraviolet light, and bacterial or candidal infection.[65, 66] Although at times the clinical picture may resemble that of impetigo or pemphigus vegetans, the disorder can be differentiated on the basis of family history (present in 70 per cent of patients with familial benign pemphigus) and the recurring nature of the disorder.

Biopsy of the advancing border of a lesion is particularly helpful in establishing the proper diagnosis. The histologic picture is characterized by vesicle formation in a suprabasal location, separation of the epidermal cells with neighboring cells still adhering loosely one to another, producing a "dilapidated brick wall" appearance, and upward protrusion of villi (papillae lined by a single layer of basal cells) into the vesicular spaces. In some instances corps ronds (large round dyskeratotic masses surrounded by a clear halo as the result of shrinkage) similar to those in Darier's disease may be seen in the granular layer or vesicular spaces. Although some dermatologists have suggested that familial benign pemphigus may represent a vesicular form of Darier's disease, differences in histologic findings, lack of response of Darier's disease to antibiotic therapy, and independent inheritance patterns appear to differentiate the two disorders.

As yet there is no effective treatment that will arrest the basic defect of familial benign pemphigus. An effort should be made to avoid the precipitating factors of heat, humidity, and the friction associated with tight or ill-fitting clothing. Although topical antibiotics may be helpful in some cases, systemic antibiotics chosen on the basis of bacterial culture and sensitivity studies appear to be most effective in the treatment of this disorder.[67] Topical and systemic corticosteroids may also be effective in some cases. Systemic corticosteroids, however, are not recommended since the disorder frequently recurs when the dosage levels are reduced. In persistent cases when patients have been disabled by painful eroded plaques unresponsive to other therapeutic measures, excision of the involved regions, followed by split-thickness skin grafts, has been helpful.[68]

HERPES GESTATIONIS

Herpes gestationis is an uncommon blistering disorder that occurs during pregnancy and the postpartum period and tends to recur in subsequent pregnancies. Its cause is unknown and its pruritic eruption consists of grouped erythematous edematous papules and plaques, grouped vesicles on erythematous bases, and tense bullae. The onset of the eruption most commonly occurs during the fourth or fifth month of gestation, but has occurred as early as two weeks after conception and as late as the day before delivery, and even during the first few weeks of the postpartum period. The course of herpes gestationis is cyclic but generally tends to abate spontaneously during the last few weeks of gestation. Although the eruption tends to clear in the majority of patients within a few days of delivery, the eruption can persist for many months after delivery, and mild recurrences occasionally have been noted to appear at the time of menstruation and again with recurrent pregnancies.

Speculations regarding the cause of herpes gestationis vary. In view of its clinical and histologic resemblance to erythema multiforme, the possibility that this may represent a hypersensitivity or toxic reaction to fetal or placental products or to hormones or their metabolites must be considered. The immunopathologic hallmark of herpes gestationis is the presence of the third component of complement (C_3), with or without IgG, in a linear band-like distribution along the basement membrane zone.[69] A circulating factor in the serum of patients with this disorder, termed the herpes gestationis factor (HGF), can cause the deposition of C_3 in the same region (this factor has recently been shown to be IgG).[70]

The histopathologic features of this disorder, although resembling those of dermatitis herpetiformis and erythema multiforme, are said to be distinctive and are characterized by a subepidermal vesicle with a dense perivascular infiltrate containing lymphocytes, histiocytes, and numerous eosinophils.[69]

Owing to the relative rarity of herpes gestationis (1 in 4000 to 10,000 cases of pregnancy), the question of whether or not there is an increased fetal morbidity and mortality in women with this disorder varies from estimates of little to no fetal risk to studies suggesting an incidence of morbidity as high as 30 per cent.[70, 71] The course of herpes

gestationis is characterized by alternating exacerbations and remissions. The pruritus is not relieved by sedatives, antihistamines, or sulfones. When therapy for this disorder is prescribed, the possibility of drug-induced fetal damage, particularly during the first trimester of pregnancy, must be carefully considered. Systemic corticosteroids are the most reliable mode of therapy and, with certain precautions, generally are considered safe for both mother and fetus. In order to avoid potential risk of fetal developmental abnormality, however, they should be withheld, if possible, during the first trimester of pregnancy. Prednisone (in dosages of 20 to 40 mg daily) or its equivalent, is generally effective and well tolerated. The patient, however, should be monitored, particularly in regard to weight gain, hypertension, and possible fluid retention. Alternate-day dosage, if possible, is preferable to daily treatment, and in order to avoid adrenal suppression to the fetus, dosages should be reduced to a minimum during the final weeks of pregnancy.

Pyridoxine also has been reported to be effective in some patients. One advantage of this form of therapy is the fact that pyridoxine can be administered safely without risk of fetal damage within the first trimester of pregnancy. Initially it may be administered intravenously or intramuscularly in dosages of 50 mg once or twice a day. Oral pyridoxine, in dosages of 100 to 400 mg, may be administered simultaneously, and after good control has been achieved, the parenteral administration may be discontinued and oral pyridoxine continued in dosages varying from 25 to 400 mg daily. If there is no response to pyridoxine within 10 days, it is wise to abandon this form of therapy in favor of another modality. It must be remembered that no form of therapy, to date, has been curative, and therefore whatever mode of treatment is prescribed, it must be continued throughout the time of pregnancy and during the first few postpartum weeks.

References

1. Pearson RW: Studies on the pathogenesis of epidermolysis bullosa. J. Invest. Derm. 39:551–575, 1962.

   Electron microscopic examination reveals distinct pathologic features in epidermolysis bullosa with pathogenetic hypotheses based upon these data.

2. Pearson RW: The mechanobullous diseases — Epidermolysis bullosa. In Fitzpatrick TB et al. (Eds.): Dermatology in Practice, McGraw-Hill Book Company, New York, 1971, 621–643.

   A thorough discussion of present concepts of epidermolysis bullosa based on light and electron microscopy, pathogenesis, and clinical patterns.

3. Gorlin RJ, Pindborg JJ, and Cohen MM Jr: Epidermolysis bullosa. In Syndromes of the Head and Neck, 2nd ed. McGraw-Hill Book Company, New York, 1976, 281–288.

   A description of the clinical signs of epidermolysis bullosa with emphasis on the head and neck.

4. Bart BJ, Gorlin RJ, Anderson VE, et al.: Congenital localized absence of the skin, blistering and abnormality of nails. Arch. Dermatol. 93:296–304, 1966.

Congenital localized defects of the skin, mechanoblisters, and nail deformities described in a large kinship suggest a distinct mechanobullous disorder of autosomal dominant inheritance with variable penetrance.

5. Smith SZ, Cram DL: A mechanobullous disease of the newborn. Bart's syndrome. Arch. Dermatol. *114*:81–84, 1978.

A female infant with absent areas of skin on the hands, legs, and feet with associated nail dystrophy.

6. Baxter DL: Epidermolysis bullosa. In Demis DJ, Dobson RL, and McGuire J: Clinical Dermatology, Unit 2. Harper and Row, Hagerstown, Maryland, 1977, 6:6, 1–14.

A thorough discussion of epidermolysis bullosa, its pathogenesis and clinical characteristics.

7. Briggaman RA, Wheeler CA Jr: Epidermolysis bullosa dystrophica-recessive: a possible role of anchoring fibrils in the pathogenesis. J. Invest. Dermatol. *65*:203–211, 1975.

A review of ultrastructural defects and the role of anchoring fibrils in the pathogenesis of recessive epidermolysis bullosa dystrophica.

8. Eisen AZ: Human skin collagenase: localization and distribution in normal human skin. J. Invest. Dermatol. *52*:442–448, 1969.

The isolation of collagenolytic enzyme suggests its role in the mechanism of collagen degradation.

9. Eisen AZ: Human skin collagenase: relationship to the pathogenesis of epidermolysis bullosa dystrophica. J. Invest. Dermatol. *52*:449–453, 1969.

Additional studies on collagenase activity in patients with dystrophic epidermolysis bullosa suggest overproduction of collagenase in the role of blister formation.

10. Bauer EA: Recessive dystrophic epidermolysis bullosa. Evidence for an altered collagenase in fibroblast cultures. Proc. Natl. Acad. Sci. USA *74*:4646–4650, 1977.

Studies in two patients with recessive dystrophic epidermolysis bullosa suggest that the altered collagenase present in patients with this disorder may be the result of a structural gene mutation, a defect in post-translational modification of the enzyme, or mutation in a gene that regulates the normal degradation of collagenase.

11. Lazarus G: Collagenase and connective tissue metabolism in epidermolysis bullosa. J. Invest. Dermatol. *58*:242–249, 1972.

Studies of 19 patients with various types of epidermolysis bullosa suggest that increased local levels of collagenase may merely represent a secondary tissue reaction to chronic injury.

12. Jarratt M: Current concepts in diagnosis. Diagnosis and treatment of epidermolysis bullosa. So. Med. J. *69*:113–117, 1976.

A comprehensive review of the clinical and histologic features and management of epidermolysis bullosa.

13. Solomon LM, Esterly NB: Epidermolysis bullosa. In Neonatal Dermatology. W. B. Saunders Co., Philadelphia, 1973, 142–147.

A discussion of epidermolysis bullosa with particular reference to the disease and its management during the newborn period.

14. Moynahan EJ: Epidermolysis bullosa affecting the buccal and pharyngeal mucosae. Proc. Royal Soc. Med. *56*:885–887, 1963.

A review of seven cases of dystrophic epidermolysis bullosa treated with corticosteroids.

15. Reed WB, College J Jr, Frances MJV: Epidermolysis bullosa dystrophica with epidermal neoplasms. Arch. Dermatol. *110*:894–902, 1974.

Twenty-one patients with carcinoma in scars of dystrophic epidermolysis bullosa (all were over 20 years of age and most were over age 35).

16. Moynahan EJ: Epidermolysis bullosa. In Maddin S (Ed.): Current Dermatologic Management. C. V. Mosby Co., St. Louis, 1970, 110–111.

A discussion of the management of epidermolysis bullosa, with emphasis on systemic steroids and their role in severe dystrophic forms of this disorder.

17. Smith EC, Michener WM: Vitamin E treatment of dermolytic bullous dermatosis. Arch. Derm. *108*:254–256, 1973.

Controlled double-blind crossover studies in two sisters with mild recessive dystrophic epidermolysis bullosa demonstrate reduced blister formation while on 1600 IU daily of vitamin E (DL-alpha-tocopherol).

18. Pearson RW: Advances in the diagnosis and treatment of blistering diseases: a selective review. In Malkinson FD, Pearson RW (Eds.): Yearbook of Dermatology, 1977, 7–52.

A critical review of current concepts of blistering disorders.

19. Katz J, Gryboski JP, Rosenbaum HM, et al.: Dysphagia in children with epidermolysis bullosa. Gastroenterol. *52*:259–262, 1967.

The authors conclude that steroids appear to be helpful in some patients for the control of bulla formation, but they caution that steroids should be used only for the most severely affected patients.

20. Orlando RC, Bozymski EM, Briggaman RA, et al.: Epidermolysis bullosa: gastrointestinal manifestations. Ann. Int. Med. *81*:203–206, 1974.

In patients with esophageal involvement, if conservative management fails to maintain weight, bougienage, surgery, or both, should be considered.

21. Absolon KB, Finney LA, Waddill GM Jr, et al.: Esophageal constriction — colon transplant — in two brothers with epidermolysis bullosa. Surgery *65*:832–836, 1969.

Colon transplants in the esophagus were successful in two patients unresponsive to conservative management and bougienage.

22. Eisenberg M, Stevens LH, Schofield PJ: Epidermolysis bullosa: new therapeutic approaches. Australian J. Dermatol. *19*:1–8, 1978.

Parenteral diphenylhydantoin, an apparently effective form of therapy for two children with dystrophic epidermolysis bullosa.

23. Shmunes E, Shu S: Bullous disease of childhood, report of a case demonstrating antibasal cell antibody. Arch. Dermatol. *113*:325–327, 1977.

Immunofluorescent studies in a 5-year-old boy with a bullous disorder that developed one week after a penicillin injection suggests drug reaction as a possible factor in the etiology of juvenile bullous pemphigoid.

24. Bean SF, Jordon RE, Winkelman RK, et al.: Chronic non hereditary blistering disease in children. Am. J. Dis. Child. *122*:137–141, 1971.

Immunofluorescent staining techniques suggest benign chronic bullous dermatosis of childhood (CEDC) to be a distinct disorder rather than a variant of bullous pemphigoid or a bullous form of childhood dermatitis herpetiformis.

25. Bean SF, Jordon RE: Chronic non-hereditary blistering disease in children. Arch. Dermatol. *110*:941–944, 1974.

Immunofluorescent studies help clarify the classification of dermatitis herpetiformis and bullous pemphigoid in childhood.

26. Esterly NB, Furey NL, Krschner BS, et al.: Chronic bullous dermatosis of childhood. Arch. Dermatol. *113*:42–46, 1977.

Studies of two boys with chronic bullous dermatosis of childhood.

27. Kim R, Winkelmann RK: Dermatitis herpetiformis in children: a relationship to bullous pemphigoid. Arch. Dermatol. *83*:895–902, 1961.

In a report of 22 children with dermatitis herpetiformis, the patients were divided into two groups on the basis of papular and bullous lesions.

28. Chorzelski TP, Jablonska S, Beutner EH, et al.: Juvenile dermatitis herpetiformis versus "benign chronic bullous dermatosis of childhood": Are these immunologic diseases of childhood? J. Invest. Dermatol. 65:447–450, 1975.

Studies demonstrate that on the strength of clinical, histologic, immune criteria, as well as response to sulfapyridine and sulfones, bullous disorders of childhood can be classified as dermatitis herpetiformis or bullous pemphigoid.

29. Ackerman AB, Tolman MM: Papular dermatitis herpetiformis in childhood. Arch. Dermatol. 100:286–290, 1969.

Clinical, histologic, and therapeutic evaluation of a 6-year-old girl with a vesiculobullous disorder lends support to the hypothesis that dermatitis herpetiformis is fundamentally the same disease in children as it is in adults.

30. Hertz DC, Katz SI, Aaronson C: Juvenile dermatitis herpetiformis: an immunologically proven case. Pediatrics 59:945–948, 1977.

A 2 1/2-year-old boy, both clinically and histologically, fits the classification of juvenile bullous pemphigoid; therapeutic response to dapsone and the presence of IgA at the basement membrane or normal and perilesional skin, however, are characteristic of the adult-type small blister variety of dermatitis herpetiformis.

31. Seah PP, Fry L: Immunoglobulins in the skin in dermatitis herpetiformis and their relevance in diagnosis. Br. J. Dermatol. 92:157–166, 1975.

Immunofluorescent studies of 50 patients confirm that detection of IgA in uninvolved skin of patients with dermatitis herpetiformis appears to be the most reliable means of diagnosis.

32. Jablonska S, Chorzelski TP, Beutner EH, et al.: Dermatitis herpetiformis and bullous pemphigoid: intermediate and mixed forms. Arch. Dermatol. 112:45–48, 1976.

Immunofluorescent studies of nine cases of dermatitis herpetiformis with features of bullous pemphigoid reveal the presence of mixed and intermediate forms of these disorders.

33. Marks J, Shuster S, Watson AJ: Small bowel changes in dermatitis herpetiformis. Lancet 2:1280–1282, 1966.

Patients with dermatitis herpetiformis are frequently noted to have villous flattening in the small intestine similar to the histologic findings seen in patients with gluten-sensitivity enteropathy.

34. Marks J, Shuster S: Dermatitis herpetiformis: the role of gluten. Arch. Dermatol. 101:452–457, 1970.

Although some patients with dermatitis herpetiformis have an enteropathy that responds to a gluten-free diet, in this study the cutaneous eruption does not appear to be altered.

35. Katz SI, Hertz KC, Rogentine GN, et al.: The association between HLA-B8 and dermatitis herpetiformis in patients with IgA deposits in skin. Arch. Dermatol. 113:155–156, 1977.

A discussion of the relationship of leukocyte HL-A-B8 antigen, dermatitis herpetiformis, and gluten-sensitive enteropathy.

36. Seah PP, Fry L, Kearney JW, et al.: Comparison of histocompatibility antigens in dermatitis herpetiformis and adult celiac disease. Br. J. Dermatol. 94:131–138, 1976.

Significantly elevated incidences of HL-A8 and HL-A1 suggest a common etiology in the pathogenesis of dermatitis herpetiformis and adult celiac disease.

37. Kahn G: Vesiculobullous disorders. In Gellis SS, Kagan BJ (Eds.): Current Pediatric Therapy 8. W. B. Saunders Co, Philadelphia, 1978, 481–484.

A discussion of the therapeutic management of childhood blistering disorders.

38. Shuster S, Watson AJ, Marks J: Coeliac syndrome in dermatitis herpetiformis. Lancet 1:1101–1106, 1968.

Small-bowel abnormalities, varying from mild to severe, are described in 61 per cent of patients with dermatitis herpetiformis.

39. Bean SF, Good RA, Windhorst DB: Bullous pemphigoid in an 11-year-old boy. Arch. Dermatol. 102:205–208, 1970.

Clinical course and immunologic changes in a child with bullous pemphigoid suggest an immune reaction followed by antibody reactivity at the dermal-epidermal junction as a factor in the etiology of this disorder.

40. Gould WM, Zlotnick DA: Bullous pemphigoid in infancy: a case report. Pediatrics 59:942–945, 1977.

Improvement on systemic prednisone in a 3 1/2-month-old infant with bullous pemphigoid.

41. Robison JW, Odom RB: Bullous pemphigoid in children. Arch. Dermatol. 114:899–902, 1978.

Report of a 3-year-old boy with bullous pemphigoid and a review of the literature.

42. Ramsdell W, Jarratt M, Fuerst J, et al.: Bullous disease of childhood. Am. J. Dis. Child. In press.

A report of four children (12 months to 11 years of age) with a review of the literature suggests bullous disease of childhood to be a specific disorder distinct from bullous pemphigoid and juvenile dermatitis herpetiformis.

43. Jacqueline L, Schmitt D, Thirrolet J, et al.: Benign chronic bullous dermatosis of childhood: an immunologic and ultrastructural study. Ann. Dermatol. Venereol. 104:795–804, 1977.

Findings in a 3-year-old boy appear to differentiate benign chronic dermatosis of childhood from dermatitis herpetiformis and bullous pemphoid.

44. Prystkowsky S, Gilliam JN: Benign chronic bullous dermatosis of childhood. Linear IgA and C_3 deposition on the basement membrane. Arch. Dermatol. 112:837–838, 1976.

A 2 1/2-year-old boy with deposition of IgA and C_3 on the basement membrane classified as having chronic bullous disease of childhood.

45. Dabrowski J, Chorzelski TP, Jablońska S, et al.: The ultrastructural localization of IgA deposits in chronic bullous disease of childhood (CBDC). J. Invest. Dermatol. 79:291–295, 1979.

Immunoelectronmicroscopic studies lend support to the view that bullous disease of childhood is the counterpart of dermatitis herpetiformis in adults. (They both have the same linear localization of IgA deposits.)

46. Lever WF: Pephigus and pemphigoid. A review of the advances made since 1964. J. Am. Acad. Dermatol. 1:2–27, 1979.

A comprehensive review of pemphigus and pemphigoid with emphasis on clinical patterns, diagnosis, and therapy.

47. Lehman R, Landau JW, Newcomer VC: Pemphigus vulgaris in a 12-year-old boy. J. Pediatr. 67:264–269, 1965.

Report of a case of pemphigus vulgaris in a 12-year-old boy stresses prompt recognition and institution of corticosteroid therapy in the treatment of this disorder.

48. Jordan RE, Ihrig JJ, Perry HO: Childhood pemphigus vulgaris, report of a case. Arch. Dermatol. 99:176–179, 1969.

A case of pemphigus vulgaris, proven by histopathologic and immunofluorescent studies, in a 13-year-old boy and summary of four other cases report in the literature.

49. Murphy PJ, Harrel ER: Pemphigus vulgaris in childhood. Am. J. Dis. Child. 123:70–71, 1972.

A nine-year-old girl with pemphigus vulgaris started with blisters in her mouth. As in many other cases, the correct diagnosis was delayed owing to the low index of suspicion for this disease in a young patient.

50. Elias PM, Jarratt M, Zalitis IE, et al.: Childhood pemphigus vulgaris. N. Engl. J. Med. 287:758–760, 1972.

This report of a 13-year-old Negro girl with pemphigus

vulgaris emphasizes the importance of early mucous membrane biopsy and the efficacy of alternate-day steroids.

51. Berger BW, Maier HS, Kantor IW, et al.: Pemphigus vulgaris in a 3 1/2-year-old boy. Arch. Dermatol. 107:433–434, 1973.

Diagnosis of pemphigus vulgaris in a 3 1/2-year-old boy was confirmed both by histologic picture and immunofluorescent pattern.

52. Paltzik RL, Laude TA: Childhood pemphigus treated with gold. Arch. Dermatol. 114:768–769, 1978.

A 4-year-old girl with pemphigus responded favorably to chrysotherapy. The exact mechanism of action of gold in the treatment of this disorder is unknown.

53. Lever WF: Pemphigus and its variants. In Madden S (Ed.): Current Dermatologic Management. The C. V. Mosby Co, St. Louis, 1970, 178–181.

A review of pemphigus and its therapy.

54. Schroeter A, Sams M Jr, Jordan RE: Immunofluorescent studies of pemphigus foliaceus in a child. Arch. Dermatol. 100:736–740, 1969.

Experience in management of a 3-year-old boy with pemphigus foliaceus suggests that immunofluorescent studies, in addition to aiding in diagnosis, helps predict relapses before the appearance of clinical lesions.

55. Kahn G, Lewis HM: True childhood pemphigus. Pemphigus foliaceus in an 18-month-old child: immunofluorescence as a diagnostic aid. Am. J. Dis. Child. 121:253–256, 1971.

Report of an 18-month-old with pemphigus foliaceus treated with topical high-potency steroids.

56. Usher B: Pemphigus erythematosus — forty years later. Cutis 3:230, 1967.

Forty years after its original description, the disease called pemphigus erythematosus (Senear-Usher Syndrome) appears to be a localized form of pemphigus foliaceus.

57. Brown MF: Fogo selvagem (pemphigus foliaceus). Arch. Derm. Syph. 69:589–599, 1954.

In Brazil, the terms fogo selvagem and pemphigus foliaceus are considered to be synonymous.

58. Sneddon IB: Pemphigus. In Rook A, Wilkinson DS, Ebling FJG (Eds.): Textbook of Dermatology, Vol. 2. Blackwell Scientific Publications, Oxford, 1972, 1306–1315.

A comprehensive review of pemphigus and its variants.

59. Sneddon IB, Wilkinson DS: Subcorneal pustular dermatosis. Br. J. Dermatol. 63:385–394, 1956.

Six patients with subcorneal pustular dermatosis are reported with a description of the clinical features and a review of the literature.

60. Johnson SAM, Cripps DC: Subcorneal pustular dermatosis in children. Arch. Dermatol. 109:73–77, 1974.

Of two 3-year-old children with subcorneal pustular dermatosis, one appeared to have the onset of disease at seven weeks of age.

61. Hailey H, Hailey H: Familial benign chronic pemphigus. Arch. Derm. Syph. 39:679–685, 1939.

The first description of a previously unrecognized disorder characterized by chronic and recurring eruptions in the neck and axillae.

62. Schneider W, Fischer H, Wiehl R.: Zur Frage der Schleimhautbeteiligung beim pemphigus benignus familiaris chronicus. Arch. Klin. Exp. Derm. 225:74–81, 1966.

Oral lesions in a mother and daughter with familial benign pemphigus.

63. Palmer DD, Perry HO: Benign familial chronic pemphigus. Arch. Derm. 86:493–502, 1962.

A review of 23 patients with benign familial chronic pemphigus.

64. Gottlieb SK, Lutzner MA: Hailey-Hailey Disease. An electron microscopic study. J. Invest. Dermatol. 54:368–376, 1970.

Electron microscopic examination of 18 lesions from four patients reveal a genetic defect in adhesion of epidermal cells one to another.

65. Montes LF, Narkates AJ, Hunt D, et al.: Microbial flora in familial benign chronic pemphigus. Arch. Dermatol. 101:140–144, 1970.

Studies confirm the fact that bacterial infection due to Staphylococcus aureus can act as a precipitating factor in the etiology of familial benign chronic pemphigus.

66. Cram DL, Muller SA, Winkelmann RK: Ultraviolet-induced acantholysis in familial benign chronic pemphigus. Detection of the forme fruste. Arch. Dermatol. 96:636–641, 1967.

Ultraviolet light induces histologic acantholysis in patients with familial benign pemphigus.

67. Shelley WB, Pillsbury DM: Specific systemic antibiotic therapy in familial benign chronic pemphigus. Arch. Dermatol. 80:554–556, 1959.

Bacterial cultures and sensitivities are essential to appropriate antibiotic therapy in this disorder.

68. Thorne FL, Hall JH, Mladick RA: Surgical treatment of familial chronic pemphigus (Hailey-Hailey disease). Arch. Dermatol. 98:522–524, 1968.

Excision and grafting proved to be helpful in the management of a 29 year-old-male with severe persistent familial benign pemphigus.

69. Hertz KC, Katz SI, Maize J, et al.: Herpes gestationis: clinicopathologic study. Arch. Dermatol. 112:1543–1548, 1976.

Herpes gestationis in three patients verified by immunofluorescence of IgG and C_3 deposits along the basement membrane zone.

70. Lawley TJ, Stingl G, Katz SI: Fetal and maternal risk factors in herpes gestationis. Arch. Dermatol. 114:552–555, 1978.

Review of 41 cases of immunologically proven herpes gestationis suggest a definite increased risk of fetal morbidity and mortality.

71. Keaty C, Jones PE, Lamb JH: Progesterone therapy in dermatoses of pregnancy (herpes gestationis). Arch. Derm. Syph. 63:675–686, 1951.

A review of 10 patients with herpes gestationis suggests a tendency to recurrence with increased severity in successive pregnancies and possible grave prognosis to the fetus.

16

DISORDERS OF PIGMENTATION

Although chiefly of cosmetic significance, disorders of pigmentation are among the most conspicuous and, at times, among the most cosmetically and psychologically annoying and persistent of cutaneous disorders.

Melanin is the black or brown pigment that is responsible for the color in hair and for the natural and, at times, abnormal pigmentation of the skin. Its presence in the epidermis helps protect against ultraviolet radiation and associated cutaneous damage, of which the most serious is skin cancer. The synthesis of melanin occurs in melanocytes, specialized dendritic secretory cells derived from the neural crest, which migrate to the basal layer of the epidermis during embryogenesis.

The amino acid tyrosine is the substrate inside the melanocytes from which melanin is formed. In the presence of tyrosinase and a small amount of oxygen, tyrosine is converted into another amino acid, dihydroxyphenylalanine (dopa). This is then oxidized to dopaquinone and, through a complex series of steps, is eventually converted to melanin. Although the mechanism by which melanin is transferred from epidermal melanocytes to keratinocytes is uncertain, it appears to be brought about through active phagocytosis of the distal processes of melanocytes by keratinocytes. The cell walls of the phagocytized dendritic processes then disappear, and the melanin particles are dispersed throughout the cytoplasm of keratinocytes.

Normal skin color is dependent upon the

342

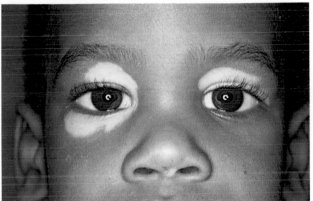

Figure 16–1 Vitiligo. Completely depigmented oval ivory-white areas with convex hyperpigmented borders.

deposition of melanin in epidermal cells, the thickness of the stratum corneum, the presence of carotene in the epidermis, and variations in blood flow. Pigmentation of the skin involves the formation and packaging of melanin within the melanosomes of the epidermal cells. The intensity of skin coloration is determined by the size and total number of melanosomes present within the keratinocytes and melanocytes of the epidermis, by the rate of melanogenesis within the melanocytes, and by the rate of transport within the keratinocytes.

There are two major classes of hormones that affect pigmentation: (1) sex steroids, especially estrogen and progestational agents, and (2) peptide hormones, including alpha- and beta-melanocyte stimulating hormone (MSH) and adrenocorticotropic hormone (ACTH). Genetic factors play a primary role in the degree of normal pigmentation for each individual and the capacity of his melanocytes to respond to local stimuli that influence melanogenesis.

In all races the dorsal and extensor surfaces are relatively hyperpigmented, and the ventral surfaces are less pigmented. This is most evident in dark races (Blacks and Mongoloids). The separation of the dorsal and ventral pigmentation is most conspicuous on the extremities and more or less follows Voight's lines. Termed Futcher's or Ito's line, this differentiation of dorsal and ventral pigmentation is present from infancy and occurs ten times more frequently in males than in females.[1, 2]

DISORDERS OF HYPOPIGMENTATION

Disorders of hypopigmentation may be grouped into two major classifications as follows: (1) genetic or developmentally controlled disorders in which normal amounts of melanin were never present in affected areas and (2) disorders associated with depigmentation or loss of previously existing melanin. Congenital diseases of hypopigmentation include tuberous sclerosis, nevus achromicus, hypomelanosis of Ito, and partial or total albinism. Acquired disorders of hypo-

pigmentation include vitiligo, postinflammatory hypopigmentation, pityriasis alba, and tinea versicolor. Hypopigmentary disorders may be further divided into patterned or unpatterned groups. Patterned forms of leukoderma include pityriasis alba, tinea versicolor, postinflammatory hypopigmentation, leprosy, pinta, tuberous sclerosis, hypomelanosis of Ito, vitiligo, partial albinism, and the Waardenburg and Vogt-Koyanagi syndromes. Unpatterned disorders include albinism and the leukoderma seen in association with nevus achromicus, phenylketonuria, kwashiorkor, hypopituitarism, the Chediak-Higashi and Alezzandrini syndromes, incontinentia pigmenti, chemically induced hypopigmentation, and sarcoidosis.

Vitiligo

Vitiligo is a common genetically determined patterned loss of pigmentation that follows the destruction of melanocytes and is characterized by oval or irregular ivory-white patches of skin surrounded by a well-demarcated or hyperpigmented, often convex, border (Figs. 16–1 and 16–2). Seen in at least 1 to 2 per cent of the population, or approximately two million people in the United States and forty million in the entire world, the disorder appears to be inherited as an autosomal dominant trait of variable penetrance. One-fourth of affected individuals have a history of leukoder-

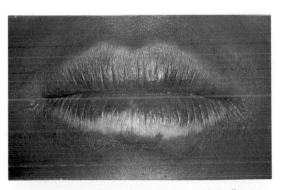

Figure 16–2 Vitiligo. Depigmentation of the lips.

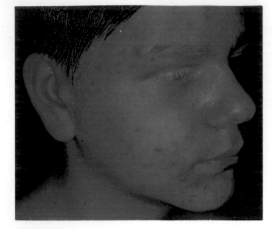

Figure 16–3   Segmental vitiligo of the eyebrow and eyelashes.

ma, and at least one-half of affected persons have a positive family history of vitiligo, halo nevi, traumatic depigmentation of the skin, or markedly premature graying of the hair.[3, 4, 5]

Although the etiology of vitiligo is unknown, three different hypotheses have been advanced to explain the cause of this disorder. In one theory, melanocytes are destroyed by an autocytotoxic process. In another, the immune system is the destructive source, and in the third, neurochemical factors, such as an increase in acetylcholine in the vicinity of pigment cells, are implicated.

The immune hypothesis implicates an autoimmune process in the cause of vitiligo and is based on many clinical associations of vitiligo. The incidence of vitiligo in patients with some form of autoimmune disease may be as high as 10 to 14 per cent, compared to 1 per cent in the general population. Patients with various abnormalities of the immune system such as lymphomas, thymomas, myasthenia gravis, and mucocutaneous candidiasis tend to develop vitiligo.[5]

Most patients with vitiligo are in good general health. The incidence of this disorder, however, is higher (8 to 20 per cent) in individuals with disorders such as hyperthyroidism, thyroiditis, adrenocortical insufficiency, pernicious anemia, and certain types of uveitis, including Vogt-Koyanagi and Harada's syndromes; and the incidence of vitiligo in patients with sympathetic

ophthalmia and adult-onset and juvenile-type diabetes appears to be higher than that in the general population. Vitiligo and alopecia areata also appear to be linked. Patients with scleroderma or morphea have an increased incidence of vitiligo; approximately 50 per cent of patients with vitiligo have halo nevi; and, perhaps most significant of all, there appears to be a link between vitiligo and melanoma (20 per cent of patients with melanoma have vitiligo).[4, 6] Since vitiligo often appears in patients with melanoma who have been ill and have an advanced stage of their disorder, the onset of vitiligo in such patients may suggest a poor prognostic sign. Actually, most patients with melanoma who develop vitiligo have had their melanoma for a long period of time. The onset of vitiligo in such patients, therefore, may actually imply an immunologic response, with an attempt at the destruction of all melanocytes within the individual system.

Vitiligo may begin at any age. Its onset is most common in young adults, and in about half of the patients it begins prior to the age of twenty years. Although relatively uncommon during infancy, patients with congenital vitiligo have been observed.[6] In 75 per cent of affected individuals the first lesions occur as depigmented spots on exposed areas such as the dorsal surfaces of the hands, the face, and neck. Other sites of predilection include the body folds (the axillae and groin), body orifices (the eyes, nostrils, mouth, navel, areolae, genitalia, and perianal regions), and areas over bony prominences such as the elbows, knees, knuckles, and shins.

The location, size, and shape of individual lesions vary considerably, yet the overall picture is characteristic. Lesions appear as partially or completely depigmented ivory-white macules or patches, usually with well-defined, frequently hyperpigmented, convex borders. They frequently have an oval or linear contour and vary in size from several millimeters or less to large, occasionally segmental areas or almost total depigmentation of the body. The latter form is termed universal or total vitiligo.[4] Although usually considered to be a bilateral disorder, vitiligo is often asymmetrical and frequently may be confined to an area supplied by a nerve segment (this variant is termed segmental vitiligo) (Figs. 16–3, 16–4, 16–5).

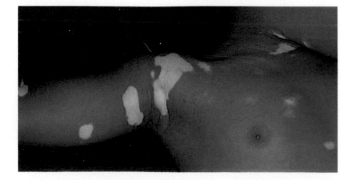

Figure 16–4   Segmental vitiligo on the arm, neck, and chest. Note areas of spontaneous follicular repigmentation.

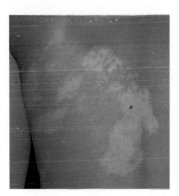

Figure 16-5 Segmental vitiligo on the left upper back with partial spontaneous repigmentation.

Many patients date the onset of their disorder to an exposure to the sun, and 15 per cent of patients relate sunburn as a factor in the initiation or as a cause of the disorder. Other individuals associate the onset of vitiligo with periods of severe physical or emotional trauma. In instances in which the onset of vitiligo appears to follow a sunburn or intense tan, the possibility exists that vitiligo may have been present and became apparent only after the patient developed a tan in the surrounding area, thus accentuating the contrast with the depigmented area. It appears, however, that sunburn with vesiculation frequently will precipitate vitiligo. Therefore, although ultraviolet exposure is used in the treatment of this disorder, patients must be forewarned to initiate sunlight or ultraviolet exposure judiciously in an effort to avoid excessive sunburn reactions, particularly in depigmented areas where protective melanin pigment is absent.

Ordinarily the diagnosis of vitiligo is not difficult, especially when there is symmetrical hypopigmentation about the eyes, nostrils, mouth, nipples, umbilicus, or genitals.[4] In fair-skinned individuals it may be difficult to differentiate areas of vitiligo from the adjacent normal skin. In such cases examination under Wood's light in a dark room may help to delineate a contrast between normal and hypopigmented skin. When the diagnosis is in doubt, the distribution of lesions, the age of onset, the presence of a convex hyperpigmented border, and the characteristic sites of predilection may help establish the correct diagnosis.

Lesions of postinflammatory hypopigmentation reveal irregular mottling of hyperpigmentation and hypopigmentation (Fig. 16-6). Pityriasis alba may be differentiated by its distribution on the face, upper arms, neck, and shoulders; its characteristic light-pink color; and its fine adherent scale (Figs. 16-7 and 16-8). Lesions of tinea versicolor may be differentiated by their fine scales, and typical distribution on the trunk, neck, and upper arms (Figure 13-18), and by the demonstration of hyphae on microscopic examination of epidermal scrapings.

Albinism, either generalized or partial, may be difficult to distinguish from total vitiligo. The diagnosis of albinism, however, may be established by its presence at birth and by the facts that normal eye color is retained in vitiligo (whereas the pigment may be diluted in albinism) and that hair on glabrous skin in the vitiliginous patient tends to retain pigment (Figs. 16-9 and 16-10). In partial albinism the diagnosis can be more difficult (Figs. 16-11 and 16-12). The presence of a white forelock and the pattern of hypopigmentation suggests a diagnosis of partial albinism.[4]

The hypopigmented macules of tuberous sclerosis lack the characteristic milk-white appearance of lesions of vitiligo, are present at birth or during the early neonatal period, do not change with age, and have a normal number of melanocytes (with reduction in size of melanosomes and melanin granules within them) in contrast to the absence or decrease in number of melanocytes in patients with vitiligo.[7]

Biopsies taken from the depigmented skin of vitiligo reveal a partial to total loss of epidermal pigment cells, and at the borders of lesions the melanocytes are often large and have long dendritic processes.[5] On electron microscopic examination the number of Langerhans' cells seems to be increased, and many are found in the basal portion

Figure 16-6 Postinflammatory hypopigmentation following resolution of guttate psoriasis.

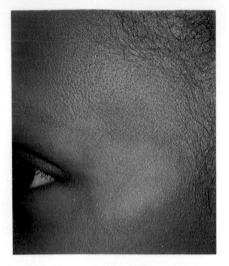

Figure 16–7 Pityriasis alba. Ill-defined hypopigmented oval patches. Generally seen on the face, upper arms, neck, and shoulders of affected individuals. This disorder can be differentiated from vitiligo by its fine adherent scale, partial hypopigmentation, and distribution.

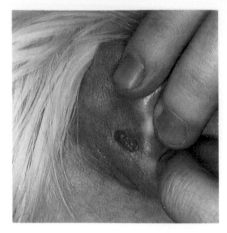

Figure 16–9 Albinism. Light skin, yellowish-white hair, and a lack of pigmentation in nevi (Department of Dermatology, Yale University School of Medicine).

of the epidermis rather than in the mid-epidermis.

The course of vitiligo is variable. Long periods of quiescence may be interrupted by periods of extension or partial improvement. Extension of vitiliginois areas, however, frequently tends to occur when the patient experiences severe stress of either emotional or physical nature. Complete spontaneous repigmentation is unusual. Some temporary and partial repigmentation, however, may be detectable in vitiliginous lesions less than two years old (particularly in children) during the summer months. In such cases small freckle-like spots of repigmentation may appear in the white patches during periods of prolonged sun exposure, but occasionally may fade again during the winter months. Complete repigmentation of all involved areas, however, is the exception rather than the rule, and recurrences are common.

Although there is no completely satisfactory treatment of vitiligo, repigmentation can occasionally be accomplished by the administration of psoralen compounds followed by gradually increasing exposure to sunlight or long-wave ultraviolet light (UVA)[8-10] (Fig. 16–13). Since treatment of vitiligo is long and difficult, only those patients who are highly motivated and completely informed about their chances for improvement should begin such therapy.[10] This therapy is most effective in young patients, particularly those who have a relatively short history of the disorder. Trimethylpsoralen tablets, 5 mg (Trisoralen, Elder), or 8-methoxypsoralen capsules, 10 mg (Oxsoralen, Elder), may be administered two hours prior to sunlight or long-wave ultraviolet exposure. Normal sunlight (particularly between the hours of 11:00 A.M. and 4:00 P.M.) is by far the best source of ultraviolet light for this form of therapy. If sunlight is impractical or unavailable, black-light bulbs or fluorescent tubes, though less efficient, are rich in wavelengths from 320 to 400 nm (the action spectrum of the psoralens) and may be utilized.[11] Ordinary commercial sun lamps are deficient in this wavelength and accordingly frequently ineffective for this purpose. The usual recommended dose of trimethylpsoralen is one to four tablets (5 to 20 mg) and that for 8-methoxypsoralen is one or two capsules (10 to 20 mg) two hours before ultraviolet exposure. With such therapy reasonably good repigmentation may occur in up to one-third of cases, some repigmentation may occur in one-third of cases, and poor results occur in the other third. Patients should be forewarned that sunburn may develop, particularly in areas of depigmentation, during the early phases of therapy. The duration of exposure, accordingly, should be initiated gradually and increased as tolerated. Although repigmentation may begin after a few weeks, significant results frequently take as long as six months or more, and treatment during the summer months may have to be continued for periods of two years or more.

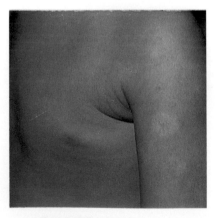

Figure 16–8 Pityriasis alba.

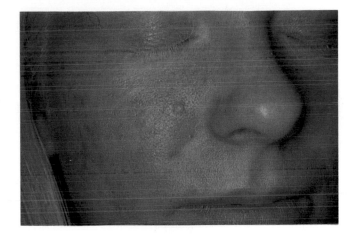

Figure 16–10 Albinism. (Department of Dermatology, Yale University School of Medicine.)

It should be noted that when trimethylpsoralen was first introduced during the 1950's, some laboratory animals showed abnormalities of liver function tests. The manufacturers of this preparation accordingly include a warning of possible hepatic damage and recommend that these preparations be avoided in the treatment of children under age 12. Extensive use of psoralens in children as well as adults, however, has failed to reveal evidence of liver toxicity, and there have been no reported adverse effects, even in young children.[9]

If vitiligo is localized to a small area, topical application of methoxsalen lotion (Oxsoralen lotion, 1 per cent) followed by short exposure to ultraviolet light (after waiting 45 minutes to one hour) or black light (UVA) may be considered.[11] Since sunburn may follow such therapy, this approach should be initiated with extreme caution, and it is advisable that patients be treated only under the careful supervision of the physician. It should be emphasized that after treatment the area should be washed with soap and water and that the topical therapy be closely supervised by the physician.

When treatment of vitiligo is unsatisfactory, lesions can be hidden by the use of cosmetic makeups or aniline dye stains such as Neo-Dyoderm or Vita-Dye. In those few cases in which vitiligo has progressed to such an extent that more than 50 per cent of the body is involved (particularly in those individuals in whom only a few islands of normal skin remain), an attempt at depigmentation with 20 per cent monobenzyl ether or hydroquinone (Benoquin ointment, Elder) may be utilized.[4] Such patients should be reminded to use appropriate sunscreens and to avoid excessive sun exposure, since, once treated, they lack their usual melanin protection and are more susceptible to sunburn.

Albinism

Albinism is an uncommon inherited disorder manifested by congenital hypopigmentation of the skin, hair, and eyes, and occurs in two forms: oculocutaneous and ocular. The oculocutaneous form affects both sexes equally, occurs in all races, and is inherited as an autosomal recessive disorder. The ocular form is a rare X-linked recessive condition in which the affected male has a deficiency of retinal pigment but lacks the cutaneous

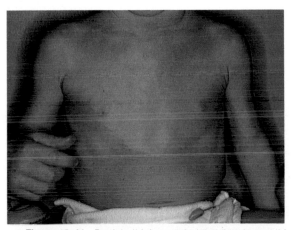

Figure 16–11 Partial albinism and piebaldism in a child with tuberous sclerosis.

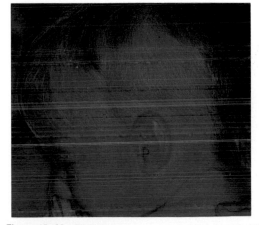

Figure 16–12 Partial albinism and piebaldism (same child as in Figure 16–11).

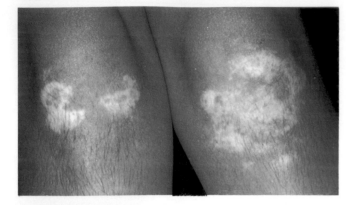

Figure 16–13 Partial repigmentation (at the periphery and center of lesions) of vitiligo one month following initiation of treatment with trioxsalen (Trisoralen) and summer sunlight.

findings seen in the oculocutaneous form of this disorder.

Human oculocutaneous albinism (OCA) represents a heterogeneous group of at least four distinct disorders.[12] Seen in one in 5000 to one in 25,000 individuals (once in every 20,000 births in the United States), the highest incidence (1 to 7:100) occurs in the Cuna tribe of Indians on the San Blas Islands off the coast of Panama.[13] The disorder is characterized by varying degrees of unpatterned reduction of pigment in the skin and hair, translucent irides, hypopigmented ocular fundi, and an associated nystagmus. Melanocytes and melanosomes are present in the affected skin and hair in normal numbers, but although they are tyrosine positive, they fail to produce normal amounts of melanin in the areas of leukoderma or poliosis.

The two most common forms of oculocutaneous albinism have been separated into two forms. The two forms, termed tyrosinase-negative and tyrosinase-positive, have been separated on the basis of pigment production in plucked hair incubated in tyrosine. Two less common forms of oculocutaneous albinism are the Hermansky-Pudlak syndrome (oculocutaneous albinism with a hemorrhagic diathesis associated with von Willebrand's pseudohemophilia)[14] and a yellow mutant form of oculocutaneous albinism.[12]

In Caucasians with oculocutaneous albinism the skin may be milk-white, the hair is white to yellow or light-brown in color, the pupils are pink, the irides are gray or blue, and photophobia and photosensitivity are common (Fig. 16–9 and 16–10). In Blacks the skin color may be tan or may resemble that of Caucasians; freckles can appear on exposure to light; the hair is blond to red; and the eyes are blue or hazel. Patients have a typical appearance, not only because of the decrease in skin color, but also because of a typical facial expression that results from photophobia, central scotomata, and the associated tendency to habitual squinting and nystagmus. Although the degree of pigment dilution in affected individuals is variable, the diagnosis is easily established in those who have striking pigment loss or relative pigment dilution when compared to unaffected siblings or parents.

The incidence of oculocutaneous albinism is much higher among the Cuna Indians of the San Blas Islands off the east coast of Panama than it is among the general population. This form of oculocutaneous albinism appears to be transmitted by a non-sex–linked autosomal recessive gene, and although the true incidence in this group is not established, it has been estimated to approach 1:100 to 7:100. Affected children have been called "moon children" because they have marked photosensitivity and photophobia and prefer to go outdoors only at night.

The skin of Cuna "moon children" becomes freckled, wrinkled, and easily blistered by the tropical sunshine. Malignant skin tumors are common, and life expectancy is short. Actinic keratoses, atrophy, telangiectasia, and actinic cheilitis appear early, and actinic keratoses occur in most Cuna Indian children, unless carefully protected from the sun, by seven years of age. Malignant changes generally occur by age 30 and often prove fatal, and few Cuna albinos live beyond 40 years of age.[13]

Other abnormalities reported in association with albinism include congenital deafness, small stature, retardation, spasticity, and coagulation disorders. The Tietz syndrome is a rare autosomal dominant disorder characterized by albinism, complete deaf-mutism, hypoplasia or absence of the eyebrows, and normal eye color. Since the irides of the eyes have normal pigmentation, photophobia and nystagmus are not seen as features of this disorder.[15] An oculocerebral syndrome with hypopigmentation (the Cross-McKusick-Breen syndrome), characterized by oculocutaneous albinism, microphthalmus, spasticity, and mental retardation, also has been reported,[16] and von Willebrand's pseudohemophilia has been described in association with oculocutaneous albinism. In the latter disorder affected individuals show a variable bleeding tendency with a prolonged bleeding time but normal platelet count. When ceroid-containing macrophages are present in the bone marrow, this constellation of findings has been termed the Hermansky-Pudlak syndrome.[14, 17]

Ocular Albinism. Ocular albinism, first recognized by Nettleship in 1909, is a rare sex-linked recessive disorder, probably with linkage of the loci for ocular albinism and Xg.[18] It presents the same ocular features of oculocutaneous albinism but lacks the cutaneous findings. Affected males have translucency of the iris, photophobia, nystagmus, and head-nodding similar to that seen in patients with oculocutaneous albinism. Affected females and female carriers have a milder clinical picture, with decreased pigmentation of the iris and posterior fundus and typical retinal changes (stippling, alternating dark and light patches, giving a salt and pepper, grouped, mottled, or striped appearance to the retina, and easily visible choroid vasculature).[19] Except for the frequent presence of myopia, visual acuity in affected individuals is generally normal.

TREATMENT. Except for contact lenses and tinted glasses to ameliorate photophobia there is no effective treatment for patients with ocular forms of albinism. Since early actinic changes, keratoses, basal cell tumors, and squamous cell carcinomas are common, even in children and adolescents, those with cutaneous albinism must learn to avoid sunlight exposure and to use protective clothing and sunscreen preparations on exposed surfaces.

Partial Albinism (Piebaldism)

Partial albinism, also termed piebaldism, is an uncommon but widely distributed dominantly inherited disorder. Commonly associated with a white lock of hair above the forehead (the white forelock) in 85 to 90 per cent of affected individuals, this disorder is characterized by congenital patterned areas of depigmentation and varying shades of normal skin color that are usually present at birth. Partial albinism occasionally may occur without a white forelock; a white forelock without some degree of leukoderma of the underlying scalp or other parts of the body, however, has not been reported in this disorder (Figs. 16–11 and 16–12).

The clinical manifestation of partial albinism may be explained either by incomplete migration of melanoblasts from the neural crest to the ventral midline or by a defect in the differentiation of ventral melanoblasts to melanocytes.[20] The most striking features of partial albinism include distinctive patterns of hypopigmentation or depigmentation, which generally persist unchanged throughout life. These include a hypopigmented triangular patch on the scalp and forehead (widest at the forehead, with the apex pointing backward) and hypopigmented or depigmented areas on the chin, anterior neck, anterior portion of the thorax and abdomen, and, at times, on both the anterior and posterior aspects of the midarm to the wrist and the midthigh to midcalf. At times there may be islands of normal pigment within the hypomelanotic areas, and the borders and small islands of pigmentation within the unpigmented areas may be hyperpigmented.

In many individuals the areas of unpigmented

skin on the forehead include the whole or inner portions of the eyebrows and eyelashes and extend to the root of the nose. The leukoderma may begin again on the chin or front of the chest and abdomen, and it often spreads to the flanks and back in the form of scattered white patches.[20] The occiput, back of the neck, dorsal aspect of the trunk, and the hands and feet are less commonly involved, and there is little tendency to symmetry of the hypopigmented areas.

The patterns of hypopigmentation of partial albinism can be differentiated from those of vitiligo by their usual presence at birth, lack of convex borders, and predilection for ventral surfaces as opposed to exposed areas, body orifices, areas of trauma, and intertriginous regions. The clinical features that distinguish partial albinism from oculocutaneous albinism are its dominant mode of inheritance, lack of ocular manifestations, and characteristic distribution of lesions, with a predilection for the ventral areas.

Electron microscopic examination of lesions of partial albinism reveals an absence of melanocytes, with markedly deformed melanosomes, Langerhans' cells in the amelanotic areas, and an increase of melanin granules in the hyperpigmented borders.

Treatment consists of cosmetic masking of areas of leukoderma with aniline dyes (as in the treatment of vitiligo), the protection of hypopigmented and depigmented areas from sun damage by proper clothing, and the use of appropriate sunscreen preparations on exposed surfaces.

Chediak-Higashi Syndrome

The Chediak-Higashi syndrome is a rare autosomal recessive, lethal disorder characterized by diffuse oculocutaneous hypopigmentation, photophobia, hepatosplenomegaly, abnormal granulation of leukocytes, and recurrent pyogenic infections. Patients with this condition have fair skin, pale retinae, translucent irides, light-blond, frosted, or silvery hair, recurrent respiratory and cutaneous infections, and hematologic, neurologic, and renal abnormalities.

A disorder of giant lysosomal inclusion bodies found in all circulating granulocytes, as well as in many other cells of the body, and the large size of the inclusion bodies reflect a functional abnormality that leads to improper handling or distribution of normal lysosomal enzymes.[21] Characteristic cytoplasmic inclusions resembling lysosomes within nerve cells, muscle weakness, and progressive cranial and peripheral neuropathy have been seen in individuals with this disorder, and a lymphoma-like phase with hepatosplenomegaly, lymphadenopathy, and widespread organ infiltrates has been noted.[22]

Most patients die in early childhood of overwhelming infection, hemorrhage, or a lymphoma-like process, over 50 per cent succumbing before the end of the first decade of life.[22] The management of this disorder accordingly consists of supportive measures to prevent recurrent infection. Combined prednisone and vincristine therapy has been suggested in the management of the accelerated lymphoma-like phase, and ascorbic acid (possibly combined with a cholinergic agent) appears to be beneficial. Ascorbic acid appears to help, not because of a possible nutritional deficiency but because of a lowering effect on cyclic AMP and an associated improvement in leukocyte function.[23]

The Waardenburg Syndrome

The Waardenburg (also termed Klein-Waardenburg) syndrome is a rare autosomal dominant disorder characterized by congenital deafness, lateral displacement of the medial canthi and lacrimal puncta of the lower eyelids (dystopia cantharum), broad nasal root, white forelock, and heterochromia irides.[24] Other features include excessive and occasionally confluent eyebrows, hypoplasia of the ala nasi, mild mandibular prognathism, impaired speech with or without cleft lip or cleft palate, and a variety of skeletal deformities.

Measurements of the interocular distance can help determine the presence or absence of dystopia cantharum, a highly diagnostic feature of this disorder, which is seen in 69 per cent of patients with the Waardenburg syndrome. If the inner canthal distance divided by the interpupillary distance is greater than 0.6, this lateral displacement of the inner canthi may help confirm the diagnosis.[25]

Tuberous Sclerosis

Partially depigmented white macules (the earliest cutaneous feature) are present in 78 to 90 per cent of individuals affected with tuberous sclerosis (Figs. 18–43, 18–44, 18–45). Since these hypopigmented spots are present at birth or first noted in the neonatal period, they may permit an early diagnosis of tuberous sclerosis in a child with seizures or mental retardation, long before the development of the usual recognized cutaneous and radiologic signs.[7]

In 1968, Fitzpatrick and his associates called attention to oval or lance-ovate white macules as the earliest sign of this disorder. The lance-ovate configuration was observed to resemble the shape of the leaf of the mountain ash tree, hence the term ash leaf spots.[26] Although these lesions are highly characteristic of tuberous sclerosis, it should be noted that only 18 per cent of the hypopigmented lesions of tuberous sclerosis have this configuration.[7] The hypopigmented macules of tuberous sclerosis are seen on the trunk, arms, and legs, and generally spare the face, palms, and soles. Most lesions average 1 to 3 cm in diameter; they may number one to several hundreds and are usually oval with irregular margins. Occasionally there may be numerous small freckle-sized hypopig-

mented lesions ("white freckles") on the anterior aspects of the legs.[7] Although the white spots of tuberous sclerosis have been termed "vitiliginous" by many authors, they are unrelated to vitiligo and can be differentiated from it by many characteristics (see discussion under vitiligo). Of further interest is the fact that in addition to the characteristic hypopigmented macules, there also appears to be an increased incidence of tuberous sclerosis in patients with partial albinism.[27, 28] In fair-skinned individuals the detection of characteristic hypopigmented macules is aided by a powerful Wood's light in a completely darkened room. This procedure may be of value in the differentiation of lesions of tuberous sclerosis from the less discrete hypopigmentation of postinflammatory hypomelanosis and pityriasis alba (see Chapter 18 for a more detailed discussion of tuberous sclerosis).

Incontinentia Pigmenti

Incontinentia pigmenti (Bloch-Sulzberger syndrome) is a hereditary disorder affecting the skin, central nervous system, eyes, and skeletal system. Although the genetics of this disorder have not been delineated, it appears to be an autosomal dominant or X-linked dominant disorder, prenatally lethal to males (see Chapter 18 for a more detailed discussion of incontinentia pigmenti).

In addition to the well-recognized vesiculobullous, verrucous, and highly characteristic pigmentary stages of this disorder (Figs. 18–49, 18–50, 18–51, 18—52), a fourth manifestation, consisting of depigmented lesions, has recently been reported.[29] Observed as isolated lesions or seen in conjunction with other dermatologic manifestations, they have been reported on the arms, thighs, and trunk. More characteristically, however, they appear on the calves of children as well as adults with this disorder. Although the histologic features of these hypopigmented lesions are poorly defined and their incidence and pathogenesis are unknown, the presence of streaked hypopigmented macules in family members related to children with incontinentia pigmenti may provide clues to the hereditary pattern and may play a role in the genetic counseling of families of individuals with this disorder.[29]

NEVOID TYPES OF HYPOPIGMENTATION

Incontinentia Pigmenti Achromians

Among nevoid causes of hypopigmentation, incontinentia pigmenti achromians (hypomelanosis of Ito) is a neurocutaneous syndrome characterized by distinctive macular, linear, or irregular whorls and swirls of hypopigmentation (Fig. 18–55). Unrelated to incontinentia pigmenti, the loss of pigment begins spontaneously during infancy or early childhood and is of particular significance because of the fact that approximately 50 per cent of patients have associated internal manifestations (seizure disorders, delayed development, musculoskeletal anomalies, or ocular disturbances.[30-34] Microscopic examination of affected areas reveals normal numbers of melanocytes. The melanocytes contain less melanin, are less dopa-positive, and have smaller melanosomes than the adjacent normal skin. Since the hypopigmented lesions appear early, the appearance of hypopigmentation in a whorled or swirled pattern should alert physicians to the possible association with systemic disease[32, 33, 34] (see Chapter 18).

Nevus Achromicus

Nevus achromicus is a congenital disorder characterized by single macular lesions, bands, or bizarre streaks of hypopigmentation (Fig. 16–14).[35] Affected areas may be quite small or may cover large segments of the body, and present at birth, they grow only with the growth of the individual. This disorder may be seen in association with hemihypertrophy and severe mental retardation.[36]

Probably seen more frequently than the literature indicates, the hypopigmented areas are usually confined to one side of the body and are most often located on the trunk. They are generally irregular in shape, frequently tend to occur in long bands or streaks, and show varying degrees of melanin deficiency and a reduced number of functional melanocytes.

Nevus Anemicus

Nevus anemicus is a developmental anomaly characterized by a circumscribed round or oval patch of pale or mottled skin. Appearing at birth or in early childhood, the area of involvement appears to be pale owing to a decreased sensitivity of the vessels to endogenous vasodilatory mediators such as acetylcholine, histamine, and serotonin.[37] When the diagnosis is in doubt, rubbing makes the pale area stand out in contrast to the adjacent vasodilated normal skin. Although there is no effective therapy other than cosmetic makeups,

the lesion is usually in a covered are and generally is so slight that treatment is rarely required.

OTHER TYPES OF HYPOPIGMENTATION

Vogt-Koyanagi Syndrome

The Vogt-Koyanagi syndrome (Vogt-Koyanagi-Harada syndrome) is a rare, possibly autoimmune, disorder characterized by bilateral uveitis, alopecia, vitiligo, poliosis (which may be limited to the eyebrows and eyelashes or may also involve the scalp and body hair), dysacousia (a condition in which certain sounds produce discomfort), and deafness. Usually seen in adults in the third and fourth decades of life, the disorder also occurs in children and adolescents. Although the etiology is unknown, it has been hypothesized that this syndrome is associated with an abnormal host response to an infective agent, possibly a virus, with an allergic sensitization to uveal melanocyte antigens and destruction of melanin in the hair and skin.[38] The Vogt-Koyanagi and the Vogt-Koyanagi-Harada syndromes appear to be one and the same, except that meningeal irritation or encephalitic symptoms are described in association with the latter condition. In this variant a prodromal febrile episode, with encephalitic or meningeal symptoms, lymphocytosis, and increased pressure of the cerebrospinal fluid, is followed by bilateral uveitis (often with choroiditis and optic neuritis).

In all patients there is a bilateral uveitis, which is self-limiting in its course. As the uveitis begins to subside, poliosis (in 80 to 90 per cent), temporary auditory impairment, vitiligo, usually symmetrical (in 50 to 60 per cent), and alopecia (in 50 per cent of affected individuals) develop. The hearing usually returns to normal, but the pigmentary changes, which generally appear about three weeks to three months after the onset of the uveitis, tend to be permanent. The uveitis generally takes a year or more to clear, and although most cases show some recovery of visual acuity, only partial recovery may occur at times, and some individuals may be left with a residual visual defect.

The Alezzandrini Syndrome

The Alezzandrini syndrome is a rare disorder of unknown origin primarily seen in adolescents and young adults. Possibly related to the Vogt-Koyanagi syndrome, it is characterized by unilateral degenerative retinitis with visual impairment, which is followed, at times, after an interval of months or years, by bilateral deafness and unilateral vitiligo and poliosis, which appear on the same side of the face.

Chemically Induced Hypopigmentation

A number of chemical agents are known to cause depigmentation. Among these compounds, the rubber antioxidant monobenzyl ether of hy-

Figure 16–14 Nevus achromicus, achromic nevus (a congenital area of partial hypopigmentation which remains unchanged throughout life). This disorder is probably more common than the literature indicates.

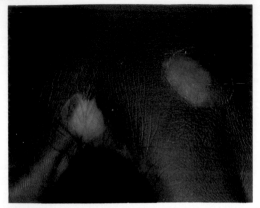

Figure 16-15 Chemical depigmentation due to a germicidal detergent. Patients with this disorder usually improve after discontinuation of the offending agent (Department of Dermatology, Yale University School of Medicine).

droquinone, phenolic germicidal agents (paratertiary butylphenol and amylphenol), hydroxyanisole, and 4-tertiary butyl catechol (an additive to polyethylene film) have been recognized as causes of leukoderma (Fig. 16–15).[39] The biochemical mechanism by which phenolic chemicals induce such hypopigmentation appears to be the competitive inhibition of tyrosinase[40] or the release of toxic metabolites that produce injury to the melanocytes.

Postinflammatory Hypopigmentation

Postinflammatory leukoderma may be associated with a wide variety of inflammatory dermatoses or infections. This relative pigmentary deficiency may be noted following involution of certain inflammatory skin disorders, particularly burns, bullous disorders, infections, eczematous or psoriatic lesions, and pityriasis rosea (Fig. 16–6). The inflammatory reactions in some secondary syphilitic lesions and pityriasis lichenoides (Mucha-Habermann) in particular have a propensity for postinflammatory hypopigmentation. In the inflammatory dermatoses the intensity of the inflammatory reaction may bear little relationship to the development of postinflammatory leukoderma, and such hypopigmentation is generally self-limiting.

Although the pathophysiology of postinflammatory hypopigmentation is unclear, it is postulated that the hypopigmentation is caused when keratinocytes injured by the inflammatory process are temporarily unable to accept melanosomes from the melanocyte dendrites. Since the defect is primarily epidermal, postinflammatory hypopigmentation generally improves with time, without need for active therapy.

Sarcoidosis

In addition to the characteristic yellowish-brown, flesh-colored, pink, red, and reddish-brown to black or blue lesions, subcutaneous nodules, and infiltrated plaques (see Chapter 18), the spectrum of sarcoidal skin lesions has been extended to include hypomelanotic macules and papules. Measuring up to 1.0 to 1.5 cm in diameter, these depigmented lesions reveal sarcoid-type granulomas on cutaneous biopsy and accordingly have been suggested as another cutaneous manifestation of this disorder.[41]

Leprosy

Leprosy (Hansen disease) is generally classified into three types: (1) lepromatous, (2) tuberculoid, and (3) intermediate. Lepromatous leprosy generally is manifested by symmetrically arranged lesions, which, at first macular in nature, develop nodules or diffuse infiltrates (especially on the eyebrows and ears), resulting in a leonine facies. Tuberculoid leprosy, conversely, shows characteristic well-defined anesthetic hypopigmented lesions and thickened and palpable peripheral nerves. Intermediate leprosy, an early stage of the latter, is manifested by one or a few macules or edematous papules that are erythematous and may show loss of pigment. (This disorder is discussed in more detail in Chapter 10.)

When the diagnosis is indeterminate, the presence of thickened tender superficial nerves, anesthetic hypopigmented macules, a granulomatous infiltrate on microscopic examination of cutaneous lesions, and demonstration of the acid-fast bacillus *Mycobacterium leprae* on cutaneous smear or biopsy generally help confirm the diagnosis.[42, 43]

Pinta

Pinta, a treponemal infection caused by *Treponema carateum,* seen almost exclusively among the colored population of Cuba, Central and South America, is frequently seen in children of parents afflicted with this disorder.

The cutaneous manifestations may be divided into primary, secondary, and tertiary stages (these are described in Chapter 10). The late dyschromic stage takes several more years to develop. These lesions have an insidious onset and usually appear during adolescence or young adulthood. They consist of slate-blue hyperpigmented lesions, which, after a period of years, become widespread and are replaced by depigmented macules resembling those seen in patients with vitiligo. Located chiefly on the face, waist, and areas close to bony prominences (elbows, knees, ankles, wrists, and the dorsal aspect of the hands), these depigmented lesions of pinta can be differentiated from those of vitiligo by the presence of the other pigmented lesions, microscopic examination of cutaneous lesions, and isolation of *Treponema careteum* by serologic testing and darkfield examination. The histopathologic features consist of atrophy of the epidermis, with absence of melanin and liquefactive degeneration of the basal layer in the hypomelanotic lesions, and plasma cell, lymphohistiocytic, and neutrophilic infiltrates in the dermis and epidermis of the hyperpigmented lesions.

DISORDERS OF HYPERPIGMENTATION

Disorders of pigmentation may be external or internal in origin. The diagnosis and therapy of some of these disorders are described below.

Postinflammatory Melanosis

Postinflammatory melanosis (postinflammatory hyperpigmentation), one of the most common causes of hyperpigmentation, is characterized by an increase in melanin formation following cutaneous inflammation. Ordinary postinflammatory hyperpigmentation is of relatively short duration and tends to persist for several weeks or months after the original cause has subsided. Examples include the pigmentation following physical trauma, friction, primary irritants, eczematoid eruptions, lichen simplex chronicus, and dermatoses such as pityriasis rosea, psoriasis, dermatitis herpetiformis, fixed drug eruptions, photodermatitis, and pyoderma (Fig. 16–16). Individuals with dark complexions and those who tan easily following ultraviolet exposure show the greatest degree of this form of melanosis. In cases in which the dermo-epidermal junction and basal layer become disrupted (lupus erythematosus, lichen planus, lichenoid drug eruptions) melanin incontinence occurs. The melanin tends to drop from its normal epidermal position and passes into the melanophages of the epidermis, and the discoloration is frequently longer lasting and more pronounced.

If areas of postinflammatory hyperpigmentation can be protected from further ultraviolet exposure, fading gradually occurs over a period of months. In blacks and other heavily melanized individuals, however, the disorder may persist for longer periods of time. In cases in which hyperpigmentation is prolonged and therapy is desired, a low-potency steroid (hydrocortisone in a 1.0 per cent concentration) may be helpful. In patients who desire more active therapy, a hydroquinone cream (available commercially as Artra in a 2 per cent concentration as an over-the-counter preparation or as Eldoquin, Elder) may hasten improvement. Eldopaque and Eldopaque Forte (Elder) contain hydroquinone in 2 per cent and 4 per cent concentrations, respectively, in an opaque base, which excludes light. These hydroquinone preparations may be rubbed into the involved areas twice daily, but because of the possibility of hydroquinone sensitivity, patients should be advised to discontinue their use at the first sign of irritation.

If these preparations do not achieve the desired result, higher concentrations of hydroquinone may be utilized. Benoquin ointment (20 per cent monobenzyl ether of hydroquinone) is frequently helpful. Since the incidence of sensitization to this preparation is high (13 per cent), a mixture of Benoquin with an equal amount of a water-washable base (such as Unibase) is advisable in the early stages of therapy. Again, the patient must be warned to discontinue the use of this preparation immediately when signs of irritation develop. It should be noted that irreversible depigmentation can occur with the use of 20 per cent monobenzyl ether of hydroquinone. This preparation, therefore, should be used with extreme caution and probably should be reserved for the depigmentation of residual areas of normal pigment in patients with extensive vitiligo (that involving 50 per cent or more of the cutaneous surface).

Two other formulations frequently found to be helpful for the treatment of postinflammatory hyperpigmentation, melasma, and, in some instances, even freckles, may be prepared as follows: (1) 2 per cent salicylic acid and 5 per cent hydroquinone in 1 per cent hydrocortisone cream,[9] or (2) tretinoin (0.1 per cent Retin-A cream), 5 per cent hydroquinone, and 0.1 per cent dexamethasone in a hydrophilic ointment.[44]

Hydroquinones act by the inhibition of tyrosinase. These preparations, therefore, act slowly and frequently require periods of three to four months before a therapeutic effect is achieved. Since the ability of the sun to darken areas of postinflammatory hyperpigmentation is greater than the lightening effect of hydroquinones, ultraviolet exposure should be avoided and appropriate sun blocking agents should be utilized.

Melanosis of the Face and Neck

Melasma. Melasma (formerly referred to as chloasma) is a term applied to a patchy dark-brown to black hyperpigmentation located primarily on

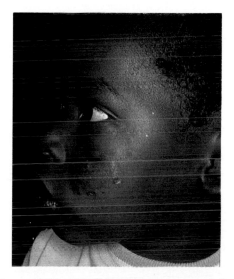

Figure 16–16 Postinflammatory hyperpigmentation following resolution of lymphocytoma cutis on the cheek of a black child.

the cheeks, the forehead, and occasionally the temples, upper lip, and neck. Seen in up to 20 per cent of women who take anovulatory drugs or who are pregnant, this disorder has been termed "the mask of pregnancy." Since sun exposure tends to trigger and intensify this hyperpigmentation, the disorder characteristically becomes more prominent in the summer months.

Typical melasma also can occur in males and in individuals who are neither pregnant nor taking oral contraceptives. Occasionally it may also appear in patients of both sexes taking diphenylhydantoin (Dilantin) or its derivatives.[45] Dermatoses considered in the differential diagnosis of melasma include berloque dermatitis, postinflammatory hyperpigmentation, Riehl's melanosis, poikiloderma of Civatte, and cases of vitiligo in which the depigmented skin may appear to be normal while the surrounding normal skin may appear to be abnormal or "hyperpigmented."

The histopathologic features of melasma include increased melanization of the epidermis without melanocytic proliferation. When induced by oral anovulatory preparations, a mild perivascular and perifollicular lymphocytic infiltrate may be present.

Once melasma has developed it generally tends to persist for long periods of time, and treatment is generally not very satisfactory. Melasma of pregnancy usually clears within a few months after delivery, only to recur with subsequent pregnancies. Oral contraceptive pill-induced melasma, however, rarely clears after cessation of oral intake of the anovulatory preparation, and pigmentation may persist for periods of up to five years after discontinuation of the medication. The treatment of melasma consists of discontinuation of potentially responsible medications, protection from sun or ultraviolet exposure by the use of appropriate clothing and sunscreen preparations, and the topical application of hydroquinones (as described for the treatment of postinflammatory hyperpigmentation).

Riehl's Melanosis. Riehl's melanosis represents a spotty hyperpigmentation of the face and occasionally of the neck and arms. Primarily seen in adult women with a history of exposure to cosmetics, it may also appear in men and children of all ages. Approximately half the reported cases result from the use of cosmetics containing coal tar derivatives. Other possible etiologic factors include avitaminosis, malnutrition, and contact with hydrocarbons (especially impure mineral oil).

The disorder is characterized by a distinctive brownish-gray spotty pigmentation on the forehead and malar areas, behind the ears, on the sides of the neck, and, at times, on other sun-exposed areas of the scalp, arms, chest, forearms, and hands. Although most cases appear to be associated with a photocontact-type reaction, pigmentation on covered parts of the body (e.g., the anterior axillary folds and umbilicus) exposed to friction has also been associated with this disorder.

Histopathologic examination of affected areas reveals liquefactive degeneration of the basal layer of the epidermis in the early stages, large amounts of melanin within melanophages located in the dermis, and a perivascular band-like dermal infiltrate. Treatment is dependent upon identification of the cause of the dermatosis, the use of suitable sunscreen preparations, and, if desired, the topical application of hydroquinone preparations.

Poikiloderma. The term poikiloderma (poikiloderma atrophicans vasculare) is used to describe a triad of telangiectasia, atrophy, and dyschromia (hyperpigmentation and hypopigmentation). The disorder may be seen in patients with poikiloderma congenitale (Rothmund Thomson syndrome), xeroderma pigmentosum, congenital telangiectatic erythema and stunted growth (Bloom syndrome), dyskeratosis congenita, connective tissue disorders, lymphomatous diseases, and myocosis fungoides. It may also be seen as cutaneous changes associated with actinic, thermal, or x-ray damage.

Poikiloderma of Civatte (thought by many to be a variant of Riehl's melanosis) appears over light-exposed areas in females of middle age or older. Characterized by uneven, frequently reticulated, reddish-brown pigmentation, superficial telangiectasia, and atrophy in irregular, more or less symmetrical patches on the cheeks, sides of the neck, and upper chest, the disorder persists indefinitely. Photosensitivity is believed to be involved in the pathogenesis of this disorder.

Histopathologic examination of areas of poikiloderma reveals varying degrees of epidermal hyperkeratosis and atrophy, hydropic degeneration of the basal layer, varying numbers of pigment-laden melanophages, and a lymphocytic band-like or perivascular infiltration in the dermis. Management consists of early recognition, avoidance of sun exposure, and the use of protective clothing and topical sunscreen preparations in an attempt to arrest progression of the dermatosis.

Erythema Dyschromicum Perstans

Erythema dyschromicum perstans (dermatosis cenicienta, ashy dermatosis) is a chronic, progressive bluish to ash-gray hyperpigmentation first described in patients in San Salvador in 1957, but also recently described in Central and South America and the United States.[46, 47] This disorder affects individuals of both sexes from childhood through adulthood. Although nearly all reported patients have been dark-complexioned Spanish or Indian subjects from Central America, reports of fair-skinned individuals suggest that this condition may be more widespread than previously recognized and that mild variants of the disorder probably occur. The etiology is unknown.

Lesions usually begin as erythematous macules and gradually assume a slate-gray hue and a thin slightly raised erythematous border. Generally seen on the face, trunk, and upper limbs, lesions may also occur on other areas, with the exception of the scalp, mucous membranes, palms, and soles. Lesions vary in size from a few millimeters to many centimeters in diameter, and larger lesions, formed by the merging of small macules, may cover extensive areas.

This disorder must be differentiated from lesions of tinea versicolor, erythema annulare centrifugum, melasma, poikiloderma, fixed drug eruption, leprosy, and pinta by its characteristic slate-gray macular lesions with a peripherally spreading erythematous border and characteristic but not diagnostic histologic features of spongiosis, microvesicle formation, hydropic degeneration of epidermal cells, and pigmentary incontinence. The dermatosis is asymptomatic but chronic. There are frequent exacerbations, with extension into previously uninvolved areas, and there is no known effective therapy.

Familial Progressive Hyperpigmentation

Familial progressive hyperpigmentation is an uncommon but distinctive dominantly inherited gonodermatosis that presents at birth as irregular patches and streaks of hyperpigmentation, which increase in size, number, and confluence with age. Hyperpigmentation later appears in the conjunctivae and buccal mucosa and, with time, extensive areas of the skin and mucous membrane become involved.[48] The most distinctive histopathologic manifestation consists of heavy melanization of the basal cell layers, particularly the tips of the rete ridges, and a diffuse scattering of pigmented granules throughout the epidermal layers, including the stratum corneum.

Metabolic Causes of Hyperpigmentation

Cutaneous changes frequently are helpful in the diagnosis of underlying metabolic or endocrine disorders. Hepatobiliary disorders, hemochromatosis, Addison's disease, hyperthyroidism, hypothyroidism, acromegaly, and Cushing's syndrome are prime examples of metabolic disorders in which hyperpigmentation may be seen as a cutaneous manifestation.

Hepatobiliary Hyperpigmentation. More than two-thirds of patients with chronic hepatic disease (cirrhosis or prolonged bile duct obstruction) have some degree of cutaneous hyperpigmentation. Of these, diffuse darkening of the skin is perhaps the most common. Blotchy areas of brown hyperpigmentation occasionally may be seen, and accentuation of normal freckling and areolar hyperpigmentation may appear. Although the actual cause of hyperpigmentation associated with chronic liver disease is uncertain, it appears to be associated with humoral mechanisms that result in stimulation of melanogenesis, such as is seen with ACTH, MSH, or endocrine abnormalities,[49] or perhaps hepatic dysfunction may lead to biochemical abnormalities of the epidermal melanin unit with a resultant increase in pigment.[50]

Adrenal Insufficiency (Addison's Disease). Addison's disease (chronic adrenocortical insufficiency) is characterized by weakness, anorexia, hypotension, loss of body hair, low values of serum sodium and chloride, high levels of serum potassium, and melanin hyperpigmentation of the skin and mucous membranes. Hyperpigmentation, apparently the result of increased production of melanocyte stimulating hormone (MSH) by the pituitary gland (a compensatory phenomenon associated with decreased cortisol production by the adrenals), is most intense in the flexures, at sites of pressure and friction, in creases of the palms and soles, in sun-exposed areas, and in normally pigmented areas such as the genitalia and areolae. Pigmentation of the conjunctivae and vaginal mucous membranes is common, and pigmentary changes of the oral mucosae include spotty or streaked blue-black to brown hyperpigmentation of the gingivae, tongue, hard palate, and buccal mucosa.

The diagnosis of chronic adrenocortical insufficiency is suggested by the clinical features and may be confirmed by serum electrolyte studies and cortisol level determinations following stimulation by ACTH (the ACTH-stimulating test).

Hyperthyroidism. The cutaneous changes in hyperthyroidism consist of warm, moist, smooth, and elastic skin, and, in some patients, increased hyperpigmentation (thought to be caused by increased MSH secretion from the pituitary).[51] Vitiligo develops in about 7 per cent of thyrotoxic individuals, and pretibial myxedema, due to the presence of long-acting thyroid stimulating substance (LATS), may also be seen in patients with this disorder.

Pretibial myxedema is manifested by plaques on the shins, exophthalmos, and clubbing, with or without associated osteoarthropathy. Hyperpigmentation, seen in about 10 per cent of patients with primary thyrotoxicosis, is usually diffuse and generally appears in a pattern similar to that seen in patients with Addison's disease, except that the eyelids may occasionally be conspicuously hyperpigmented and involvement of the mucous membranes, areolae, and genitalia is less prominent.[51]

Hyperpituitarism. The excessive secretion of growth hormone by pituitary tumors produces gigantism in children whose epiphyses have not yet closed and acromegaly in adults whose normal bone growth has ceased.[51]

Acromegaly is rare in children, but transitional acromegalic features at times may be seen in adolescents. In addition to cutis verticis gyrata (coarse furrowing of the skin on the posterior aspect of the neck and the vertex of the scalp), a large and sometimes deeply furrowed tongue, thick lips, large nose, lantern jaw, broad spadelike hands with squatty fingers, hirsutism, and hyperpigmentation in a pattern similar to that observed in patients with Addison's disease may be seen in approximately 40 per cent of patients with acromegaly. Although the cause of hirsutism is not well understood, the hyperpigmentation appears to be related to increased secretion of melanocyte stimulating hormone (MSH).[51]

Cushing's Syndrome. Addison-like pigmentation (particularly on the face and neck) has also been noted in 6 to 10 per cent of individuals with Cushing's syndrome. Other associated features include a characteristic plethoric "moon" facies, with telangiectasia over the cheeks; patchy cyanosis over the upper arms, breast, abdomen, buttocks, thighs, and legs; increased presence of fine lanugo hair on the face and extremities; fatty deposits over the back of the neck ("buffalo hump"); increased fat deposits on the torso with a contrasting thinning of the arms and legs; purplish atrophic striae at points of tension such as the lower abdomen, thighs, buttocks, upper arms, and breasts; fragility of dermal blood vessels with increased tendency to bruisability and ecchymoses at sites of slight trauma; poor wound healing; frequent and recurrent pyoderma; and steroid acne (see Chapter 6).

Hemochromatosis. Hemochromatosis, occasionally termed bronze diabetes, is a familial iron storage disorder characterized by cutaneous hyperpigmentation, hepatic cirrhosis, diabetes mellitus, and, at times, cardiac failure. An uncommon disorder generally seen in males between 40 and 60 years of age, but also occasionally seen in childhood (particularly during adolescence), the pathogenesis is uncertain but appears to be associated with an increase in iron absorption attributable perhaps to an as yet undemonstrated enzymatic defect.

Thought to be inherited as a Mendelian dominant trait with incomplete penetrance, hyperpigmentation is seen in almost every patient and is the presenting sign in 25 to 40 per cent of affected individuals. The increased pigmentation is produced by melanin and not by the deposition of iron in the skin.[52, 53] It appears initially in the exposed areas before it becomes diffuse and is most intense in the skin of the face, arms, body folds, and genitalia. Mucous membranes (the gums, palate, and buccal mucosa), and sometimes the conjunctivae, are involved in 15 to 20 per cent of affected individuals. The skin is soft, dry, thin, shiny, and of fine texture. Spider angiomas are present in 60 to 80 per cent of affected individuals; icterus is unusual; palmar erythema is common; hypogonadism may be present; and facial, axillary, thoracic, and pubic hairs are scant or absent.[51, 54]

Secondary hemochromatosis (hemosiderosis) may be seen in patients with anemia who receive numerous blood transfusions. This disorder occurs in individuals of both sexes and all ages. In such instances, visceral fibrosis is unusual, diabetes mellitus is uncommon, and hypogonadism is not present.

The diagnosis of metabolic hemochromatosis is suggested by the presence of cutaneous hyperpigmentation in patients with hepatic cirrhosis and a history of diabetes mellitus. Elevated serum iron and saturation of serum iron-binding globulin help confirm the diagnosis. The demonstration of parenchymal iron distribution by skin, liver, and gastric biopsies, and the presence of hemosiderin in urinary sediment are particularly helpful. Histopathologic examination of involved skin is characterized by a normal epidermis, increased melanin in the basal layer, and deposition of iron in the upper cutis (especially in macrophages, endothelial cells of capillaries, and the propria of eccrine glands).

The clinical course of untreated hemochromatosis is characterized by tissue destruction, malfunction of involved organs, and eventual death. Symptomatic treatment of the diabetes, liver dysfunction, and cardiac symptoms and repeated phlebotomies, when initiated early, frequently result in clinical and pathologic improvement. Dietary restriction of iron is impractical, and chelating agents to date have been of little value. Since individuals with hemochromatosis accumulate about 3 mg of iron daily in excess of body losses, in order to maintain normal iron balance, quarterly phlebotomies of about 500 ml are generally necessary throughout life.

Hypermelanosis in Other Systemic Disorders. Increased pigmentation may also appear as an inconstant feature of a wide variety of other systemic disorders. In most instances the mechanism is obscure, and a number of factors may be involved.[55]

Pigmentation may occur in chronic infections. Whether the hyperpigmentation is due to the infection, associated malnutrition, or other factors, however, is uncertain. Pigmentation also may be seen as a manifestation of lymphomas and may be noted in 10 per cent of cases of Hodgkin's disease and in 1 or 2 per cent of cases of lymphosarcoma or lymphatic leukemia. It has been noted that attacks of asthma may be preceded by three or four days of diffuse darkening of the skin and an increase in the size and number of melanocytic nevi. Rheumatoid arthritis, particularly the juvenile variety (Still's disease), also may be associated with a generalized cutaneous hyperpigmentation.

Generalized hyperpigmentation may also be noted in patients with progressive systemic sclerosis or dermatomyositis (accompanying or following the cutaneous lesions) and on light-exposed skin in about 10 per cent of patients with systemic lupus erythematosus.

Polycystic kidney disease and other forms of chronic renal disease with nitrogen retention may also be accompanied by pruritus and, at times, a diffuse yellowish-brown discoloration of the skin. It is most pronounced on the face and hands, and although urinary chromogens and carotenemia may be implicated, melanin pigmentation also has been implicated as a cause of this discoloration.[55]

Exogenous Pigmentation

Hyperpigmentation Due to Heavy Metals. The systemic absorption of chemicals can also cause discoloration of the skin. Although the incidence of hyperpigmentation due to exogenous heavy metals has decreased in recent years, limited exposure to such preparations still occurs, and metallic hyperpigmentation still may be seen in children as well as adults.

Argyria is a localized or wide-spread bluish-gray or slate-colored discoloration of the skin produced by the deposition of silver within the dermis. The condition is more pronounced on exposed parts of the body, namely the face, forearms, and hands, but may also occur in the sclerae, oral mucous membranes, and lunulae of the nails. Most cases develop as a result of long-continued use of nose drops (Argyrol) or ophthalmic preparations containing silver, the degree of discoloration being proportional to the duration of exposure to the preparation and the duration and intensity of light exposure to the areas of involvement.

The diagnosis of argyria is based upon clinical examination and history of exposure, and may be confirmed by cutaneous biopsy of affected areas. Histopathologic examination is characterized by fine, small round refractive silver granules, which may be seen throughout the dermis, particularly the hyaline basement zone and membrana propria surrounding eccrine glands. In addition to silver, increased amounts of melanin may be seen in the basal layer of the epidermis and also within macrophages in the upper dermis. Treatment of argyria depends upon recognition of the disorder, discontinuation of the use of the silver-containing preparation, and avoidance of sunlight exposure.

Chrysiasis (gold-induced hyperpigmentation) is a rare cutaneous disorder induced by the administration of gold salts followed by exposure to ultraviolet light. The pigmentation is bluish-gray or purplish in color and is similar to that seen in argyria except that the pigmentation is more prominent around the eyes, is limited to areas of sunlight exposure, and does not affect the sclerae and oral mucous membranes. Other cutaneous manifestations are seen in up to 20 per cent of individuals on gold therapy. These include morbilliform, eczematous, urticarial, bullous, purpuric, lichen planus-like, and pityriasis rosea-like eruptions.[56] The histopathologic features of gold-induced pigmentation consist of small, black, round or oval irregularly shaped gold particles that are located in a perivascular distribution and in dermal histiocytes.

Mercury-induced pigmentation also may result in the deposition of the metal in the dermis, with a slate-gray pigmentation in areas of topical application. The discoloration is exaggerated in the areas of skinfolds, and the resulting pigmentation is permanent.[57]

Drug-Induced Hyperpigmentation. Hyperpigmentation may be induced by chronic long-term chlorpromazine (thorazine) administration (dosages of 300 to 500 mg per day for periods of three to five years or more).[58] The bluish-gray discoloration is most prominent about the face, particularly the tip of the nose, malar prominence, forehead, and cheeks, the V of the neck, the dorsal

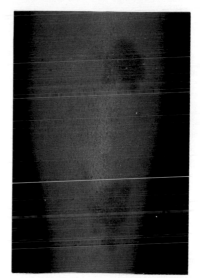

Figure 16–17 Fixed drug eruption. This disorder tends to recur in the same areas on readministration of the offending drug.

aspect of the hands, and exposed areas of the legs (Fig. 16–17). A brownish pigmentation of the conjunctivae occurs in only a small percentage of patients and has been described primarily in those on long-term therapy, such as might be seen in mental hospitals. Although the mechanism is uncertain, it has been suggested that chlorpromazine may have a specific affinity for melanin-containing tissues.

About 25 per cent of patients receiving antimalarial preparations (quinacrine, chloroquine, or hydroxychloroquine) for long periods of time develop a bluish-gray pigmentation of the face, neck, oral mucous membranes (particularly the soft palate), forearms, legs and nail beds.[59] Of interest and occasional diagnostic significance is the fact that antimalarials (chloroquine) may at times produce a silvery or white bleaching at the eyebrows, eyelids, or temples of redheaded, blond, or fair-haired individuals.

Circumscribed plaques of purplish to purplish-red pigmentation, usually round or oval, sometimes bullous, are commonly associated with fixed drug eruptions. Drug-induced hyperpigmentation tends to recur in the same location following the readministration of certain drugs, particularly phenolphthalein, barbiturate derivatives, and antineoplastic agents such as bisulfan and cytoxan. Other occasionally incriminated drugs include aspirin, phenacetin, diphenylhydantoin, gold, arsenic, sulfonamides, and tetracycline.

The diagnosis of a drug eruption is based almost entirely on history and physical examination. Histopathologic examination of lesions reveals subepidermal bullae with degeneration of the detached portion of the epidermis in early lesions. The late hyperpigmented stage is characterized by an increase in the amount of melanin in the basal layer of the epidermis and within macrophages of the upper dermis.

Carotenemia. Carotenemia is a yellowish-orange discoloration of skin due to the ingestion of excessive quantities of carotene-containing foods, particularly carrots, squash, pumpkins, yellow turnips, sweet potatoes, peaches, apricots, papaya, or egg yolk. Seen primarily in infants, occasionally in older children and adults, the color is most prominent on the palms and soles, in the nasolabial grooves, on the forehead, chin, upper eyelids, postauricular areas, anterior axillary folds, and over areas of pressure such as the elbows, knees, knuckles, and ankles. Lack of involvement of the sclerae and mucous membranes, coupled with the absence of pruritus and lack of color change in the urine or stool, helps rule out the presence of hepatic or biliary jaundice. Lycopene, a red-colored carotenoid pigment found in fruits and vegetables, especially ripened tomatoes, beets, chili beans, and various fruits and berries, may cause a reddish-yellow discoloration of the skin (lycopenemia).

The diagnosis of carotenemia is confirmed by the presence of high carotene levels in the presence of normal serum bilirubin. Reduction of dietary intake of carotene-containing foods to normal levels results in gradual improvement (usually within a period of four to six weeks). A few persons have been found in whom carotenemia develops despite a normal vegetable intake; these patients appear to have a genetic inability to convert carotenoids into vitamin A to the same degree as normal persons. For patients who cannot convert carotenoids to vitamin A, the vitamin should be given if its serum levels are found to be below the normal range. In such individuals control of the carotenodermia may be difficult. Such patients, under the supervision of a dietician, should try to decrease red and yellow vegetables and fruit intake, making sure that the diet is otherwise well balanced.[60]

References

1. Futcher PH: A peculiarity of pigmentation of the upper arms of Negroes. Science 88:570–571, 1938.

   A distinctly darker dorsolateral and lighter anteromedial pigmentation noted on the upper arms (bilaterally in 17.5 per cent and unilaterally in 2.0 per cent of 200 Negroes) of dark-skinned individuals.

2. Ito K: The peculiar demarcation of pigmentation along the so-called Voigt's line among the Japanese. Dermatologia Internationalis. 4:45–47, 1965.

   A pigmentary peculiarity (similar to that described by Futcher in 1938 and Matsuomoto in 1913) is seen in 130 of 3000 Japanese; this peculiarity appeared 10 times more frequently in females than in males.

3. Lerner AB: Vitiligo. J. Invest. Dermatol. 32:285–310, 1959.

   A classic reference for vitiligo, a chronic disorder of depigmentation affecting two million people in the United States.

4. Lerner AB: Vitiligo: Progress in Dermatology 6:1–6, 1972.

   Theories of pathogenesis, clinical features, differential diagnosis, and management of vitiligo.

5. Nordlund JJ, Lerner AB: Vitiligo: its relationship to systemic disease. *In* Moschella SL (Ed.): Dermatology Update. Review for Physicians. 1979 edition. Elsevier North Holland, Inc. New York, 1979, 411–432.

   A review of the pathogenesis of vitiligo and its relationship to other disorders.

6. Lerner AB, Nordlund JJ: Vitiligo. What is it? Is it important? JAMA 239:1183–1187, 1978.

   An update of the clinical features, classification, and physiology of vitiligo.

7. Hurwitz S, Braverman IM: White spots in tuberous sclerosis. J. Pediatr. 77:587–594, 1970.

   Hypopigmented macules, the earliest sign of tuberous sclerosis: their clinical variations and differentiation from lesions of vitiligo.

8. El-Mofty AM: The treatment of vitiligo with a combination of psoralens and quinolines. Br. J. Dermatol. 76:56–62, 1964.

   Psoralens and quinolone derivatives produced good to excellent repigmentation (over 50 per cent) in 84 per cent of 55 patients with vitiligo.

9. Kenny JA Jr: Pigmentary disturbances. *In* Conn HF (Ed.): Current Therapy, 1978. W. B. Saunders Co., Philadelphia, 1978, 641–643.

   A practical approach to the therapy of pigmentary disorders.

10. Parrish JA, Fitzpatrick TB, Shea C, et al.: Photochemotherapy of vitiligo. Use of orally administered psoralen and a high-intensity long-wave ultraviolet system. Arch. Dermatol. 112:1531–1534, 1976.

    An artificial light source that provides high-intensity ultraviolet light (UVA, 300 to 400 nm) to the entire body, with orally administered psoralen as an adjunct to the treatment of patients with vitiligo.

11. Fulton JE, Leyden JE, Papa C: Treatment of vitiligo with topical methoxsalen and blacklight. Arch. Dermatol. 100:224–229, 1969.

    Fourteen of 15 patients with vitiligo respond to topical application of 10 per cent methoxsalen in hydrophilic ointment followed by exposure to long-wave ultraviolet light.

12. King RA, Witkop CJ Jr: Hairbulb tyrosinase activity in oculocutaneous albinism. Nature 263:69–71, 1976.

    An assay for quantifying tyrosinase activity in human hairbulbs and application of this technique to human oculocutaneous albinism.

13. Jeliffe DB, Jeliffe EFP: The children of the San Blas Islands of Panama. J. Pediatr. 59:271–285, 1961.

    A comprehensive analysis of the children of the San Blas Islands from birth to four years of age.

14. Hermansky F, Pudlak P: Albinism associated with hemorrhagic diathesis and unusual pigmented reticular cells in the bone marrow. Report of two cases with histochemical studies. Blood 14:162–169, 1959.

    Two unrelated patients with oculocutaneous albinism with prolonged bleeding time and unusual pigment-containing macrophages in the bone marrow suggest a syndrome of pseudohemophilia and albinism.

15. Tietz W: A syndrome of deaf-mutism associated with albinism showing dominant autosomal inheritance. Am. J. Hum. Genet. 15:259–264, 1963.

    A family pedigree of 14 individuals combining the features of albinism with deaf-mutism as an autosomal dominant disorder.

16. Cross H, McKusick J, Breen W: A new oculocerebral syndrome with hypopigmentation. J. Pediatr. 70:398–406, 1967.

    A family with three siblings affected with mental retardation, spastic diplegia, hypopigmentation with many characteristics of true albinism, and multiple ocular anomalies appear to comprise a unique autosomal recessive syndrome.

17. Logan LJ, Rapaport SI, Maher I: Albinism and abnormal platelet function. N. Engl. J. Med. 284:1340–1345, 1971.

Family studies suggest that the coexistence of albinism and primary dysfunction of platelet-adenosine diphosphate release results from a mutation involving closely linked recessive genes, one affecting tyrosinase activity and the other affecting platelet function.

18. Pearce WG, Sanger R, Race RR: Ocular albinism and Xg. Lancet 1:1282–1283, 1968.

Studies in a kindred of eight sons and one daughter of two women known to be heterozygous for ocular albinism and Xg confirm earlier evidence that the locus responsible for ocular albinism is within measurable distance of that for Xg.

19. Falls HF: Sex-linked ocular albinism displaying typical fundus changes in the female heterozygote. Am. J. Ophthal. 34:41–50 (May), 1951.

Ophthalmic examination in two families with sex-linked ocular albinism reveals typical retinal changes in the heterozygote female carrier.

20. Comings DE, Odland GF: Partial albinism. JAMA 195:111–115, 1976.

Partial albinism in 24 individuals of a family of six generations.

21. Windhorst DB, Zelickson AS, Good RA: Human pigmentary dilution based on heritable subcellular structural defect: Chediak-Higashi syndrome. J. Invest. Dermatol. 50:9–18, 1968.

A failure in the control of the size of melanin granules relates to the color defect in the giant granules seen in leukocytes, leukocyte precursors, and other cells of children with the Chediak-Higashi syndrome.

22. Blume RS, Wolff SM: The Chediak-Higashi syndrome. Studies in four patients and review of the literature. Medicine 51:247–280, 1972.

A thorough analysis of the Chediak-Higashi syndrome with a description of four patients and review of 59 cases from the literature.

23. Boxer LA, Wanatabe AM, Rister M, et al.: Correction of leukocyte function in Chediak-Higashi syndrome by ascorbate. N. Engl. J. Med. 295:1041–1045, 1976.

The effect of ascorbic acid on cyclic AMP in leukocytes of patients with the Chediak-Higashi syndrome may be associated with differences in leukocyte membrane structure.

24. Waardenburg PJ: A new syndrome combining developmental anomalies of the eyelids, eyebrows and nose root with pigmentary defects of the iris and head hair with congenital deafness. Am. J. Hum. Genet. 3:195–253, 1951.

A clinical description of 161 individuals with the Waardenburg syndrome.

25. Reed WB, Stone VM, Boder E, et al.: Pigmentary disorders in association with congenital deafness. Arch. Dermatol. 95:176–186, 1967.

Review of 16 patients with typical features of the Klein-Waardenburg syndrome and eight others without dystopia cantharum.

26. Fitzpatrick TB, Szabo G, Hori Y, et al.: White leaf-shaped macules, earliest visible sign of tuberous sclerosis. Arch. Dermatol. 98:1–6, 1968.

Of 31 individuals with tuberous sclerosis, 10 had white leaf-shaped macules as the only cutaneous manifestation of their disorder.

27. Nickel WR, Reed WB: Tuberous sclerosis. Arch. Dermatol. 85:209–226, 1962.

In 40 of 61 patients with tuberous sclerosis who had associated areas of leukoderma or poliosis, 29 had leukoderma alone, 2 had poliosis alone, and 9 had a combination of both.

28. Hurwitz S: Discussion on Tuberous Sclerosis, Society Transactions. Arch. Derm. 104:336–337, 1971.

A patient with partial albinism, hypopigmented macules, and a discussion of leukoderma in tuberous sclerosis.

29. Wiley HE III, Frias JL: Depigmented lesions in incontinentia pigmenti. A useful diagnostic sign. Am. J. Dis. Child. 128:546–547, 1974.

Streaked hypopigmented macules on the calves or other areas in relatives of individuals in families with incontinentia pigmenti serve as a clue to the familial genetic pattern of patients with this disorder.

30. Ito M: Studies on melanin. I. Incontinentia pigmenti achromians: a singular case of nevus depigmentosus systematicus bilateralis. Tohoku J. Exp. Med. (Suppl I) 55:57–59, 1952.

Description of a woman with a distinctive, depigmented, systematized, bilateral "nevus" that took the form of bizarre irregular hypopigmented patches on the trunk and extremities.

31. Hamada T, Saito T, et al.: Incontinentia pigmenti achromians (Ito). Arch. Dermatol. 96:673–676, 1967.

A 3-month old Japanese girl with incontinentia pigmenti achromians.

32. Rubin MB: Incontinentia pigmenti achromians. Arch. Dermatol. 105:424–425, 1972.

Multiple cases of incontinentia pigmenti achromians in a family suggests an autosomal dominant mode of inheritance.

33. Jelinek JE, Bart RS, Schiff GM: Hypomelanosis of Ito ("Incontinentia Pigmenti Achromians"). Report of three cases and review of the literature. Arch. Dermatol. 107:596–601, 1973.

Three children with hypopigmented asymmetric whorls and streaks in a marble-cake pattern representing a negative picture of incontinentia pigmenti.

34. Schwartz MF, Esterly NB, Fretzin DF, et al.: Hypomelanosis of Ito (incontinentia pigmenti achromians): a neurocutaneous syndrome. J. Pediatr. 90:236–240, 1977.

The identification of 10 patients with hypomelanosis of Ito within a relatively brief period suggests that this entity probably is more common than the literature would indicate.

35. Coupe RL: Unilateral systematized achromic nevus. Dermatologica. 134:19–35, 1967.

Congenital systematized hypopigmentation — an embryonic error of melanocytic migration from the neural crest.

36. Solomon LM, Esterly NB: Pigmentary abnormalities, nevus achromicus. In Neonatal Dermatology. W. B. Saunders Publishing Co., Philadelphia, 1973, 106.

The authors note the case of an infant with an achromic nevus, hemihypertrophy, and retardation.

37. Fleisher TL, Zeligman I: Nevus anemicus. Arch. Dermatol. 100:750–755, 1969.

Nevus anemicus may be due to a defect at the motor end plate or smooth muscle effector cell of blood vessels associated with increased stimulation of vasoconstrictor or inhibition of vasodilator fibers of arterioles.

38. Hammer H: Lymphocyte transformation test in sympathetic ophthalmitis and the Vogt-Koyanagi-Harada syndrome. Br. J. Ophthalmol. 55:850–852, 1971.

Lymphocyte transfer tests in two patients with Vogt-Koyanagi syndrome and three with sympathetic ophthalmitis stimulated with bovine uveal pigment suggests that delayed autoaggressive allergic response to uveal pigment plays a role in the pathogenesis of these disorders.

39. Kahn G: Depigmentation caused by phenolic detergent germicides. Arch. Dermatol. 102:177–187, 1970.

Eighteen patients with patchy depigmentation from contact with paratertiary butyl phenol or paratertiary amyl phenol in commercial disinfectants.

40. McGuire J, Hendee J: Biochemical basis for depigmentation

of skin by phenolic germicides. J. Invest. Dermatol. 57:256–261, 1971.

The depigmentation caused by phenol-containing germicides appears to be due to competitive inhibition of tyrosinase by phenolic compounds.

41. Cornelius CE III, Stein KM, Hanshaw WL, et al.: Hypopigmentation and sarcoidosis. Arch. Dermatol. 108:249–251, 1973.

Microscopic examination of cutaneous biopsies of hypopigmented lesions in patients with sarcoidosis suggests hypopigmentation as another cutaneous clue to the diagnosis of this disorder.

42. Rodriguez JM, Stevens DM: Leprosy: a report of two cases in children. J. Pediatr. 93:192–195, 1978.

Two children with leprosy and a review of the diagnosis and management of this disorder.

43. Lauer BA, Lilla JA, Golitz LE: Experience and reason: Leprosy in a Vietnamese adoptee. Pediatrics 65:335–337, 1980.

A 10-year-old Vietnamese adoptee with tuberculoid leprosy serves as a reminder that leprosy, a common infection (3 to 5 cases per 1000 population) in Vietnam, because of a long incubation period of two to six years or more, may not be manifested for several years.

44. Kligman AM, Willis I: New formulation for depigmenting human skin. Arch. Dermatol. 111:40–48, 1975.

A new formulation containing 0.1 per cent tretinoin (vitamin A acid), five per cent hydroquinone, 0.1 per cent dexamethasone, and hydrophilic ointment effective in the management of cosmetically objectionable freckles, postinflammatory hypopigmentation, and melasma.

45. Kuske H, Krebs A: Hyperpigmentation of chloasma-type after treatment with hydantoin preparations. Dermatologica 129:121–139, 1964 (in German).

Chloasma-type hyperpigmentation developed in 13 patients on hydantoin and its derivatives (particularly mesantoin).

46. Knox JM, Dodge BG, Freeman RG: Erythema dyschromicum perstans. Arch. Dermatol. 97:262–272, 1968.

Six patients from Houston, Texas, with erythema dyschromicum perstans.

47. Byrne DA, Berger RS: Erythema dyschromicum perstans: report of two cases in fair-skinned patients. Acta Derm. Venereol. 54:65–68, 1974.

Erythema dyschromicum perstans on the trunk, arms, neck, and thighs of two fair-skinned 12-year-old girls suggests that this condition may be more widespread than generally recognized and that relatively mild variants of this disorder apparently occur.

48. Chernosky ME, Anderson DE, Chang JP, et al.: Familial progressive hyperpigmentation. Arch. Dermatol. 103:581–598, 1971.

Four patients in a Negro family with irregular patchy areas of hyperpigmentation which progressed in number, size, and confluence with the patients' increasing age.

49. Lerner AB, McGuire JS: Melanocyte stimulating hormone and adrenocorticotrophic hormone. N. Engl. J. Med. 270:539–564, 1964.

Homogeneous pig ACTH and alpha MSH given separately in large quantities to a bilaterally adrenalectomized patient resulted in true pigment darkening of the skin.

50. Tisdale WA: Cutaneous manifestations of hepatobiliary disease. In Fitzpatrick TB, et al. (Eds.): Dermatology in General Medicine. McGraw-Hill Book Co., New York, 1971, 1339–1347.

A review of pigmentary and other cutaneous manifestations of hepatobiliary disease.

51. Braverman IM: Skin Signs of Systemic Disease. W. B. Saunders Co., Philadelphia, 1970, 350–397.

Chapter 13 contains a review of endocrine and metabolic disorders and their effect on the skin.

52. Cawley EP, Hsu T, Wood BT, et al.: Hemochromatosis and the skin. Arch. Dermatol. 100:1–6, 1969.

The cutaneous pigmentation in patients with hemochromatosis is related to epidermal thickening and the amount of epidermal melanin not iron.

53. Perdrup A, Poulsen H: Hemochromatosis and vitiligo. Arch. Dermatol. 90:34–37, 1964.

A patient who had both vitiligo and hemochromatosis vividly demonstrates that melanin rather than iron is the cause of hyperpigmentation in hemochromatosis.

54. Cherant-Breton J, Simon M, Bourel M, et al.: Cutaneous manifestations of idiopathic hemochromatosis: study of 100 cases. Arch. Dermatol. 113:161–165, 1977.

Skin pigmentation, one of the earliest signs of hemochromatosis.

55. Ebling FJ, Rook A: Disorders of skin color. Hypermelanosis in other systemic disorders. In Rook A, Wilkinson DS, Ebling FJG (Eds.): Textbook of Dermatology, 2nd ed. Blackwell Scientific Publications, Oxford, 1972, 1262–1265.

A review of various systemic disorders that may result in hypermelanosis of the skin.

56. Penneys NS, Ackerman AB, Gottlieb NL: Gold dermatitis. Arch. Dermatol. 109:372–376, 1974.

Review of 37 patients with skin eruptions that developed while on gold therapy for rheumatoid arthritis or pemphigus.

57. Lamar LM, Bliss BO: Localized pigmentation of the skin due to topical mercury. Arch. Dermatol. 93:450–451, 1966.

Lichen planus-like and pityriasis rosea-like eruptions in patients on topical mercuric preparations.

58. Hays GB, Lyle CB Jr, Wheeler CE: Slate-gray color in patients receiving chlorpromazine. Arch. Dermatol. 90:471–476, 1964.

Five white women in a mental hospital who had taken large amounts of chlorpromazine (500 to 3000 mg daily for periods of one to five years) developed a bluish discoloration on exposed areas resembling the slate-gray discoloration seen in patients with argyria.

59. Tuffanelli D, Abraham RK, Dubois EJ: Pigmentation from antimalarial therapy. Arch. Dermatol. 88:419–426, 1963.

Localized cutaneous blue-black pigmentation on the pretibial, facial, and subungual areas in 8 per cent (25) of 300 patients receiving antimalarial therapy.

60. Mathews-Roth MM: Answer to a question on carotenemia. JAMA 241:1835, 1979.

Although overindulgence in carotenoid-containing vegetables, fruit, and fruit juices is the most common cause of carotenemia, hypothyroidism, diabetes, renal failure, and a genetic inability to convert carotenoids into vitamin A also should be considered as possible causes of this disorder.

DISORDERS OF HAIR AND NAILS

HAIR

Hair is a protein byproduct of follicles that are distributed everywhere on the body surface except the palms, soles, vermilion portion of the lips, the glans penis, penile shaft, the nail beds, and the sides of the fingers and toes. Although hair is of minimal functional benefit to man, the psychological effects of disturbances of hair growth are frequently a source of great concern to children, adolescents, and their parents.

In the human fetus, groups of cells appear in the epidermis at about the eighth week of gestation. These differentiate to form the hair follicles, and hair begins to develop between the eighth and twelfth weeks of fetal life. This growth continues throughout pregnancy, and although there are indications that some hair is lost during gestation and at the time of birth, the majority of hairs on the newborn infant are approximately five to six months old.[1]

Although the terms lanugo and vellus are frequently used synonymously, lanugo hairs, except in the rare hereditary syndrome hypertrichosis lanuginosa, are seen only in fetal and neonatal life. They are fine, soft, unmedullated, and poorly pigmented, and they appear as a fine dense growth over the entire cutaneous surface of the fetal infant. Lanugo hair is normally shed in utero in the seventh or eighth month of gestation but may cover the entire cutaneous surface of the newborn premature infant. Postnatal hair may be divided into vellus and terminal types. Vellus hairs are the fine, lightly pigmented hairs seen on the arms and faces of children and faces of women. Terminal hairs are the mature thick dark hairs on the scalp, eyebrows, eyelashes, and areas of secondary sexual hair distribution.

The hair root is characterized by three definable cyclic stages of growth — anagen, catagen, and telogen (Table 17–1). The anagen or active growth phase lasts for periods of two to six years, with an average of about three years. The follicle then undergoes a short period of partial degeneration (the catagen phase). This generally lasts for a period of 10 to 14 days and is immediately followed by a resting or telogen phase, which lasts for three to four months.[2] What triggers the resumption of the active growing stage is yet to be determined.

Neonatal Hair

The first crop of terminal scalp hairs are in the actively growing anagen phase at birth, but within the first few days of life there is a physiologic conversion to the telogen phase. Consequently, a high proportion of neonatal scalp hairs are shed during the first four months of life. This telogen shedding (telogen effluvium of the newborn) may occur as a sudden hair loss, leading to almost complete alopecia or, in a more common gradual form, may be scarcely perceptible. Whether sudden or gradual, replacement of the first terminal hairs is generally completed before the first six months of life.[2] Some infants do not become significantly bald. Presumably these individuals retain the telogen club hairs until anagen replacement takes over. The neonatal hairline frequently extends along the forehead and temples to the lateral margin of the eyebrows. These terminal hairs gradually convert to vellus hairs during the first year of life (the influence at birth on vellus hair, however, is not fully explained).

Premature infants are frequently covered by lanugo hairs, which are more densely distributed on the face, limbs, and trunk. This probably is related to the cyclic activity in utero and the normal shedding of telogen vellus hairs in the fetus during the last few weeks of gestation.[3] The thickness of infant scalp pelage varies among individuals and, depending upon habits such as hair rubbing or head banging, is determined by how rapidly trauma results in destruction of terminal hairs and the rate at which telogen hairs are rubbed away.

Congenital Disorders

A variety of congenital and hereditary disorders are associated with abnormalities of hair growth. These include a congenital triangularly patterned alopecia seen at the frontotemporal as-

Table 17–1 CYCLIC STAGES OF HAIR GROWTH

1. Anagen phase (active growth phase) lasts 2 to 6 years (average 3 years)
2. Catagen phase (stage of partial degeneration) lasts 10 to 14 days
3. Telogen phase (resting stage) lasts 3 to 4 months

pect of the hairline;[4] aplasia cutis, acrodermatitis enteropathica, and Leiner's disease (discussed in Chapter 2); Rothmund-Thomson syndrome (discussed in Chapter 4); the hereditary ectodermal dysplasias and progeria (discussed in Chapter 7); and the Hallerman-Streiff syndrome, hereditary trichodysplasia (Marie-Unna hypotrichosis), and the oral-facial-digital syndromes I and II (OFD I and II), which are discussed below.

Hallerman-Streiff Syndrome

The Hallerman-Streiff syndrome (oculomandibulocephaly) is characterized by dwarfism, beaked nose, and brachycephaly, often accompanied by frontal and parietal bossing, mandibular hypoplasia, microphthalmia, low-set ears, thin and small lips, high-arched palate, congenital cataracts, blue sclerae, motor and occasionally mental retardation, supernumerary teeth, and hypotrichosis of the scalp, eyebrows, and eyelids. Alopecia is most prominent about the frontal and occipital areas and is especially marked along suture lines. Axillary and pubic hair also may be scant, and cutaneous atrophy, largely limited to the scalp and nose, may be seen as thin taut skin and prominence of underlying blood vessels.

Hereditary Trichodysplasia

Hereditary trichodysplasia (Marie-Unna hypotrichosis) is a rare autosomal dominant disorder manifested by almost complete congenital absence of scalp hair, eyebrows, and eyelashes; decreased body hair; and widespread facial milia. In early childhood hair growth may occur, but the hair soon becomes coarse, flattened, or twisted. During puberty the hair becomes very sparse, particularly on the vertex and scalp margins, resulting in a high frontal and nuchal hairline. Scattered follicular horny plugs may be associated with this disorder, and histologic examination of cutaneous biopsy of involved areas reveals an abnormal proliferation of the internal root sheath in many of the follicles. When examined under the dissecting microscope, abnormal hairs are seen as flat, twisted, and ribbon-like. Electron microscopic examination of hair may reveal peeling of the cuticle, increased interfibrillar cortical matrix, and intracellular fractures of the cuticular cells, cortical cell fibrils, and medullary cells.[5]

Oral-Facial-Digital Syndromes

The oral-facial-digital syndrome consists of two distinct disorders (OFD I and OFD II). OFD I was originally described as a condition of hypoplasia of nasal cartilages, lobulated cleft tongue, cleft lip and palate, maldeveloped frenula, hypertelorism, trembling, mental retardation, and various malformations of the hands. It is a rare dominant X-linked disorder limited to females and lethal to males. It occurs in approximately one in 50,000 live births and is characterized by a distinctive facies with frontal bossing, a hooked pug-nose with hypoplasia of the nasal cartilages, lateral displacement of the inner canthi (dystopia canthorum), micrognathia, cleft lip, a high-arched or cleft palate, lobulated clefts of the tongue, hyperplasia of the frenulum with thick bands in the lower buccal fold, dental abnormalities, mental retardation, hydrocephalus, kyphoscoliosis, equinovarus, conductive hearing loss, and various malformations of the hands (brachydactyly, syndactyly, clinodactyly, polydactyly). Cutaneous abnormalities seen in association with this disorder include alopecia (secondary to a decrease in the number of hair follicles) and coarse, lusterless hair.

Oral-facial-digital syndrome II, an autosomal recessive trait that affects both sexes, may be differentiated from OFD I by a broad bifid nasal tip, occasional flaring of the alveolar ridge, a tendency toward hexadactyly, bilateral polysyndactyly of the halluces, and a lack of cutaneous or appendageal changes.[6]

NON-SCARRING ALOPECIA

Hair loss disorders can be divided into non-scarring (non-cicatricial) or scarring (cicatricial) groups (Table 17–2). Causes of non-scarring alopecia include alteration of the hair growth cycle, structural abnormalities of the hair, and inflammatory cutaneous disease.[7]

Telogen Effluvium

It is calculated that the average human scalp contains 100,000 hairs. The average growth rate of terminal hair is approximately 2.5 mm per week (1 cm per month). The hair shaft itself is a non-living structure and is not susceptible to biologic activity once it has formed. Although the hair shafts are the clinical focus of interest, it is the follicle itself that is responsible for the changes seen in most abnormalities of hair growth. The human hair follicle

Table 17–2 CLASSIFICATION OF HAIR LOSS

1. Scarring (cicatricial)
   a. Developmental defects
   b. Infectious disorders
   c. Chemical or thermal injury
   d. Dermatologic disorders

2. Non-scarring (non-cicatricial)
   a. Male pattern alopecia
   b. Telogen effluvium (physiologic)
   c. Hair shaft abnormalities
   d. Inflammatory disease
   e. Traumatic alopecia

has a fairly long phase of regular growth (the anagen phase). It then undergoes a period of involution (the catagen phase), lasting about three weeks, followed by a resting (telogen) club phase. The telogen phase of the follicle lasts for about three months. At the end of this time new growth is initiated, and as new hairs grow, they push out the old club hairs that have remained in the resting follicles. In healthy individuals, 80 to 90 per cent of the scalp is in the actively growing (anagen) stage, 5 per cent is in the brief transitional (catagen) stage, 10 to 15 per cent is in the resting or telogen stage, and 50 to 100 hairs are shed and simultaneously replaced each day.[2]

During the period of hair growth, the normal cyclic pattern may be interrupted by a variety of different stimuli and may result in a highly characteristic form of alopecia termed telogen effluvium. Second in incidence only to male-pattern baldness, this disorder represents the most common type of alopecia. The stimuli capable of producing an interruption in the normal growing (anagen) phase of the hair follicles include febrile illness (Fig. 17–1), parturition, surgical shock, crash diets,[8] injury, emotional stress, anticoagulant drugs, excessive ingestion of vitamin A (hypervitaminosis A) (Fig. 17–2), and discontinuation of an estrogen-dominated oral contraceptive. The proportion of follicles affected and the severity of the subsequent alopecia depend upon the duration and severity of the stress and individual variations in susceptibility.

It must be remembered that about 50 to 100 hairs are lost from the average scalp per day, that 25 per cent (25,000 hairs) must be shed before unmistakable thinning becomes apparent, and that club hairs do not fall out but are pushed out as new hairs drive their way through the anchoring fibrils. Accordingly, the shedding seen in telogen effluvium actually marks the end, not the beginning, of the disorder.[2]

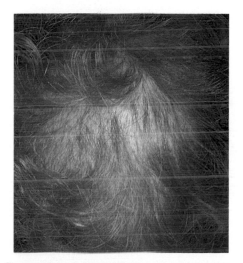

Figure 17–1 Telogen effluvium. Temporary diffuse alopecia initiated by a stressful situation (a severe viral infection) in a 4-year-old girl

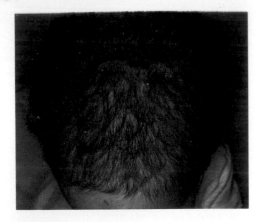

Figure 17–2   Toxic alopecia in a 2 1/2-year-old boy caused by the ingestion of excessive amounts of vitamin A.

The diagnosis of telogen effluvium may be suggested by a history of a stressful event preceding the onset of alopecia by 6 to 16 weeks (generally two to four months), and can be confirmed by counting the number of hairs shed each day and by determining the percentage of telogen hairs in the scalp. Daily hair counts can be accomplished by counting the number of hairs lost each day (broken hairs without roots should not be included). Loss of over 100 hairs a day can be considered excessive. The ratio of resting to growing hairs (the "telogen-anagen" ratio) can be determined by gently plucking approximately 50 hairs from the patient's temporoparietal scalp and examining them under a hand lens or low-power microscope. This can be accomplished by clamping approximately 50 hairs about one centimeter from the skin surface with a hemostat (the jaws of which have been covered by rubber tubing to prevent trauma to the hair shafts) followed by a gentle but short tug.

Hairs thus obtained can be placed on a microscope slide and examined under low magnification. Anagen hair roots can be recognized by the fact that the outer and inner hair sheaths are intact, with or without a portion of the dermal papilla adherent to the tip of the root. Telogen hair roots have uniform shaft diameters, contain no pigment, and are club-shaped, much like the tip of a cotton applicator. The ratio of telogen to anagen hairs varies from one person to another, with an average telogen count of 15 per cent and an anagen count of 85 per cent. A telogen count of 25 per cent or more is considered to be diagnostic of telogen effluvium.

There is no effective treatment for telogen effluvium, and since spontaneous regrowth is characteristic of this disorder, unless the stressful event is repeated, complete regrowth takes place almost invariably within about six months. Exceptionally prolonged illness with high fevers, however, may destroy some follicles completely, so that in some cases only partial recovery may be possible. Careful explanation of the cause of this disorder and its favorable prognosis, with careful instructions to the patient to avoid manipulation such as vigorous shampooing, combing, and brushing until new growth has occurred, is generally all that is required.

Anagen Effluvium

Anagen effluvium is a far less common disorder of hair loss that follows the use of antimitotic agents such as those used in the therapy of cancer or leukemia. These agents include folic acid antagonists (aminopterin and amethopterin), purine antagonists such as 6-mercaptopurine, alkylating agents (cyclophosphamide and nitrogen mustard), and natural alkaloids such as vincristine. In addition, anagen effluvium may be associated with excessive x-ray radiation to the scalp and the ingestion of various chemicals such as lead, thallium, arsenic, bismuth, and coumadin. During the period of drug administration, the follicle remains in a modified growth phase, and in contrast to telogen effluvium, the disorder occurs with follicles in the anagen growing stage.

The clinical features of anagen alopecia depend upon the degree of toxicity created by the causative agent. Since an average of 85 per cent of scalp hairs in a healthy individual are in the anagen stage at a given time, severe toxicity may result in profound hair loss. The usual change in the hair root is quite characteristic in this disorder and consists of tapered hair root tips and sharp thinning or constriction of the hair shaft (at which point the hairs simply separate). With lower doses there may be only segmental thinning or narrowing, without actual fracture of the hair shaft.[2] A careful history, documented evidence of hair loss, microscopic examination of spontaneously shed and manually epilated hairs, and appropriate physical and toxicologic examinations help establish the correct diagnosis. Cessation of the responsible drug generally results in regrowth of hair.

There is no effective treatment for anagen effluvium except removal of the precipitating cause. The use of a simple occlusive scalp tourniquet, however, frequently is effective in protecting against this disorder during the intravenous use of vincristine (as in the treatment of children with acute leukemia, Wilms' tumor, neuroblastoma, lymphoma, and rhabdomycosarcoma). With this technique, a specially constructed scalp tourniquet placed around the head just above the ears and inflated to 10 mm of mercury above systolic pressure immediately before injection of the drug frequently helps minimize the toxic effects of vincristine on the hair follicles of the scalp.[9]

Alopecia Areata

Alopecia areata is a common disorder, with an incidence of 17.2 per 100,000 population, characterized by the sudden appearance of sharply defined round or oval patches of hair loss. Although the condition occurs at all ages, the first attack usually appears in patients under twenty-five years of age, and there is a history of familial occurrence in 10 to 20 per cent of affected individuals. Although occasional reports of simultaneous occurrence in identical twins have been published, the genetic status of this disorder is unclear at this time.

The cause of alopecia areata remains unknown, but various causes have been proposed. Recent evidence suggests an immune mechanism (an auto-immunologic process) as a possible cause of this disorder. In support of this hypothesis several studies indicate an interrelationship with chronic lymphocytic thyroiditis (Hashimoto's disease), pernicious anemia, adrenal disease, vitiligo, diabetes, and atopy.[10] An increased incidence has also been noted in patients with Down's syndrome, and there also seems to be more than a coincidental association with cataracts.

CLINICAL MANIFESTATIONS. The typical clinical picture of alopecia areata generally consists of a sudden (frequently overnight or over a period of several days) appearance of one or more round or oval well-circumscribed and clearly defined patches of hair loss (Figs. 17–3, 17–4). Occasionally, particularly in children, the initial patches may be atypical, may lack a regular outline, and, at times, may demonstrate scattered long hairs within the bald areas. In other instances the initial loss may be diffuse, with patches of alopecia only being apparent after one or two weeks, if at all. The primary patch may appear on any hairy cutaneous surface but usually occurs on the scalp. Characteristically the skin is smooth, soft, ivory-white, and almost totally devoid of hair. Rarely, slight erythema or edema may be found at an early stage, and older patches frequently contain depigmented hair shafts, simulating poliosis (Fig. 17–5). Discrete islands of hair loss sometimes are separated by completely uninvolved or partially in-

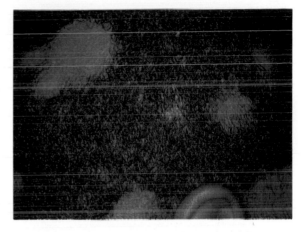

Figure 17–4 Multiple lesions of alopecia areata. Short stubby "exclamation-mark" hairs may be plucked out and identified under low-power microscopic examination.

volved scalp, and around the margins of patches of alopecia, pathognomonic "exclamation-mark" hairs may be detected. These loose hairs, with attenuated bulbs and short stumps, are easily plucked out of the scalp. Examination of such hairs under a low-power microscope reveals an irregularity in diameter and a poorly pigmented, attenuated bulb (due to atrophy of the hair root) rather than the club-shaped tips of telogen hairs.

A clinical form of alopecia termed ophiasis occasionally occurs, particularly in children. This unusual form of alopecia begins as a bald spot on the posterior occiput and extends anteriorly and bilaterally in a one to two inch wide band above the ear, at times extending to meet on the anterior aspect of the scalp.

It is stated that alopecia totalis (loss of all scalp hair) may ultimately develop in 5 to 10 per cent of cases of partial alopecia. This figure may be high in view of the fact that a high percentage of cases of mild alopecia resolve spontaneously,

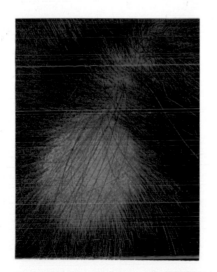

Figure 17–3 Alopecia areata with sharply defined oval patches of hair loss.

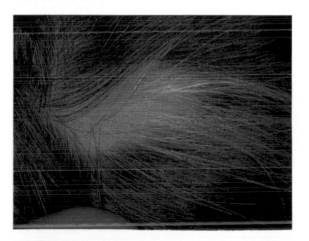

Figure 17–5 Alopecia areata with depigmented hairs simulating poliosis.

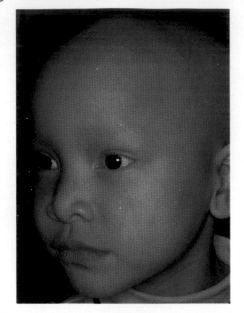

Figure 17–6 Alopecia universalis. Loss of scalp hair, eyebrows, and eyelashes in a 5-year-old boy.

thus never being seen by a physician. Progression to the totalis form occurs more slowly, but more frequently in children than in adults. If, in addition, there is complete or virtually complete loss of body hair, the disorder is termed alopecia universalis (Fig. 17–6).

Nail defects are seen in 10 to 20 per cent of cases. While it is true that the more extensive the disease, the more likely the possibility and severity of nail involvement, some patients may have gross nail dystrophy with little hair change. The most characteristic nail abnormality is a fine grid-like stippling, regularly arranged in horizontal or vertical rows or both, with pits smaller than those seen in patients with psoriasis. Ridging and dystrophy may, at times, be quite marked but, when present, are generally confined to only a few nails.

DIAGNOSIS. The diagnosis of alopecia areata is based upon its clinical picture. The sudden appearance and circumscribed non-scarring, patterned nature of hair loss frequently will distinguish it from other disorders of alopecia. Trichotillomania typically is associated with bizarre, irregular patches of hair loss, with areas of broken hairs of different lengths. The absence of signs of inflammation and scaling will generally help distinguish this disorder from that of tinea capitis. Alopecia due to secondary syphilis may be recognized by its moth-eaten appearance, irregular borders, incomplete loss of hair within individual patches, and a predilection for the posterior scalp. When the diagnosis is in doubt, microscopic examination of hairs with potassium hydroxide, fungal cultures, serological testing, and cutaneous punch biopsy frequently will help establish the proper diagnosis.

In newly formed patches of alopecia areata

the vast majority of hair follicles are in telogen phase. When a patch of alopecia has been present for a period of many months, however, most hairs are in the anagen phase. Histopathologic examination of affected areas is characterized by small hair structures and hair bulbs located higher in the scalp than normally seen. The most characteristic microscopic feature consists of a non-specific inflammatory infiltrate of the hair follicles and a round cell "swarm of bees" infiltration surrounding the hair bulbs.

The course of alopecia areata is variable and difficult to predict. Extension may continue for a few weeks. Frequently new patches of hair loss appear within a period of four to six weeks, and occasionally, after a period of four to ten months, spontaneous regrowth may occur. In general, when the process is limited to a few patches, the prognosis is good, with complete regrowth occurring within one year in 95 per cent of children; the earlier the onset, however, the poorer the prognosis. When the disorder is extensive or total, the possibility of complete and permanent recovery is poor, and about 30 per cent of patients will have future episodes of alopecia areata.

THERAPY. The therapy of alopecia areata consists of topical corticosteroids alone or under occlusion (such as may be achieved under a wig, bathing cap, or Saran wrap)[11, 12] or multiple intradermal corticosteroid injections, which frequently results in regrowth in tufts at injection sites within a period of four to six weeks. When an intralesional corticosteroid is used, a syringe with a 30-gauge needle or jet-injection may be utilized. All anti-inflammatory insoluble corticosteroids are effective. However, triamcinolone acetonide in concentrations of 5 to 10 mg per ml is the most practical for acute cases, with a maximum of 1 or 2 cc total at four to six week intervals (no more than

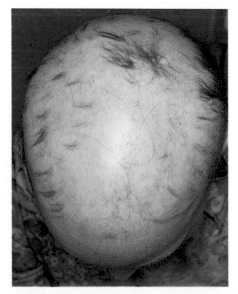

Figure 17–7 Alopecia totalis. Early regrowth of hair following intradermal corticosteroid injections.

one injection per site per month) (Fig. 17–7). Intradermal corticosteroid therapy usually results in a more rapid regrowth of hair in a high percentage of cases, but there is little evidence that this method of therapy alters the final outcome of the disorder.[13]

Although not recommended for general use, systemic steroids may be considered for carefully selected patients with severe involvement and an associated psychological handicap who do not respond to topical and intralesional steroid therapy. In such instances, prednisone, in dosages of 20 to 30 mg daily for periods of four to six weeks, followed by alternate-day therapy, may be beneficial and cause relatively few significant side effects. It must be emphasized that close follow-up evaluation is indicated in such cases and that the potential side effects associated with systemic corticosteroid therapy must be explained to the patient and his or her parents.[10, 14]

Recent experimental studies suggest a possible therapeutic approach utilizing contact sensitization with weekly applications of dinitrochlorobenzene (DNCB) sufficient to produce a mild contact dermatitis. Although the mechanism of the therapeutic effect is unknown, it has been suggested that the induced contact dermatitis may produce an accumulation of suppressor cells that neutralize the effects of lymphocytes surrounding the hair bulbs (an "antigenic-competitive phenomenon"). Studies suggest a possible mutagenic response to DNCB. This form of therapy, therefore, remains experimental and cannot be recommended for general use until further investigative evaluation is complete.[15, 16]

Traumatic Alopecia

Traumatic alopecia results from the forceful extraction of hair or the breaking of hair shafts by friction, traction, or other physical trauma. The

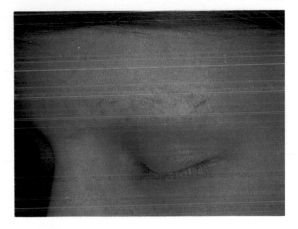

Figure 17–9 Trichotillomania of the eyebrow with characteristic short broken hairs.

usual causes are trichotillomania (a self-induced alopecia caused by plucking, pulling, or cutting the hair in a bizarre manner) and cosmetic practices, such as tight braiding or pony-tails; the use of tight rollers, barrettes, head bands, or rubber bands; hair straightening practices such as teasing or pulling, or frequent brushing with nylon bristles; and the use of hot combs and petrolatum (Figs. 17–8 to 17–12). Other common causes of traumatic alopecia include pressure, such as is seen on the occiput of infants who lie on their backs or are in the habit of "head-banging"; prolonged bed rest in one position in chronically ill persons; thermal or electric burns; repeated vigorous massage; a severe blow to the scalp; and avulsion, such as may occur after hair-pulling (Fig. 17–13).

Traction Alopecia. Traction alopecia is characterized by oval or linear areas of hair loss at the margins of the hair line, along the part, or scattered through the scalp, depending upon the type of traction or trauma. Peripheral scalp hair loss may occur in individuals who wear their hair in pony-tail style, and the hair loss from hair rollers is usually most conspicuous in the frontocentral area or around the margins of the scalp. Hot comb alopecia, seen primarily in black individuals who

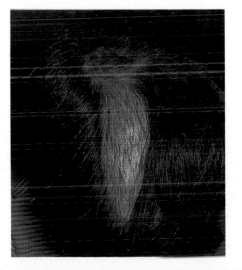

Figure 17–8 Trichotillomania of the scalp. A self-induced traumatic alopecia.

Figure 17–10 Traumatic alopecia produced by tight braiding of hair.

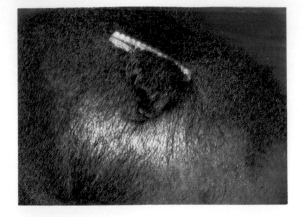

Figure 17–11   Traction alopecia caused by frequent use of hair curlers.

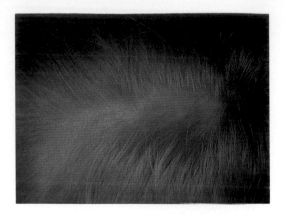

Figure 17–13   Traumatic alopecia. Alopecia induced by a severe blow to the scalp.

straighten their hair for cosmetic purposes, generally occurs on the vertex or marginal areas of the scalp. In severe chronic forms, however, the entire scalp may be involved.

Trichotillomania.   Trichotillomania is a self-limiting form of traction alopecia produced either consciously or subconsciously as the result of habit. Seen in children and young adults of both sexes, it is most commonly seen in children between four and ten years of age and young adolescents. The scalp is the most common site of involvement, but the eyebrows and eyelashes may also be affected as the patient plucks, twirls, or rubs hair-bearing areas, resulting in the epilation or breakage of hair shafts.

The habit is usually practiced in bed before the child falls asleep (when the parent does not notice the habit) or when the child is reading, writing, or watching television. In young individuals the condition is frequently associated with a habit of finger or thumb sucking. Although many authors emphasize severe psychological problems in patients with this disorder, most affected individuals are merely under varying degrees of emotional stress or have developed a habit that generally can be managed by a sympathetic physician and understanding parent.

Trichotillomania usually begins insidiously

as an irregular linear or rectangular area of partial hair loss. Affected areas are generally single, often frontal, frontotemporal, or frontoparietal in location, and frequently appear on the contralateral side of right- or left-handed individuals. The affected patches have irregularly shaped angular outlines and are never completely bald. Within the involved regions the hair is short or stubbly and broken off at varying lengths (Fig. 17–8).

If one maintains a high index of suspicion, traction alopecia can generally be distinguished from other forms of hair loss by its characteristic configuration and distribution. Occasionally the diagnosis can be confirmed by the finding of wads of hair under the pillow or bed, or by observation of the habit by a parent, teacher, or physician. When the diagnosis is suspected, regrowth of hair in a carefully shaved or occluded path of scalp in the involved area (in order to prevent manipulation) frequently will confirm the correct diagnosis. Clinical differentiation from alopecia areata is usually based upon the bizarre configuration, irregular outline, and presence of short stub-like broken hairs. Differentiation from tinea capitis may require Wood's light examination, microscopic examination of plucked hairs with potassium hydroxide (occasionally revealing node-like swellings of the hair shaft and broken hairs), and fungal culture (see Chapter 13). Of particular significance is the fact that the broken hairs of trichotillomania, unlike those of certain forms of tinea capitis, remain firmly rooted in the scalp, and the cutaneous surface is normal and stubbled rather than erythematous or scaly.

If the diagnosis remains in doubt, biopsy of the involved area is frequently helpful. The histopathologic features of trichotillomania consist primarily of catagen hairs, evidence of traumatic damage, the presence of keratin plugs and dilated follicular infundibula, the replacement of some hair follicles by fibrosis, and absence of significant inflammation or scarring.[17, 18] In taking biopsy specimens from suspected patients with trichotillomania it is best to carefully select the precise site of most recent hair loss.

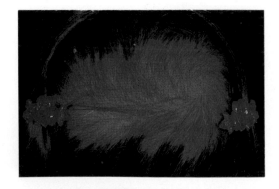

Figure 17–12   Traction alopecia caused by barettes.

The management of trichotillomania is often difficult and requires a strong doctor, patient, and parent relationship. Although patients occasionally will admit to touching the affected areas, they frequently will deny plucking, rubbing, or excessive manipulation. Direct confrontation and accusation frequently is detrimental and rarely helpful. Psychopathologic changes are said to be present in some 50 to 75 per cent of affected individuals. They are usually mild and require no special management. Deep emotional and psychological disorders occur in fewer than 5 per cent of cases of trichotillomania.

If patients are reassured, given an opportunity to express their emotional needs, and offered a reasonable therapeutic regimen such as a mild shampoo and scalp lotion (perhaps hydrocortisone in a 1.0 per cent concentration as a placebo or to "relieve pruritus or possible irritation"), the tic will frequently disappear. For those individuals with persistent or severe emotional problems, however, professional psychological assistance should be considered and, in those with a persistent habit, particularly nervous young females with long hair, the possibility of trichophagia and trichobezoar should be considered.[19]

Male Pattern Alopecia

Androgenic male pattern alopecia (male pattern baldness) occurs in both men and women and appears to be inherited as an autosomal dominant trait with variable expression. The onset of this androgenically induced disorder has been noted as early as 14 years of age; the earlier the onset, the more profound the subsequent alopecia.[7]

The mildest and often earliest form of androgenic baldness is seen as a symmetrical triangular recession of the hairline in the frontoparietal and occasionally frontal scalp margins. Uniform recession of the frontal hairline is seen during

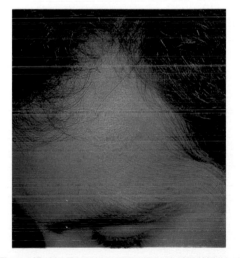

Figure 17-14 Triangular recession of the hairline in the frontotemporal scalp margin, the earliest and mildest form of male pattern alopecia (seen in 5 per cent of males before age 20).

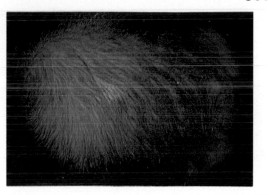

Figure 17-15 Androgenic male pattern baldness on the crown of the scalp of an adult male.

adolescence in 96 per cent of males and in about 80 per cent of females; it does not represent the first stage of male pattern alopecia and does not signify the onset of profound or premature baldness (Fig. 17-14). In 5 per cent of Caucasian males, alopecia is first observed before the age of 20, usually as symmetrical frontotemporal recession. It is generally not until the third or fourth decade that the incidence of this pattern increases and is associated with some loss of hair in the crown of the scalp (Fig. 17-15). In women the loss in rare instances progresses to the total crown involvement of males but otherwise appears to be a diminutive form of the disease as seen in males.

In a young male the onset of male pattern alopecia frequently causes severe distress and anxiety. Careful examination and repeated reassurance are required in order to discourage recourse to expensive and ineffective proprietary therapeutic regimens. Unfortunately modern medicine to date has found no effective therapy for male pattern androgenetic baldness. Massage and topical stimulating agents have no value, and the use of estrogenic creams and other hormonal approaches are ineffective or potentially hazardous.[20] Until recently treatment has been limited to reassurance or to the recommendation of artificial hair pieces. Currently, radical plastic surgery techniques and attempts at implantation of nylon filaments have been replaced by the multiple-punch autografting hair transplant technique.[21] Punch-graft hair transplants can be performed in the physician's office, and although not a panacea, when properly performed by an experienced dermatologist or plastic surgeon, a cosmetically satisfactory redistribution of hair generally can be achieved (Fig. 17-16).

SCARRING ALOPECIA

Scarring or cicatricial alopecia is the end result of a wide number of inflammatory processes in and about the pilosebaceous units, resulting in irreversible destruction of tissue and consequent permanent scarring alopecia of the affected areas. The scarring may be the result of a developmental

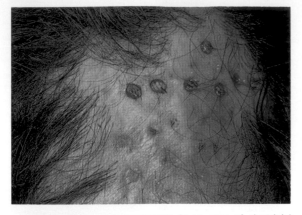

Figure 17–16   Hair transplants in an area of cicatricial alopecia.

defect (aplasia cutis) (Fig. 17–17); inflammatory changes of infective origin, such as severe bacterial, viral, or fungal infection; physical trauma (x-ray, trichotillomania practiced over a long period of time, thermal or caustic burns); neoplastic disorders; various dermatoses (lichen planus, lupus erythematosus, localized or systemic scleroderma); or various dermatologic syndromes, such as keratosis pilaris atrophicans, folliculitis decalvans, dissecting cellulitis of the scalp, acne keloidalis, pseudopelade, and alopecia mucinosa. This latter group of dermatologic disorders is described below.

Keratosis Pilaris Atrophicans

Numerous terms have been used to describe a group of interrelated syndromes characterized by atrophic variants of keratosis pilaris. These include keratosis pilaris atrophicans faciei (also known as ulerythema ophryogenes, atrophoderma vermiculata, and keratosis pilaris decalvans. These disorders occur sporadically and are presumed to be the result of inborn defects. The major histologic features include plugging and distension of hair follicles, dilatation of dermal vessels, perifollicular and perivascular lymphocytic infiltration, dermal atrophy, and horn cysts.[22]

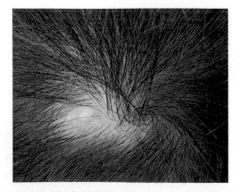

Figure 17–17   Cicatricial alopecia due to aplasia cutis.

Ulerythema Ophryogenes.   Ulerythema ophryogenes (keratosis pilaris atrophicans faciei) is a disorder primarily affecting infants, boys, and young men and is characterized by persistent reticular erythema, small horny papules, atrophy, and permanent loss of the involved hairs in the outer halves of the eyebrows. Occasionally the disorder extends to include the adjacent skin, adjacent scalp, and cheeks. To date there is no effective therapy for this disorder.

Atrophoderma Vermiculata.   Atrophoderma vermiculata (folliculitis ulerythema reticulata) is a variant of keratosis pilaris atrophicans, which usually has its onset between 5 and 12 years of age, occasionally later. This disorder is characterized by the formation of numerous tiny symmetrical atrophic and, at times, erythematous pits on the cheeks. Generally measuring 1 to 2 mm across and 1 mm deep, these cribriform lesions are separated one from another by narrow ridges of normal-appearing skin. Although there is no effective treatment for this disorder, dermabrasion frequently can improve the cosmetic appearance of affected individuals.

The variant termed *keratosis pilaris decalvans* occurs in infancy or early childhood. It is characterized by numerous milia and prominent follicular plugs on the nose and cheeks, and later, on the limbs and neck. Various exfoliants and keratolytics have been utilized for this disorder, but with limited success.

Folliculitis Decalvans

Folliculitis decalvans is a rare form of cicitricial alopecia characterized by erythematous scaling and small rounded or oval patches of scarring surrounded by perifollicular pustules. The etiology is unknown, but it appears to be associated with a long history of seborrheic dermatitis and a low-grade pustular reaction in hair follicles of the scalp, occasionally of the bearded, axillary, pubic or other cutaneous areas, resulting in a peripherally spreading inflammatory disease and alopecia. Although a bacterial folliculitis, such as caused by *Staphylococcus aureus*, at times is associated with this disorder, virulent pyococcal organisms frequently are not demonstrated. In many forms of this disorder the condition tends to persist indefinitely, and although the inflammation and cosmetic disability is frequently limited, severe forms, especially in males, may be particularly disfiguring.

In the pustular phase the histologic picture is characterized by polymorphonuclear microabscesses in the upper half of the pilosebaceous follicle and a perifollicular infiltrate that contains numerous plasma cells. In the atrophic phase the histology of the disorder is frequently indistinguishable from that seen in the atrophic phase of lichen planus or lupus erythematosus.

The treatment of folliculitis decalvans consists of topical antibiotics, systemic antibiotics, and, in severe or protracted cases, a combination of topical, intralesional, and systemic corticosteroids and long-term antibiotics. Unfortunately, in many individuals the disorder persists and may result in severe alopecia and scarring despite long-term and intensive therapy.

Dissecting Cellulitis of the Scalp

Dissecting cellulitis of the scalp, also termed perifolliculitis capitis abscedens et suffodiens, is a rare dissecting cellulitis of the scalp that leads to the formation of burrowing abscesses and fluctuant nodules connected by tortuous ridges or elevations. Seropurulent drainage may persist indefinitely, and cicatricial alopecia and keloid formation frequently develop. Seen primarily in individuals between 18 and 40 years of age, the disease occurs in Caucasians and Blacks, with a greater incidence in the latter, and men are affected more frequently than women.

The disease appears to have a slightly increased incidence in patients with chronic hidradenitis or acne conglobata. There is no specific therapy for this disorder. Local and systemic antibiotics, intralesional steroids, incision and drainage of abscesses, and x-ray therapy have been used with varying results, but the course is generally chronic, with remissions and relapses over many years.

Acne Keloidalis

Acne keloidalis (folliculitis keloidalis) is a chronic scarring folliculitis and perifolliculitis of the nape of the neck (occasionally the bearded area) that leads to the formation of keloidal papulels, nodules, and plaques.

Seen most frequently in postpuberal males, especially Blacks between the ages of 14 and 25, it has also been noted in Caucasian males and Black women. Although the precise cause of this disorder is not clear, it appears to be related to a persistent infection (frequently but not necessarily streptococcal or staphylococcal), with a tendency toward granulomatous change followed by eventual destruction of normal structures and their replacement by hypertrophic connective tissue and plasma cell infiltrate.

Treatment of this disorder is difficult and consists of topical antiseptic agents, long-term systemic antibiotics, intralesional corticosteroids, and, in some cases, perhaps x-ray therapy. In long-term cases with severe scarring, excision and plastic repair occasionally are beneficial.

Pseudopelade

Pseudopelade is a non-specific scarring form of alopecia of the scalp generally seen in adults. It is characterized by multiple small, round, oval, or irregularly shaped hairless cicatricial patches of varying sizes. Affected areas are shiny, ivory-white, or slightly pink in color and atrophic. Interspersed between the patches may be a few hair-containing dilated hair follicles. The etiology is unknown, and the onset of the disorder is insidious and asymptomatic. Lesions generally appear at the vertex of the scalp. They frequently coalesce to form finger-like projections and have been compared to "footprints in the snow."

The histopathologic examination of involved areas reveals perifollicular and perivascular infiltrates composed almost entirely of lymphocytes and a few histiocytes. Slight follicular hyperkeratosis may be present, and in late stages, extensive fibrosis of the dermis predominates.

There is no specific or effective therapy for this disorder. Infiltration of triamcinolone acetonide in a 2.5 mg per ml concentration into active areas at six to eight week intervals may be temporarily beneficial and, in persistently unresponsive cases, a reasonable cosmetic improvement frequently can be achieved by the multiple-punch autograft technique of hair transplantation.

Alopecia Mucinosa

Alopecia mucinosa (follicular mucinosis) is an inflammatory disorder characterized by sharply defined follicular papules or infiltrated plaques, with scaling, loss of hair, and accumulation of mucin (acid mucopolysaccharide) in sebaceous glands and the outer root sheaths of affected hair follicles. A relatively uncommon condition affecting children as well as adults, the disorder presents three morphologic forms: flat rough patches consisting of grouped follicular papules, scaly plaques formed through the coalescence of follicular papules, and nodular boggy infiltrated plaques with overlying erythema and scaling. Distributed primarily on the face, scalp, neck, and shoulders (occasionally the trunk and extremities), lesions are usually devoid of hair. Except in the scalp or eyebrows, this generally is not a conspicuous feature.

The cause of follicular mucinosis is unknown. In the majority of cases (those under age 40) it is a benign idiopathic condition. In persons above age 40, however, the presence of boggy infiltrated plaques of alopecia mucinosa may be the first sign of an accompanying reticulosis, usually mycosis fungoides (an uncommon neoplastic disorder of the lymphoreticular system generally affecting adults and but rarely seen in childhood).

In the benign form, lesions of alopecia mucinosa generally appear as grouped skin-colored papules or firm and coarsely rough plaques of erythema measuring 2 to 5 cm in diameter, sometimes larger, with prominent follicles and fine scaling. In patients with solitary or few lesions, clearing usually occurs spontaneously within a period of two years. In the chronic form, lesions are more numerous and more widely distributed, and the plaques may be flat, domed, or elevated. Destruction of follicles may give rise to permanent alopecia, and the disorder may persist, with new lesions continuing to appear over a period of many years.

Alopecia mucinosa must be differentiated from lichen spinulosus, pityriasis rubra pilaris, tinea infection, pityriasis alba, granulomatous diseases, and the papulosquamous group of disorders. When the diagnosis remains in doubt, cutaneous biopsy of an affected area is generally confirmatory. The histopathologic picture is characterized by intracellular edema, loss of cohesion between cells, formation of cystic spaces, and accumulation of mucin within the external root sheaths and sebaceous glands. This substance shows metachromatic staining with Giemsa stain, is PAS-negative, stains with alcian blue, and is digested by hyaluronidase.

Generally, especially in children and young adults, lesions of alopecia mucinosa involute spontaneously. Although some cases appear to benefit from topical or intralesional corticosteroids or x-ray therapy, such claims are difficult to evaluate,[23] since spontaneous healing is the rule.

HAIR SHAFT ABNORMALITIES WITH INCREASED FRAGILITY

Variations in the structure of the hair shaft are a common occurrence and, at times, may provide clues to other pathologic abnormalities. Because each hair shaft anomaly has a distinctive morphology, the diagnosis frequently can be established in the office by microscopic examination of preferably snipped rather than pulled hairs.

Monilethrix

Monilethrix (beaded hair) is a rare autosomal dominant disorder affecting both sexes equally. It is characterized by variation in hair shaft thickness, with small node-like deformities that produce a beaded appearance, internodal fragility, breakage, and partial alopecia.

In this disorder, normal neonatal lanugo hairs are shed during the first few weeks of life, and subsequent hair growth, generally at about the second month of life, becomes dry, lusterless, and brittle, failing to grow to any appreciable length. In severe cases the infant may remain bald, or the scalp hair may be sparse, easily fractured, and stubble-like. Although generally a disorder of scalp hair, body hairs may also be affected.[7] Occasionally this disorder is not apparent during infancy, only to become apparent later in childhood or during adult life.

The cause of monilethrix is unknown. It is not characteristic of any systemic disease or metabolic defect, but may be seen in association with keratosis pilaris, brittle nails, cataracts, or dental abnormalities. Although argininosuccinic aciduria has been reported in patients with this disorder, this association requires confirmation. A tendency to spontaneous improvement or remission may occur at puberty or during pregnancy and, in some cases, may continue during adult life. In some individuals, however, the disease may persist unchanged throughout adulthood. Prognosis, accordingly, is guarded, and there is no effective therapy for this disorder.

Trichorrhexis Nodosa

Trichorrhexis nodosa, the most common hair shaft anomaly, is a distinctive disorder manifested by increased fragility due to the presence of grayish-white nodules, which, under a light microscope, give the appearance of two interlocking brushes or brooms, an appearance based upon segmental longitudinal splitting of fibers without complete fracture.

The disorder features dry lusterless short hair that is easily fractured and may be seen in a congenital or familial form. In affected individuals scalp hair breaks easily and leaves short stubby broken ends, areas of partial alopecia, and may be associated with tooth or nail abnormalities. The occasional association of congenital or familial forms of trichorrhexis nodosa in mentally retarded children with argininosuccinic aciduria is of particular import. In such cases the amino acid arginine can be measured in the red blood cells as well as skin fibroblasts, and marked elevations of argininosuccinic acid may be detected in the urine, blood, and cerebrospinal fluid. It must be remembered that this is a relatively uncommon disorder, and most patients with trichorrhexis nodosa have no underlying disease.[24]

The most common type of hair loss secondary to structural hair shaft abnormality is that seen in patients with *acquired* forms of trichorrhexis nodosa. This disorder is seen in two clinical varieties, proximal trichorrhexis nodosa (a common condition seen in the black population) and distal trichorrhexis nodosa (a disorder observed mostly in Caucasians and Orientals).

Proximal trichorrhexis nodosa appears to be associated with a genetic predisposition and trauma from hair straightening, tight caps, or harsh brushing and combing techniques. Distal trichorrhexis nodosa is a disorder that occurs in otherwise normal hair as a result of cumulative cuticular damage (vigorous combing and brushing, repeated salt-water bathing, prolonged sun exposure, and frequent shampooing). Cream rinses and protein conditioners are helpful, and if hair straightening procedures, vigorous grooming habits, and thermal and chemical trauma to the hair are discontinued, the acquired forms of trichorrhexis nodosa generally improve within a period of two to four years.[25, 26]

Trichorrhexis Invaginata

Trichorrhexis invaginata (bamboo hair) is a peculiar nodular defect caused by abnormal intussusception or telescope-like invagination along the

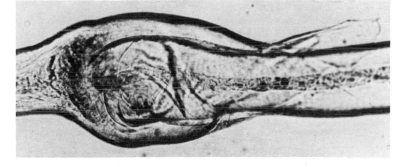

Figure 17–18 Trichorrhexis invaginata (bamboo hair). A nodular defect caused by intussusception of the hair shaft (Hurwitz S, Kirsch N, McGuire J: Arch. Dermatol. *103*:266, 1971).

hair shaft, which microscopically resembles the ball-and-cup joints of bamboo (Fig. 17–18). A relatively rare disorder, it is more common in females than in males, may involve all body hairs, and clinically is characterized by dry, lusterless, easily fractured sparse and short hair (Fig. 17–19). This disorder has been found in a rare, apparently autosomal recessive genodermatosis known as Netherton's disease, a combination of trichorrhexis invaginata, various forms of ichthyosis, and, at times, atopy, manifested by flexural eczema, allergic vasomotor rhinitis, asthma, angioneurotic edema, urticaria, or anaphylactic reaction. Although ichthyosis linearis circumflexa (see Chapter 7) is the form of ichthyosis most frequently seen in patients with this disorder, studies suggest that the original patient reported by Netherton probably had a form of lamellar ichthyosis.[27, 28]

The hair defect in trichorrhexis invaginata appears in infancy, and all hair is affected to some degree. No specific therapy is available for this hair abnormality. Although spontaneous remission of the hair defect can occur (generally between 6 and 15 years of age), many cases will persist into adulthood.[28]

Pili Torti

Pili torti (twisted hairs) is an autosomal dominant congenital hair defect of variable expression characterized by dry, fragile, twisted hairs. It affects females (chiefly blondes) more often than males and generally is observed in infancy as a patchy or diffuse hair loss. Although twisted hairs may be found in some individuals, the hair of children with classic pili torti, in contrast to those with pili torti associated with copper deficiency (Menkes' kinky hair syndrome), is clinically normal at birth, but by the age of two or three years or later is replaced by brittle hair. The hairs shimmer in reflected light, and the twisted feature of this disorder often creates a "spangled" appearance. Other ectodermal defects often present are keratosis pilaris, dental abnormalities, dystrophic nails, and corneal opacities. Reports of patients with pili torti and sensorineural hearing loss suggest early auditory testing for patients with this disorder.[29]

The scalp hair in patients with pili torti becomes more normal with time, and although twisted hairs can still be found in the adult scalp, the cosmetic appearance may be normal by puberty. Those who still manifest the disorder at puberty, however, are unlikely to show significant improvement with age.

The diagnosis of pili torti is confirmed by microscopic examination of snipped hairs. Although a dry mount frequently is satisfactory, immersion of the hairs in water or a weak solution of potassium hydroxide (10 per cent) often allows swelling of the hairs, which may assist in the microscopic differentiation of abnormal from normal hairs. Other than reduction of trauma to reduce breakage, there is no effective treatment for this disorder.

Menkes' Kinky Hair Syndrome

Menkes' kinky hair syndrome (trichopoliodystrophy) is a rare, sex-linked recessive neurodegenerative disorder that affects infant males and is characterized by coarse facies, pili torti, temperature instability, seizures, psychomotor retardation, arterial intimal changes, low or absent plasma copper and ceruloplasmin, growth failure, increased susceptibility to infection, and death, generally by age three or four years.[30, 31, 32] Clinical features often include premature birth, hypothermia, and relatively normal development until two to six months of age, when drowsiness and lethargy are noted, intractable seizures begin, and growth and

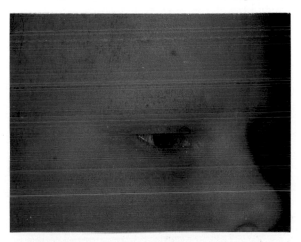

Figure 17–19 Alopecia in a patient with trichorrhexis invaginata.

development cease. Usually the hair is fine, dull, sparse, and poorly pigmented in infancy, stands on end, and looks and feels like steel wool. Additional features include a seborrheic rash, which may be coincidental; tortuous cerebral and other medium-sized arteries; osteoporosis; frequent subdural hematomas; widening of the metaphyses, with spurring; and frequent fractures, at times simulating the radiologic findings characteristic of patients with the battered child syndrome. Although pili torti is generally a prominent feature of this disorder, other less frequently reported hair abnormalities include monilethrix and trichorrhexis nodosa.

The combination of clinical features, bone abnormalities, and low plasma copper and ceruloplasmin levels establishes the correct diagnosis in patients with this disorder. Since the demonstration of a defect in intestinal absorption and utilization of copper, parenteral copper and ceruloplasmin therapy have been attempted, with results varying from a temporary arrest to clinical worsening of the disorder. Although treatment has raised plasma copper and ceruloplasmin levels to normal, possible irreversible damage prior to diagnosis (presumably in utero) cautions against undue optimism in using intravenous copper therapy for this disorder.[32]

HAIR SHAFT ABNORMALITIES WITHOUT INCREASED HAIR FRAGILITY

Fragilitas Crinium

Splitting of the hair shaft along its long axis (fragilitas crinium, trichoptilosis) is a common condition occurring particularly in the hair of girls and women who subject their hairs to various chemical and physical agents in the course of cosmetic treatment.[3] Although the disorder may occur anywhere along the length of the shaft, splitting and fraying at the ends of dry and heavily bleached hair is a particularly common manifestation of this disorder.

The condition is readily distinguished by examination with a hand lens or low-power microscope, and therapy consists of gentle grooming techniques and the application of oils or cream rinses.

Pili Annulati

Pili annulati (ringed hair) is a rare familial defect of keratin synthesis involving the cortex of the hair shaft of scalp hair and is characterized by alternating bands of dark and light hair. The banding is due to an irregular distribution of air-filled cavities within the cortex of the hair shaft, which appear lighter by reflected light and darker by transmitted light.[33] The disorder is noted shortly after birth and is of equal sex distribution. The hair shaft is structurally strong and the bright rings tend to produce an attractive highlight. There are no associated defects, and therapy is unnecessary.

Pseudopili annulati is an unusual variant of normal hair in which bright bands are seen at intervals along the hair shaft. Secondary to periodic twisting or curling of the hair shaft, this banding is conspicuous only in blond hairs and represents an optical effect due to reflection and refraction of light by flattened and twisted hair surfaces. This too is generally an attractive phenomenon and does not require therapy.[34]

Woolly Hair

The subject of woolly hair is confused by the use of such terms as woolly, kinky, spun glass, crimped, frizzly, and steely to define the clinical appearance of peculiar hair that will not group in locks or lie down flat and is difficult to comb or brush.[35] The term woolly hair should be reserved to describe unruly scalp hair that curls readily in spirals but does not form locks and shows a slow twist on its long axis. It is an autosomal dominant inherited disorder in which the entire scalp hair is distinctly different from that of non-affected family members. The individual hairs of the scalp are fine and dry in texture, light in color, corrugated at intervals, and resemble the crimp found in the wool of sheep. There is no known means of altering the manner of hair growth in this disorder. Treatment, therefore, is purely symptomatic.

Woolly Hair Nevus

The woolly hair nevus is a rare condition and, in contradistinction to woolly hair of the entire scalp, is without familial correlation. It arises on the scalp as one or more patches of unruly hair that are quite different in color, shape, and consistency from the normal surrounding scalp hair. The hairs on the affected area are usually smaller in diameter and lighter in color, and appear more sparse than those on the rest of the scalp. They normally are not fragile, and when examined under a dissecting microscope, the individual hairs are noted to twist about their long axis. The majority of reported cases of woolly hair nevus have been recognized during the first few months of life, but some have appeared in young adulthood. The cause of this disorder is unknown. In about 50 per cent of cases, woolly hair nevus coexists with a linear nevus elsewhere on the skin.[35] Epidermal nevi, when present, are generally on the same side of the body as the woolly hair nevus and commonly involve the neck, shoulder, or arm. No other cutaneous or systemic disorders have been associated with this condition; nails and teeth are normal, and there is no known treatment.

HYPERTRICHOSIS AND HIRSUTISM

Excessive hairiness may be localized or diffuse, congenital or acquired, and normal or patho-

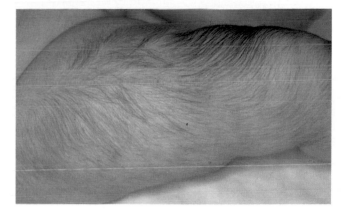

Figure 17–20 Hypertrichosis (a localized pattern of excessive hair growth) in an infant with hemihypertrophy of the right leg (Hurwitz S, Klaus S N: Arch. Dermatol. *103*:98, 1971).

logical. The terms hypertrichosis and hirsutism are frequently used inappropriately and synonymously to describe a presence of excessive hair on the body. Hirsutism implies an excessive growth of body hair in women or children (mostly females) in an adult male-pattern distribution and implies an androgen-induced hair pattern. Hypertrichosis, conversely, refers merely to localized patterns of excessive hair growth[7] (Figs. 17–20 and 17–21).

The most common form of hirsutism is not a disease. It merely represents a physiologic variant of hair growth in persons in a civilization that considers hairiness in women to be cosmetically undesirable. Endocrinopathic hirsutism, due to excessive secretion of androgenic hormone, is a relatively uncommon disorder. Complete endocrinologic workup of adolescent or adult females in whom the sole abnormality is excessive hair growth without other evidence of masculinism or menstrual abnormality, therefore, frequently is unnecessary (see Idiopathic Hirsutism below).

Congenital Hypertrichosis

Generalized hypertrichosis in the newborn generally represents a temporary normal condition. Except in the rare inherited disorder hypertrichosis lanuginosa, the first fine soft unmedullated and usually unpigmented lanugo hairs are generally shed in utero during the seventh or eighth month of gestation. Premature infants, however, frequently display this fine coat of lanugo hair, particularly on the face, limbs, and trunk. In such infants the fine lanugo hairs are shed during the first months of life and replaced by normal terminal hair growth, generally before the first six months of life.[2]

Hypertrichosis Lanuginosa. Hypertrichosis lanuginosa is an exceedingly rare heritable disorder in which there is persistence, or an acquired excessive production, of lanugo hairs. Affected infants, accordingly, may be unusually hairy at birth or may develop hirsutism in early childhood. This type of hairiness has attracted considerable attention over the years, and those afflicted by this disorder have been labeled by terms such as "dog-face men and women," "human Skye Terriers," or "monkey-men."

There are two clinical forms of congenital hypertrichosis lanuginosa. The dog-face type is transmitted as an autosomal dominant trait. In this form, affected individuals develop typical lanugo growth, reaching several inches in length over the first years of life. This persists and is associated with other congenital anomalies. The second, or monkey-face, variety is of uncertain heredity and is associated with a high incidence of infant mortality. Lanugo hair is present at birth, and surviving patients develop a simian-like facies.

In adults, acquired forms of hypertrichosis lanuginosa appear to have a strong association with internal malignancy (adenocarcinoma). Prominent red papillae on the tip and distal third of the tongue have been described and appear to be a prominent feature of the adult form of this disorder associated with underlying malignancy.[36]

The Cornelia de Lange Syndrome. The Cornelia de Lange syndrome is a congenital disorder consisting of marked hirsutism; cutis marmorata; hypoplastic genitals, nipples, and umbilicus; growth and skeletal abnormalities; mental retardation; and a characteristic low-pitched and growl-

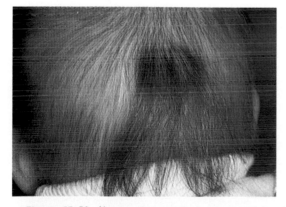

Figure 17–21 Nevoid circumscribed hypertrichosis. A congenital growth of thicker, darker, and longer hairs on the occipital scalp of a 4-month-old infant.

ing cry. Instances of affected siblings have been reported, but most cases have been sporadic and the disorder appears to be the result of a homozygous recessive mutation. The face of afflicted individuals is characterized by overgrowth of the eyebrows, long eyelashes, high upper lip, saddle-nose, and a cyanotic hue about the eyes, nose, and mouth. Children with this disorder often have recurrent respiratory infections and gastrointestinal upsets; seizures have been observed in about 20 per cent of reported cases, and most patients die before the age of six years.

Nevoid Hypertrichosis. Growth of hair abnormal in length, shaft diameter, or color for the site, size, and age of the patient may occur in association with other nevoid abnormalities or as isolated circumscribed developmental defects.[3]

Abnormal tufts of hair in the lumbosacral area (the faun-tail nevus) may be associated with duplication of a portion of the spinal cord (diastematomyelia). Although neurologic signs of this disorder generally appear during childhood, they may be delayed until the later teenage years.

Hypertrichosis may also be a characteristic of melanocytic nevi, Becker's nevus, nevoid circumscribed hypertrichosis, chronic low-grade physical trauma, chemical irritation, or hormonal stimulation. Although for years individuals have been advised not to pluck, cut, or shave areas of hypertrichosis, it now is apparent that cutting, shaving, or epilation of such areas does not produce faster or thicker growth or increased predisposition to neoplastic change.

Generalized Hypertrichosis

Generalized hypertrichosis may be associated with nervous system disorders (postencephalitic hypertrichosis, multiple sclerosis, anorexia nervosa, the Hurler syndrome, the Cornelia de Lange syndrome, and hypertrichosis lanuginosa). Other disorders that may be associated with hypertrichosis include acrodynia, hypothyroidism, dermatomyositis in some children, gross malnutrition, and various forms of drug-induced hypertrichosis. Drug-induced hypertrichosis may be seen following the administration of diphenylhydantoin (usually after two or three months of treatment); hexachlorobenzene, as in the classic epidemic of drug-induced porphyria cutanea tarda in Turkey (Chapter 4, reference 28); occasionally following the systemic use of testosterone propionate, streptomycin, cortisone, diazoxide,[37] or penicillamine; or in association with hyperpigmentation in some individuals treated with systemic psoralens and ultraviolet light exposure.

Idiopathic Hirsutism

The term idiopathic hirsutism is used to describe the presence in females of excessive body hair in a male sexual pattern (the face, particularly the upper lip, chest, abdomen, arms, and legs) in the absence of clinical evidence of disturbed endocrine or metabolic function. The pathogenesis of idiopathic hirsutism is assumed to be an increased stimulation of the hair follicles of genetically predisposed females by normal levels of androgenic hormones.[7]

The incidence of hirsutism in any population is difficult to assess, since the range of normal is quite wide, subject to individual acceptance, and includes that which is not always socially acceptable in a particular culture. Latin, Jewish, and Welsh women in general have more hair than their counterparts of Northern European, Japanese, and Indian heritage. In such cases the physician should be cognizant as to what is normal and acceptable to some individuals yet unacceptable and a source of anguish to others.

A detailed history and thorough physical examination generally will help the physician decide whether or not a full endocrinologic investigation is indicated. When hirsutism is observed in a postpuberal female without other signs of masculinity (receding hairline, deepening of the voice, or evidence of menstrual disturbance) there is little likelihood of endocrine disease. When the disorder does not appear to be physiologic in nature, abnormalities of the pituitary, adrenals, and ovaries must be ruled out. Of these, the adrenogenital, Cushing, Stein-Leventhal, and Achard-Thiers syndromes are the most frequently implicated. If endocrine abnormality is suspected, minimal laboratory testing for excessive androgen production should include urinary 17-ketosteroids, plasma testosterone levels, and morning and evening cortisol levels.

Once endocrine or local factors have been ruled out, there are several ways in which the appearance of excessive hair may be modified. Cutting with a scissors or shaving with a razor or electric shaver, although occasionally not psychologically acceptable to the patient, are the simplest methods and least likely to irritate the skin, and bleaching by a 6 per cent hydrogen peroxide solution or a commercial bleach may be used to render the objectionable hair less conspicuous. Contrary to a popular misconception, there is no evidence that cutting, plucking, or shaving leads to neoplastic potential or increases the growth or coarseness of hair.

Gentle rubbing with a pumice stone will help remove fine hairs. Plucking or wax epilation (essentially a form of widespread plucking) by application of a warm wax preparation to the affected areas, although slightly uncomfortable, is effective. Depilatories consist of sulfides of alkali metals or alkaline earths or of thioglycolate-containing agents that destroy the projecting hair shafts by degradation of disulfide bonds. Of these, the sulfide-containing preparations are more effective, but more irritating, and produce a disagreeable hydrogen sulfide odor. The thioglycolate-containing agents are less irritating, but slower in action and less effective on coarse hairs.

Electrolysis is a tedious procedure and, even in the best of hands, one can expect up to 25 per cent regrowth. Although not all patients with excessive facial hair are suitable candidates and overaggressive electrolysis may produce perceptible scarring, when done carefully by knowledgeable individuals this procedure generally offers a satisfactory approach to hair removal.

PIGMENTARY CHANGES OF HAIR

Premature Graying

Graying of human hair is caused by a reduction in the activity of melanocytes within hair follicles. Premature graying of hair, termed canities, refers to a loss of color, especially of scalp hair, at an age earlier than that generally accepted as physiological (before the age of 20 in Caucasians and 30 in Blacks).[3] It may be seen as an early sign of pernicious anemia and in hyperthyroidism and other thyroid disorders, progeria, Werner's disease, Rothmund-Thomson disease, vitiligo, alopecia areata, poliosis, tuberous sclerosis, neurofibromatosis, and the Waardenburg and Vogt-Koyanagi syndromes.

Premature graying may be readily masked, if desired, by chemical rinses and dyes. Since the possibility of carcinogenesis or chromosomal damage due to chemical hair dyes has recently been suggested,[38] the possibility of this risk may be avoided by the use of vegetable dyes.

Green Discoloration

Recent reports have described the occasional occurrence of green discoloration in the hair of light-haired (blond) individuals. After elaborate analyses of hair, pigment, and possible trace elements, it is now apparent that the discoloration is related to copper used as an algae-retardant in swimming pools[39] or to household tap water containing excessive amounts of copper.[40] In patients with copper tinting of hair from household plumbing, the introduction of fluoride into a town water supply (thus acidifying the water and causing copper to be leached from the plumbing system) or a ground wire connecting a faulty electrical apparatus to the copper water pipes (thus diverting sufficient flow of electric current through the water system to dissolve copper) have been implicated as possible causes of this condition.

Knowledgeable swimming-pool owners and swimming enthusiasts are often aware of this problem. In such cases, the use of a copper-based algicide should be discontinued, and in cases related to household tap water, electrical grounding of household plumbing and adjustment of the pH of the tap water will help prevent recurrences.

NAILS

The nails are convex horny structures originating from a matrix that develops from a groove formed by epidermal invagination on the dorsum of the distal phalanges during the ninth week of fetal life. At 10 weeks a smooth shiny quadrangular area can be recognized on the distal dorsal surface of each digit, and formation is completed by the twentieth week of gestation. While the nail plate is translucent and essentially colorless, most of the exposed nail appears pink, as the result of transmission of color from the adherent richly vascular underlying nail bed. Usually in the thumbs, and in a variable number of digits, a white crescent-shaped lunula may be seen projecting from under the proximal nail folds. The white color of the lunula is thought to be the result of incomplete keratinization of this portion of the nail plate and the looseness of the underlying connective tissue in this region of the nail bed.[41]

Unlike hairs, the nails grow continuously throughout life and normally are not shed. Although the nails of individual fingers grow at different rates, the normal rate of growth of fingernails varies between 0.5 and 1.2 mm (approximately 1.0 mm) per week; the rate of toenail growth is one-third to one-half that of the fingernails. Many dermatoses that characteristically involve the skin and hair may also affect the nails. These include disorders such as eczema, psoriasis, lichen planus, Darier's disease, alopecia areata, onychomycosis, ectodermal dysplasia, dyskeratosis congenita, and epidermolysis bullosa.

CONGENITAL AND HEREDITARY DISEASES

Atrophic nails range from complete absence of the nail to nails that are poorly or partially developed. They frequently result from generalized congenital disorders but also may develop as the result of trauma, infection, or acquired cutaneous conditions.

Median Nail Dystrophy

Median nail dystrophy (dystrophia unguium mediana canaliformis) (Fig. 17–22) is an uncommon temporary nail disorder in which a split or canal-like dystrophy develops in one or more

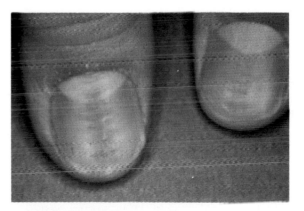

Figure 17–22 Median nail dystrophy (dystrophia unguium mediana canaliformis). An uncommon disorder in which a canal-like dystrophy develops in one or more nails.

nails, usually those of the thumb. The cause is unknown but appears to be related to some temporary defect in the matrix that interferes with nail formation. The split occurs at the cuticle, generally slightly off the midline, and proceeds outwards as the nail grows. Other than avoidance of trauma, there is no effective treatment for this disorder.

Fragile Nails

Fragile, brittle, or split nails (fragilitas unguium) are a common complaint of children (particularly adolescent females) and women (frequently housewives who often have their hands in soap and water). There is evidence that the underlying defect is an architectural abnormality that frequently is aggravated by excessive manicuring and the frequent use of solvents to remove nail polish. Although gelatin administration (Knox gelatin, one envelope daily, mixed with water, juice, or some other beverage), or other forms of gelatin (such as those available in capsule forms) have been recommended, there is no evidence that this form of therapy helps the disorder. The regular use of an emollient hand cream to the cuticle, avoidance of excessive manipulation, and the use of several layers of nail polish in an effort to splint the nail, with avoidance of all but oily polish removers, although not curative, appears to be somewhat beneficial.

Twenty-Nail Dystrophy

Twenty-nail dystrophy is an idiopathic nail dystrophy of all 20 nails that begins insidiously in early childhood (Fig. 17–23). Characterized by excessive ridging, with longitudinal striations and opalescent discoloration, the disorder is first observed between 1½ and 12 years. Apparently a self-limiting condition of childhood, treatment other than regular manicuring and application of nail lacquer to improve the appearance is unrewarding. The patient and parents should be advised of the self-limiting and reversible nature of the condition and of the fact that there are no reports of adults with this disorder.[42]

Nail-Patella Syndrome

The nail-patella syndrome, also termed the nail-patella-elbow syndrome or osteo-onycho-dysplasia, is characterized by the absence or hypoplasia of the patella and nails, subluxation of the radial heads, and, in some pedigrees, renal dysplasia, which presents as a chronic glomerulonephritis (Figs. 17–24, 17–25). Other bone features include thickened scapulae, hyperextendable joints, and iliac horns. It is inherited as an autosomal dominant disorder of variable expressivity, with high penetrance and linkage between the loci controlling the syndrome and ABO blood groups.[43]

The nail dystrophy may vary from nothing more than a triangular lunula, especially of the thumbs and index fingers, to moderate to severe dysplasia of the medial and distal aspects of the index and thumb nails; occasionally nails of other fingers and sometimes the toes may also be affected (Fig. 17–24). The nail changes, seen in 98 per cent of affected patients, consist of triangle-shaped lunulas, softening, spooning, discoloration, central grooving, splitting and cracking, narrowing, and, less commonly, thickening.[44] The thumbnails and great toenails, and occasionally the nails of the index fingers, are the most severely affected, often with severe hypoplasia or partial or total absence of the nails of the thumbs and index fingers. The remaining nails, if involved, are progressively damaged, from index to little finger, and the hands show symmetrical nail involvement.[45]

The renal involvement has been reported in up to 42 per cent of patients with this disorder.[45] Patients with renal lesions are asymptomatic and show proteinuria, reduced renal clearance, and hematuria. Although many affected individuals

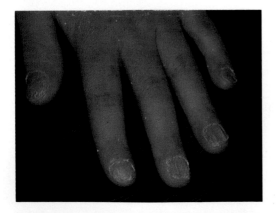

Figure 17–23 Twenty-nail dystrophy. Opalescent discoloration, excessive ridging, and longitudinal striations of all 20 nails in childhood.

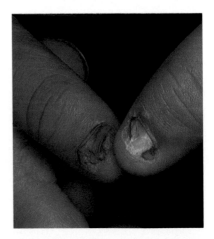

Figure 17–24 Nail-patella syndrome (osteo-onycho-dysplasia). Triangular-shaped lunulas and severe dystrophy of the thumb nail.

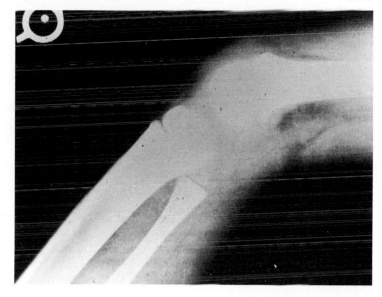

Figure 17–25 Nail-patella syndrome. Absence of the patella as seen on X-ray. Reproduced with permission from Taybi, H.: Radiology of Syndromes. Copyright © 1975 by Year Book Medical Publishers, Inc., Chicago.)

with this complication do well, the prognosis remains guarded.

Pachyonychia Congenita

Pachyonychia congenita (the Jadassohn-Lewandowsky syndrome) is an unusual congenital and sometimes familial disorder, inherited in an autosomal dominant fashion, and characterized by dyskeratosis of the fingernails and toenails, hyperkeratosis of the palms and soles, follicular keratosis (especially about the knees and elbows), hyperhidrosis of the palms and soles, and oral leukokeratosis. Frequently not all features of the disorder are present in affected individuals.[46]

Finger and toenail changes, usually present at birth or during the first year of life, consist of thickened, tubular, and hard nails, the undersurface being filled with a horny, yellowish-brown material that causes the nail to project upwards from the nail bed at the free margin. Paronychial inflammation and recurrent loss or shedding of nails are common.

Hyperhidrosis of the palms and soles nearly always occurs, and the rest of the skin is frequently quite dry and often described as ichthyotic in nature. Hyperkeratosis of the palms and soles, seen in up to 65 per cent of cases, generally appears during the first few years of life. Bullae frequently appear, particularly during warm weather, on the toes, heels, sides of the feet, and occasionally palms.

Pinhead-sized grayish-black follicular papules appear in over 50 per cent of cases in areas of trauma, on the extensor surfaces of the extremities, and on the popliteal fossae, lumbar region, and buttocks, and less commonly on the face and scalp. The hair is frequently noted to be dry, and when the follicular papules are numerous, alopecia has been seen in association with this disorder. In some cases there may be malformation of the teeth manifested by natal teeth with poor dentition.

Early oral lesions are frequently present in the form of opaque white or grayish-white plaques (leukokeratosis) on the dorsum of the tongue or the buccal mucosa at the interdental line or as neonatal teeth. Less frequently associated findings include cheilitis, scrotal tongue, corneal dystrophy, hoarseness, and steatocystoma multiplex, which is manifested as large epidermal cysts of the head, neck, and upper chest (a complication not readily evident until puberty).[46, 47]

The differential diagnosis includes the hereditary mucosal syndromes that produce leukokeratotic lesions of the oral mucosa. Of these, dyskeratosis congenita and Darier's disease, in particular, should be ruled out. The characteristic nail changes and associated findings generally allow proper identification of this disorder. Histopathologic examination of the leukokeratotic oral lesions show thickening of the oral epithelium and extensive intracellular vacuolization, similar to that seen in the white sponge nevus.

Lesions persist for life, and treatment is directed toward relief of the hyperkeratosis by the use of oral vitamin A in large doses (potentially toxic and not universally successful); 20 per cent urea in an emollient cream, available as Carmol-20 (Ingram); 60 per cent propylene glycol in water under occlusion; or 6 per cent salicylic acid in a gel containing propylene glycol (Keralyt gel, Westwood), which aids in the debridement of the excessive keratin. The nails may be treated by surgical avulsion, with scraping of the matrix to prevent regrowth, and in severe cases, drastic amputation of the distal phalanges has been resorted to in an effort to restore function.

OTHER NAIL DYSTROPHIES

Habit-tic Dystrophy. Injuries to the base of the nail and nail matrix may result in longitudinal ridging or splitting of the nail. A common form of nail injury is that caused by a habit or tic. Habit-tic

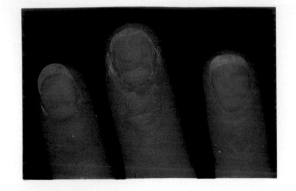

Figure 17-26   Dystrophy, central depression, and numerous horizontal ridges of the nails, seen in association with paronychia due to a habit-tic.

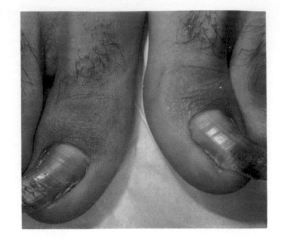

Figure 17-28   Onychogryphosis. A hypertrophic nail deformity in which the nails become thick and circular in cross section. Failure to cut the nails at regular intervals frequently results in a curved ram's horn deformity.

dystrophy is caused by continuous picking of the nail cuticle of the affected digit with a finger (usually the index finger) of the same hand and generally is characterized by a depression down the center of a nail with numerous horizontal ridges extending across it (Fig. 17–26).

Beau's Lines.   Beau's lines are transverse grooves or furrows which originate under the proximal nail fold (Fig. 17–27). They develop as a non-specific reaction to any stress that temporarily interrupts nail formation and become visible on the surface of the nail plate several weeks or more after onset of the disease that caused the condition. They first appear at the cuticle, move forward with the growth of the nail, and since normal nails grow at a rate of approximately one millimeter per week, the duration and time of the illness frequently can be estimated by the width of the furrow and its distance from the cuticle.

Onychogryphosis.   Onychogryphosis is a hypertrophic nail deformity most commonly seen in the toenails. Some cases of nail hypertrophy are developmental, the nails becoming thick and circular in cross section instead of flat (thus re-

sembling a claw). In more severe forms of onychogryphosis one or more nails become grossly thickened, and with failure to cut the nails frequently and at regular intervals, increase in length results in a curved ram's horn type of deformity (Fig. 17–28). Treatment requires regular paring or trimming, usually by a podiatrist using files, nail clippers, or mechanical burrs.

Spoon Nail.   Spoon nail (koilonychia) is a common deformity in which the normal contour of the nail is lost. The nail is thin, depressed, and concave from side to side, with turned-up distal and lateral edges. Often a congenital or hereditary disorder, this condition is occasionally associated with the Plummer-Vinson syndrome (a disorder of middle-aged women characterized by dysphagia, glossitis, hypochromic anemia, and spoon nails). Although hypochromic anemia occasionally does predispose to this disorder, this relationship is probably exaggerated, and in a few cases spoon

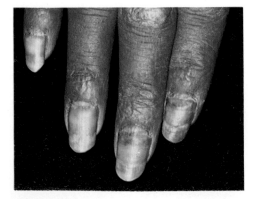

Figure 17-27   Beau's lines. Transverse grooves originate under the nail plate and move forward with the growth of the nail (this was caused by a drug-induced toxic epidermal necrolysis) (Department of Dermatology, Yale University School of Medicine).

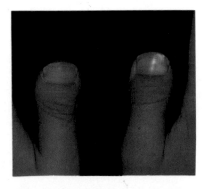

Figure 17-29   Racket nails. An abnormality of the thumbs in which the distal phalanx is shorter and wider than normal. The nails are correspondingly short and wide, with a loss of normal curvature.

nails may persist into adult life without any evidence of associated disease.

Racket Nail. The term racket nail refers to an abnormality of the thumbs in which the phalanx is shorter and wider than normal. The nail is correspondingly short, wide, and fatter than normal, and there is loss of curvature (Fig. 17–29). This disorder is dominantly inherited, may be bilateral or unilateral, and is more common in females than in males.

INGROWN NAILS

Ingrown toenails are a common disorder in which the lateral edge of the nail is curved inward and penetrates the underlying tissue, with resulting erythema, edema, pain, and, in chronic forms, the formation of granulation tissue. Generally seen on the great toes of affected individuals, the main cause of the deformity is compression of the toe from side to side by ill-fitting footwear and improper cutting of the nail (in a half-circle rather than straight across). Treatment consists of the wearing of properly fitting footwear, allowing the nail to grow out beyond the free edge, control of acute infection by compresses, topical, and, at times, systemic antibiotics, and in many instances (once the infection has subsided) surgical treatment. In recurring cases, excision of the lateral aspect of the nail under local anesthesia followed by curettage or chemical destruction of the nail matrix with liquid phenol will prevent regrowth of the offending portion of the nail.

DISORDERS OF PIGMENTATION

Abnormal nail pigmentation may be seen in systemic diseases or in association with the ingestion of various chemicals or medications.

Brown pigmentation of nails may be associated with the ingestion of phenolphthalein, as a reaction to antimalarials or gold therapy, or as a manifestation of Addison's disease. In argyria the lunulae show a distinctive slate-blue discoloration, and in hepatolenticular degeneration (Wilson's disease) the lunulae may present an azure-blue discoloration. When onycholysis is present, a

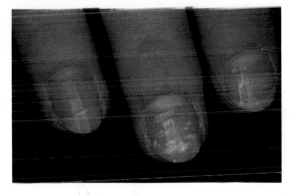

Figure 17–31 Leukonychia striata. Punctate white discoloration of the nails caused by local trauma (excessive manipulation and grooming techniques).

green discoloration in the onycholytic area may occur as the result of an infection with *Pseudomonas aeruginosa.*

The term leukonychia (white nails) is used to describe a disorder in which a portion or all of the nail becomes white (Fig. 17–30). The white color may be seen as punctate, leukonychia striata (believed to be due to local trauma such as might be seen from frequent or excessive manipulation or grooming techniques) (Fig. 17–31); as paired narrow white bands (seen in patients with cirrhosis and hypoalbuminemia); as transverse 1 to 2 mm white bands (Mees bands), suggestive of arsenic or heavy metal poisoning; or as the half-and-half nail, a disorder characteristic of renal disease and azotemia in which the proximal nail bed is white and the distal half red, pink, or brown.

The yellow nail syndrome is a disorder associated with severe long-term lymphedema and, at times, with chronic bronchitis, pleural effusion, and persistent hypoalbuminemia.[48] The condition, most often seen in middle-aged individuals, has also been described in young children. It is characterized by a pale-yellow or greenish-yellow discoloration of the nails associated with slow growth, thickening, and excessive curvature of the

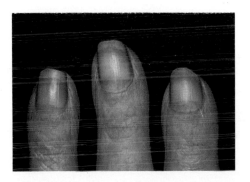

Figure 17–30 Leukonychia (white nails) in a patient with hepatic cirrhosis.

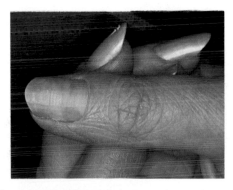

Figure 17–32 Yellow nail syndrome. A yellowish discoloration of the nails associated with slow growth, thickening, excessive curvature, and an absence of lunulas and cuticles, as seen in patients with lymphedema, bronchitis, pleural effusion, and hypoalbuminemia.

nail from side to side (on its long axis); absence of lunulae and cuticles; and swelling of the periungual tissues, as might be seen in patients with chronic paronychia (Fig. 17–32). Although the nail changes, once established, are usually permanent, complete spontaneous reversion to normal may occur at times.[48]

References

1. Saadat, M, Khan M, Gutberlet, RL, et al.: Measure of hair in normal newborns. Pediatrics 57:960–962, 1976.

   Studies of morphology and physiology of hair roots and hair shafts in 63 newborn infants.

2. Kligman AM: Pathologic dynamics of human hair loss. 1. Telogen effluvium. Arch. Dermatol. 83:175–198, 1961.

   A review of the dynamics of hair growth and the general problems encountered in analysis of hair loss.

3. Munro, DD: Disorders of hair. In Fitzpatrick TB, Arndt KA, Clark, WH, Jr, et al. (Eds.): Dermatology in General Medicine. McGraw-Hill Book Co., New York, 1971, 297–330.

   An excellent review of hair and hair growth disorders.

4. Kubba R, Rook A: Congenital triangular alopecia. Br. J. Dermatol. 95:657–659, 1976.

   Three cases of congenital triangular alopecia.

5. Solomon LM, Esterly NB, Medenica M: Hereditary trichodysplasia: Marie-Unna's hypertrichosis. J. Invest. Dermatol. 57:389–400, 1971.

   Light and electron microscopic findings in patients with Marie-Unna hypotrichosis (hereditary trichodysplasia).

6. Solomon LM, Fretzin D, Pruzansky S: Pilosebaceous dysplasia in the oral-facial-digital syndrome. Arch. Dermatol. 102:598–602, 1970.

   Eight female patients with OFD 1 and delineation of the cutaneous features of this disorder.

7. Bergfeld WF: Hair disorders. In Solomon LM, Esterly NB, Loeffel ED (Eds.): Adolescent Dermatology. W. B. Saunders Co., Philadelphia, 1978, 347–366.

   A clinical review of hair disorders as manifested in childhood.

8. Goette DK, Odom RB: Alopecia in crash dieters. JAMA 235:2622–2624, 1976.

   Nine patients develop profuse telogen effluvium two to five months after they started a vigorous 25 to 55 pound weight reduction program.

9. O'Brien R, Zelson JH, Schwartz AO, et al.: Scalp tourniquet to lessen alopecia after vincristine. N. Engl. J. Med. 238:1496, 1970.

   A simple tourniquet technique to prevent alopecia in children treated with intravenous vincristine therapy.

10. Kern F, Hoffman WH, Hambrick GW Jr, et al.: Alopecia areata, immunologic studies and treatment with prednisone. Arch. Dermatol. 107:407–412, 1973.

    Twenty-seven patients with alopecia areata who received alternate day steroid therapy demonstrated a significant hair growth and relatively few adverse effects.

11. Pascher F, Kurtin S, Andrade R: Assay of 0.2 per cent fluocinolone acetonide cream for alopecia areata and totalis. Dermatologica 141:193–202, 1970.

    Paired comparisons of fluorinated steroid and a blank vehicle applied topically on opposite areas of the scalp in patients with alopecia areata and alopecia totalis revealed a satisfactory response to therapy in 17 of 28 patients.

12. Montes, LF: Topical halcinonide in alopecia areata and alopecia totalis. J. Cutan. Pathol. 4:47–50, 1977.

    Dramatic results in ten patients with alopecia areata treated twice daily with topical applications of halcinonide cream in a 0.1 per cent concentration with and without occlusion.

13. Abell E, Munro DD: Intralesional treatment of alopecia areata with triamcinolone acetonide by jet injector. Br. J. Dermatol. 88:55–59, 1973.

    Of 84 patients treated by intradermal steroid injection, 71 per cent of patients with limited alopecia and 28 per cent of those with extensive alopecia, achieved hair regrowth in 12 weeks.

14. Unger WP, Schemmer RJ: Corticosteroids in the treatment of alopecia totalis. Systemic effects. Arch. Dermatol. 114:1486–1490, 1978.

    Seven of 15 patients with alopecia totalis or alopecia universalis treated with a combination of topical, intralesional, and oral corticosteroids with relatively insignificant side effects regrew all or virtually all of their scalp hair and were able to discontinue oral corticosteroids without recurrence of the alopecia for periods of three months to seven and one half years.

15. Happle R, Echternacht K: Induction of hair growth in alopecia areata with DNCB. Lancet 2:1002–1003, 1977.

    Thirty-three of 43 patients treated experimentally by weekly topical application of dinitrochlorobenzene (DNCB) in acetone showed significant regrowth of hair.

16. Happle R, Cebulla K, Echternacht-Happle K: Dinitrochlorobenzene therapy for alopecia areata. Arch. Dermatol. 114:1629–1631, 1978.

    Eight-nine per cent of 90 patients develop hair regrowth within eight weeks of topical DNCB: of these, 80 per cent had persistent response.

17. Muller SA, Winkelmann RK: Trichotillomania. A clinicopathologic study of 24 cases. Arch. Dermatol. 105:535–539, 1972.

    Observations in 24 patients with trichotillomania and a description of histopathologic findings helpful in the diagnosis of trichotillomania.

18. Mehregan AH: Trichotillomania: clinicopathologic study. Arch. Dermatol. 102:129–133, 1970.

    Clinical and histopathologic features of trichotillomania.

19. Hurwitz S, McAlleney PF: Trichobezoar in children. Review of the literature and report of two cases. AMA J. Dis. Child. 81:753–761, 1951.

    Two patients with trichobezoars (hairballs), a disorder generally seen in nervous young girls who have an uncontrollable habit of biting or chewing the hair.

20. Gabrilove JL, Luria M: Persistent gynecomastia resulting from scalp inunction of estradiol. A model for persistent gynecomastia. Arch. Dermatol. 114:1672–1673, 1978.

    Increased growth of scalp hairs, decrease in libido, inability to perform sexually, and persistent gynecomastia in a male due to topical application of an estrogenic cream for the treatment of baldness.

21. Orentreich N: Autografts in alopecias and other selected dermatologic conditions. Ann. N.Y. Acad. Sci. 83:463–479, 1960.

    Multiple punch autografts afford a new approach to the therapy of male pattern and other forms of alopecia.

22. Ebling FJG, Rook A: Disorders of Keratinization, keratosis pilaris atrophicans. In Rook A, Wilkinson DS, Ebling FJG (Eds.): Textbook of Dermatology, 2nd ed. Blackwell Scientific Publications, London, 1972, 1168–1169.

    A classification and description of the uncommon atrophic forms of keratosis pilaris.

23. Emmerson RW: Follicular mucinosa. A study of 47 patients. Br. J. Dermatol. 81:395–413, 1969.

    Of 47 patients with follicular mucinosis, 22 had spontaneous clearing with varying degrees of hair regrowth after a period of two months to two years.

24. Price VH: Disorders of the hair in children. Pediatr. Clin. North Am. 25:305–320, 1978.

A current review of hair disorders of infants and children.

25. Owens DW, Chernosky ME: Trichorrhexis nodosa. In vitro production. Arch. Derm. 94:586–588, 1966.

A characteristic picture of trichorrhexis nodosa was produced in normal appearing scalp hair by trauma in a laboratory setting.

26. Papa CM, Mills, OH Jr, Hanshaw W: Seasonal trichorrhexis nodosa. Role of cumulative damage in frayed hair. Arch. Dermatol. 106:888–892, 1972.

A report of seasonal trichorrhexis nodosa (occurring in two successive summers) with in vitro studies confirming the theory of cumulative hair damage in the pathogenesis of this disorder.

27. Netherton EW: A unique case of trichorrhexis nodosa "bamboo hairs." Arch. Dermatol. 78:483–487, 1958.

Description of a patient with ichthyosis and bamboo hair. Although the ichthyosis was originally thought to be ichthyosis linearis circumflexa, in retrospect it now appears that this patient actually had lamellar ichthyosis.

28. Hurwitz S, Kirsch N, McGuire J: Reevaluation of ichthyosis and hair shaft abnormalities. Arch. Dermatol. 103:266–271, 1971.

Report of a case of trichorrhexis invaginata associated with ichthyosis linearis circumflexa and a review of 25 patients with ichthyosis and/or structural abnormalities of the hair shaft.

29. Robinson GC, Johnston MM: Pili torti and sensory neural hearing loss. J. Pediatr. 70:621–623, 1967.

A five-year-old girl with characteristic twisting (pili torti) and profound bilateral sensorineural hearing loss.

30. Menkes JH, Alter M, Steigleder GK, et al.: A sex-linked recessive disorder with retardation of growth, peculiar hair, and focal cerebral and cerebellar degeneration. Pediatrics 29:764–779, 1962.

The first description of a syndrome characterized by slow growth, progressive cerebral degeneration, pili torti, x-linked inheritance, and death, usually before age three years.

31. Danks DM, Campbell PE, Stevens BJ, et al.: Menkes's kinky hair syndrome, an inherited defect in copper absorption with widespread effects. Pediatrics 50:188–201, 1972.

The recognition of seven patients with Menkes' syndrome born in five families during a three-year period suggests that this disease is not as rare as believed and that babies with this disorder may die undiagnosed.

32. Bucknall WE, Haslam RHA, Holtzman NA: Kinky hair syndrome: response to copper therapy. Pediatrics 52:653–657, 1973.

Failure of clinical response to purified human ceruloplasmin and oral and intravenous copper administration suggests irreversible damage, possibly in utero.

33. Price VH, Thomas RS, Jones FT: Pili annulati, optical and electron microscopic studies. Arch. Dermatol. 96:640–644, 1968.

Light and electron microscopic studies demonstrate air-filled cavities in affected hair shafts as the cause of this disorder.

34. Price VH, Thomas RS, Jones FT: Pseudopili annulati. An unusual variant of normal hair. Arch. Dermatol. 102:354–358, 1970.

Pseudopili annulati: flattened external surfaces of twisted hair shafts act as mirrors and variable cylindrical lenses, which reflect, refract, and focus incident light on the posterior or wall of the hair shaft.

35. Lantis SDH, Pepper MC: Woolly hair nevus. Two case reports and a discussion of unruly hair forms. Arch. Dermatol. 114:233–238, 1978.

Two case reports of woolly hair nevus with discussion of the features distinguishing this disorder from other types of unruly hair.

36. Hegedus SI, Schorr WF: Acquired hypertrichosis lanuginosa and malignancy. Arch. Dermatol. 106:84–88, 1972.

A review of hypertrichosis lanuginosa and description of two adults displaying the acquired form of this disorder as a cutaneous sign of internal malignancy.

37. Burton JL, Schutt WH, Caldwell IW: Hypertrichosis due to diazoxide. Br. J. Dermatol. 93:707–711, 1975.

Hypertrichosis as a side effect of diazoxide administered to individuals with seizure disorders.

38. Kirkland DJ, Lawler SD, Venitt S: Chromosomal damage and hair dyes. Lancet 2:124–127, 1978.

A report of possible direct genotoxic effects of hair dyes in women supports previous laboratory studies which suggest that hair dye substances may have mutagenic and carcinogenic properties.

39. Lampe RM, Henderson AL, Hansen GH. Green hair. JAMA 237:2092, 1977.

A report of two children with green discoloration of the hair acquired from swimming in pools, due to copper, not chlorine.

40. Nordlund JJ, Hartley C, Fister J. On the cause of green hair. Arch. Dermatol. 113:1700, 1977.

Two postgraduate nursing students with green hair from tap water containing excessive amounts of copper.

41. Sammon PD. The nails. In Rook A, Wilkinson DS, Ebling FJG (Eds.): Textbook of Dermatology, 2nd ed. Blackwell Scientific Publications, London. 1972, 1642–1671.

An authoritative discourse on the nail.

42. Hazelrigg DE, Duncan WC, Jarratt M: Twenty nail dystrophy of childhood. Arch. Dermatol. 113:73–75, 1977.

Six children with dystrophy of all nails (20-nail dystrophy), a self-limited disorder occasionally seen in children but, to date, not reported in adults.

43. Lucas GL, Opitz JM: The nail-patella syndrome. Clinical and genetic aspects of five kindreds with 38 affected family members. J. Pediatr. 68:273–288, 1966.

A review of the nail-patella syndrome, with discussion of the genetic and clinical aspects of this disorder.

44. Daniel CR, III, Osment LS, Noojin RO: Triangular lunulae. A clue to the nail-patella syndrome. Arch. Dermatol. 116:448–449, 1980.

A review of nail abnormalities associated with the nail-patella syndrome (NPS) and a reminder that although trauma and various other causes of matrix damage may cause triangular lunulae, the presence of triangular lunulae, especially with a sharp apex pointing distally, should suggest a diagnosis of NPS and prompt the physician to look for other associated abnormalities.

45. Carbonara P, Alpert M. Hereditary osteo-onycho-dysplasia (HOOD), Am J Med. Sc. 248:139–151, 1964.

Review of 60 well-documented and two personal cases of the nail-patella-syndrome (hereditary osteo-onycho-dysplasia).

46. Joseph HL: Pachyonychia congenita. Arch. Dermatol. 90:594–603, 1964.

Report of a newborn and four family members with pachyonychia congenita and an attempt to explain the pathogenesis of the nail deformity.

47. Valesquex JP, Bustamante J: Sebocystomatosis with congenital pachyonychia. Int. J. Derm. 11:77–81, 1972.

A study of the clinical and hereditary findings in three families with several generations of steatocystoma multiplex (sebocystomatosis) in association with pachyonychia.

48. Marks R, Ellis JP: Yellow nails. A report of six cases. Arch. Dermatol. 102:619–623, 1970.

Yellow nails reported in six patients, one of whom has severe lymphedema, pleural effusion, and persistent hypoalbuminemia.

18

THE SKIN AND SYSTEMIC DISEASE

The ability to diagnose internal disease by means of cutaneous signs is a challenging aspect of clinical diagnosis. A number of dermatologic signs, symptoms, and disorders can be invaluable as markers of systemic disease. This chapter is prepared in an effort to familiarize physicians with the value of cutaneous disorders as a key to the recognition of internal and systemic conditions that affect infants and children.

HYPERSENSITIVITY SYNDROMES

The important dermatologic disorders of hypersensitivity are urticaria, erythema nodosum, and erythema multiforme. Diagnosis of these disorders is relatively simple, but difficulties arise in determining their etiology because each entity is associated with an incredible number of underlying factors.[1]

Urticaria

Urticaria, a systemic disease with cutaneous manifestations, occurs at some time in the life of about 15 per cent of the population.[2, 3] It is characterized by the appearance of transient well-circumscribed wheals that are seen as erythematous, intensely pruritic elevated swellings of the skin (Fig. 18–1) or mucous membranes.

The etiology of urticaria is often not well understood and may be related to a multitude of factors. Therefore it can be thought of as a symp-

384

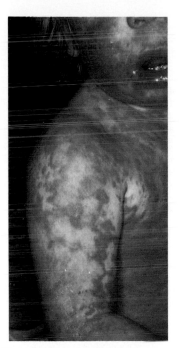

Figure 18–1 Urticaria. Transient well-circumscribed erythematous wheals.

tom complex in which multiple factors can cause and perpetuate the condition. Individual lesions are due to extravasation of fluid from small blood vessels, as a reflection of increased permeability of capillaries and small venules. Various pharmacologically active agents appear to be capable of mediating these changes (kinins, prostaglandins, serotonin, and histamine).

CLINICAL MANIFESTATIONS. Typical lesions have a white palpable center of edema with a variable halo of erythema. They vary in size from pinpoint papules to large lesions several centimeters in diameter. Central clearing, peripheral extension, and coalescence of individual lesions result in a clinical picture of oval, annular, or bizarre serpiginous configurations. They may be localized to one small area or may become so extensive and generalized as to cover almost the entire skin surface. Subcutaneous extension may result in large giant wheals. In infants and young children, swelling of the distal extremities with acrocyanosis may be a prominent feature of the urticarial reaction. Occasionally, particularly in infants and young children, bullae may form in the center of the wheal, usually on the legs and buttocks.[4] Individual wheals rarely persist longer than 12 to 24 hours. Those lasting more than 24 hours are probably not true urticaria and may represent another vascular pattern, such as vasculitis or erythema multiforme.

The terms angioedema, giant urticaria, and Quincke's edema occasionally are used to describe large giant wheals and diffuse swellings of the eyelids, hands, genitalia, and mucous mem-

branes (the lips and tongue). Although angioedema may occur on its own, it often accompanies and shares a common etiology with ordinary urticaria.

For convenience, urticaria of less than six weeks' duration is considered acute. Acute urticaria due to food or drugs is generally of brief duration (a few days to weeks). Urticaria that recurs frequently and lasts longer than six weeks is termed chronic. The exact etiology in a particular patient is often unknown and may be associated with hypersensitivity to a multitude of possible agents such as foods, drugs, infections, serum injections, insect bites, inhalant or contact allergens, and psychogenic factors. Many physicians still regard urticaria as characteristically and almost invariably allergic in origin.[2] Although an allergic cause can be determined in many cases, in 70 to 80 per cent of patients, particularly those with chronic urticaria, no definite etiology can be established.[2, 3]

Though seldom life-threatening, chronic urticaria has been noted to be an important sign of underlying systemic disease. It may occur in association with malignancy or may be an important sign of connective tissue disease. It may be seen as the first sign of Still's disease (juvenile rheumatoid arthritis); in 7 to 23 per cent of cases of lupus erythematosus;[5] in 10 per cent of patients with acute rheumatic fever; and when observed in a patient with arthralgia and fever of unknown origin, it should alert the physician to the possibility of serum hepatitis.[6] Diagnosis and treatment of a patient with chronic urticaria, therefore, demand a complete history and physical examination, appropriate laboratory evaluation, and an awareness of possible underlying disease.

Histopathologic examination of urticarial lesions reveals dilatation and engorgement of venules and capillaries, edema, and perivascular infiltration of the dermis composed of round cells, polymorphonuclear leukocytes, and a variable number of eosinophils. Urticarial wheals are characterized by edema of the dermis; in lesions of angioneurotic edema the edema extends into the subcutaneous tissue.

TREATMENT. Effective treatment of urticaria is dependent upon identification of the etiologic factor and its elimination whenever possible. Symptomatic treatment consists of antihistamines, of which hydroxyzine (Atarax or Vistaril) appears to be the most effective and the drug of choice. When antihistamines are used, they should not be stopped prematurely. In an effort to prevent recurrences and the development of chronic urticaria, it appears best to continue antihistamines for a period of one to two weeks after all signs of urticaria have cleared. The subcutaneous administration of 0.1 to 0.5 ml of epinephrine (1:1000) or 0.1 to 0.3 ml of Sus-Phrine (1:200) is often effective and particularly beneficial in patients with angioedema and acute or severe urticaria. Although frequently effective in patients with severe or persistent urticaria, because of the side effects associated with prolonged steroid therapy, administration of systemic steroids should be reserved for those patients who are unresponsive to other modes of therapy.

Cholinergic Urticaria

Cholinergic urticaria (micropapular urticaria) is a very distinctive type of urticaria. It usually starts in adolescence and is associated with heat, exertion, or emotional stress. Seen in' 5 to 7 per cent of the cases of urticaria, it is considered to be a physical allergy and not a sign of systemic disease.[4] Cholinergic urticaria is characterized by a generalized eruption, usually on the trunk and arms, which consists of discrete, papular wheals, 1 to 2 mm in diameter with or without a surrounding area of erythema (Fig. 18–2). The duration of the eruption varies from a period of 30 minutes to several hours.

Acetylcholine, released through some unknown mechanism (perhaps liberated when sweat glands are stimulated by heat, exertion, emotional, or taste stimuli), may stimulate histamine release, thus causing the lesions.[6, 7] The diagnosis is made on the basis of history and the appearance of the eruption several minutes after exercise. Once cholinergic urticaria occurs, the condition may recur for periods of months to years, and then tends toward spontaneous improvement and resolution. Treatment consists of systemic antihistamines, particularly cyproheptadine (Periactin) or hydroxyzine (Atarax or Vistaril), awareness of potential precipitating factors, and avoidance of heat, excessive exertion, and excitement whenever possible. After a severe attack of cholinergic urticaria further exertion frequently fails to cause urticaria for periods of 24 hours or more. Some patients thus find that they can induce attacks by exercise or hot showers and in this way achieve freedom from symptoms for varying periods of time.

Aquagenic Urticaria

Aquagenic urticaria, a disorder that resembles but is not identical to cholinergic urticaria, occurs most frequently in adolescence and is characterized by small, intensely pruritic, perifollicular papular wheals with surrounding axon reflex erythema (with sparing of the palms and soles). The disorder is precipitated by contact with water or perspiration (irrespective of temperature). Exercise and other cholinergic factors do not precipitate this disorder, and patients can drink water without adverse reaction.[8] Although the etiology remains unknown, aquagenic urticaria may be related to a toxic substance created by a combination of water and sebum, resulting in local histamine release from the perifollicular mast cells.[9] The administration of antihistamines by mouth seems to reduce the whealing tendency and lessen the severity of the disorder.

Solar Urticaria

Solar urticaria is a rare disorder in which minimal exposure to sunlight at different wavelengths in the visible or ultraviolet light range provokes an almost immediate localized urticarial reaction, with "burning" followed by erythema, wheal, and flare sharply confined to light-exposed sites. Urticaria is usually seen within a few minutes of exposure to sunlight. Although the reaction generally fades within 15 or 30 minutes to an hour or two, scratching and rubbing may lead to secondary eczematization with persisting cutaneous changes.[7]

Solar urticaria is a chronic disease and may appear in individuals from 3 to 52 years of age. It appears to be a disorder of multiple etiologies. The cause is unknown, and the wavelength of light causing the urticarial response varies considerably from person to person.[10] Although therapy generally is unsatisfactory, oral antihistamines occasionally may be helpful for individuals with this disorder. Repeated gradual exposure to sunlight may produce tolerance in some patients, and measures should be directed toward diminishing exposure to sunlight. Sunscreen preparations, occasionally beneficial when the precipitating wavelengths are in the sunburn range, appear to be the most consistently helpful form of therapy available at this time.

Figure 18–2 Cholinergic urticaria (induced by heat, exertion, or emotional stress). Discrete micropapular wheals and a wide area of surrounding erythema.

Cold Urticaria

Cold urticaria is a disorder characterized by localized or generalized urticaria that develops within a few minutes or hours of exposure to cold air or water. In highly sensitive persons, in whom whealing may be widespread or severe, cold showers or swimming in cold water may produce hypotension and, on occasion, syncope, loss of consciousness, and drowning.[11] If the cold extends to the mucous membranes, respiratory symptoms such as nasal stuffinesss, cough, and dyspnea, and gastrointestinal symptoms such as swelling of the lips, swelling of the oral mucous membranes, dysphagia, and abdominal cramps may occur.

Cold urticaria can be divided into two forms: a rare congenital or familial type inherited on an autosomal dominant basis and a more common acquired form. Although not sex-linked, familial cold urticaria is more common in females. The disorder may be present at birth or may occur during infancy, and usually develops in early childhood. It is characterized by an urticarial or papular eruption, fever, chills, arthralgia, headache, malaise, muscle tenderness, and, at times, a significant leukocytosis.[12] Although the tendency to familial cold urticaria generally persists for life, the severity of symptoms may decrease with advancing age. The urticarial reaction is usually induced by a generalized body cooling, more often in cold air than cold water. It generally develops after a latent period of several hours and, once it develops, may persist for up to 48 hours.

The acquired form of cold urticaria often appears suddenly, usually in children, but may occur at any age and has an equal incidence in both sexes. Once symptoms develop they are generally short-lived and, although they may persist indefinitely, usually disappear after a few months or years.

Secondary forms of cold urticaria may also be associated with cold hemolysin and cold agglutinin syndromes. These forms, generally seen in adults, cause Raynaud's phenomenon, acrocyanosis, and cutaneous ulcers. Some cases of cold urticaria manifested by itching, erythema, purpura, atypical Raynaud's phenomenon, and ulceration due to cryoglobulins may also be associated with multiple myeloma, leukemia, kala-azar, systemic lupus erythematosus, and melanoma.

The diagnosis of cold urticaria requires a careful history and investigation for other possible etiologic factors. When the diagnosis remains in doubt, patients should be evaluated for other systemic diseases, particularly lupus erythematosus, cryoglobulinemia, and hereditary angioneurotic edema. Diagnosis of cold urticaria may frequently be assisted by reproduction of symptoms by local applications of an ice cube for periods of two to ten minutes. The best areas for this testing are the face, neck, and in particular the arms. Some patients fail to respond to ice but do respond to cold water or generalized cooling of the body.[13]

Patients with a severe or widespread urticarial reaction should be forewarned of the risk of drowning following loss of consciousness when swimming or bathing in cold water. The treatment of cold urticaria is aided by oral administration of antihistamines, particularly cyproheptadine (Periactin).[14] For those unresponsive to systemic antihistamines, desensitization to cold may be attempted by gradual cooling an extremity in cold water for 5 to 10 minutes a day with a gradual increase in the time of exposure and decrease of the temperature over a period of weeks or months. This treatment is not regularly effective and must be done cautiously in an effort to minimize the risk of systemic reaction.[4]

Hereditary Angioneurotic Edema

Hereditary angioneurotic edema (HANE, hereditary angioedema) is a serious but rare autosomal dominant form of urticaria characterized by recurrent episodes of edema of the subcutaneous tissue, particularly of the hands, feet, and face and of the gastrointestinal or upper respiratory tracts. The defect is due to a deficiency of the alpha 2 globulin inhibitor of the activated first component of complement (C_1-esterase inhibitor), which results in transient episodes of increased vascular permeability.[15] Although the pathogenesis of this disorder is not fully understood, it appears that a kinin-like permeability factor generated by the action of C_1-esterase on C_4 and C_2, the episodic activation of Hageman factor working through a kinin-forming system of plasma or plasmin, and an elevated capillary filtration rate in affected areas may be physiologic mediators of attacks.[16, 17, 18]

Two genetic variants of hereditary angioneurotic edema have been described. In the more common type, seen in an estimated 85 per cent of affected kindreds, serum levels of C_1-esterase inhibitor are extremely low because of decreased synthesis in the liver.[19] In the variant form, normal or elevated levels of C_1-esterase inhibitor are present, but the inhibitor is apparently nonfunctional.[16]

CLINICAL MANIFESTATIONS. The earliest symptoms of hereditary angioneurotic edema often begin in infancy or early childhood, usually before the age of 10, rarely as late as the third decade of life. The frequency and severity of attacks are typically exacerbated during adolescence and subside in the fifth decade.[20] Mottling of the skin often occurs early in life and may be the first evidence of the disorder. Affected individuals are prone to sudden attacks of circumscribed subcutaneous edema. The swelling evolves very quickly. It usually affects the face or an extremity, may be severe enough to cause remarkable disfiguration of the affected parts, and generally subsides within one to five days. The skin and mucosal lesions may appear spontaneously or may be precipitated by minor trauma, especially extraction of teeth, strenuous exercise, or emotional excitement. There is no pitting, discoloration, redness, pain, or itching associated with the edema, and a rash similar to erythema marginatum is noted in some patients, particularly children.

Gastrointestinal involvement, second in order of frequency, is marked by nausea, vomiting, or diarrhea, sometimes with recurrent colic and severe abdominal pain simulating a surgical emergency. Involvement of the mucous membranes of the hypopharynx and larynx, although seen less often, may be particularly severe and result in asphyxiation, the leading cause of death in patients with this disorder. This complication, usually seen in the third decade of life, may occur in 25 per cent of patients.

TREATMENT. Diagnosis of hereditary angioneurotic edema can be confirmed by the findings of lower levels of C_4 or C_1 esterase activity, or both. The development of effective treatment lags behind the advances in understanding the pathophysiology of this disease. Antihistamines and corticosteroids have not been effective in the management of patients. Epinephrine is beneficial in the control of swelling in only a very few patients. Intravenous administration of diuretics such as meralluride (Mercuhydrine) or ethacrynic acid is helpful in halting the progression of severe angioedema. Tracheostomy frequently is lifesaving in patients with laryngeal obstruction. Although methyltestosterone linguets (in dosages of 10 to 25 mg once daily) may prevent attacks in one-third to one-half of patients, it can produce masculinization in women patients and its use is not recommended for children.

Epsilon aminocaproic acid (EACA) inhibits the conversion of plasminogen to plasmin (a known C_1 activator).[21] Its safety in long-term therapy has not been established; in short-term use its major side effect has been muscle weakness with associated elevation of creatine phosphokinase and aldolase and an increased predisposition to thrombosis and phlebitis. Its analogue tranexamic acid, not yet released by the FDA, in doses of 1 to 3 gm orally per day, has been effective in aborting attacks of angioedema and has few side effects.

Danazol appears to act on the disease by increasing levels of C_1-esterase inhibitor. This appears to represent one of the first examples of correction of an inherited abnormality by drug therapy. Whether it increases C_1-esterase inhibitor production, increases its release into serum, or reduces its catabolism is unknown. It has fewer androgenic side effects than methyltestosterone, but cannot be used in children and should not be administered to pregnant women.[22]

Annular Erythemas

The annular erythemas (erythema marginatum, erythema annulare centrifugum, and erythema chronicum migrans) represent a group of oval, annular, arcuate, or polycyclic lesions with individual characteristics that allow differentiation into distinctive clinical categories. Although it is not yet proved, it appears that these disorders may be related to cell-mediated urticarial reactions. Their individual appearances and behaviors are characteristic and, therefore, frequently helpful in the clinical diagnosis of various systemic disorders.

Erythema Marginatum and Rheumatic Fever. Erythema marginatum is a distinctive form of annular erythema that occurs on the trunk (especially on the abdomen) and the proximal extremities in about 10 per cent of patients with active rheumatic fever and occasionally in patients with juvenile rheumatoid arthritis. Lesions appear as evanescent pink macules or papules that fade centrally (leaving a pale or sometimes pigmented center) and rapidly expand to form non-pruritic rings or segments of rings with elevated reticular, polycyclic, or serpiginous borders.

Often easily overlooked, erythema marginatum is associated with active carditis. It is seen more frequently in children than adults with rheumatic fever, frequently follows the onset of migratory arthritis by a few days, but at times may also occur many months after the carditis.[23, 24] Lesions are evanescent (fading in a few hours to several days), spread rapidly, and may recur in crops in different areas. Unlike the characteristic rash of juvenile rheumatoid arthritis, lesions of erythema marginatum are larger, spread centrifugally with central clearing, and are limited to the trunk and sometimes the proximal limbs. Although the eruption seldom lasts more than several weeks, occasionally it may recur at sporadic intervals for several months to years.

Another type of erythema seen in rheumatic fever consists of small red macules and urticarial papules that occur on the arms and elbows, buttocks, and knees. These lesions do not form rings. They develop in crops and persist for a length of time similar to that of erythema marginatum.[1]

Subcutaneous nodules, seen in about 20 per cent of patients with this disorder, present as another characteristic cutaneous manifestation of rheumatic fever. Most numerous in children with extensive cardiac involvement, subcutaneous nodules can coexist with erythema marginatum and are a late manifestation of rheumatic fever. They usually portend serious disease and are observed in no other diseases except granuloma annulare and rheumatoid arthritis. The nodules of rheumatic fever are smaller than those seen in rheumatoid arthritis and last for shorter periods of time, usually less than one month. They tend to occur in crops and often appear in a symmetrical distribution on the extensor tendons of the hands, feet, knees, and scapulae, on the occiput, and on the spinous processes of the vertebrae. They are never painful and vary in size from 2 mm to 2 cm in diameter. Lying deep in the connective tissue over bony prominences with freely movable skin over them, they are more readily felt than seen, and, unless a careful search is made, are frequently easily overlooked.

Erythema Annulare Centrifugum. Erythma annulare centrifugum is an eruption characterized

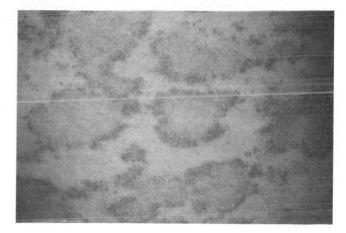

Figure 18–3 Erythema annulare centrifugum. Slowly expanding annular lesions with dusky centers and palpable scaly erythematous borders.

by persistent erythematous annular rings, each with a clear center and a raised, thin, wall-like border, which slowly enlarges centrifugally (Fig. 18–3). At times the palpable border may show scaling, suggesting a diagnosis of ringworm (tinea corporis).

The cause of erythema annulare centrifugum is unknown. Although it often occurs without apparent cause, most cases appear to be related to hypersensitivity to an underlying inflammatory or neoplastic disease. In infants it may be associated with autoimmune disorders in their mothers.[25] Erythema annulare centrifugum, therefore, may occur as a cutaneous sign of hypersensitivity to drugs, molds, foods, fungus infection, blood dyscrasia, immunologic disorder, or neoplastic disease.

Primary lesions tend to be single or multiple erythematous edematous papules with a predilection for the trunk, buttocks, thighs, and legs. They are asymptomatic except for occasional mild pruritus. The rings extend peripherally, usually slowly, 1 to 3 mm per day, sometimes up to 4 cm in a week. New lesions may form within the original circle. The resulting overall shape may be irregular, oval, circinate, semi-annular, target-like, or polycyclic. The borders may eventually reach a size of 10 cm or more in diameter. The duration of the disease is extremely variable and may go on for weeks or months and, with new lesions appearing in successive crops, frequently for years.

Erythema annulare centrifugum must be differentiated from lesions of pityriasis rosea, erythema multiforme, tinea corporis, early lesions of lupus erythematosus, granuloma annulare, and erythema chronicum migrans. Fungal infections can be distinguished by their more pronounced epidermal changes, with vesiculation or scaling or both at the edge of the lesions, by microscopic examination of skin scrapings, and fungal culture. When the diagnosis is indeterminate, histopathologic examination of cutaneous lesions showing focal infiltration of lymphocytes around the blood vessels and dermal appendages in a "coat-sleeve" arrangement may help establish the true nature of the disorder.

Since erythema annulare centrifugum represents a hypersensitivity reaction, treatment depends upon the determination and removal of the underlying cause. Antihistamines produce variable and usually incomplete relief. Although systemic steroids may aid the temporary resolution of lesions, the disorder frequently recurs as soon as medication is discontinued.

Erythema Chronicum Migrans and Lyme Arthritis. Erythema chronicum migrans is a poorly understood disorder characterized by a raised erythematous expanding lesion with advancing indurated borders and central clearing. Although common in Europe, only one case had been reported in the United States by 1970.[26] Since 1972, this disorder has also been seen in Connecticut, Rhode Island, Cape Cod, Massachusetts, Long Island, New York, New Jersey, Delaware, Maryland, Georgia, Oregon, and California.[27-30a]

The etiology of erythema chronicum migrans is unknown. In Europe the vector of transmission is usually thought to be the sheep tick, *Ixodes ricinus.* However, the lesion has been reported in areas of Scandinavia that do not have ticks; in those cases, a mosquito vector has been suspected.[29] In Wisconsin and the eastern United States the disease is associated with the tick *Ixodes dammini;* on the west coast it is associated with *Ixodes pacificus.*[30a] The mechanism of formation of lesions of erythema chronicum migrans remains unknown, but studies suggest that the disorder may be associated with a microbiological agent, transmitted by the tick bite and mediated by an immunological reaction.

The typical lesion of erythema chronicum migrans begins as an erythematous macule or papule that occurs 4 to 20 days after the tick bite and clears in three days to eight weeks. The borders of the lesion then expand to form a red ring as great as 20 to 30 cm in diameter, with central clearing (Fig. 18–4). Lesions may be single or multiple. Occasionally secondary rings may form within the original one, as in erythema multiforme. The lesion often itches, stings, or burns, and may be accompanied by fever, headache, vomiting, fatigue, and regional adenopathy.

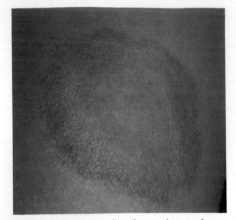

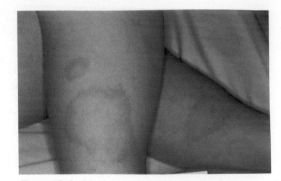

Figure 18–6   Multiple lesions of erythema chronicum migrans in a child with Lyme arthritis (Courtesy of Steere A C, Malawista S E, Hardin J A, et al.: Ann. Int. Med. *86*:685, 1977).

Figure 18–4   Erythema chronicum migrans. An expanding ringed lesion with central clearing caused by a tick bite (this disorder has been linked with Lyme arthritis).

Lesions of erythema chronicum migrans can be differentiated from those of erythema annulare centrifugum and tinea corporis by rapid peripheral expansion, lack of vesiculation and scaling along the peripheral border, microscopic examination of skin scrapings, and fungal culture. Histologically the initial lesions are consistent with an arthropod bite and reveal a primarily lymphocytic perivascular infiltration, occasionally with some eosinophils (Fig. 18–5). They differ from lesions of erythema annulare centrifugum in which the infiltrate tends to be organized around blood vessels. Unlike lesions of vasculitis, they lack polymorphonuclear leukocytes, dermal hemorrhage, and fibrinoid necrosis. No causative agents have been cultured from skin biopsies, and serologic tests to date have been negative.

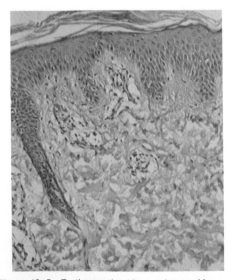

Figure 18–5   Erythema chronicum migrans. Mononuclear, primarily lymphocytic, perivascular infiltration (occasionally eosinophils may also be noted).

Of significance is the fact that erythema chronicum migrans appears to herald the onset of a new syndrome that, for want of a better name, has been termed "Lyme arthritis," or "Lyme disease" after the community in southeastern Connecticut where the initial cases were first noted (Fig. 18–6). Between 1972 and 1976 this syndrome affected over 51 individuals, 39 of them children, 12 of them adults.

The disorder is characterized by the sudden onset (in the summer or fall) of a swollen joint (one usually, occasionally several), most often the knee (70 per cent), accompanied by fever, malaise, nausea, vomiting, weakness, headache and myalgia, and, in some individuals, Bell's palsy. The initial attack generally lasts a week to a month; the duration, however, varies and recurrences are common. Other manifestations of Lyme disease include neurologic abnormalities, myocardial conduction defects, elevated erythrocyte sedimentation, decreased levels of C_3 in the serum, and, in many cases, increased IgM and IgG cryoprecipitates in the sera of patients during acute attacks.[27, 29]

Although Lyme disease was initially described in Connecticut, it is significant that *Ixodes* can be found along the eastern coast of the United States, from Massachusetts to Florida, in Wisconsin, and as far west as Texas, Utah, and the west coast.[30a] Of further importance is the fact that this disorder has been recognized in a child in Tampa, Florida, who spent summer vacations in southern Connecticut (J. Florida Medical Association, March, 1979) and in three campers who were bitten by ticks in a woodland area in northwestern Minnesota.[30] Such cases serve to emphasize the fact that Lyme arthritis is not merely a disorder restricted to Connecticut and its adjoining states, but one that has national, and with our current wide traveling society, even a possible worldwide significance.

Although Lyme arthritis has been described only as an occasional nuisance, chronic arthritis occurs in 10 per cent of patients and severe disability requiring synovectomy has been a signifi-

Zantac® 300

ranitidine HCl/Glaxo 300 mg tablets

Once-a-night
h.s. therapy for active
duodenal ulcers

Glaxo/ ROCHE ®

Before prescribing, see complete Product Information on last pages.

cant feature in a small number of patients. Patients with erythema chronicum migrans who have cryoglobulin containing IgM associated with high serum IgG levels appear to be at risk for developing arthritis.[30b] The severity of erythema chronicum migrans does not correlate with the severity of joint disease, and some patients with Lyme arthritis reportedly had no rash. Although the etiology of this disorder remains unknown, an increased prevalence of B-cell alloantigen DRw2 in seven of ten patients (as compared to 22 percent of nonaffected individuals) suggests an immunologic susceptibility of affected patients to a disordered or inappropriate immune response to a possible infectious antigen.[31]

The treatment of erythema chronicum migrans and Lyme arthritis is not clear. Aspirin prescribed for the arthritis during attacks gives symptomatic relief but does not seem to suppress joint effusion or prevent recurrences. Although the disease may fluctuate, it appears that penicillin and, alternatively, tetracycline (except below age 8) shorten the duration of erythema chronicum migrans and may prevent or attenuate subsequent arthritis.[31a]

Erythema Nodosum

Erythema nodosum represents a delayed hypersensitivity syndrome characterized by red tender nodular lesions, usually on the tibial surface of the legs (Fig. 18–7). Although etiologic causes are many, the most common are beta streptococcal infection, sarcoidosis, and tuberculosis. In children streptococcal and other respiratory infections and primary tuberculosis are the most common causes of erythema nodosum. Other disorders that may cause erythema nodosum include leprosy, coccidioidomycosis, histoplasmosis, leishmaniasis, cat scratch fever, and fungal infection. Non-infectious disorders that cause erythema nodosum are ulcerative colitis, regional ileitis, and reactions to various drugs, particularly sulfonamides, diphenylhydantoin (Dilantin), and contraceptive pills containing ethinyl estradiol and norethynodrel.[32]

The disease has its greatest incidence in the spring and fall, and is less common in summer. Although most cases occur in the third decade of life, the disorder may be seen in children, particularly those above ten years of age.[33] During childhood girls are affected slightly more than boys, but in adult life women are affected three to four times as often as men.[1] Lesions, 1 to 5 cm in diameter, occur symmetrically, usually on the pretibial areas, occasionally the knees, ankles, thighs, extensor aspects of the arms, the face, and neck. Initially they appear as bright to deep-red, warm and tender, oval, slightly elevated nodules. After a few days they develop a brownish-red or purplish bruise-like appearance (this has been termed erythema contusiformis). The eruption usually lasts three to six weeks but may recede earlier if the patient remains in bed. Recrudescences may occur over a period of weeks to months, but attacks are seldom recurrent[34] and arthralgias may precede, coincide with, or follow the eruption in as many as 90 per cent of cases.

Erythema nodosum has a characteristic clinical picture, and diagnosis generally can be made on the basis of physical examination alone. Although diagnosis usually is not difficult, common bruises, cellulitis or erysipelas, deep fungal infections (such as Majocchi's granuloma or sporotrichosis), insect bites, deep thrombophlebitis, angiitis, erythema induratum, and fat-destructive panniculitides can be confused with this disorder. When the diagnosis is in doubt, bacterial and fungal cultures and histologic examination of skin biopsies generally will help to clarify the diagnosis.

The principal histologic changes of erythema nodosum are located in the deep dermis and subcutaneous tissue. They consist primarily of lymphocytes and neutrophils (with histiocytes, giant cells, and at times plasma cells) in the fibrous septa between fat lobules as well as in individual fat cells. The dermis shows a moderate degree of perivascular infiltrate composed primarily of lymphocytes.[35]

The treatment of erythema nodosum is directed at the cause of the disorder. Bed rest, with elevation of the patient's legs, helps reduce pain and edema. When pain, inflammation, or arthralgia is prominent, salicylates may be helpful. In chronic or recurrent cases detailed investigations must be performed in order to uncover the underlying cause. Intralesional corticosteroids frequently cause rapid involution of individual lesions and in persistent or recurrent eruptions oral corticosteroids may be beneficial.

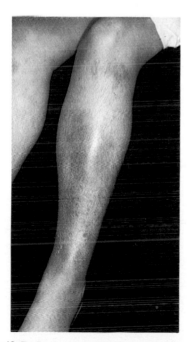

Figure 18–7 Erythema nodosum. Tender red oval nodules on the extensor aspect of the leg.

Erythema Multiforme and Stevens-Johnson Disease

Another systemic disorder highlighted by cutaneous manifestations is *erythema multiforme*, a distinctive acute hypersensitivity syndrome, again with any number of etiologies: hypersensitivity to viral, bacterial, protozoal, fungal, or *Mycoplasma pneumoniae* (Eaton agent) infections; sensitivity to food or drugs; immunizations; or connective tissue disorders. Whereas drug reactions and malignancies are important causes of erythema multiforme in older persons, infectious diseases are an important etiology in children and young adults. The most common cause of erythema multiforme appears to be the virus of herpes simplex, with a history of cold sores preceding the development of other lesions by about 3 to 14 days. Recurrences are particularly common with this form of erythema multiforme.[36]

CLINICAL MANIFESTATIONS. The clinical spectrum of erythema multiforme ranges from a localized eruption of the skin and mucous membranes to a severe multisystem disorder. The disease occurs at any age, with the most severe forms occurring most frequently in chidren and young adults. The disorder may occur at any time of year, but appears to have its highest incidence in the spring and fall. The eruption is symmetrical and may occur on any part of the body, with a predilection for the palms and soles, backs of the hands and feet, and extensor surfaces of the arms and legs. As the disorder progresses, lesions often extend to the trunk, face, and neck. Oral lesions may occur alone or in conjunction with cutaneous lesons. Seen in 25 per cent of cases, they first appear as bullae (that break soon after formation), with swelling and crusting of the lips and development of erosions of the buccal mucosa, gums, and tongue (Fig. 18-8).

The term erythema multiforme is often confusing to non-dermatologists and should not be applied indiscriminately to any polymorphic eruption. Erythema multiforme is a specific hypersensitivity syndrome with a distinctive clinical pattern, the hallmark of which is the erythematous ring (the so-called iris or target lesion) (Fig. 18-9). Although a single type of lesion might predomi-

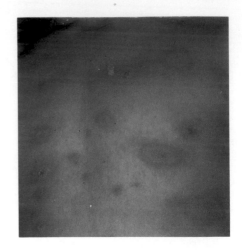

Figure 18-9 Erythema multiforme. Target lesions and marginated wheals with central vesicles.

nate during a particular attack, the basic lesions of erythema multiforme are macular, urticarial, and vesiculobullous; the clinical diagnosis can be made readily if these characteristics are kept in mind.[1] The evolution and resolution of individual lesions lasts about a week, but the eruption may continue to appear in crops for as long as two or three weeks, thus contributing to the multiform appearance of the eruption.

The primary lesion of erythema multiforme is a dull-red to dusky flat macule, or a sharply marginated wheal, in the center of which a papule or vesicle develops, thus creating the multiformity of lesions. The central area then flattens and develops clearing. As a result it is not unusual to see iris or target lesions consisting of concentric circles whose bright red rings alternate with cyanotic or violaceous ones. Although occasionally seen in erythema annulare centrifugum, target lesions are highly characteristic of erythema multiforme. Careful inspection of the eruption in erythema multiforme may disclose fine petechiae, the clinical feature that distinguishes lesions of erythema multiforme from those of urticaria and erythema annulare centrifugum.

Systemic manifestations of simple erythema multiforme, when present, are mild and consist of low-grade fever, malaise, and myalgia. Severe forms of bullous erythema multiforme with mucocutaneous involvement have been labeled Stevens-Johnson disease.[37] Stevens-Johnson disease is merely an extremely severe form of bullous erythema multiforme (Figs. 18-10, 18-11), with high fever, pronounced constitutional symptoms, and widespread bullae, which involve the mucous membranes, conjunctivae, and anogenital areas. The disorder is characterized by a sudden onset and a prodromal period of 1 to 14 days, which can consist of fever, malaise, cough, coryza, sore throat, vomiting, diarrhea, chest pain, myalgia, and arthralgias.

The mucous membranes of the lips, eyes, nasal mucosa, genitalia, and rectum show exten-

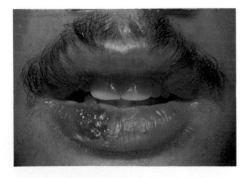

Figure 18-8 Blisters, crusting, and swelling of the lower lip in a patient with erythema multiforme.

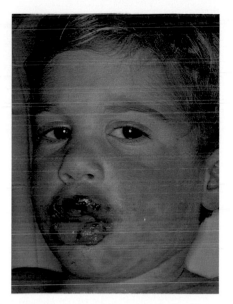

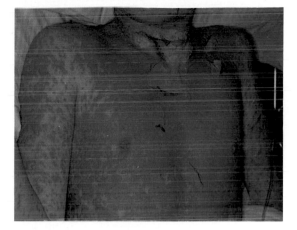

Figure 18–11 Bullous erythema multiforme (Stevens-Johnson syndrome). Confluent erythema, target lesions, blisters, and exfoliation of the epidermis.

Figure 18–10 Stevens-Johnson syndrome. Mucous membrane involvement with severe swelling and hemorrhagic crusting of the lips.

sive bullae with a grayish-white membrane, characteristic hemorrhagic crusts, and superficial erosions and ulcerations. The eye changes may be particularly serious, with severe conjunctivitis, corneal ulcerations, keratitis, uveitis or panophthalmitis. Sequelae may be grave, with a possibility of corneal ulceration and partial or even complete blindness. Pulmonary involvement may occur as an extension from the oral pharynx and tracheobronchial tree, or may be due to pneumonitis associated with an initiating viral infection or secondary infection. Renal involvement, with hematuria, nephritis, and, in some cases, progressive renal failure may result.

The cutaneous lesions of erythema multiforme appear in various forms but all have an identical histologic picture; the severity of the histologic reaction determines the clinical appearance of lesions. Microscopic examination of skin lesions reveals edema just below the epidermis, which when mild or moderate, produces urticarial lesions; when the edema is severe, bullae are formed.[38] Other histologic features consist of dilatation of blood vessels, accompanied by a perivascular infiltration composed mainly of lymphocytes, nuclear dust resulting from disintegration of neutrophils and eosinophils (leukocytoclasis), edema, and extravasation of erythrocytes (Fig. 18–12). Whereas previous immunofluorescent examinations of erythema multiforme lesions have been uniformly negative, recent studies document a high prevalence of deposits of C_3, alone or associated with IgM, in the vessels of the papillary dermis when biopsies are obtained early in the course of the lesions. These findings appear to confirm the theory of immune complexes in the etiology of erythema multiforme.[39]

MANAGEMENT. The management of erythema multiforme and Stevens-Johnson syndrome depends upon the clinical state of the patient. A thorough search for the identification and elimination of the underlying cause is imperative. If a drug is suspected, it should be discontinued. Mild cases may subside spontaneously or occasionally respond to antihistamines. Local therapy depends

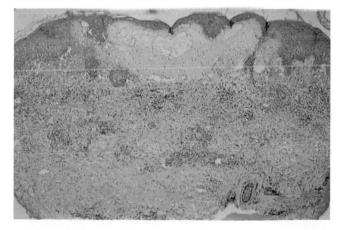

Figure 18–12 Bullous erythema multiforme. Dilatation of blood vessels, perivascular round cell infiltration, extravasation of erythrocytes, and edema of the upper dermis with subepidermal blister formation.

on the type and extent of the lesions. Simple erythema usually requires no treatment. Vesicular, bullous, or erosive lesions may be treated with wet compresses. Colloidal baths may be helpful.

Severe oropharyngeal involvement often necessitates frequent mouthwashes, local application of diphenhydramine (Elixir of Benadryl), or the topical use of diclonin (Dyclone) or lidocaine (Xylocaine Viscous) as an anesthetic. Liquid diet and replacement intravenous therapy may be required in extreme cases. Fluid loss through the skin must be considered and, when extensive, should be handled in a manner similar to that of patients with extensive burns. Dehydration and shock, electrolyte imbalance, and pulmonary, ocular, and renal involvement should be carefully monitored. Skillful cooperation from ophthalmologists should be sought, and the eyes should be cleansed frequently wth separation of the eyelids and topical antibacterial agents to prevent secondary infection. Topical steroids are contraindicated in this area, as they may produce thinning of the cornea and eventual ulceration or perforation.

Although their use is still controversial, most authors feel that steroids in high dosages are indicated in cases with severe skin or mucous membrane involvement, or when there is appreciable systemic toxicity. From 30 to 60 milligrams of prednisone or its equivalent may be given in severe cases, with gradually tapering dosages over a period of two to four weeks. The possibility of secondary infection, however, must be considered, and appropriate antibiotics initiated when indicated. Recent studies, however, suggest that the accepted therapeutic efficacy of systemic steroids in Stevens-Johnson syndrome requires further evaluation.[40]

Henoch-Schönlein Purpura

Henoch-Schönlein purpura, also known by its synonym *anaphylactoid purpura*, is a well-defined systemic disorder of children and young adults. An inflammatory disorder of multiple causes, it appears to represent a diffuse vasculitis caused by hypersensitivity to a variety of etiologic factors. Although the nature of the immunological reaction is not completely clear, a history of frequent antecedent upper respiratory infections preceding the onset of symptoms suggests a hypersensitivity phenomenon resulting in localized or widespread vascular damage. Bacterial or viral infections appear to be the most frequently implicated precipitating causes; drugs, food, insect bites, and chemical toxins also have been suggested as possible etiologic factors.

CLINICAL MANIFESTATIONS. The clinical picture of Henoch-Schönlein vasculitis is distinctive. Mainly a disease of children and young adults (particularly those between three and ten years of age), the disorder is characterized by a distinctive rash (erythematous papules followed by purpura), abdominal pain, and joint symptoms.

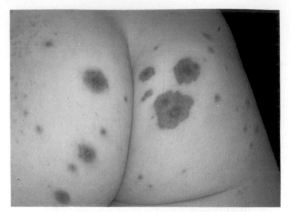

Figure 18–13   Henoch-Schönlein purpura (anaphylactoid purpura). Hemorrhagic macules, papules, and urticarial lesions in a symmetrical distribution over the buttocks of a young child.

Renal disease occurs frequently, but other organ involvement is relatively less common. Generally the disease subsides within a few weeks, with frequent recurrences often related to an upper respiratory infection or re-exposure to the offending agent. The disorder appears to represent a variety of leukocytoclastic angiitis initiated by deposition of immune complexes, which produces a vasculitis of the capillaries and pre- and post-capillary vessels in the upper dermis, gastrointestinal tract, synovial membranes, renal glomeruli, and lungs.[41]

Cutaneous Lesions. The skin lesions of Henoch-Schönlein purpura consist of small hemorrhagic macules, papules, and/or urticarial lesions, which appear in a symmetrical distribution over the buttocks (Fig. 18–13) and the extensor surfaces of the extremities (particularly the elbows and knees) (Fig. 18–14).[42] In more severe cases, hemorrhagic, purpuric, or necrotic lesions may be prominent. The disease usually consists of a single

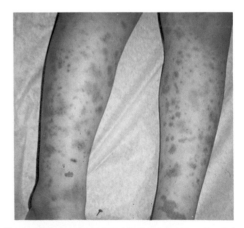

Figure 18–14   Henoch-Schönlein purpura. Small hemorrhagic symmetric papules on the lower extremities. Edema and extravasation of erythrocytes give individual lesions their diagnostic palpable and purpuric appearance.

episode, which may last for several days to several weeks. In some cases, however, recurrent attacks may occur at intervals for weeks or months.

Individual lesions occur in crops, tend to fade after about five days, and eventually are replaced by areas of brownish pigmentation, purpura, or ecchymoses. New crops of lesions frequently occur over the fading lesions of a previous episode, thus giving a polymorphous appearance to the disorder. Although the lesions may be misinterpreted as drug reactions, erythema multiforme, or urticaria, the presence of *palpable purpura* (the hallmark of leukocytoclastic angiitis) will usually clarify the true nature of the disorder. This characteristic finding, created by edema and extravasation of erythrocytes, gives individual lesions their diagnostic palpable and purpuric appearance.[1]

Rarely, the face, mucous membranes of the mouth and nose, and the anogenital regions may show petechial involvement. Children less than three years of age often have an associated edema of the scalp, hands, feet, scrotum, and periorbital tissues. This edema occurs in the absence of renal or cardiac disease and appears to reflect an increased capillary permeability due to the underlying vasculitis.

When the diagnosis remains in doubt, histopathologic examination of a cutaneous biopsy generally helps clarify the nature of the eruption. Histopathologic changes of Henoch-Schönlein purpura are characterized by leukocytoclastic vasculitis, with fibrinoid degeneration of vessel walls and a perivascular infiltrate consisting of neutrophils, some eosinophils, and only a few lymphocytes. Extravasation of erythrocytes is present in purpuric lesions, with deposits of hemosiderin in lesions of long duration. A highly characteristic feature is the presence of scattered nuclear fragments (nuclear dust), which result from the disintegration of the neutrophils.

Systemic Manifestations. Systemic involvement is seen in up to two-thirds of children with severe forms of Henoch-Schönlein purpura. Since proper diagnosis depends upon the characteristic cutaneous eruption, a significant diagnostic challenge occurs when systemic manifestations appear alone or precede the appearance of skin lesions.[43] The degree of systemic involvement may vary, with arthritis or gastrointestinal symptoms reportedly seen in as many as two-thirds of affected children. Gastrointestinal symptoms are common. They usually include colicky abdominal pain and, in severe cases, may consist of vomiting, intussusception, hemorrhage, or shock.[42] Intussusception, seen in up to 2 per cent of patients, is more frequently seen in males, particularly those about 6 years of age. Since intussusception (when not associated with Henoch-Schönlein purpura) generally occurs in young children under two years of age, when seen in older children, Henoch-Schönlein purpura must be strongly considered as a diagnostic possibility.[44]

Arthritis, when present, is characterized by warm, tender, painful swelling of joints, with or without overlying purpura. Although the ankles and knees are most frequently affected, arthropathy of the elbows, hands, and feet may also be seen in association with this disorder.

Renal involvement is probably the most frequent and serious complication of anaphylactoid purpura. It occurs in 25 per cent of children under two and in 50 per cent of those above two years of age.[45] Nephritis may be demonstrated by gross or microscopic hematuria, with or without casts and proteinuria. Although often self-limited, if hematuria persists, it may progress to advanced glomerular disease and a poor prognosis.

Other systemic manifestations may include hepatosplenomegaly. Central nervous system involvement may result in headache and diplopia, and rarely subarachnoid hemorrhage may occur, with coma, seizures, and/or paresis.[46] Respiratory involvement, also uncommon, may range from an asymptomatic pulmonary infiltrate to recurrent episodes of pulmonary hemorrhage.

MANAGEMENT. The prognosis for most patients with Henoch-Schönlein vasculitis is excellent, with full recovery without residue in most patients. In younger children the disease is generally milder, of shorter duration, with fewer renal and gastrointestinal manifestations, and fewer recurrences.[42]

There is no specific therapy for Henoch-Schönlein purpura. Bed rest and general supportive care are helpful. Throat cultures and appropriate antibiotics are indicated if a specific respiratory illness is identified. Since many cases of chronic glomerulonephritis in adults may be related to anaphylactoid purpura during childhood, serial urinalyses are indicated. The efficacy of corticosteroids is debatable. Although there is little evidence that corticosteroids influence the prognosis of Henoch-Schönlein purpura, they suppress the acute manifestations and may be justified for short periods in severe cases, particularly those with significant gastrointestinal complications.

TOXIC EPIDERMAL NECROLYSIS

Toxic epidermal necrolysis (TEN, scalded skin syndrome) is a specific exfoliative dermatitis that consists of two separate and distinctive entities. The overwhelming majority of cases in infants and children are caused by an exfoliative toxin — "exfoliatin" — produced by coagulase-positive Group II staphylococci, usually phage type 55 or 71, and rarely by certain phage Group I staphylococci.[46-51] This form is often termed staphylococcal scalded skin syndrome (SSSS).[49] Bullous impetigo is considered by some investigators to be one of the forms of staphylococcal scalded skin syndrome.[48] In older children and adults toxic epidermal necrolysis is usually, but not necessarily, related to a hypersensitivity to drugs: phenylbutazone, phenolphthalein, procaine, sulfonamides, penicillin, other antibiotics, barbiturates, tranquilizers, vaccines, salicylates, aminopyrine, and diphenylhydantoin (Dilantin).[52]

The reason for the increased incidence of staphylococcal scalded skin syndrome (SSSS) in infants and young children as opposed to adults appears to be related to the fact that adults and 85 per cent of children over 10 years of age have specific staphylococcal antibody that allows the development of localized staphylococcal bullous impetigo but limits widespread bloodstream dissemination of lesions in older individuals. The reason for the decreased incidence of drug-induced toxic epidermal necrolysis (TEN) in infants and young children remains unknown (personal communication, Marian E. Melish).

CLINICAL MANIFESTATIONS. The staphylococcal type of toxic epidermal necrolysis often begins with a prodromal period of malaise, fever, and irritability; a generalized erythema with a fine, stippled sandpaper appearance; and exquisite tenderness to the skin. From the intertriginous and periorificial areas and trunk, the erythema and tenderness spread over the entire body, but usually spare the hairy parts. Children are extremely irritable, uncomfortable, and difficult to hold, owing to the extreme tenderness of the skin. Within two or three days, frequently in a few hours, the upper layer of the epidermis may become wrinkled or may be removed (often peeling off like wet tissue paper) by light stroking, the characteristic Nikolsky sign (Fig. 18–15). The Nikolsky sign is not specific for toxic epidermal necrolysis and may be seen in other bullous disorders (pemphigus, Stevens-Johnson disease, and epidermolysis bullosa). Shortly thereafter the pa-

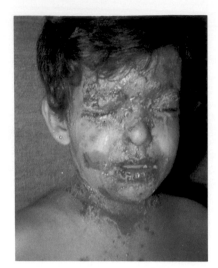

Figure 18–16 Scalded skin syndrome. Characteristic facies with crusting about the eyes, nose, and mouth.

tient develops flaccid bullae and eventual exfoliation of the skin.

During this period the patient develops a highly characteristic pathognomonic facies with crusting, perioral erythema with fissures, and rhagades (deep clefts and fissures) about the nasolabial folds and corners of the mouth (Fig. 18–16). In some cases the skin appears pushed together as though rolled onto itself (resembling planed wood shavings), owing to edema in the epidermis (Figs. 10–10 and 10–11). This may slough off, leaving a moist epidermis resembling a second degree burn. In severe cases the skin of the entire body may peel off.

Although an occasional patient may be desperately ill, when treated properly most have surprisingly little difficulty, except for extreme irritability and skin tenderness. Healing of the involved skin is complete in 10 to 14 days and, if uncomplicated, proceeds without scarring. The mortality rate, if untreated, is highest in children under one year of age and relatively low in those from one to six years of age. Death, when it occurs, has usually been the result of sepsis and fluid and electrolyte imbalance.

Although the staphylococcal scalded skin syndrome is seen primarily in children under 10, drug-related TEN in children and staphylococcus-induced disease in adults have been reported. Since there are clear etiologic and pathologic differences between the two types of toxic epidermal necrolysis, appropriate therapy requires definitive etiologic diagnosis. Diagnosis of staphylococcal scalded skin syndrome can be verified by isolation of coagulase: positive Group II staphylococcus aureus, most frequently types 55 and 71, occasionally Group I, type 52. In patients with this disorder, cultures from intact bullae are usually sterile,[49] but the organism can be recovered from pyogenic foci on the skin, conjunctivae, ala nasi, nasopharynx, stool, and occasionally the blood.

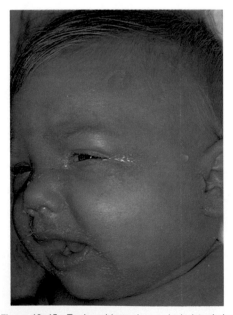

Figure 18–15 Toxic epidermal necrolysis (staphylococcal scalded skin syndrome). Generalized erythema with a fine sandpaper appearance; tenderness of the skin; crusting around the eyes, nose, and mouth; and a positive Nikolsky's sign.

History of ingestion of a drug known to provoke toxic epidermal necrolysis in an older child or adult is suggestive evidence for the drug-induced form of TEN (Lyell's disease). When the diagnosis is indeterminate, the two disorders can be differentiated on histopathologic examination by a simple skin biopsy. In the staphylococcal disorder the disruption shows cleavage in the epidermis; in the drug-induced disorder the separation is seen in the upper dermis below the basement membrane (as in bullous erythema multiforme).[52]

TREATMENT. Treatment of staphylococcal scalded skin syndrome requires prompt initiation of antistaphylococcal therapy in all patients, to eradicate the focus of infection and eliminate further toxin production. One of the penicillinase-resistant antistaphylococcal agents (e.g., dicloxacillin) is preferred, since most of the organisms are resistant to penicillin and some are resistant to erythromycin. Corticosteroids appear to be contraindicated, as they seem to enhance susceptibility of the host to infection.[48] In the late desquamatous phase the skin may be lubricated with bland ointments or lubricating lotions. Topical antibiotics are unnecessary and should be avoided.

In patients with drug-induced TEN, all drugs administered prior to onset of the eruption should be discontinued. Systemic corticosteroids may be life-saving in this form of the disorder. In patients where the true cause of the disorder is indefinite, systemic corticosteroid coverage with appropriate antibiotics may be necessary until an infectious etiology can be excluded.

Although statistics reveal a high mortality in patients with staphylococcal scalded skin syndrome (20 per cent), today this figure is considerably reduced owing to recognition of the true nature of this disorder. In older patients with drug-induced forms of toxic epidermal necrolysis, however, mortality may reach as high as 50 per cent.

KAWASAKI DISEASE

Kawasaki disease (mucocutaneous lymph node syndrome, MCLS, MLNS) is a disorder of unknown etiology affecting infants and young children since around 1950. Mucocutaneous lymph node syndrome was first reported by a Japanese pediatrician, Dr. Tomisaku Kawasaki, in 1967.[53] The Center for Disease Control in Atlanta, Georgia, currently prefers to call it "Kawasaki disease" in honor of the Tokyo physician who contributed so much to our recognition of the syndrome. Patients with this multisystem disease have been described in most other parts of the world.[54-59] The first cases in the United States were seen in Hawaii and reported by Melish in 1974.[60-62] Since then over 650 cases have been reported in the United States between July 1976 and August 1980, and over 24,000 cases have been

Table 18–1 PRINCIPAL SIGNS AND SYMPTOMS OF KD

1. Fever (lasting 1–3 weeks)
2. Cervical adenopathy
3. Bilateral congestion of ocular conjunctivae
4. Reddening of lips and oral mucosa
5. Strawberry tongue
6. Dryness, erosion, and fissuring of lips
7. Polymorphous maculopapular eruption
8. Swelling of hands and feet
9. Desquamation of fingers and toes
10. Transverse nail grooves (Beau's lines)

recorded in Japan (personal communication, Tomisaku Kawasaki, August 1980).

CLINICAL MANIFESTATIONS. Patients with Kawasaki disease (KD) exhibit a unique spectrum of six clinical findings that are distinctive and diagnostically helpful: (1) fever lasting more than five days; (2) bilateral conjunctival injection; (3) dry, red, and fissured lips, strawberry tongue, and redness of the oropharynx; (4) erythematous rash; (5) indurative edema of the hands and feet, followed by desquamation of the fingertips; and (6) non-purulent cervical lymphadenopathy. At present the diagnosis of this disorder is based upon strict adherence to clinical criteria together with exclusion of other clinically similar disease and is considered to be established by the presence of fever and four of the five remaining criteria.[61] A summary of signs and symptoms is presented in Table 18–1.

Fever. To make a diagnosis of Kawasaki disease the patient should have a fever lasting more than five days (with no other reasonable explanation of the illness). Fever, the first sign and principal symptom of this disorder, begins abruptly without prodromal signs. Seen in most patients (95 per cent), it has a remittent pattern with several spikes in temperature up to 104° C each day, does not respond to antibiotics or intermittent doses of antipyretics, and lasts one to three weeks (five to twenty-three days, with an average duration of eleven days).

Conjunctival Injection. Discrete bilateral

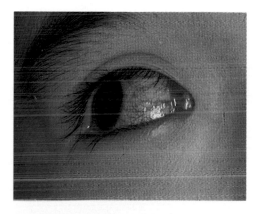

Figure 18–17 Congestion of bulbar conjunctivae in a patient with mucocutaneous lymph node syndrome (Kawasaki disease) (Courtesy of Dr. Tomisaku Kawasaki).

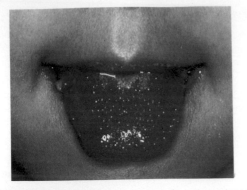

Figure 18–18 Strawberry tongue in mucocutaneous lymph node syndrome (Kawasaki disease) (Courtesy of Dr. Tomisaku Kawasaki).

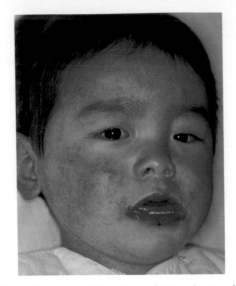

Figure 18–19 Kawasaki disease (mucocutaneous lymph node syndrome). Characteristic facies with congestion of the bulbar conjunctivae and hemorrhagic crusts and erosions of the lips (Courtesy of Dr. Tomisaku Kawasaki).

injection of the bulbar conjunctivae (seen in 88 per cent of patients) generally appears within two days of the onset of fever and persists for a period of one to three weeks (throughout the febrile course of the illness) (Fig. 18–17). This is not a true conjunctivitis and consists chiefly of discrete dilatation of the bulbar conjunctival vessels without evidence of exudative discharge or corneal ulceration.

Oral Cavity Changes.   Changes in the mouth consist of erythema, fissuring, and, at times, bleeding and severe crusting of the lips. The lip changes (seen in 90 per cent of patients) may last for a period of one to three weeks. Erythema and protruberance of the papillae of the tongue (seen in 77 per cent of patients) produces a "strawberry tongue" appearance. When present, strawberry tongue and erythema of the oropharynx appear within one to three days after the onset of fever (Figs. 18–18 and 18–19).

Exanthem.   On the third to fifth day of illness a macular erythematous skin eruption appears (in 92 per cent of patients) (Fig. 18–20). Usually occurring simultaneously with or soon after the onset of fever, it generally begins with pronounced reddening of the palms and soles and gradually spreads to involve the entire trunk and extremities within a period of two days. The rash is polymorphous in nature and usually begins on the extremities as erythematous macules measuring 5 mm or more in diameter. Individual lesions become increasingly larger and often coalescent. Although frequently pruritic, the eruption is never accompanied by vesicles, bullae, or crusts. Deeply erythematous and widespread, the rash may be maculopapular or morbilliform, urticarial, scarlatiniform, or erythema multiforme–like[63] and generally persists for the duration of the fever. In some patients, scattered areas of desquamation may appear sometime between the tenth and fifteenth days of the illness.

Changes in the Extremities.   Reddening of the palms and soles (seen in 90 per cent of patients) and a firm indurative edema of the hands and feet develop (in 75 per cent of patients). The edema is characterized by deeply erythematous to violaceous brawny swelling of the palms and soles, fusiform swelling of the digits, and tightly

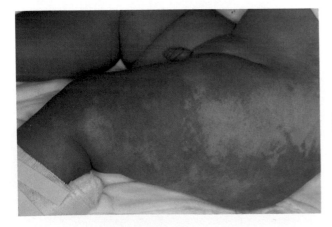

Figure 18–20 Urticaria-like rash in mucocutaneous lymph node syndrome (Kawasaki disease) (Courtesy of Dr. Tomisaku Kawasaki).

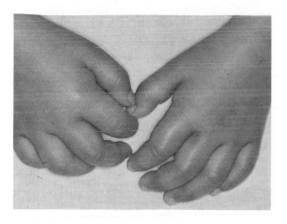

Figure 18–21 Indurative edema of the hands in mucocutaneous lymph node syndrome (Kawasaki disease) (Courtesy of Dr. Tomisaku Kawasaki).

stretched skin on the dorsal aspect of the hands and feet (Fig. 18–21).

Generally 14 to 20 days after the onset of fever a highly characteristic pattern of desquamation begins. Seen in 94 per cent of patients it lasts approximately one week. The desquamation generally begins at the tips of the fingers and toes at the junction of the nails and skin (just beneath the tips of the nails) and, over a period of ten days, gradually progresses to include the fingers, toes, and areas of the palms and soles (Fig. 18–22).

As with many other severe illnesses, Beau's lines (transverse furrows on the nail surface) may develop one or two months after the onset of the illness. This horizontal groove, although seen in almost all patients with Kawasaki disease, is not diagnostic of this disorder; these horizontal grooves develop as a nonspecific reaction to any stress that temporarily interrupts nail growth and become visible on the surface of the nail several weeks later (Table 18–1).

Lymphadenopathy. Cervical lymphadenopathy (the least reliable clinical feature of this disorder) is said to occur in 70 per cent of patients with Kawasaki disease in Japan and in 50 to 86 per cent of patients seen in the United States.[61, 63]

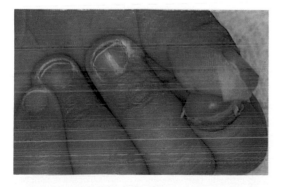

Figure 18–22 Desquamation of the fingers in a patient with mucocutaneous lymph node syndrome (Kawasaki disease) (Courtesy of Dr. Tomisaku Kawasaki).

When present it is unilateral and is generally seen as a single enlarged lymph node in the cervical region. Measuring more than 1.5 cm in diameter, the enlarged node is usually not warm, red, tender, or fluctuant, and in most cases, the lymphadenopathy disappears as the fever subsides.

OTHER CLINICAL FEATURES. Although occasional cases of Kawasaki disease may be seen in adults and children over ten years of age, most patients (85 per cent) are under five and 50 per cent are under 2½ years of age.[53] Associated features include cardiac manifestations, central nervous system involvement (extreme irritability, lethargy, and aseptic meningitis), pyuria, rheumatic complications (arthritis and arthralgia), and gastrointestinal manifestations. The prognosis of mucocutaneous lymph node syndrome is good in most cases, with improvement usually beginning about the 14th day of the illness. ECG abnormalities (prolongation of the PR and QT intervals, and ST segment and T-wave changes), however, have been found in 70 to 90 per cent of children with this disorder, and 27 per cent of patients have shown abnormalities in coronary angiography one to six months after the onset of the disease.

Coronary Occlusion. Of even greater significance is the fact that sudden death due to coronary occlusion occurs in 1 to 2 per cent of patients, generally young infants with this disorder. Male infants are at special risk, since 80 per cent of fatalities have been in boys. Although death due to coronary occlusion has been noted a short time after apparent recovery from the illness, most deaths (90 per cent) occur suddenly between three and seven weeks after the onset of the disease, and several deaths have been reported two to four years after apparent recovery from this disorder.[57] Children at high risk of sudden death or carditis are boys less than one year of age, particularly those who have prolonged or recurrent fever and rash, extreme elevation of the erythrocyte sedimentation rate, and cardiac signs such as gallop rhythm, arrhythmia, cardiomegaly, and ECG abnormality.[61] It should be noted, however, that these factors are only a guide and are not always reliable in predicting the prognosis for patients with Kawasaki disease. The causes of sudden death are myocarditis, inflammation of the A-V conduction system, ischemic heart disease, and rupture of aneurysms.[59]

Central Nervous System Effects. Central nervous system effects are seen in nearly all patients with KD. They consist of negativistic behavior, sleep disturbances, severe irritability, and frequent episodes of crying and whining. Approximately one-third of patients have severe lethargy, semi-coma, or coma during the acute febrile stage. One-fourth of patients are found to have an associated aseptic meningitis.[61]

Pyuria. Pyuria, seen in 70 per cent of patients, occurs in the acute stage of the disease. It appears to be urethral in origin, and although a small portion of patients may have a transient hematuria, proteinuria is not a feature of the disease. A number of boys have also been found to have small meatal ulcers during the acute stage of the illness.

Arthritis and Arthralgia. Arthritis and arthralgia (seen in 20 and 40 per cent of patients respectively) occur later in the febrile stage of the illness, or shortly thereafter. Large joints such as the knees, hips, and elbows are the most commonly affected. Although ultimately self-limiting, arthritis and effusion may last for periods of two to four weeks.

Gastrointestinal Manifestations. Gastrointestinal manifestations (diarrhea and abdominal pain) are seen in approximately one-fourth of affected patients, and hepatitis, with modest to moderate bilirubin elevation and moderate elevations of serum SGOT and SGPT, is seen in about 10 per cent of patients during the acute febrile stage of the illness. Acute hydrops of the gallbladder has also been reported. Appearing late in the acute febrile phase of the illness, or early in convalescence, this complication may manifest as a mass in the right upper quadrant of the abdomen. Ultrasound examination is useful in the diagnosis and monitoring of this frequently severe but apparently self-limiting phenomenon.

PATHOGENESIS. Despite the thousands of well-documented case histories accumulated since this disorder was first described, the etiology of Kawasaki disease remains unknown. Rickettsia-like antibodies in biopsy specimens have suggested a rickettsial etiology, but negative serologic studies and failure of response to tetracycline fail to substantiate this possibility. An abnormal host reaction to a variety of different infections and chemical factors has been suggested. Generalized vasculitis, circulating immune complexes, occasional hypocomplementemia, elevated IgE, and a higher incidence of allergic phenomena in patients and their families lend support to this hypothesis. Because this disease appears to be most prevalent in Japan and the incidence is much higher in Japanese than in Caucasians or Blacks, a unique genetic susceptibility is suspected. This appears to be supported by an increased frequency of HLA-BW22 and HLA-BW22J2 (antigens that have a higher incidence in Japanese than in other people) in patients with Kawasaki disease.[64]

From a pathologic viewpoint, Kawasaki disease is an arteritis involving the small and medium-sized arteries, with a predilection for involvement of the main coronary arteries. Histopathologic findings reveal an arteritis involving small and medium-sized vessels, marked edema of the dermal connective tissue, swelling of endothelial cells in postcapillary venules, dilatation of small blood vessels, and lymphocytic and monocytic perivascular infiltrates. Pathologic examination of the hearts of patients who died of Kawasaki disease reveals acute perivasculitis of the arterioles, capillaries, and venules of the small arteries, acute perivasculitis and endarteritis of the three major coronary arteries, myocarditis, coagulation necrosis, lesions of the conduction system, pericarditis, and endocarditis with vasculitis. The

causes of sudden death in such individuals are myocarditis, inflammation of the A-V conduction systems, rupture of aneurysms, and ischemic heart disease.[59]

Kawasaki disease resembles infantile periarteritis nodosa in many respects. Although it has been suggested that the small number of reported cases and the high rate of mortality of infantile periarteritis nodosa appear to distinguish this disorder from mucocutaneous lymph node syndrome, it now appears that infantile periarteritis nodosa may merely represent a fatal form of this disorder.[65] The link between Kawasaki disease and periarteritis nodosa is also interesting, since hydrops of the gallbladder has been seen in association with both conditions. Infantile periarteritis nodosa should not be confused with the adult form of periarteritis nodosa. These two conditions differ in their clinical presentations, pathologic manifestations, and laboratory findings (see Chapter 9).

LABORATORY STUDIES. Laboratory tests show leukocytosis, polycythemia, a mild anemia, normal flora in the throat and stools, and sterile cultures of the blood and cerebrospinal fluid. Thrombocytosis is a universal laboratory finding in Kawasaki disease, and it appears to coincide with the period of highest risk of coronary thrombosis. Unlike the sedimentation rate and white blood count, platelet counts are usually normal during the acute febrile phase of the illness. Thrombocytosis generally rises after the tenth day of illness, reaches a peak of 600,000 to 1,800,000 between the fifteenth and twenty-fifth days, and then falls to normal values by the thirtieth day of the disorder.[61]

Febrile agglutinins, hemagglutination titers for rubella and toxoplasmosis, and complement fixation titers for ECHO virus, Coxsackie virus, Rocky Mountain spotted fever, rubeola, typhus, rickettsial pox, Q-fever, and *Mycoplasma pneumoniae* reveal no significant changes. There may be white blood cells and protein in the urine. Cerebrospinal fluid may show mononuclear pleocytosis with slightly elevated protein, and bilirubin determinations may reveal a slightly increased indirect fraction. Other laboratory findings noted to date may include an increased erythrocyte sedimentation rate, positive C-reactive protein, increased serum alpha$_2$ proteins, elevated IgM and IgE levels, reduced serum protein levels with reversal of the A/G ratio, and transient elevation of SGOT and pyruvic transaminase (Table 18–2).

Table 18–2 OTHER SIGNIFICANT SYMPTOMS AND FINDINGS OF KD

1. Gastrointestinal manifestations	9. Elevated alpha$_2$ globulins
2. Arthritis	10. Elevated IgM and IgE
3. Urinary findings	11. Positive CRP
4. Aseptic meningitis	12. Hepatic abnormalities
5. EKG changes (70%)	13. Rickettsia-like bodies
6. Leukocytosis, mild anemia	14. Infantile polyarteritis
7. Thrombocytosis	a. coronary thrombosis
8. Increased sed rate	b. coronary aneurysms

DIFFERENTIAL DIAGNOSIS. Differential diagnosis of Kawasaki disease includes scarlet fever, viral exanthems, erythema multiforme and Stevens-Johnson syndrome, rickettsial disease, atypical measles, juvenile rheumatoid arthritis, systemic lupus erythematosus, toxic epidermal necrolysis, herpetic stomatitis, drug reactions, acrodynia, and staphylococcal toxic shock syndrome of childhood.

MANAGEMENT. To date there is no effective or definitive treatment for this disease or its catastrophic sequelae. Currently the most important problem in the management of patients with Kawasaki disease appears to be the ability to detect and prevent coronary aneurysm and myocardial infarction. Although coronary angiography and, at times, coronary by-pass surgery is often recommended for children who develop myocardial infarction,[58] bi-planer echocardiography is suggested as an effective non-invasive technique for the detection of aneurysms, mitral valve dysfunction, myocardiopathy, and pericardial effusion.[66, 67]

Present treatment is supportive and requires a careful program of repeated clinical and laboratory evaluation in an attempt to detect and manage serious cardiac and vascular complications.[61] Heparin, steroids, antibiotics, azathioprine, and cyclophosphamide have not been very effective. Anti-inflammatory therapy with aspirin, however, appears to be beneficial. In addition to shortening the febrile stage in some patients, it may have an effect on platelet adhesiveness and platelet-endothelial interaction, and thus may help prevent coronary thrombosis.

At present aspirin, in dosages of 80 to 100 mg/kg/day, appears to shorten the duration of the fever. Approximately two-thirds of patients become afebrile within two days of treatment, and in the remaining one-third of cases the temperature remains elevated for several days. Once the patient has become afebrile, if there is no evidence of arthritis or arthralgia, the dosage of aspirin may be reduced to 20 to 30 mg/kg/day and, in patients without complications, aspirin should be continued until the sedimentation rate has become normal (this usually occurs approximately 6 to 10 weeks after the onset of illness).[61] Although systemic corticosteroids have been suggested for the treatment of Kawasaki disease, recent studies suggest that corticosteroids are contraindicated since there appears to be a higher incidence of coronary aneurysms in patients so treated.[68]

SARCOIDOSIS

Sarcoidosis, a systemic granulomatous disorder of unknown etiology with widespread manifestations, is rarely seen in children. The greatest incidence of this disorder is in patients between 20 and 40 years of age. Although the youngest reported patient was a two-month-old infant, of the relatively few childhood cases in the literature, most have occurred in the preadolescent or ado-

lescent age group (between 9 and 15 years of age).[69]

The disease occurs in Blacks, Mongoloids, and Caucasians. It appears to be most common among Scandinavians, American Blacks, and Caucasians of the southeastern United States. It is rarely seen in African Blacks and does not occur in the American Indian. Although there have been case reports involving Caucasian children of Northern European ancestry, most cases of childhood sarcoidosis in the United States have been in Blacks from the "sarcoid belt" of the southeastern states.[69-74]

CLINICAL MANIFESTATIONS. The signs and symptoms of sarcoidosis are due primarily to local tissue infiltration and injury from pressure and displacement by sarcoidal lesions. The skin, lungs, eyes, liver, spleen, lymph nodes, bones, muscles, nervous system, and exocrine glands may be involved, with clinical manifestations of the disorder dependent upon the organ or system involved and its degree of involvement.[70]

Arthralgias, low-grade fever, and abdominal pain are the most frequent symptoms in children with sarcoidosis.[70] Pulmonary involvement, the earliest and most frequently seen in adults, also occurs in most childhood forms of this disorder. Symptoms referable to the lungs are usually mild and often consist of a dry hacking cough, with or without mild to moderate dyspnea.[69] The most common roentgenographic finding in children is that of bilateral hilar lymph node enlargement, with or without detectable lung changes.[70, 71] Ocular involvement, too, is extremely common in children. Uveitis and iritis constitute the most frequently observed lesions, but keratitis, retinitis glaucoma, and involvement of the eyelids and lacrimal glands may also occur. (Fig. 18–23). Although examination of the world literature suggests that eye lesions in children are not usually severe, involvement of the eye, with resultant partial or total blindness, occurs in a relatively high percentage of children with sarcoidosis.[69, 72]

Facial nerve paralysis and central nervous

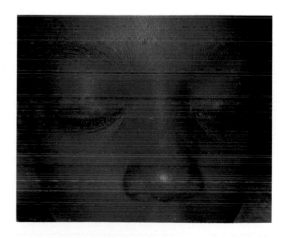

Figure 18–23 Granuloma annulare of upper eyelid resembling sarcoidosis.

system involvement, although common in adults, are rare in children. Osseous involvement is also rarely seen in children. When present, however, the metacarpals, metatarsals, and phalanges are the bones most frequently affected. Uveoparotid fever (a combination of uveitis, parotitis, and Bell's palsy) and Sjögren's syndrome without arthritis (keratoconjunctivitis sicca and enlargement of the parotid and lacrimal glands), though often seen in adults, are quite rare in children. Parotid gland enlargement and peripheral adenopathy are commonly seen in children. Hepatic and splenic involvement, though clinically uncommon, are frequently seen at necropsy.

Although the incidence of skin lesions noted in patients with sarcoidosis depends upon the observer and therefore varies in different series, of the 113 children with sarcoidosis reviewed by McGovern and Merritt, 57 patients (50 per cent) were noted to have skin lesions.[70] Cutaneous lesions can arise anywhere on the body, and although they do not have a pathognomonic clinical morphology, they exhibit highly characteristic features that should strongly suggest the presence of the disease.[1]

Cutaneous Lesions. Cutaneous lesions of sarcoidosis include papules, nodules, infiltrated plaques, subcutaneous tumors, and scaly erythematous patches with little or no palpable infiltration. The most common lesions are soft, red to yellowish-brown or violaceous flat-topped papules, with a predilection for the face. Although the extremities, neck, and trunk may be affected, an annular configuration of these lesions around the nares, lips, and eyelids is highly characteristic of this disorder. Frequently these lesions will present a waxy or translucent appearance. Occasionally the mucous membranes may be involved as well. If the cutaneous lesions are pressed out with a glass slide (diascopy), a characteristic yellowish-brown or "apple-jelly" color may be demonstrated.

Other forms of sarcoidosis in the skin have received special designations, which are becoming obsolete. One of these is *lupus pernio,* a variant in which soft infiltrated violaceous plaques are located on the nose, cheeks, ears, forehead, dorsa of the hands, fingers, or toes. *Angiolupoid* is a term used to describe purplish infiltrated plaques or nodules, particularly on or around the nose, with a characteristic telangiectatic vascular component. *Erythrodermic sarcoidosis* is a term used to describe a relatively rare variant of this disorder. Characterized by extensive, sharply demarcated, brownish-red scaly patches with little or no palpable infiltration, these lesions often involute spontaneously. Another form of skin involvement is a nodular vasculitis with a granulomatous infiltrate largely confined to the subcutaneous tissue. This variant has been termed the *Darier-Roussy* type of sarcoidosis. These skin-colored or violaceous, round or oval, deep-seated nodules appear primarily on the trunk and legs, usually without subjective symptoms. Since lesions often have a non-specific inflammatory etiol-

ogy, this eponym probably should be abandoned.

Erythema nodosum, occasionally seen in association with sarcoidosis, is a striking but not diagnostic finding; it represents a hypersensitivity phenomenon and is not specific for this disorder.

DIAGNOSIS.   There is no single fully reliable test for sarcoidosis. Since the clinical picture may be mimicked by other diseases, histologic proof in the form of either a biopsy or a positive *Kveim* test is essential. The Kveim test consists of intradermal injection of a 10 per cent suspension of human sarcoidal tissue in normal saline. During the following weeks a small papule may develop at the site of injection. Biopsy of the papule four to six weeks after the injection reveals specific distinctive sarcoidal granulomas. In general, the frequency of a positive response to the Kveim test is greatest in early cases of sarcoidosis. Because of loss of reactivity as the disease progresses, this test has been found to have prognostic as well as diagnostic value. Tuberculin, histoplasmin, coccidioidin, and cat-scratch antigen tests also should be performed, as these conditions may closely resemble sarcoidosis in children. The diagnosis often is hindered by a lack of the classic laboratory findings of hyperglobulinemia, hypercalcemia, leukopenia, and eosinophilia. Although occasionally found, they rarely prove to be reliable features of this disorder in childhood.[70]

The natural course of sarcoidosis in childhood is insidious, follows a smoldering course, and often regresses completely after many years. Mortality is reported to be about 5 per cent, and tuberculosis has been estimated to occur in 10 per cent of children with sarcoidosis.[70]

Since the etiology of sarcoidosis is unknown, specific therapy is not available. Corticosteroids, however, can suppress the acute manifestation of sarcoidosis. Because of the well-known hazards of prolonged systemic corticosteroid therapy, the indications for treatment are determined by the specific organ system involved and the severity of the involvement. Corticosteroids should be used in patients with hypercalcemia, ocular involvement, severe or debilitating lung disease, or lung disease that is progressing rapidly, and for the management of ocular sarcoidosis. In ocular sarcoidosis, corticosteroid ophthalmic preparations may be utilized in conjunction with the systemic therapy. In children the dose of prednisone is 1 mg/kg of body weight, with gradual reduction to the lowest dosage that will suppress the symptoms and signs of the disorder. The course of treatment is usually about six months, but the duration of therapy is determined by the response to therapy and the type and severity of involvement.

DISORDERS ASSOCIATED WITH DIABETES

Necrobiosis Lipoidica Diabeticorum

Necrobiosis lipoidica diabeticorum (NLD) is a degenerative disorder of the dermal connective

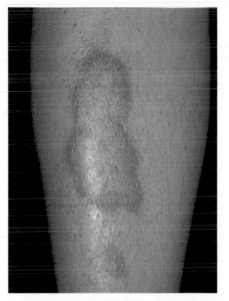

Figure 18–24   Necrobiosis lipoidica diabeticorum. A yellowish-red oval atrophic plaque with a waxy translucent surface, telangiectatic vessels, and a characteristic violaceous margin.

tissue, often seen in patients with diabetes mellitus, characterized by atrophic plaques on the anterior surface of the lower legs (Fig. 18–24). Although the etiology of this disorder is unknown, it appears to be related to an alteration of dermal collagen due to angiopathy of small vessels (possibly a diabetes-related endarteritic obliterative vascular occlusion).[75, 76]

Necrobiosis lipoidica diabeticorum precedes the onset of diabetes in 20 per cent of patients. More than half the patients have active diabetes mellitus, and an abnormal glucose tolerance test is demonstrable in from 50 to 87 per cent of patients with this disorder.[1] Although statistics vary, NLD occurs in 0.1 to 0.3 per cent of diabetics. It appears to be relatively more frequent in children than in adults and occurs three times more often in women than in men.[77] In 90 per cent of patients it is localized to one or both pretibial areas; in the remaining individuals it may occur on the trunk, face, scalp, arms, palms, or soles.[1] The disorder may occur at any age. It was noted at birth in one patient, but usually develops in the third or fourth decade of life and has a peak incidence in persons between 50 and 60 years of age.[1, 77]

A typical lesion of necrobiosis diabeticorum begins as an erythematous papule or nodule with a sharply circumscribed border. It gradually enlarges and slowly develops into an oval yellowish-red sclerotic plaque with an irregular outline and a violaceous margin. The center of the plaque is often depressed or atrophic and shows a waxy translucent surface coursed by telangiectatic vessels. Lesions are usually asymptomatic. Trauma to the atrophic skin is poorly tolerated and ulceration, although rare in childhood, may occur in up to 30 per cent of patients with this disorder.[78]

The treatment of necrobiosis diabeticorum is, in general, not very satisfactory. Since trauma may produce stubborn painful ulcerations, protection of the legs, elastic stockings, and bed rest may be useful. Although patients may be seen without evidence of diabetes, the presence of lesions should alert one to this possibility, and an appropriate search for frank diabetes, latent diabetes, or a prediabetic state should be initiated.

Lesions of NLD are usually symptom free and often are only of diagnostic or cosmetic importance. Cosmetic makeup or dark hose may help hide lesions. Topical corticosteroids (alone or under occlusion) or intralesional steroid injection may improve and clear some lesions. Since patches of necrobiosis are ordinarily atrophic, caution must be exercised to prevent further atrophy or ulceration. Ulcerative lesions are best treated conservatively with compresses and topical antibiotics. Extensive ulcerations may require excision and full-thickness skin grafts. Poor healing due to vascular damage and recurrences in and around grafts, however, is not uncommon.

Diabetic Dermopathy

Diabetic dermopathy, first described in 1964 by Melin, is a characteristic dermatosis seen in 50 per cent of patients with diabetes mellitus.[79] Seen most frequently in males, the initial lesions are round or oval, red or reddish-brown papules that slowly evolve into discrete, sharply circumscribed atrophic, hyperpigmented, or scaly patches; sometimes only depressed areas with normal skin color are seen. Lesions generally measure one centimeter or less in diameter, and although they may occur on the scalp, forearms, or trunk, they usually appear on the anterior aspect of thighs and shins of affected individuals.[80]

The histologic picture of this disorder suggests a possible relationship to diabetic microangiopathy.[79, 81] Although the exact pathogenesis is still undetermined, the presence of these characteristic lesions can serve as a clue to the diagnosis of diabetes mellitus. More studies on the vascular and dermal changes, however, are required to help elucidate the true pathogenesis of this disorder.

Lesions of diabetic dermopathy are in large part uninfluenced by treatment. Individual lesions tend to disappear spontaneously after a period of one and a half to two years. The development of new lesions, however, often creates an impression that individual lesions persist for longer periods of time. Treatment should emphasize protection of the shins from trauma, and bed rest, open wet compresses, and topical antibiotics should be utilized to assist healing of inflammatory and crusted lesions.

Bullous Dermatosis in Diabetes Mellitus

Bullosis diabeticorum is a rare disorder that consists of large asymptomatic bullous lesions that

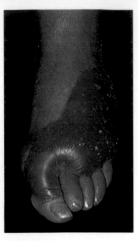

Figure 18–25 Bullous dermatosis in diabetes mellitus (bullosis diabeticorum). Painless bullae on the dorsal aspect of the foot of a patient with diabetes mellitus (Department of Dermatology, Yale University School of Medicine).

develop rapidly on the distal extemities, especially the hands and feet (Fig. 18–25).[82, 83] Although many of the patients have peripheral neuropathy, this complication of diabetes is not present in all.[1] The bullae are painless, clear, and non-inflammatory. They develop rapidly, without evidence of trauma, ultraviolet exposure, or vascular insufficiency and heal slowly and spontaneously.[83]

The etiology of bullosis diabeticorum is not known. Treatment consists of aseptic aspiration or incision and drainage and the use of topical antibiotics to prevent secondary infection.

GRANULOMA ANNULARE

Granuloma annulare is a relatively common cutaneous disorder characterized clinically by papules or nodules that are grouped in a ring-like or circinate distribution. Although granuloma annulare may occur on any part of the body, it usually begins on the lateral or dorsal surfaces of the hands or feet. Females are affected twice as frequently as males. Granuloma annulare may occur at any age. Children and young adults, however, are most commonly affected, with over 40 per cent of cases appearing in children under 15 years of age.[84]

The cause of granuloma annulare is unknown. Various studies have shown latent diabetes to be present in a third of patients with this disorder.[85] Although still open to controversy, this finding (demonstrated in some adults but not in children) suggests that the underlying defect may be related to diabetes and to vascular changes associated with the diabetic state.[85, 86] In some individuals granuloma annulare has been noted following trauma or insect bites. These theories, although

attractive, still remain unsubstantiated and require further confirmation.[87]

Early lesions of granuloma annulare begin as smooth, flesh-colored or pale-red papules that slowly undergo central involution and peripheral extension to form rings with clear centers and elevated borders of continuous papules or nodules (Fig. 18–26). The rings are oval or irregular in outline and vary in size from 1 to 5 cm in diameter. Lesions may be single or multiple; multiple lesions are more common in young children than in older patients, but numerous widely disseminated lesions can occur at any age. Subcutaneous forms, most often seen on the legs, scalp, palms, and buttocks, have a similar clinical and histological appearance and often are confused with rheumatoid nodules. Rheumatoid nodules, however, are usually larger and subcutaneous rather than intradermal in location.

Lesions of granuloma annulare usually disappear spontaneously, often within a period of several months to several years. Although 73 per cent of lesions disappear within a period of two years (with no residual scarring), recurrences are common and may be seen, usually at the original site, in up to 40 per cent of patients.[84] At times, as simple a procedure as intralesional saline or a small biopsy may be followed by complete involution.

Although topical corticosteroids, corticosteroids under occlusion, and intralesional steroids are beneficial and hasten resolution of lesions, because of the potential risk of dermal atrophy associated with such therapy, reassurance of eventual spontaneous resolution may be all that is necessary for treatment of the cosmetic aspect of this disorder. Since we recognize the fact that patients with granuloma annulare (particularly adults) may be candidates for diabetes mellitus, it is reasonable that all patients with granuloma annulare be investigated for this possibility.

Figure 18–26 Granuloma annulare. Flesh-colored papulonodular lesions in an annular configuration.

CONNECTIVE TISSUE DISORDERS (COLLAGEN DISEASES)

The connective tissue or collagen diseases are often grouped together because they are characterized by inflammatory changes of the connective tissue in various parts of the body. The etiology of these disorders and the pathogenesis of their inflammation, to date, remain unknown. Of these disorders, juvenile rheumatoid arthritis, lupus erythematosus, and dermatomyositis exhibit a variety of cutaneous findings, which indicate the presence of connective tissue disease and act as specific markers for the individual disorders.[1]

Juvenile Rheumatoid Arthritis

Juvenile rheumatoid arthritis (Still's disease) is a common generalized systemic disease of unknown etiology and may occur at any age in childhood. The disorder occurs almost twice as frequently in females as in males. The most common age of onset is between two and four, with another peak in frequency in girls during adolescence. Although the age of onset is rarely under one year, it has been reported as early as the first week of life.[88]

CLINICAL MANIFESTATIONS. The onset of juvenile rheumatoid arthritis may be sudden and fulminating, with a high spiking fever (which may last for weeks or months), adenopathy, splenomegaly, and anemia, with or without arthralgia; or it may begin slowly, with insidious involvement of a single joint for weeks or months before other joints are affected. The type of onset, to a considerable extent, is related to the age of the patient — the younger the patient, generally the more prominent the systemic manifestations. When the onset is abrupt, with combined constitutional and joint symptoms, the disorder is termed Still's disease.

A highly characteristic rash may be the first clue to the diagnosis of juvenile rheumatoid arthritis. Seen in 25 to 50 per cent of patients, it may precede other manifestations by up to three years. The eruption, generally seen at the height of fever, appears as flat to slightly elevated macules or papules that measure from 2 to 6 mm in diameter. Lesions vary in color from salmon-pink to red and display a characteristic slightly irregular or serpiginous margin (Fig. 18–27).[89] Some lesions may be slightly raised, edematous, and urticarial in nature, but, unlike true urticaria, they do not itch, migrate, or change in shape. They are often surrounded by a zone of pallor, and larger lesions frequently have a pale center.

The eruption is usually intermittent, is often evanescent, and frequently subsides during periods of remission. The rash may appear at any time during the course of the disease and is associated in particular with spikes in fever, splenomegaly, and lymphadenopathy. Accentuated in areas of local heat or trauma, it may be precipitated by emotional, infectious, or surgical stress. Individual lesions often coalesce to form large plaques 8 to 9 cm in diameter and, in severely affected individuals, the eruption may persist for periods of one week to several years.

Histologic examination of the cutaneous eruption reveals edematous collagen fibers and perivascular cell infiltrate in the upper portion of the corium, with polymorphonuclear leukocytes and, to a lesser extent, plasma cells and histiocytes.[88]

Children with juvenile rheumatoid arthritis characteristically have an anxious or worried facial expression and an intense desire to be left alone, perhaps owing to their extreme discomfort and an attempt to guard their joints against movement. Thirty to 50 per cent of affected children have involvement of only one joint for a time, usually the knee or ankle, but eventually almost all manifest polyarthritis. When multiple joint involvement occurs, it usually is symmetrical and may involve any synovial joint in the body (with the possible exception of joints of the lumbothoracic spine). Joints of the lower extremities are usually affected first, especially the knee joint, which is involved in 90 per cent of patients. Finger joints are involved in approximately 75 per cent and the ankles and wrists in approximately two-thirds of all patients. There is limitation of motion, usually due to pain; the joints may be warm but not tender; and redness is not marked. The skin, especially over the affected joint of the extremi-

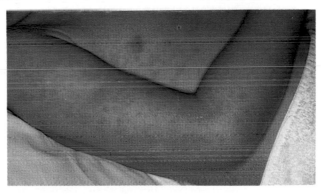

Figure 18–27 A salmon-pink to red maculopapular eruption with irregular or serpiginous margins seen in a child with juvenile rheumatoid arthritis.

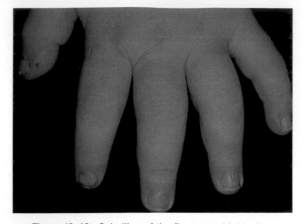

Figure 18-28 Spindling of the fingers—a highly diagnostic feature of juvenile rheumatoid arthritis. The spindle-shaped deformity is related to the fact that the proximal interphalangeal joints are affected more severely than the distal ones.

ties, becomes atrophic, smooth, and glossy. The thenar and hypothenar eminences may be red; the palms, however, usually remain cold and damp.

Spindling of the fingers (Fig. 18-28), one of the earliest objective signs of joint involvement, is seen in more than 50 per cent of children with juvenile rheumatoid arthritis. The spindle-shaped deformity of the fingers develops because the proximal interphalangeal joints are affected more severely than the distal joints. This finding, rarely seen in any other childhood disease, is highly characteristic and carries considerable diagnostic significance.

Subcutaneous nodules are seen in 6 to 10 per cent of children with rheumatoid arthritis at some time during the course of the disease. Barely palpable to several centimeters in size, they may be the first presenting sign of juvenile rheumatoid arthritis. Their most common location is near the olecranon process on the ulnar border of the forearm. Less commonly they may occur on the dorsal aspect of the hands, on the knees and ears, and over pressure areas such as the scapulae, sacrum, buttocks, and heels. In the areas of fingers and toes, subcutaneous nodules are only a few millimeters in size. Subcutaneous nodules are firm and non-tender, and may be attached to the periarticular capsules of the fingers. In contrast to lesions of granuloma annulare they may be deep in the dermis or in the subcutaneous tissue. Subcutaneous nodules are associated with severe exacerbation of the disease but are not related to prognosis.

About 5 per cent of patients with rheumatoid arthritis have cuticular telangiectases, a characteristic sign of connective tissue disease also seen in patients with lupus erythematosus, scleroderma, and dermatomyositis. This finding is seen as linear wiry vessels perpendicular to the base of the nail in the overlying cuticular and periungual

skin. Cuticular telangiectases are usually bright red; not caused by trauma; and when thrombosed, appear to be black. Cuticular telangiectases are rarely seen in normal individuals and are particularly helpful in the diagnosis of connective tissue disease.[1]

The natural course of juvenile rheumatoid arthritis is variable. The disease may end after a few months and never recur, or it may recur after months or years of remission. The active process often improves by puberty, but about 10 per cent of patients are severely crippled by this disorder.

TREATMENT.   There is no specific or curative treatment for this disorder. Aspirin (acetylsalicylic acid) is the drug of choice for early treatment, with an attempt to maintain serum salicylate levels between 25 and 30 mg per 100 ml. Once active disease is suppressed, aspirin must be continued for months before it is gradually withdrawn. Corticosteroids (0.5 to 1.0 mg per kg of prednisone or its equivalent) are indicated only for the seriously ill child or when disease threatens life or sight. Corticosteroids are vital for protracted iridocyclitis and vasculitis. Intrasynovial steroid injections are helpful in severe joint involvement.

Gold therapy, with weekly doses of 1 mg per kg of the salt for a total of 500 mgm, may be useful for patients with non-responsive polyarthritis. Careful examination, however, for leukopenia, thrombocytopenia, eosinophilia, proteinuria, hematuria, severe pruritus, or cutaneous eruption, particularly exfoliative dermatitis, should be performed at frequent intervals. Corticosteroid drops in association with mydriatics are helpful in the management of iridocyclitis. Appropriate rest, splinting, exercise, and physical therapy are important for the prevention and correction of deformity. Although severe deformities can be corrected by surgery, surgical treatment (synovectomy for removal of granulation tissue) should be considered only after a fair trial of medical therapy has been undertaken. Children six years of age or younger are poor surgical risks, however, because of their inability to cooperate effectively with postoperative measures.[90]

Dermatomyositis

Dermatomyositis is an inflammatory disorder that primarily affects the skin and striated muscles. In cases in which cutaneous changes are absent or insignificant the term polymyositis is used. Since the clinical and pathological features of involved skin and muscles are similar, dermatomyositis and polymyositis are felt to be variants of the same disease process.

The etiology of dermatomyositis is unknown. Recent studies suggest that the pathogenesis involves an immunologic reaction directed at blood vessels and skeletal muscle. Although vascular deposits of immunoglobulins and complement have been demonstrated in blood vessel walls of skeletal muscle of involved children and it has been suggested that they are antigen-antibody complement, their pathogenic role remains uncertain.[91]

Dermatomyositis occurs twice as frequently in females as in males. Although it may occur at any age, about 25 per cent of those afflicted are less than 18 years of age at the time of onset.[92] In adults the disorder occurs most commonly between 50 and 70; in childhood the highest incidence is between 5 and 12, the youngest case reported being that of a 4-month-old infant. Malignancy is associated with adult dermatomyositis in about 20 per cent of cases.[93] Although malignancy has been reported twice in children with dermatomyositis, in contrast to adults, no relationship between malignancy and this disorder appears to occur in childhood.[94-96]

CLINICAL MANIFESTATIONS.   The onset of dermatomyositis is usually insidious, with muscle weakness and fatigue. Children often present with fever. Characteristic cutaneous lesions include a violaceous erythema of the upper eyelids (Figs. 18–29 and 18–30) and extensor joint surface. They may come after polymyositis or may precede muscle disease by an interval of a few weeks to three years. When skin markings precede polymyositis, the interval is generally between three and six months.[1]

A variety of cutaneous findings may be noted in dermatomyositis. The dermatitis may be the most striking feature of the illness, or it may be so minor as to be easily overlooked. The rash in most cases is distinctive and highly suggestive, but not pathognomonic.[90] A purplish-red erythema occurs on the face, especially on the eyelids, upper cheeks (Fig. 18–29), forehead, and temples. Frequently associated with photosensitivity, it is often described as a heliotrope erythema, from the flower of the reddish-purple plant bearing this name. When present, this color is highly distinc-

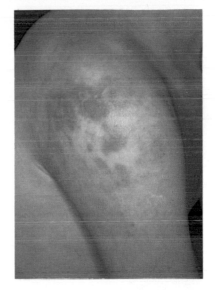

Figure 18–30   Heliotrope eruption on the shoulders and upper arm of an 11-year-old boy with dermatomyositis.

tive and often diagnostic. Sometimes the facial lesions are very edematous, leading to a periorbital edema with the reddish or purplish heliotrope color. Within a few weeks a confluent, violaceous, often edematous erythema with fine scaling may also appear over the hairline of the scalp, nape of the neck, extensor surfaces of the arms and shoulders (Fig. 18–30), elbows, knees, and dorsal interphalangeal joints (often suggesting a diagnosis of contact dermatitis or photosensitivity).

Again, in almost every case, there is erythema of the cuticles at the base of the nails, with accompanying cuticular linear telangiectasia (Fig. 18–31). Hypertrichosis and hyperpigmentation, independent of corticosteroid therapy, may complicate previously involved skin, particularly in

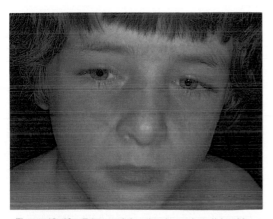

Figure 18–29   Edema of the cheeks and eyelids with a purplish-red heliotrope erythema on the eyelids and cheeks of a child with dermatomyositis.

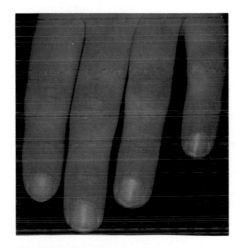

Figure 18–31   Violaceous flat-topped papules (Gottron's papules) on the dorsal interphalangeal joints and erythema and telangiectasia of the cuticles in a patient with dermatomyositis.

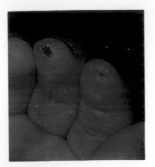

Figure 18–32 Angiitis with ulcerations on tips of the index and third fingers in a young child with acute dermatomyositis.

children. Ulcerations of the fingertips (Fig. 18–32), probably associated with angiitis, may also be seen in acute forms of this disorder.

A pathognomonic sign in dermatomyositis is the *Gottron papule,* a violaceous flat-topped lesion over the dorsal interphalangeal joints, which usually occurs late in the disease (in about one-third of patients).[1] When the papule resolves, atrophy, telangiectasia, or hypopigmentation may persist.

The mucous membranes may also be involved in dermatomyositis. Erythema of the palate and buccal mucosa, with or without ulceration; erythema of the gum margin; and whitish patches on the tongue and buccal mucosa have been observed.[1]

A sequel to the inflammatory phase of the disease is the occurrence of calcinosis. Cutaneous calcinosis, more characteristic of juvenile rather than adult-onset dermatomyositis, is seen in 44 to 70 per cent of children as compared with 20 per cent of adults with dermatomyositis.[94, 95] Most commonly seen on the buttocks and about the shoulders and elbows, subcutaneous calcium deposits may produce local pain, and can be extruded, leading to ulcers, sinuses, or cellulitis. Calcinosis, although often resulting in impaired function, is associated with a longer survival time and, accordingly, is viewed as a favorable prognostic sign. Sometimes patients may present with widespread calcification without apparent preceding illness. In such cases it is suspected that calcinosis may be the result of an old dermatomyositis.

The course of dermatomyositis in children differs from that in adults. Children rarely have Raynaud's phenomenon, malignancies are not present, and the mortality rate is lower; but morbidity is higher, and functional recovery is less. Whereas in adults the disease usually begins in a healthy-appearing individual, in children respiratory illness often precedes the onset of dermatomyositis.[96, 97]

DIAGNOSIS. The diagnosis of dermatomyositis is made on clinical grounds and depends upon the typical cutaneous manifestations and evidence of muscle involvement and weakness. It is confirmed by electromyography, elevated serum enzyme levels — serum aldolase, serum glutamic oxaloacetic transaminase (SGOT), lactic dehydrogenase (LDH), and serum creatine phosphokinase (CPK), and biopsy from a muscle of the shoulder or pelvic girdle (preferably a muscle that is tender).[97] The muscles most commonly biopsied are the deltoid, supraspinatus, and quadriceps.

Tests for rheumatoid factor may be positive in about 10 per cent of cases of dermatomyositis, lupus erythematosus (LE) cells may be seen occasionally, and a positive antinuclear factor may be found in about one-third of cases of dermatomyositis.

TREATMENT. The course of dermatomyositis is highly variable. Acetylsalicylic acid is of value in reducing the pain, tenderness, and inflammatory activity of this disorder. Without specific therapy, about one-third of affected children recover completely, usually within one year of onset;[98] with modern steroid management, however, the death rate has been reduced from about 33 per cent to less than 10 per cent.[99] Long-term follow-up of chronically affected children indicates that in most instances, the disease subsides after about three years, leaving various degrees of disability. If the child can be kept alive for three to five years, although calcinosis and mild manifestations of disease may persist, all medication can often be discontinued.

Hospitalization is advisable in the acute stages, as the disease processes may involve the muscles of respiration or deglutition and necessitate tracheotomy or the use of a mechanical respirator. A physical therapy program aimed at prevention of deformities and increasing muscle strength should be initiated early. Physical rest is extremely important during active phases of dermatomyositis. It may permit control on much lower steroid dosages than otherwise would be possible. When palato-respiratory muscles are affected, great care is required to prevent aspiration and to ensure adequate respiration.

Severe dermatomyositis may be accompanied by diffuse cardiomyopathy. Although this is a rare complication, non-specific electrocardiographic abnormalities are found in about 20 per cent of cases. In severely affected patients, respiratory insufficiency must be watched for carefully. When direct measurements of ventilation or arterial pCO_2 indicate that this is occurring, it is usually necessary to perform a tracheostomy. Tube feedings or intravenous maintenance may be required when dysphagia is present. In those instances in which prompt vigorous therapy is begun, palatal-respiratory function is monitored, adequate physical therapy is actively pursued, and meticulous long-term follow-up is maintained, successful outcome occurs in over two-thirds of the cases.

Most childhood forms of dermatomyositis require high-dosage corticosteroid therapy. The initial dose of prednisone is 1.5 to 2.5 mg per kg of body weight per day, usually a dose of 60 mg of prednisone or its equivalent (up to 90 to 100 mg every day if that proves insufficient). As soon as a response is attained, as judged by muscle enzyme levels, the dosage may be reduced by decrements of about 15 per cent (at intervals of about two weeks) over a period of 10 to 12 months.

Some patients may fail to respond even to very large doses of corticosteroids. Cytotoxic agents such as azathioprine (Imuran) in dosages of 1 to 3 mg per kg of body weight (up to 200 mg a day) or biweekly injections of methotrexate (2 to 3 mg per kg per dose) may be used as ancillary therapeutic agents in severe life-threatening forms of dermatomyositis, or when the disease cannot be adequately managed with prednisone alone.[100]

Although areas of calcinosis frequently disappear spontaneously, for patients with severe calcinosis, disodium etidronate (EHDP) or a diet low in phosphorus and calcium in conjunction with aluminum hydroxide gels (15 ml to 30 ml 4 times a day) appears to lower serum phosphorus and aids in the removal of cutaneous calcification.[101, 102]

During the active phase of dermatomyositis, children are particularly at risk for sudden, overwhelming gram-negative sepsis secondary to aspiration due to weak palatal-respiratory function or perforation of a viscus. This risk is intensified by the masking effects of corticosteroids. A high index of suspicion, therefore, must be maintained for these complications, and early aggressive therapy must be instituted when necessary.[103]

Scleroderma

Scleroderma can be classified into two categories, a variety limited to the skin (morphea and linear scleroderma) and the multisystem disease, systemic scleroderma (progressive systemic sclerosis). Cutaneous scleroderma is discussed in chapter 19. Systemic scleroderma is a generalized disorder of connective tissue affecting the skin, lungs, heart, gastrointestinal tract, joints, and kidneys. Seen in all age groups, it is relatively uncommon in childhood and occurs three times more frequently in women than in men. The pathogenesis of progressive systemic sclerosis is thought to be related to genetic factors, vascular abnormalities, abnormal collagen metabolism, and immunologic abnormalities. Of major importance is the excessive deposition of collagen and fibrosis, possibly due to a defect at the fibroblast level, vasospastic phenomena involving digital, pulmonary, and renal vessels, and cell-mediated hypersensitivity.[104]

Initially, scleroderma was divided into two forms, acrosclerosis and diffuse scleroderma. Diffuse scleroderma begins with cutaneous sclerosis over the central portion of the body and gradually spreads to the extremities. Raynaud's phenomenon is invariably absent and sex distribution is equal. Acrosclerosis, accounting for 95 per cent of all cases of scleroderma, is characterized by cutaneous sclerosis of the digits (sclerodactyly) and Raynaud's phenomenon. It was generally thought that diffuse scleroderma was rapidly fatal, and that

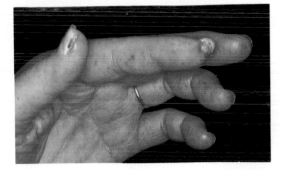

Figure 18–33   Scleroderma. Calcinosis on the fingertips and flat mat-like telangiectatic vessels on the fingers.

acrosclerosis generally seemed to have a relatively long and benign course. This concept now appears to be incorrect. The only value of this classification is that it describes the mode of onset and the distribution of lesions.[1]

Raynaud's phenomenon is present in almost every case of acrosclerosis and varies from mild vasospasm, without permanent changes in the skin, to severe vascular insufficiency, with small pitted scars on the fingertips and, in severe cases, even gangrene.

Scleroderma, although relatively uncommon in childhood, has been reported in children as young as two years of age.[105, 106] Raynaud's phenomenon, extremely uncommon in childhood, is frequently the first sign of systemic scleroderma in this age group. Even in the prepuberal years there is a preponderance of female patients. The appearance of the face is characteristic. The forehead is smooth and cannot be wrinkled, and atrophy and tightening of the skin give a characteristic appearance due to a fixed stare, pinched nose, prominent teeth, pursed lips, and perpetual grimace. The hands become shiny, with tapered finger ends and restricted movement. Subcutaneous calcification and ulceration (Fig. 18–33) may be seen, as well as telangiectases (Fig. 18–34) and hypo- and hyperpigmentation (common cutaneous signs of scleroderma).

Three varieties of telangiectasia are characteristic of scleroderma. These include linear telangiectasia of the cuticles similar to that seen in other connective tissue disorders (Fig. 18–34), sharply defined telangiectatic macules of linear, oval, square, and multiangular configurations that vary in size from 1 to 6 mm in diameter (telangiectatic mats), and in a very small percentage of patients, telangiectasia similar to that seen in patients with Rendu-Osler-Weber disease (see Chapter 9).[1]

Polymyositis and involvement of the esophagus probably are the most common extracutaneous sites of sclerotic change in scleroderma. Other gastrointestinal disturbances include constipation, regurgitation, weight loss, and malabsorption. Although cardiovascular, respiratory, and renal involvement have been described, these do not

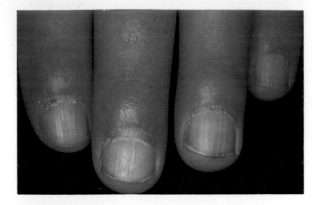

Figure 18–34 Thrombosed cuticular telangiectases without cuticular erythema. In contrast to other connective tissue diseases, cuticular hyperemia is relatively uncommon in scleroderma.

appear to be prominent in childhood forms of this disorder.

No specific therapy is available and management is mainly supportive. General measures include avoidance of factors producing vasospasm (tension, fatigue, stress, and cold weather) and minimizing trauma to the hands. Rest is important and, if polyarthritis is present, salicylates may be beneficial. Treatment of gastrointestinal symptoms includes small frequent feedings, with elevation of the head of the bed, bland diet, and antacids. Corticosteroids, because of complications from long-term therapy, should be reserved for those with debilitating arthritis not controlled by aspirin and for patients with extensive cutaneous edema with severe recurring digital ulcerations and acute toxic phases of the disease. Corticosteroids do not appear to help the sclerodermatous process and, according to many authorities, in many cases may even be harmful.

Lupus Erythematosus

Lupus erythematosus is a chronic inflammatory disorder that may affect the skin as well as most other organ systems. Although the etiology of lupus erythematosus is unknown, current evidence suggests an autoimmune basis to the disorder. Familial cases of lupus erythematosus are numerous. Data concerning hereditary mechanisms are lacking, however, and the role of genetic factors, if any, is as yet undertermined.[107]

Typically a disease of young women, the disorder is seen in all age groups. Up to one-fourth of all cases of systemic lupus erythematosus (SLE) occur within the first two decades of life.[108] The onset in adults usually is during the third and fourth decades of life; in childhood the peak incidence occurs between the 11th and 13th years.[109] Although several cases of lupus erythematosus have been described in newborns, except for neonatal lupus, it rarely is seen before the age of three years.[110]

Clinically two forms of lupus erythematosus are described. Cutaneous manifestations affect most patients at some time during the course of their disease. The cutaneous features of cutaneous (often referred to as "discoid") and systemic lupus erythematosus suggest that both forms of this disorder are variants of the same disease. Cutaneous lupus erythematosus (often termed discoid lupus erythematosus [DLE]), a disorder of the skin without systemic manifestations, is seen at the benign end of the spectrum. Systemic lupus erythematosus (SLE), on the other hand, is a chronic multisystem disease. Most authors agree that affected females outnumber males by a ratio of 8 or 9 to 1. Fifteen to twenty per cent of cases of SLE begin in children, usually in girls over eight years of age. Cutaneous or discoid LE is rare in children, and most childhood cases are systemic in nature, with widespread involvement of multiple organ systems.[111] The disease is more acute and of greater severity in children than in adults; the younger the patient, the more acute the disorder.

CLINICAL MANIFESTATIONS.   Although the incidence of cutaneous (discoid) lupus erythematosus is rare in childhood, the cutaneous lesions of children and adults are similar. About 80 per cent of patients with systemic lupus erythematosus have cutaneous involvement at some time; in up to 25 per cent of patients cutaneous lesions are the initial presenting sign of the disorder. A butterfly rash often appears over the cheeks and bridge of the nose. This so-called malar or "butterfly" rash, however, is neither a specific nor the most frequent sign of lupus erythematosus.[1]

The classic discoid lesion of LE is a red to purplish plaque with adherent scale (Fig. 18–35), fine telangiectasia, and areas of atrophy.[109] Discoid lesions can be asymmetrical on the head and face, scalp, arms, legs, hands, fingers, back, chest, or abdomen. At times the openings of hair follicles are dilated and plugged by an overlying scale. If the scale is thick enough, it can be lifted off in one piece. The undersurface then reveals follicular projections that resemble carpet tacks, a characteristic sign of lupus erythematosus.[1]

Another common lesion of LE is the reddish-purple urticarial plaque, which is relatively fixed in shape and does not undergo atrophy or scaling. This lesion, often associated with photosensitivity, represents another characteristic cutaneous manifestation suggestive of lupus erythematosus (Fig. 18–36). Although cutaneous lesions and pho-

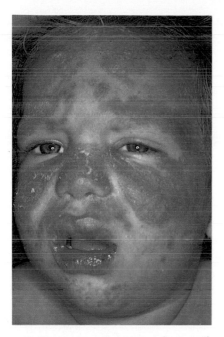

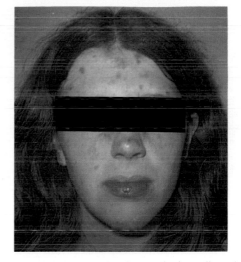

Figure 18–37 A crusted lesion on the lower lip and discoid LE plaques on the face of a 16-year-old girl with systemic lupus erythematosus.

Figure 18–35 Lupus erythematosus. Scaly erythematous urticarial plaques on the face, with scaling and crusting of the lips in a 2-year-old boy with systemic lupus erythematosus.

tosensitivity are of diagnostic and cosmetic significance, photosensitivity reactions have also been known to precipitate fatal exacerbations of the disease. When untreated, lesions may go on to develop permanent areas of hyper- or hypopigmentation with atropy — another commonly seen cutaneous manifestation of lupus erythematosus.

Mucosal membrane lesions (gingivitis, mucosal hemorrhage, erosions, and small ulcerations) are seen in 3 per cent of patients with cutaneous LE and in from 10 to 15 per cent of patients with the systemic form of the disorder. A silvery whitening of the vermilion border of the lips is highly characteristic and pathognomonic of lupus erythematosus. The lips are often involved, with slight thickening, roughness, and redness, with or with-

out superficial ulceration and crusting. One must never neglect, therefore, to examine the nose and mouth of patients for evidence of silvery-white scaling and ulcerations (Fig. 18–37). The gingivae may also appear red, edematous, friable, and eroded, or they may exhibit silvery-white changes similar to those on the nasal or buccal mucosa.

Scarring alopecia, another important marker of lupus erythematosus, may be seen as single or multiple well-demarcated patches (Fig. 18–38) that exhibit erythema, scaling, telangiectasia, atrophy, and plugging (the classic changes of LE).[109] Increased fragility of the hair in LE may produce broken hairs several millimeters from the roots, with a resulting receding hairline with an unruly appearance due to the short broken hairs ("lupus hair").

Livedo reticularis, a peculiar blotchy bluish-red discoloration of the skin due to vasospasm of the arterioles, although often normal when seen in young children, may be the earliest sign of lupus erythematosus, rheumatoid arthritis, or rheumatic

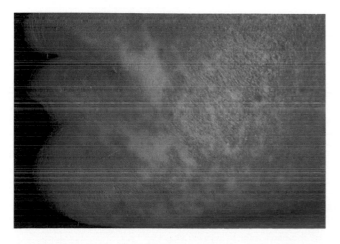

Figure 18–36 Reddish-purple plaques on the face following sun exposure in a 17-year-old patient with systemic lupus erythematosus.

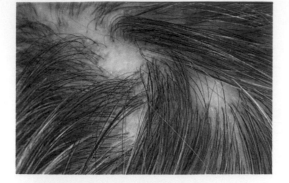

Figure 18–38   Scarring alopecia of the scalp in a patient with systemic lupus erythematosus.

fever. It can also be seen in children with leukemia, idiopathic thrombocytopenia, or neurologic abnormalities, or in those on immunosuppressive therapy. Aggravated by exposure to cold, the area becomes livid or cyanotic when the arterial supply is reduced. Livedo reticularis, when it affects the entire trunk or limbs in a continuous manner, is often a normal phenomenon. When it develops in a blotchy interrupted configuration, however, it is frequently a sign of systemic disease.

Chronic urticaria-like lesions associated with a leukocytoclastic vasculitis may be the first sign of LE.[5] The extent of hives, seen at some time in 7 per cent of patients with lupus erythematosus, frequently reflects the activity of the disease and accordingly may serve as a useful guide to therapy.[1]

Telangiectases represent another characteristic marker of connective tissue disease. Distinctive findings here include papular telangiectasia of the palms and fingers and linear telangiectasia of the cuticles and periungual skin (with or without thromboses). Cuticular telangiectasia is not specific for LE; it is also seen in patients with dermatomyositis and scleroderma, and in about 5 per cent of patients with rheumatoid arthritis. Diffuse angiitis, with or without ulceration, also occurs in about 10 per cent of patients with lupus erythematosus.

Neonatal Lupus Erythematosus.   The LE cell factor can be transmitted via the placenta to infants born to mothers with lupus erythematosus. The maternal antibodies generally disappear and the LE test reverts to negative within the first few months of life. Congenital lupus has also been reported in children of unaffected mothers.

Infants born to mothers with disseminated LE are usually normal but on occasion have been found to have some manifestations of the disease, generally transient, including a discoid lupus rash, positive LE cell preparations, lymphocyte tuboreticular inclusions, and a syndrome of leukopenia, thrombocytopenia, and Coombs test–positive hemolytic anemia.[112-115]

It now appears that neonatal LE with discoid-type lesions may not merely represent a transient disease and that systemic involvement and the development of congenital heart block or active and progressive lesions may indeed be a distinct possibility in some infants with this disorder. It has been postulated that these effects are due to immune complexes formed by transplacental passage of maternal antibodies. Brustein recently described a family in which two infants of a mother with cutaneous LE developed lupus during infancy, both cases persisting beyond the initial neonatal stage.[112] A patient noted to have discoid lupus erythematosus (DLE) as an infant eventually developed systemic lupus erythematosus (SLE) at age 19 years,[113] and congenital complete heart block recently has been noted in some infants with neonatal lupus erythematosus.[115] It is essential, therefore, that all children who have cutaneous neonatal LE be investigated for the possibility of congenital atrioventricular block and be followed for signs of active or recurring disease.

DIAGNOSIS.   The diagnosis of lupus erythematosus is chiefly clinical and based on the presence of typical cutaneous lesions, systemic manifestations, and confirmatory laboratory tests. Histologic examination of cutaneous lesions will often confirm the diagnosis. Leukopenia of less than 5000 frequently occurs, anemia and thrombocytopenia are frequently noted in patients with systemic LE, and serum gamma globulins are elevated in about 80 per cent of patients. In patients with active disease a reduced serum complement level frequently may be noted. The erythrocyte sedimentation rate is elevated in all but an occasional patient during periods of clinical disease activity. The LE cell phenomenon, usually negative in cutaneous lupus, is found in 70 to 85 per cent of patients with systemic LE.

Direct immunofluorescence is most useful in the diagnosis of lupus erythematosus. In systemic lupus erythematosus, dermo-epidermal deposition of immunoglobulin may be demonstrated by the direct method of immunofluorescence at the dermal-epidermal junction of clinically uninvolved as well as involved skin (Fig. 18–39). The presence of an immunofluorescent band in clinically normal skin suggests greater severity of the disease. In chronic cutaneous (discoid) LE, although direct immunofluorescence of clinically involved skin is positive in 90 per cent of patients, immunofluorescent studies of uninvolved skin are negative.[107]

TREATMENT.   The therapy of lupus erythematosus depends upon the extent of local and systemic involvement. Avoidance of sun exposure and a trial of sunscreens in areas of cutaneous lesions are advisable, particularly during the initial phases of therapy. Although it is the ultraviolet portion of the spectrum that is most damaging to the skin lesions, heat, trauma, and infrared exposure will also cause exacerbations.[109] Local corticosteroid preparations are a simple and effective form of therapy, particularly for early erythematous plaques. Antimalarial therapy, often useful in adults with cutaneous LE, is rarely indicated in children. Although very effective in long-term suppression of the disease, antimalarial drugs can

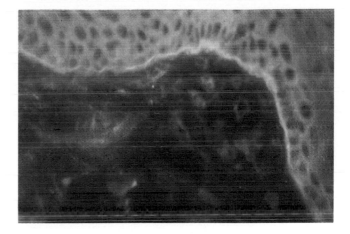

Figure 18–39 Lupus erythematosus. Direct immunofluorescence with globulin deposition at the dermal-epidermal junction (Courtesy of Irwin M. Braverman, M.D.).

result in an irreversible retinopathy due to deposition of the drug in the pigmented portion of the retina. Antimalarial therapy, accordingly, should be avoided whenever possible in the management of young children with lupus erythematosus.

Systemic lupus erythematosus must be considered a lifelong, controllable but incurable, disease. Although children with mild lupus erythematosus may respond well to mere bed rest, aspirin, and avoidance of excessive sun exposure, in general the prognosis in childhood is worse than in adulthood.[116, 117] Children, therefore, should be evaluated for major organ involvement, particularly for the presence of nephritis, the major cause of death of individuals with this disorder. In severe cases, hospitalization may be necessary for diagnostic evaluation as well as for definitive therapy of systemic LE. Prednisone in dosages of 1 to 2 mg per kg per 24 hours may be lifesaving for patients with renal complication, pericarditis, neurologic involvement, or hemolytic anemia. Once remission is induced, a minimal corticosteroid maintenance dose, preferably alternate-day therapy, is advisable. Although it appears that steroid therapy has increased the survival rate, the possibility of complications due to infections such as widespread tuberculosis, viral and bacterial pneumonia, bacterial (especially gram-negative) sepsis, and systemic fungal disease must be considered.

Since immunosuppressive agents are beneficial but carry an increased risk of neoplasia, aplastic anemia, and sepsis, when renal disease is present, the patient is best referred to a center where immunosuppressive therapy is available. The recommended dosage for azathioprine (Imuran) is 100 to 200 mg per day; for 6-mercaptopurine, 50 to 100 mg per day; for cyclophosphamide (Cytoxan), 50 mg per day; and for chlorambucil (Leukeran), 0.1 mg per kg per day, with appropriate modification depending on the size and weight of small children.[118-120]

Sjögren's Syndrome

Sjögren's syndrome is a chronic autoimmune disorder characterized by keratoconjunctivitis sicca (inflammation of the cornea and conjunctiva with dryness), xerostomia, and chronic enlargement of salivary glands, and in at least half of the cases it is associated with a connective tissue disease. Although rarely seen in childhood, the presence of chronic parotid enlargement should suggest this disorder as a possible diagnosis.

Diagnostic studies include scintigraphy; demonstration of decreased salivary flow by secretory sialography; biopsy of minor salivary glands of the lips; careful examination of the eyes, including Schirmer's test (less than 5 mm wetting of a strip of filter paper inserted under the lower eyelid); conjunctival staining with Rose Bengal solution; filamentary keratitis on slit lamp examination; and full serological workup for autoimmune disease.[121]

Mixed Connective Tissue Disease

Mixed connective tissue disease (MCTD, Sharp's syndrome) is a distinct clinical entity characterized by the combination of clinical features and laboratory data of systemic lupus erythematosus, polymyositis, and/or Sjögren's disease. Originally described by Sharp in 1972, the disorder is associated with high titers of RNAase-sensitive extract of cell nuclei, termed extranuclear antigen (ENA) and ribonucleoprotein (RNP), and epidermal nuclear staining on direct immunofluorescence of normal skin.[122-128] The cutaneous features of MCTD include cutaneous photosensitivity, a heliotrope rash over the eyelids, alopecia, malar telangiectasia or erythema or both, cutaneous lesions of lupus erythematosus, hyperpigmentation, hypopigmentation, periungual erythema, livedo reticularis, mucosal dryness, arthritis or arthralgia, sclerodactyly, and a tapered or sausage appearance of the fingers.

CLINICAL MANIFESTATIONS. The most common presenting features are joint complaints, Raynaud's phenomenon, or cutaneous lupus erythematosus.[125] Although some patients with MCTD have deforming arthritis, the most common symptom is an evanescent, non-erosive, non-deforming polyarthritis similar to that seen with systemic lupus erythematosus. The most important diagnostic features of MCTD are Raynaud's phenomenon, periungual telangiectasia, swelling of the hands, with a tapered or sausage appearance to the fingers, abnormal pulmonary function tests, myositis, disturbances of esophageal motility, joint pain, alopecia, and lesions of cutaneous lupus erythematosus. Lupus-like rashes of the face may be found in 50 per cent of untreated MCTD patients; cine-esophagogram and monometric studies of the esophagus reveal abnormalities (even in the absence of symptoms) in 70 to 80 per cent of patients; up to 80 per cent of patients have evidence of pulmonary disease on the basis of pulmonary function, roentgenographic measurements, or both; proximal muscle weakness is common, with or without tenderness or elevated levels of serum creatine phosphokinase (CPK) and aldolase; nearly all patients have polyarthralgia and three-fourths of them have frank arthritis; approximately two-thirds of children with MCTD have cardiac involvement, including pericarditis, myocarditis, congestive heart failure, and aortic insufficiency; about 10 per cent have renal disease; and about 10 per cent of affected individuals have neurologic abnormalities (trigeminal sensory neuropathy, "vascular" headaches, seizures, multiple peripheral neuropathies, and cerebral infarction or hemorrhage).[126]

Identification of children with MCTD permits their separation from other connective tissue diseases that may have a more serious prognosis and respond less well to systemic steroid therapy. When MCTD occurs in childhood, it may mimic juvenile rheumatoid arthritis. Distinct differences, however, frequently exist between adult and childhood forms of mixed connective tissue disease. Severe thrombocytopenia appears to be limited to childhood forms, and the incidence of renal involvement is higher in children than in adults.[128]

TREATMENT. The prognosis of mixed connective tissue disease in children appears to be good. Patients should be treated according to the particular systems of involvement, with high doses of steroids and, when necessary, immunosuppressive agents similar to those required in the management of patients with severe systemic lupus erythematosus. Cutaneous lesions of lupus erythematosus respond to topical steroid preparations or intralesional injections of corticosteroids.

BEHÇET'S DISEASE

The Behçet syndrome is an uncommon chronic systemic disorder characterized by a triad of oral ulcerations, genital ulcerations, and relapsing inflammatory disease of the eyes. Originally described in 1937, the spectrum of this disease has been broadened with the recognition of multiple organ system involvement, namely dermal vasculitis, arthritis, central nervous system involvement, myocarditis, colitis, phlebitis, and focal necrotizing glomerulonephritis.[129]

Three etiologic hypotheses have been proposed based upon viral, autoimmune, and defective fibrinolytic activity. Although successful culture of a responsible virus has been reported, subsequent studies have not been able to duplicate this work, and administration of serum prepared from patients during the active stage of this disorder has been ineffective in the management of the disease. While the association between Behçet disease and venous thrombosis is clear, the pathogenesis of the thrombotic process has not been fully elucidated.[130]

CLINICAL MANIFESTATIONS. Although onset in early childhood has been reported, this rare syndrome usually begins in patients between the ages of 10 and 45 years, with a marked predilection (between 3:1 and 5:1) for males. Oral lesions are an almost constant feature of this disorder and are the initial manifestation in about 60 per cent of cases. The ulcerations begin as vesicles or pustules, may occur anywhere on the oral mucosa, and present as superficial erosions indistinguishable from aphthous stomatitis or as deeply punched-out necrotic ulcers. They tend to appear in crops and are characterized by superficial grayish erosions that vary in size from a few millimeters to a centimeter in diameter. The ulcer base is covered with a yellowish-gray exudate and the margin is surrounded by a red halo. The aphthous lesions, whether in the mouth or genitalia, usually persist for periods of 7 to 14 days and usually heal without scarring. They recur at irregular intervals varying from weeks to months. Deep crateriform necrotic ulcerations with raised margins, called periadenitis mucosa necrotica recurrens (Sutton's disease), are distinctive, usually very painful, and frequently heal with scarring.

Cutaneous lesions present a varied picture. Seen in approximately 70 per cent of patients, they consist of vesicles, pustules, pyoderma, acneform lesions, furuncles, ulcerations, and angiitic lesions of the legs, suggesting a diagnosis of erythema nodosum.

Ocular lesions, seen in about 80 per cent of patients, generally begin with intense periorbital pain and photophobia. Conjunctivitis may be an early ocular finding, followed by iritis or uveitis, often with loss of vision from vitreous opacification and, eventually, hypopyon.

Fever and constitutional symptoms are variable. Other findings include recurrent thrombophlebitis of the superficial veins of the legs (in about 45 per cent of patients), arthralgia (in about 35 per cent), gastrointestinal ulceration, pericarditis, orchitis, and epididymitis. Central nervous system involvement, often the most severe prognostic feature of this disorder, is seen in 20 to 50 per cent of patients (generally an average of two to five years after the disease has begun).[131]

Diagnosis of the Behçet syndrome in a patient with the full triad of oral and genital ulcers and iritis is not difficult. However, many patients do not present with the classic triad. Diagnosis may then be established by the association of ocular or cutaneous lesions, or both, with neurological or other systemic signs.

TREATMENT. There is no entirely satisfactory treatment of the Behçet syndrome. Treatment of the aphthous ulcers with a tetracycline suspension (250 mg swished around in the mouth for two minutes and then swallowed), four times a day for a period of five to ten days, may be beneficial. Intralesional steroid injection (triamcinolone acetonide, 0.2 to 0.3 ml, in concentrations of 10 mg per ml) may give rapid relief and resolution of large ulcerations. Milder cases may be treated with topical application of silver nitrate ($AgNO_3$) or oral rinses with Elixir of Benadryl or Viscous Xylocaine. Application of a steroid (Kenalog in Orabase) to the lesions four times daily may give some symptomatic relief. Although favorable results are inconsistent, in severe cases systemic corticosteroids may suppress many of the inflammatory features of this disorder, particularly for those individuals with central nervous system involvement.

NEUROCUTANEOUS SYNDROMES

The neurocutaneous disorders consist of a group of hereditary conditions with cutaneous, nervous system, and internal manifestations. Since the skin and nervous system share a common embryological origin, it is not surprising that there are a large number of neurological conditions associated with cutaneous manifestations. Four of these, tuberous sclerosis, neurofibromatosis, incontinentia pigmenti, and incontinentia pigmenti achromians, have striking cutaneous markers.

Tuberous Sclerosis

Tuberous sclerosis is a relatively uncommon disease of irregular but dominant autosomal inheritance occurring with an incidence of about 7 in 100,000 individuals. Of these, 50 to 70 per cent of cases may arise from new mutations. Tuberous sclerosis is classified as a neurocutaneous syndrome in which the brain, eyes, skin, heart, kidneys, lungs, and bones may be affected. The full entity classically is defined by a triad of seizures, mental deficiency, and a variety of pathognomonic skin lesions. The latter include adenoma sebaceum, shagreen patches, periungual and gingival fibromas, and hypopigmented macules. Although café au lait spots have an increased incidence (26 per cent) in this disorder, they are not a true diagnostic sign of tuberous sclerosis.[132]

CLINICAL MANIFESTATIONS. Adenoma sebaceum, present in 80 to 90 per cent of cases, is the most common skin manifestation associated with this disorder. The term adenoma sebaceum is a misnomer; these lesions represent angiofibromas, hamartomas composed of fibrous and vascular tissue. The lesions usually appear as 1 to 4 mm dome-shaped nodules with a smooth surface (Figs. 8-30, 8-31, 18-40). They range from pink to red in color and often are accompanied by fine telangiectasia. Lesions of adenoma sebaceum are usually located in a bilaterally symmetrical distribution in the nasolabial folds, cheeks, and chin and sometimes on the forehead and scalp. They are rarely found on the upper lip except for the central area immediately below the nose. The lesions, rarely present at birth, usually appear sometime between the second and fifth birthdays, often not until puberty. Since only 13 per cent of children with tuberous sclerosis develop the facial lesions of adenoma sebaceum during the first year of life, it appears that this is not the best early marker of this condition.

Fibromas also develop around and under the nails of the fingers and toes (periungual and subungual fibromas) (Fig. 18-41) and on the gums (gingival fibromas). The periungual and subungual fibromas, seen in about 50 per cent of patients, appear at puberty as firm, flesh-colored growths. Because of their relatively late appearance they too are of little value in the early diagnosis of this disorder.

Shagreen patches are seen in 21 to 83 per cent of patients with tuberous sclerosis (Figs. 8-32, 18-42). They develop during early childhood, usually between the patient's second and fifth

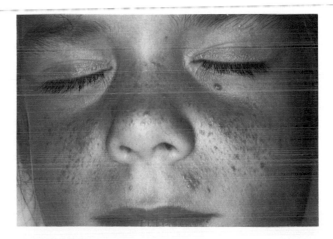

Figure 18-40 Adenoma sebaceum. Small discrete reddish-pink dome-shaped angiofibromas in a bilaterally symmetrical distribution on the cheeks, nose, and upper lip of a 5-year-old girl with tuberous sclerosis.

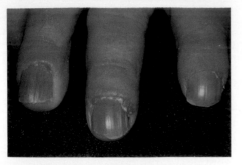

Figure 18–41 Periungual fibromas. Firm flesh-colored growths in the periungual region of a patient with tuberous sclerosis.

Figure 18–43 An irregular oval-shaped white macule (the earliest cutaneous marker) in a patient with tuberous sclerosis (Hurwitz S, Braverman I M: J. Pediatr. 77:587, 1970).

birthdays. They generally develop on the trunk (most frequently the lumbosacral area) and appear as flesh-colored to yellowish or yellowish-orange slightly elevated plaques of dermal connective tissue. Seen as single or multiple lesions measuring 2 to 10 cm or more in diameter, they frequently have an orange-peel or pigskin appearance resembling shagreen leather.

White macules, seen in 70 to 90 per cent of patients with tuberous sclerosis, are a particularly valuable early marker of this disorder. They appear at birth or shortly thereafter, and, although they may enlarge as the infant grows, persist throughout life and otherwise do not change in size or shape. Of further interest is the fact that in addition to the characteristic hypopigmented macules, there also appears to be an increased incidence of tuberous sclerosis in patients with poliosis and partial albinism (see Chapter 16), and individuals with tuberous sclerosis also appear to have an increased number of café au lait spots[132, 133, 134] (Figs. 16–11 and 16–12). Although the etiologies of hyperpigmentation and hypopigmentation are unknown, since melanocytes are derived from the neural crest and in many ways function as nerve cells, it is not surprising that these changes are found in patients with disorders involving the central nervous system.[132]

A striking feature of the white spots of tuberous sclerosis is the marked variability in size and shape of lesions. They range in size from 0.4 to 7 cm or more, with the majority of lesions measuring between 1 and 3 cm in diameter. They usually are oval or semioval in appearance and have highly irregular margins (Fig. 18–43). Although ash-leaf-shaped lance-ovate hypopigmented macules (Fig. 18–44) have been described as the characteristic lesions of tuberous sclerosis,[135] it has been noted that only 18 per cent of the white spots of tuberous sclerosis are truly ash-leaf in shape.[132]

The white spots of tuberous sclerosis have often been termed "vitiliginous" by nondermatologists, but these partially depigmented lesions are unrelated to vitiligo and can be differentiated by many characteristics. Vitiligo represents an acquired form of hypopigmentation characterized by sharply demarcated "ivory-white" macules surrounded by hyperpigmented skin. The completely depigmented ivory-white macules of vitiligo may occur at any age, but are rare in infants. Although lesions of vitiligo may appear on any part of the body, they frequently have a bilateral or symmetrical distribution, with involvement of the skin of the face and neck, of the backs of hands and forearms, over bony prominences, and in body folds and periorificial areas. They often change in size and shape, frequently spread, and occasionally may show partial to complete repigmentation. Conversely, the leukoder-

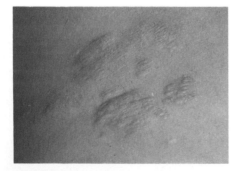

Figure 18–42 Shagreen patches. Slightly elevated flesh-colored plaques of connective tissue with an orange-peel (peau d'orange) surface on the lumbosacral area of a girl with tuberous sclerosis.

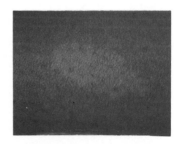

Figure 18–44 Lance-ovate ash leaf-shaped hypopigmented macule of tuberous sclerosis (only 18 per cent of white macules seen in patients with tuberous sclerosis are truly ash leaf in shape).

ma of tuberous sclerosis is usually present at birth and is located over the abdomen, back, and anterior and lateral surfaces of the arms and legs. It is a dull-white, incomplete depigmentation (in comparison to the ivory-white color of vitiligo), does not alter in shape or size with age, and appears to be related to a defect of melanosome melanization. The basic cause of this pigmentary disturbance remains obscure.

The difference between hypopigmented lesions of tuberous sclerosis and vitiligo can be demonstrated by electron microscopy. Whereas the completely depigmented lesions of vitiligo reveal an absence or decrease in the number of melanocytes, the partially depigmented macules of tuberous sclerosis have a normal number of melanocytes with a decrease in the size, synthesis, and melanization of melanosomes.[135]

Another peculiar form of speckled leukoderma in tuberous sclerosis may be seen as small 1 to 3 mm hypopigmented lesions (white freckles) in a confetti-like pattern over the pretibial area in some patients with tuberous sclerosis (Fig. 18–45). Although occasionally seen in normal individuals, they too can serve as helpful markers in the diagnosis of patients with this disorder.[132] Of further significance are the facts that there also appears to be an increased incidence of tuberous sclerosis in patients with partial albinism,[133, 134] and that the presence of one or more tufts of white hair in an infant with seizures is suggestive of a diagnosis of tuberous sclerosis.[136]

In view of the high frequency of white mac-

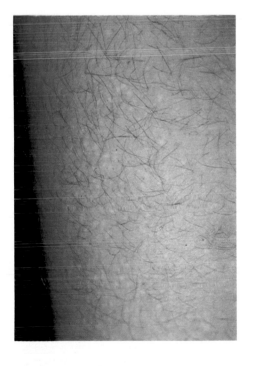

Figure 18–45 White freckles. Multiple 1 to 3 mm hypopigmented lesions in a confetti-like pattern on the leg of a patient with tuberous sclerosis (Hurwitz S, Braverman I M: J. Pediatr. 77:587, 1970).

ules present at birth in patients with tuberous sclerosis, all infants and children, particularly those with seizure disorders, should be screened for the characteristic but easily overlooked dull-white macules that are now recognized as the earliest cutaneous markers of tuberous sclerosis. In individuals with light pigmentation, however, these macules can be extremely faint. Illumination of the skin with a Wood's light in a darkened room can be helpful in detecting hypopigmented spots that contrast poorly with surrounding normal skin.

Tooth pits (seen as punctate, round or oval, 1 to 2 mm randomly arranged enamel defects), particularly in the permanent teeth, appear to be another recently recognized marker of tuberous sclerosis. Recent studies suggest that when tooth pits are seen in numbers of five or more, they may prove to be pathognomonic of this disorder.[137]

The systemic lesions of tuberous sclerosis may produce severe symptoms and possibly death. Central nervous system involvement may lead to convulsions and mental retardation. Retardation may be mild or severe and appears in 62 per cent of affected individuals, and seizures are present in more than 80 per cent of cases. Sclerotic calcification in the brain is visible as "tubers" by x-ray in approximately 50 to 75 per cent of individuals. In young children when skull x-rays are not diagnostic, computerized axial tomographic (CAT) scan findings of small calcifications, ventricular dilatations, or both, are frequently helpful in the diagnosis of this disorder.[138, 139] The kidneys may reveal tumors that are hamartomas. Rhabdomyomas in the heart may be associated with congestive heart failure, murmurs, cyanosis, or sudden death. The eyes may have characteristic retinal lesions (gliomas) referred to as phakomas. Cystic lesions in the lungs may rupture and produce spontaneous pneumothorax, often with a radiographic "honeycombed" appearance. The bones, particularly those of the hands and feet, may demonstrate the presence of cysts and periosteal thickenings.[134]

MANAGEMENT. Seizure disorders associated with tuberous sclerosis often respond to anticonvulsant therapy. Death, when it occurs, may result from status epilepticus, pulmonary or renal insufficiency, or cardiac failure. Adenoma sebaceum requires no treatment except for cosmetic reasons. Best results are seen following cryosurgery, electrodesiccation and curettage, or dermabrasion. Although surgery may be required for relief of symptoms from internal tumors of tuberous sclerosis, surgical removal is often unsatisfactory. Genetic counseling against childbearing is recommended for individuals (even those with mild forms of tuberous sclerosis), since their children may be more severely affected than they are. Since 50 to 70 per cent of patients with tuberous sclerosis may be mutations, unless there is evidence of tuberous sclerosis in other members of the family, genetic counseling is not completely effective in the prevention of new cases. Recognition of cutaneous markers, however, may help screen previously unrecognized or mildly affected individuals with *formes frustes* of the disorder.

Neurofibromatosis

Neurofibromatosis (von Recklinghausen disease) is an autosomal dominant disorder characterized by cutaneous pigmentation (café au lait spots) and tumors of the nervous system, which manifest themselves by changes in the skin, bones, endocrine system, and muscle. It is estimated to occur approximately once in 2500 to 3000 births, with no significant difference in respect to sex, race, or color.[140, 141] About 50 per cent of cases probably represent new mutations.

CUTANEOUS MANIFESTATIONS. Café au lait spots, the hallmark of neurofibromatosis, may occur anywhere on the body (Fig. 18–46). They are seen as sharply defined oval pale-brown patches. Although giant café au lait spots as large as 15 cm in diameter may be seen, they characteristically average 2 to 5 cm in length. Crowe and associates have postulated that the existence of six or more café au lait spots greater than 1.5 cm in diameter probably indicates the presence of neurofibromatosis.[141, 142] Although 10 to 20 per cent of normal individuals have one or more café au lait spots, these characteristic macules are seen in 95 per cent of patients with neurofibromatosis (78 per cent of patients with von Recklinghausen disease have six or more such lesions).[141, 142] This "six spot" criterion, while not a hard and fast rule, may be valuable, particularly in young children and adolescents before the cutaneous neurofibromas make their appearance. In children five years of age or under, smaller lesions may be significant in the diagnosis of this disorder. In this age group it appears that five or more café au lait spots 0.5 centimeter or greater indicate the presence of neurofibromatosis.[143]

Another form of café au lait pigmentation, termed axillary "freckling," may serve as a valu-

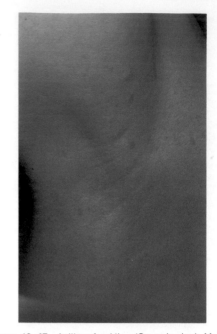

Figure 18–47 Axillary freckling (Crowe's sign). Multiple 1 to 4 mm café au lait spots in the axilla (Crowe's sign is pathognomonic of multiple neurofibromatosis).

able diagnostic aid in the early recognition of neurofibromatosis (Fig. 18–47). Seen in 20 per cent of the patients with the disease, axillary freckling appears as multiple 1 to 4 mm café au lait spots in the axillary vault. Lack of sun exposure in this area prevents confusion with true freckles. Since such axillary pigmentation is not seen in any other condition, it is highly pathognomonic of von Recklinghausen disease.[144]

Microscopic examination of café au lait spots reveals increased pigment in the basal layer of the epidermis in patients with neurofibromatosis. Giant pigment granules have been observed in the melanocytes and keratinocytes of the epidermis, particularly in the café au lait spots of patients with neurofibromatosis. These are not found in the café au lait spots of normal individuals.[145, 146] Another significant finding is the fact that in patients with neurofibromatosis there are more dopa-positive melanocytes per square centimeter in the café au lait spots than in the surrounding normal skin. In individuals without neurofibromatosis, conversely, there are fewer dopa-positive melanocytes per square centimeter in the café au lait spots than in the surrounding normal skin.[147]

Café au lait spots also occur in the Albright syndrome (polyostotic fibrous dysplasia with sexual precocity in girls). In the Albright syndrome pigmented lesions are dark-brown in color and tend to have a markedly irregular border (resembling the coast of Maine). This is in contrast to the smooth outline (resembling the coast of California) and light-brown color of the spots seen in von Recklinghausen disease. In Albright's disease

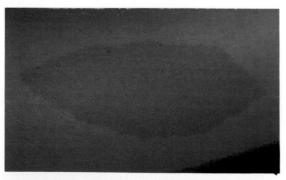

Figure 18–46 Café au lait spot. Six café au lait spots larger than 1.5 cm in diameter suggest a diagnosis of multiple neurofibromatosis (von Recklinghausen disease). In children five years of age or under, 5 or more café au lait spots 0.5 cm or greater probably indicate the presence of this disorder.

the café au lait spots tend to follow a dermatomal distribution, are more commonly seen over the neck and buttocks, and often develop over bones, stopping abruptly at the midline.[148]

Other cutaneous pigmentary changes have been noted in patients with neurofibromatosis but lack the diagnostic significance attributed to axillary freckling and multiple café au lait spots. These include minute freckle-like café au lait spots distributed in other regions of the body, areas of leukoderma, and diffuse graying or bronzing of the skin suggestive of the color seen in patients with argyria.[140]

Neurofibromas. Von Recklinghausen disease is further characterized by the development of dermal fibromas (Fig. 18–48) and dermal or subcutaneous neurofibromas of Schwann cell origin (derived from peripheral nerve sheaths). The tumors of neurofibromatosis ordinarily appear late in childhood or early adolescence — their first appearance frequently is associated with puberty. They vary in number from a few to many hundreds, with a progressive increase in size and number as the patient becomes older. Neurofibromas may occur anywhere on the body, with no specific site of predilection other than the fact that they usually avoid the palms and soles. They may appear as superficial tumors varying in size from 1 or 2 mm to several centimeters in diameter or as discrete beaded, nodular, elongated masses seen along the course of nerves, usually the trigeminal or upper cervical nerves (plexiform neuromas).

Although generally flesh-colored, neurofibromas tend to have a distinctive violaceous hue when small. As they enlarge they tend to become pink, blue, or pigmented. Small tumors may be deep-seated, sessile, or dome-shaped; as they become larger they become globular, pear-shaped, pedunculated, or pendulous. With moderate digital pressure the smaller lesions may be invaginated into an underlying dermal defect, an almost pathognomonic maneuver termed "button-holing." It should be noted that solitary neurofibromas without other cutaneous findings are not diagnostic of neurofibromatosis and may be seen in patients without evidence of this disorder.[142]

Although a benign course for neurofibromas is

usual, some of the tumors may undergo malignant change. Because of a tendency to report unusual cases, the literature reflects a high incidence of malignant transformation, which has been estimated to range between 2 and 16 per cent. A more accurate figure for this complication appears to be in the range of 2 to 3 per cent.[1] Although fibrosarcomatous malignant degeneration has occurred in early childhood, it is rare before the age of forty. Malignant degeneration may be heralded by rapid enlargement or pain. Malignant growth, however, once it develops is often slow, with few metastases. Following excision, however, local recurrences are common.

SYSTEMIC MANIFESTATIONS. The severity of cutaneous involvement is not indicative of the extent of disease in other organs. Neurological manifestations have been reported in as high as 40 per cent of patients and may involve any part of the central nervous system. The acoustic nerve (VIII) and optic nerve (II) are the most commonly involved of the cranial nerves. Deafness is common in neurofibromatosis and gliomas of the optic nerve, with exophthalmos, decreased visual acuity, or restricted ocular movements, are occasionally seen as complications of this disorder. The degree of mental deficiency, although occasionally severe, fortunately is usually mild to moderate and not progressive.

Neurologic disease occurs in more than half the cases of neurofibromatosis and includes retardation, seizure disorders, and tumors. Seizures are said to occur in 10 per cent of patients, and mental retardation, seen in 10 to 20 per cent of patients, varies from mild learning disabilities to severe retardation.[139]

As many as 50 per cent of patients with neurofibromatosis may have osseous defects associated with this disorder. All bony changes may be explained by the development of neurofibromas lying within or in close proximity to involved bone. Of these, spinal deformity, particularly scoliosis or kyphosis, are the most common and may be seen in over 10 per cent of patients.

Endocrine disorders associated with neurofibromatosis include acromegaly, cretinism, menstrual abnormalities, delayed or incomplete sexual development, gynecomastia, hyper- and hypothyroidism, infertility, Addison disease, hyperparathyroidism, and diabetes. In children the most common endocrine abnormality that occurs is sexual precocity. Of particular significance is the fact that between 5 and 20 per cent of patients with pheochromocytoma also have neurofibromatosis, but only 1 of every 223 patients with neurofibromatosis is found to have pheochromocytoma.[141]

DIAGNOSIS. The diagnosis of neurofibromatosis depends upon the number and size of café au lait spots (the earliest manifestation of this disorder), axillary freckling when present, and cutaneous neurofibromas. In individuals with inconclusive cutaneous changes, giant pigment granules or an increased number of melanocytes in the

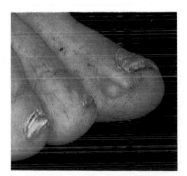

Figure 18–48   Fibromas of the toe in multiple neurofibromatosis.

café an lait macules compared to the surrounding skin can help establish the diagnosis.

TREATMENT. Reassurance for parents of children affected with neurofibromatosis is often helpful, since many patients have minor or incomplete forms of this disorder. Treatment consists of surgical excision of tumors that are disfiguring, interfere with function, or are subject to irritation, trauma, or infection. Periodic complete physical examinations are necessary, with particular attention to possible hypertension, skeletal deformities, and involvement of cranial nerves II and VIII. Although malignant degeneration of cutaneous tumors before age 50 is rare, complete surgical excision with histopathologic examination is mandatory if cutaneous neurofibromas become painful or show signs of rapid enlargement.

Incontinentia Pigmenti

Incontinentia pigmenti (Bloch-Sulzberger syndrome) is a hereditary disorder that affects the skin, central nervous system, eyes, and skeletal system. Although the genetics of this disorder have not been delineated, the familial tendency with almost exclusive involvement in females (97 per cent) suggests that transmission is either autosomal dominant or X-linked dominant, prenatally lethal to males.[149]

CLINICAL MANIFESTATIONS. The disorder generally appears at birth or shortly thereafter (90 per cent of patients have cutaneous lesions within the first two weeks of life; 96 per cent have their onset before the age of six weeks). Although the cutaneous lesions have three, possibly four, distinct phases, their sequence is irregular and overlapping of stages is common.

Phase 1. The first phase of incontinentia pigmenti begins with inflammatory vesicles (Fig. 18–49) or bullae that develop in crops over the trunk and extremities, often persisting for weeks to months. An interesting and unexplained feature of this phase of the disorder is the high degree of eosinophilia (from 18 to 50 per cent) which is present in 74 per cent of patients during the first two weeks of life. Biopsy of a small blister during

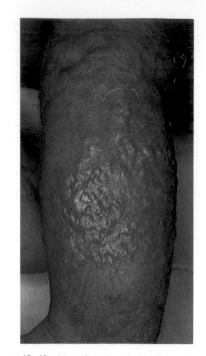

Figure 18–49 Incontinentia pigmenti (vesicular stage). Multiple vesicles and bullae, many in a linear distribution (the first phase of incontinentia pigmenti as seen on the leg of a two-week-old infant).

this vesicular stage reveals an inflammatory dermatitis with epidermal vesicles filled with eosinophils.

Phase 2. The vesicular stage is followed by an intermediate phase characterized by irregular linear warty or verrucous lesions (Fig. 18–50) on one or more extremities, usually the backs of the hands and feet. This stage, seen in 70 per cent of patients with incontinentia pigmenti, resolves spontaneously, usually within a period of several months.

Phase 3. During or shortly following this intermediate verrucous stage, the highly characteristic pigmentary state begins. The pigmentation that is the hallmark of the disease, seen in almost

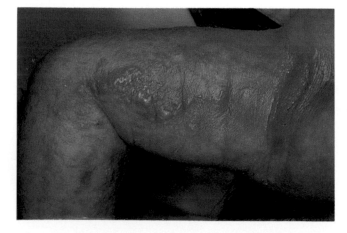

Figure 18–50 Vesicular and verrucous lesions on the thigh of the same 2-week-old infant with incontinentia pigmenti. Although incontinentia pigmenti has three (possibly four) distinct cutaneous phases, their sequence is irregular and overlapping is common.

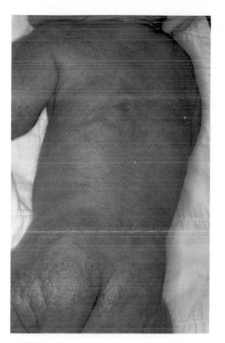

Figure 18–51   Swirl-like bands of slate-brown to blue-gray hyperpigmentation in a child with incontinentia pigmenti.

100 per cent of patients, is characterized by bands of slate-brown to blue-gray splattered Chinese-figure-like patches arranged in swirl-like formations on the extremities and trunk (Fig. 18–51, Fig. 18–52). This stage tends to increase in intensity until the patient's second year of life. It persists for many years and gradually fades and, in many cases, completely disappears by adolescence or early adulthood. It is from this pigmentary stage that the disease derives its name (because histologically melanin appears to drop down from the melanocytes into the dermis).

Although the pigmentary changes were originally considered to be a post-inflammatory phenomenon secondary to the vesiculo-bullous or verrucous stages, the pigment fails to follow the pattern, shape, or location of the bullous and verrucous lesions. Recent electron microscopic studies, however, conclude that all three stages are related to each other and that pigmentary incontinence can be explained as a phagocytic phenomenon.[150]

Phase 4. A fourth phase consisting of depigmented lesions has also recently been reported in individuals with incontinentia pigmenti.[151] Seen as isolated streaked hypopigmented lesions or in conjunction with other manifestations, they have been noted on the arms, thighs, trunk, and particularly the calves of children as well as adults. The histologic features, incidence, and pathogenesis of these hypopigmented lesions are poorly defined. Their presence, however, may serve as a clue to the hereditary pattern and may play a role in the genetic counseling of families of individuals with this disorder.

SYSTEMIC MANIFESTATIONS. Systemic manifestations are seen in a high percentage of patients with incontinentia pigmenti. Almost 80 per cent of patients have one or more abnormalities of the hair (Fig. 18–53), eyes, central nervous system, and/or structural development. Thirty per cent of patients have central nervous system involvement. Of these, 3.3 per cent have seizures, and although many individuals are bright or have normal intellect, 16 per cent have low mentality and 13 per cent have spastic abnormalities. Ophthalmic changes are present in 35 per cent of patients; 18 per cent have strabismus; and an equal number demonstrate more serious eye involvement (cataracts, optic atrophy, or retinal damage). Alopecia is seen in 38 per cent of patients; nail dystrophy is present in 7 per cent of individuals; and 64 per cent of patients have dental anomalies (delayed dentition, partial anodontia, pegged or conical teeth, Fig. 18–54).[149] Occasionally cardiac anomalies and skeletal malformations (such as microcephaly, syndactyly, supernumerary ribs, hemiatrophy, or shortening of the arms or legs) may occur.

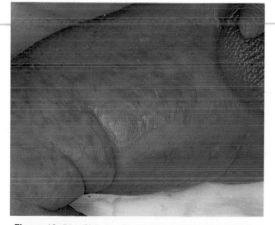

Figure 18–52   Chinese figure-like hyperpigmentation in a male newborn with incontinentia pigmenti.

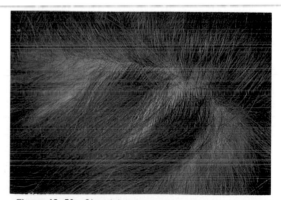

Figure 18–53   Cicatricial alopecia in a 7-year-old girl with incontinentia pigmenti (alopecia is seen in 25 to 38 per cent of patients with this disorder).

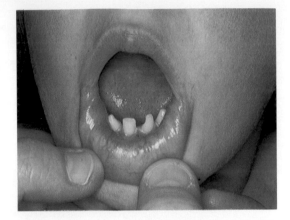

Figure 18–54 Pegged (conical) teeth. Approximately two-thirds of patients with incontinentia pigmenti have dental anomalies (anodontia, pegged or conical teeth, or delayed dentition).

The combination of bullae and linear nodular or warty lesions in a female infant is pathognomonic of this disorder; the pigmentation in older children is a hallmark of the disease. Because of the risk of involvement of other children and a potential for ocular, dental, osseous, and neurological changes, it is important that pediatricians, usually the first to see the patient, be familiar with this entity and be able to diagnose and counsel patients seen with this disorder.

No special therapy is required for the skin lesions of incontinentia pigmenti. Genetic counseling is advisable, however, since at least 50 per cent of affected children have associated congenital defects (cataracts, microcephaly, spastic paralysis, strabismus, alopecia, delayed or impaired dentition, epilepsy, or mental retardation).

Incontinentia Pigmenti Achromians

Incontinentia pigmenti achromians (hypomelanosis of Ito) is a peculiar condition of hypopigmentation first described by Ito in 1952.[152] The name was first coined because hypopigmentation of the skin appeared in a linear swirled pattern that resembled a negative image of the hyperpigmentation seen in patients with incontinentia pigmenti.[153] Histologic examination of the hypopigmented areas reveals a normal number of melanocytes. They, however, are weakly dopa-positive and contain less melanin than cells in the surrounding pigmented skin. Since there is no histologic evidence of pigment incontinence and the disorder appears to be distinct from, and unrelated to, incontinentia pigmenti, these two disorders should not be confused with one another. A more appropriate term for this disease, therefore, appears to be *hypomelanosis of Ito*.

Although multiple cases of hypomelanosis of Ito have been described in several families, its genetic pattern remains unclear.[154, 155] The disorder is often seen at birth, or early in infancy, and persists for many years. In a few patients the

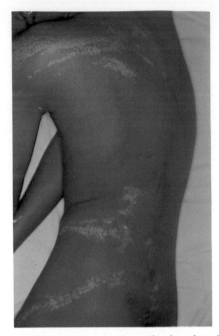

Figure 18–55 Incontinentia pigmenti achromians (hypomelanosis of Ito). Patterned macular, linear, or swirls of hypopigmentation (approximately 50 per cent of patients with incontinentia pigmenti achromians have internal manifestations).

lesions may be patchy and confined to relatively limited areas of the body; in most patients, however, the hypopigmented areas are more extensive, often bilateral, and appear to be more pronounced on the ventral surface of the trunk and the flexor surfaces of the limbs (Fig. 18–55).

Of significance is the fact that approximately 50 per cent of patients with hypomelanosis of Ito have internal manifestations. These include central nervous system dysfunction (seizure disorders and delayed development), ocular disturbances (strabismus, heterochromia iridis, microphthalmia, and nystagmus), and musculoskeletal anomalies (macrocephaly, scoliosis, asymmetry of the limbs, weakness, and hypotonicity.[153-156]

Since hypopigmented lesions appear infrequently in early infancy and young children, the appearance of such lesions, particularly in the absence of previous inflammatory skin disease, should alert the physician to possible association with systemic disease. A search for anomalies should be made, and a careful developmental evaluation should be obtained. If scoliosis or asymmetry is present, since the likelihood of seizures with this combination is high, an electroencephalogram and neurologic assessment are indicated.[154]

MUCOSAL NEUROMA SYNDROME

Mucosal neuroma syndrome (multiple mucosal neuroma syndrome) is characterized by the association of multiple mucosal neuromas, medullary thyroid carcinoma, and pheochromocytoma.[157] A relationship between carcinoma of the thyroid and pheochromocytoma was first described by Eisenberg in 1932. It was not until almost 30 years later that Sipple, in 1961, again noted this combination of findings.[158] Since then, reports of this association with other findings such as parathyroid hyperplasia and multiple mucosal neuromas have been known as the Sipple syndrome. Associated with this constellation of findings are other abnormalities; a characteristic facies, marfanoid appearance, intestinal ganglioneuromatosis, and various eye disorders. Other terms used to denote variations of this combination include multiple mucosal neuroma syndrome, medullary thyroid carcinoma syndrome, oral mucosal neuroma medullary thyroid carcinoma syndrome, and multiple endocrine neoplasia type III.

CLINICAL MANIFESTATIONS. Mucosal neuromas (seen in 80 per cent of patients with this group of disorders) may present at multiple sites (the lips, tongue, eyes, and gastrointestinal tract) and appear to represent the hallmark of this syndrome.[159] Labial involvement results in diffusely enlarged lips with a characteristic fleshy, blubbery, or Negroid appearance (Fig. 18–56). Lingual neuromas, generally limited to the anterior third of the tongue, appear as pink, sessile, or pedunculated nodules (Figs. 18–56 and 18–57). These may be congenital or may be noted in the first few years of life and often represent the first markers heralding this syndrome. Neuromas may also be seen at the limbus of the conjunctivae and at the margins of the eyelids, with thickening of the margin and displacement of the cilia (Fig. 18–58).

Intestinal ganglioneuromatosis may commonly be seen as another form of mucosal neuroma in this disorder. Here, failure to thrive, constipation, or diarrhea may lead to further evaluation and eventual demonstration of the full abnormality.[160, 161]

Physical features of these patients include a

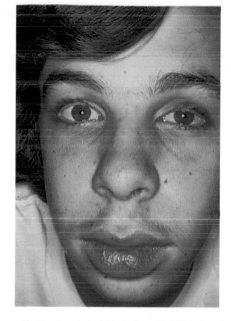

Figure 18–57 Characteristic facies with diffusely enlarged lips in multiple mucosal neuroma syndrome (Hurwitz S: Arch. Dermatol. *110*:139, 1974).

marfanoid appearance with long slender limbs and fingers, poor muscular development with very little subcutaneous fat, and skeletal defects such as kyphoscoliosis, pectus excavatum (funnel chest), and pectus carinatum (pigeon breast). Other abnormalities, such as a high-arched palate and pes cavus, may also be seen in this disorder.[160]

Medullary carcinoma of the thyroid, a malignancy seen in only 5 to 10 per cent of all thyroid cancers, is the major endocrine tumor of this syndrome. Here the perifollicular cells of the thyroid (termed "C" cells because of their secretion of calcitonin, the calcium-lowering polypeptide hormone) may also be the source of other

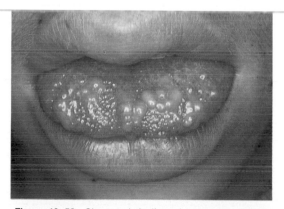

Figure 18–56 Characteristic lingual neuromas and protuberant fleshy lips in a 16-year-old boy with multiple mucosal neuroma syndrome.

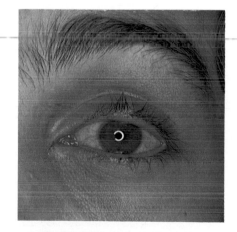

Figure 18–58 Multiple mucosal neuroma syndrome. Neuromas of the eyelid margins causing thickening of the margins and displacement of the cilia.

humoral substances such as prostaglandin and serotonin in occasional patients. Histopathologic examination of medullary carcinoma of the thyroid reveals sheets of rather uniform, round to spindle-shaped cells, often binucleated, with eosinophilic cytoplasm. The increased calcitonin released by these cells lowers serum calcium, thus stimulating a compensatory parathyroid response resulting in hyperparathyroidism or parathyroid adenoma. Parathyroid abnormalities, therefore, represent a secondary response and are not the direct result of genetic aberration.

Pheochromocytoma may be present in 38 per cent of patients with the Sipple syndrome.[159] Here the chromaffin cells of the adrenal medulla and sympathetic nerves and ganglia, also derived from primitive neural crest ectoderm, synthesize catecholamines, norepinephrine, and epinephrine, with resultant hypertension, tachycardia, anxiety, hyperhidrosis, weight loss, and/or fatigue.

TREATMENT. Early recognition and removal of medullary carcinoma of the thyroid gives the best chance for survival. Calcitonin levels are helpful in the diagnosis of this disorder, and patients with mucosal neuromas and facies characteristic of this syndrome should be evaluated for evidence of thyroid cancer and pheochromocytoma.[159-161] With early recognition an attempt should be made to excise the medullary carcinoma. Unfortunately, most patients with this disorder expire in their twenties or thirties. Adequate therapy includes thyroidectomy and a search for parathyroid hyperplasia, hypercalcinosis, and nephrocalcinosis. Pheochromocytomas and eye lesions should be sought, and since this syndrome appears to be genetic in origin, relatives should be examined and appropriately counseled.[161, 162]

HISTIOCYTOSIS IN CHILDREN

Histiocytosis X is a term originated by Lichtenstein in 1953 to identify three related clinical entities of unknown etiology characterized by histiocyte proliferation.[163] This classification includes the triad of Letterer-Siwe disease, Hand-Schüller-Christian disease, and eosinophilic granuloma. Each of these disorders presents a distinct clinical picture with overlapping transitional stages suggesting that they are all variants of the same basic disease process. Proof of the unity of the three syndromes came with recognition of the histologic similarity and with electron microscopic demonstration of Langerhans' granules in the cytoplasm of histiocytes in all three syndromes.

The X in the title only reminds us of the lack of a specific etiology for this group of disorders. Numerous etiologies have been proposed for histiocytosis. These include a disturbance of intracellular lipid metabolism, an infectious process, and a neoplastic disorder of histiocytes. Since data are insufficient to support any of these theories, the true pathogenesis remains obscure. Recent

studies of Letterer-Siwe disease in uniovular twins, reports of familial incidence, and cases of consanguinity have suggested a hereditary influence, perhaps an autosomal recessive gene with reduced penetrance.

Letterer-Siwe Disease

Letterer-Siwe disease is seen at the severe fulminating end of the histiocytosis spectrum, as the acute disseminated form of the disease. It usually occurs during the first year of life and is almost exclusively limited to children up to three years of age. In virtually all patients with Letterer-Siwe disease, skin markers may represent the first recognizable sign of the disorder. The infant may appear healthy for many months before fever, anemia, thrombocytopenia, adenopathy, hepatosplenomegaly, or skeletal tumors become apparent.

The skin eruption presents in several forms. It frequently begins with a scaly, erythematous seborrhea-like eruption on the scalp, behind the ears, and in the axillary, inguinal or perineal areas. On close inspection, the presence of basic lesions of histiocytosis (reddish-brown or purpuric papules) may identify the disorder (Fig. 18–59). In infants, vesicular or crusted papules may predominate (Fig. 18–60). Purpuric nodules on the palms and soles of infants appear to be a particularly bad prognostic sign of this disorder (Fig. 18–61). Buccal and gingival ulcerations, chronic otitis media, and ulceration of the post-auricular, inguinal, or perineal regions also represent important diagnos-

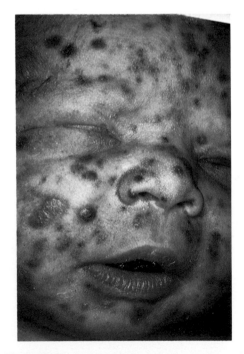

Figure 18–59 Reddish-brown purpuric papules and nodules in a newborn with congenital histiocytosis (Letterer-Siwe disease).

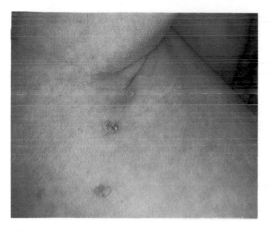

Figure 18–60 Crusted and vesicular lesions in a 1-month-old infant with congenital Letterer-Siwe disease.

tic clues. When the diagnosis is indeterminant, the character and distribution of lesions should suggest the true nature of the eruption. Diagnosis, then, can be confirmed easily by skin biopsy.[164]

This disease was considered to be an invariably fatal disorder until 1951 when Aronson reported the first incidence of recovery.[165] Since then, additional long-term survivals have been reported sporadically. Careful clinical reviews have shown that prognosis is related to age of onset, duration of symptoms, and the degree of systemic involvement. Benign and purely cutaneous forms, although rare, have been reported by Esterly, Freeman, and others.[166-168] The absence of thrombocytopenia and a lack of extensive visceral involvement favor a good prognosis.

The highest mortality is seen in patients under the age of six months, particularly those with widespread systemic involvement. Purpura of the palms, a finding seldom seen in other skin disease, early age of onset, and lung involvement appear to be signs of a particularly poor prognosis. Death, when it occurs, may be caused by pulmonary, hepatic, or splenic involvement and frequently is attributed to hemorrhage, anemia, or infection. Despite reports of long standing that Letterer-Siwe disease bears a poor prognosis, the disease course fluctuates and spontaneous remissions have been documented. Although in general Letterer-Siwe disease often implies a fatal outcome, therapy is often beneficial, spontaneous remissions have occurred, and at times the illness may evolve into a more chronic phase of histiocytosis X such as Hand-Schüller-Christian disease.[164]

Hand-Schüller-Christian Disease

This is the variant of histiocytosis generally seen between two and six years of age. Classically this syndrome consists of a triad of osteolytic defects, diabetes insipidus, and exophthalmos. The bony lesions are invariably present; only 50 per cent of patients, however, have diabetes insipidus, and a mere 10 per cent demonstrate exophthalmos. Chronic otitis media secondary to histiocytic infiltration of the mastoid is common. Histiocytic proliferation may also cause necrosis, ulcerations, and small tumors of the gums and oral mucous membranes. Roentgenograms of the skull often reveal sharply defined areas of osseous rarefaction, termed "geographic skull," or erosions of the tooth-bearing portion of the mandible, with loosening or extrusion of the teeth. The lungs and pleura represent a major cause of disability and are affected in 30 per cent of patients, with death resulting from pulmonary fibrosis, associated ventricular hypertrophy, and right-sided heart failure.

Skin lesions, seen in 30 to 50 per cent of patients, are similar to those of the Letterer-Siwe syndrome, except that in Hand-Schüller-Christian disease purpura is less common and the skin lesions are neither as vivid nor as destructive. The skin lesions consist of coalescing, scaling or crusted, brown to flesh-colored papules. Occasionally, lesions of long duration develop a shiny yellowish hue. As in Letterer-Siwe disease, granulomatous infiltrates with ulceration are also found in the axillary or anogenital areas.

Eosinophilic Granuloma

Eosinophilic granuloma represents the third and most benign form of histiocytosis. Usually seen in young adults and children over the age of six years, the onset is insidious. The patient is generally symptom-free until headaches, localized pain, tenderness, or swelling of soft tissues suggest the diagnosis. In children, eosinophilic granuloma often represents an early or transitional form of Letterer-Siwe or Hand-Schüller-Christian disease. In adults it is usually a benign, although chronic, illness. The disorder may present as single or multiple skeletal lesions and often goes undetected until a spontaneous fracture or an incidental roentgenographic examination suggests the diagnosis.

Skin lesions are relatively rare, but may be

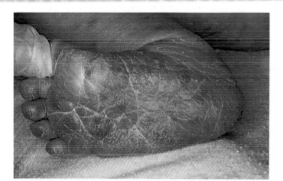

Figure 18–61 Purpuric nodules on the sole of a newborn with congenital Letterer-Siwe disease (a particularly bad prognostic sign of Letterer-Siwe disease).

identical to those seen in Letterer-Siwe or Hand-Schüller-Christian disease. Again they may consist of crusting of the scalp (suggesting seborrheic dermatitis); reddish-brown papules or nodules in the retroauricular and perineal areas; or ulcerated granulomatous lesions of the buccal mucous membranes or inguinal, perineal or vulvar regions. The course is characteristically chronic, with a strong tendency to spontaneous remission. Diabetes insipidus, pulmonary lesions, and Langerhan's granules have been reported, adding to the evidence that all three forms of histiocytosis are caused by a common disease process.

Xanthoma Disseminatum

Xanthoma disseminatum is a rare benign histiocytic proliferative disorder of unknown cause characterized by disseminated xanthomatosis in predominantly young male adults. In 30 per cent of cases the disorder begins before the age of 15.[1] Lesions consist of closely set round to oval yellowish-orange or yellowish-brown to mahogany-brown or purple papules, nodules, and plaques that are present mainly on the face, flexor surfaces of the neck, antecubital fossae, periumbilical area, perineum, and genitalia. Xanthomatous deposits have been observed in the mouth and upper respiratory tract (epiglottis, larynx, and trachea in 40 per cent of cases), occasionally leading to respiratory difficulty.[169]

Diabetes insipidus is present in 40 per cent of cases. Although the cutaneous lesions are similar in xanthoma disseminatum and Hand-Schüller-Christian disease and both diseases share the fairly common occurrence of diabetes insipidus, the question as to whether xanthoma disseminatum is a forme fruste of Hand-Schüller-Christian disease remains controversial.

The distribution of lesions, their histologic features, and the usual lack of disturbed lipid metabolism help establish the diagnosis. Histologic examination of lesions shows xanthoma cells, eosinophilic histiocytes, numerous Touton giant cells, and an inflammatory infiltrate.

Except for severe laryngeal involvement occasionally necessitating tracheostomy, the disease tends to run a chronic but benign course and the lesions have been seen to regress spontaneously. If diabetes insipidus occurs, it usually is mild and may be transient, so that continued therapy with vasopressin injections (Pitressin) become unnecessary.

Juvenile Xanthogranuloma

Juvenile xanthogranuloma, or nevoxanthoendothelioma, represents a benign self-limiting disease of infants and children characterized by a cutaneous infiltrate. Since histiocytes represent the basic cell, and internal lesions similar to those seen in Hand-Schüller-Christian disease occasionally occur, many authors consider juvenile xanthogranuloma to be an abortive cutaneous form of histiocytosis. The lesions have no relationship to nevi, and endothelial cells are not responsible for the histogenesis of this disorder. Accordingly, the earlier term, nevoxanthoendothelioma (a misnomer), has been replaced by the name juvenile xanthogranuloma.

The condition represents a benign self-limiting disorder of childhood characterized by solitary or multiple yellow to reddish-brown papules and nodules (Fig. 18–62) of the face, scalp, neck, and proximal portions of the extremities or trunk. Lesions also occur on mucous membranes or at mucocutaneous junctions (the mouth, vaginal orifice, and perianal area). Typically the lesions are present at birth (20 per cent) or during the first six to nine months of life. The lesions run a benign course, often increasing in number until about 1 to 1½ years of age, and then involute spontaneously. There may be as few as one or two lesions or as many as several hundred. They may range in size from several millimeters to one centimeter in diameter and frequently have a discrete, firm or rubbery consistency.

About 90 per cent of cases have a self-limiting cutaneous disease. This disorder, therefore, was regarded as a lesion limited to the skin until 1949, when Blank reported a lesion of the iris in a 4-month-old infant with this condition.[170] Lesions also may occur in the lung, pericardium, meninges, liver, spleen, and testes. Patients with pulmonary involvement often show spontaneous regression of lesions. Ocular tumors, however, the most frequent internal complication, often require therapy if extensive glaucoma, hemorrhage, or blindness is to be avoided. Once the proper diagnosis has been established, therapy of ocular lesions includes radiation and topical or systemic steroids; skin lesions, however, involute spontaneously and require no treatment.

MANAGEMENT OF HISTIOCYTOSIS. Therapeutic regimens for histiocytosis vary widely, and since the disease is of variable activity, evaluation of therapy is often difficult. In general, patients with diffuse systemic disease of the reticulohistio-

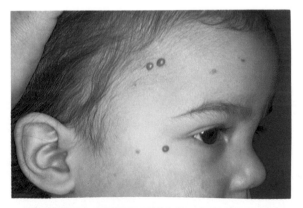

Figure 18–62   Yellow to reddish-brown papular and nodular lesions on the face of an infant with juvenile xanthogranulomas (nevoxanthoendotheliomas).

cytic system suffer impaired immunity, and, subsequently, diminished resistance to infection. Blood transfusions and antibiotics may improve the long-term outlook for such patients, in particular for those with anemia, leucopenia, or thrombocytopenia.

Immunosuppressive drugs currently appear to offer the greatest hope for survival. Simultaneous combination of drugs has been most effective. This suggests that aggressive combination regimens with good symptomatic care may achieve further long-term remissions, and possibly eventual cure. Prednisone, in dosages averaging 2 to 4 mg/kg daily, may result in complete clearing of lesions or remissions lasting from 12 to 30 months. Alkylating agents such as nitrogen mustard, Leukeran, and Cytoxan appear to be highly effective. Procarbazine offers a very limited response and a high incidence of toxicity.

Nitrogen mustard (mechlorethamine) gives a rapid effect and may be administered intravenously in dosages of 0.2 to 0.5 mg/kg body weight. For long-term therapy, chlorambucil (Leukeran) may be given orally in dosages of 0.1 to 0.3 mg/kg per day, for several months, depending upon the course of the disease. A year or more of therapy is frequently required to control histiocytosis.

The plant alkaloids vinblastine and vincristine have produced some notable successes. Vinblastine may be given in weekly or semiweekly intravenous injections of 0.1 to 0.3 mg/kg for many weeks. This drug, however, causes bone marrow suppression, neuritis, alopecia, and gastrointestinal side effects. Therapy, therefore, should be initiated in low dosages with gradual increments, as tolerated, in an effort to minimize side effects.

Methotrexate, 1.25 mg daily, alone or in combination with steroids, though potentially toxic, is also an effective mode of therapy. Intermittent dosages (once or twice a week as opposed to daily doses) may prove to be less toxic. Cyclophosphamide (Cytoxan), 3 mg/kg daily, appears to be less toxic and is especially beneficial when combined with steroids or when combined with steroids and vinblastine.

In general, patients with Hand-Schüller-Christian disease and eosinophilic granuloma are more responsive to therapy than patients with Letterer-Siwe disease. Radiation therapy, particularly when initiated early in the course of the disease, is very effective for localized skeletal lesions. Diabetes insipidus is controllable with vasopressin (Pitressin) by injection or nasal insufflation. X-ray therapy or curettage is effective for bone lesions of eosinophilic granuloma.

Histiocytosis, although still a potentially fatal disorder, particularly in young children, can be diagnosed early by characteristic cutaneous manifestations. These skin signs may appear alone or in combination with systemic symptoms. Although the disease reputedly has a poor prognostic outlook, it often presents in much less severe form, so that prognosis is often more optimistic than the literature suggests. Vigorous therapeutic approaches, with a combination of steroids, immunosuppressive drugs, and general supportive measures, appear to offer the greatest hope for survival. With accumulation of data, the fatalistic approach to the disease must be reassessed. Aggressive chemotherapy and good supportive care may allow children not only hope for long-term remission but, perhaps, even eventual complete cure.[171-174]

References

1. Braverman IM: Skin Signs of Systemic Disease. W. B. Saunders Co., Philadelphia, 1970.

   An invaluable well-written text emphasizing the cutaneous features and their role in the diagnosis of systemic disease.

2. Champion RH, et al.: Urticaria and angioedema. Br. J. Dermatol. 81:588–597, 1969.

   Clinical features, pathogenesis, and management of urticaria and angioedema.

3. Maize JD: Urticaria. In Demis DJ, Dobson RL, McGuire J (Eds.): Clinical Dermatology, Vol. 2. Harper and Row, Hagerstown, Md., 1976, 7–9.

   Urticaria, its pathogenesis, clinical features, and therapy.

4. Warin RP, Champion RH: Major Problems in Dermatology, Vol. 1: Urticaria. W. B. Saunders Co. Ltd., London, Philadelphia, 1974.

   A comprehensive and authoritative monograph on urticaria.

5. O'Laughlin S, Schroeter AL, Jordon RE: Chronic urticaria-like lesions in systemic lupus erythematosus. A review of 12 cases. Arch. Dermatol. 114:879–883, 1978.

   Twelve of 54 patients (23 per cent) with systemic lupus erythematosus had chronic urticaria-like lesions; biopsies in 9 of 11 of these patients revealed necrotizing vasculitis with leukocytoclasis as the major histologic finding.

6. Braverman IM: Urticaria as a sign of internal disease. Postgrad. Med. 41:450–454, 1967.

   Chronic urticaria can be a valuable sign of connective tissue disease, malignancy, or hepatitis.

7. Champion RH: Urticaria and angio-edema. Br. J. Hosp. Med. 3:233–238, 1970.

   A review of the various types of urticaria, their pathogeneses, and treatments.

8. Chalamidas SL, Charles R: Aquagenic urticaria. Arch. Dermatol. 104:541–546, 1971.

   Studies in a 49-year-old man with a three-year-history of hives on contact with water support the hypothesis that aquagenic urticaria probably is due to a histamine-induced phenomenon.

9. Shelly WB, Rawnsley HM: Aquagenic urticaria. JAMA 189:895–898, 1964.

   An unusual form of perifollicular urticaria caused by a toxic substance formed by a combination of water and sebum which induces degranulation of perifollicular mast cells and subsequent histamine release.

10. Harber LC, Halloway RM, Wheatley VR, et al.: Immunologic and biophysical studies in solar urticaria. J. Invest. Dermatol. 41:439–443, 1963.

    A classification of solar urticaria based upon biochemical, biophysical, and immunologic studies in five patients.

11. Juhlin L, Shelley WB: Role of mast cell and basophil in cold urticaria with associated systemic reactions. JAMA 177:371–377, 1961.

With the use of an in vitro technique, circulating basophils and cutaneous mast cells in cold urticaria patients were shown to discharge their granules upon cooling.

12. Tindall JP: Cold urticaria. Postgrad. Med. 50:133–137, 1971.

A review of acquired and familial forms of cold urticaria.

13. Sarkany I, Gaylarde PM: Negative reactions to ice in cold urticaria. Br. J. Derm. 85:46–48, 1971.

Some patients with cold urticaria who do not respond to application of ice to the skin may be diagnosed by generalized cooling of the body, or by a positive response to cold water.

14. Wanderer AF, St. Pierre J, Ellis E: Primary acquired cold urticaria. Arch. Dermatol. 113:1375–1377, 1977.

Patients unresponsive to chlorpheniramine responded to treatment with cyproheptadine (Periactin).

15. Frank MM, Gelfand JA, Atkinson JA: Hereditary angioedema: the clinical syndrome and its management. Ann. Intern. Med. 84:580–593, 1976.

A review of hereditary angioedema, the clinical syndrome, its pathophysiology, diagnosis, and management.

16. Klemperer MR, Rosen FS, and Donaldson VH: A polypeptide derived from the second component of human complement (C2) which increases vascular permeability. J. Clin. Invest. 48:44a–44b, 1969.

An esterase derived from the first component of human complement (C'1s) demonstrated increased vascular permeability when incubated with human C'4 and C'2.

17. Donaldson VH: Mechanisms of activation of C1 esterase in hereditary angioneurotic edema plasma in vitro: the role of Hageman factor, a clot promoting agent. J. Exp. Med. 127:411–429, 1968.

Studies of C'1 esterase activity in plasma obtained from individuals with hereditary angioneurotic edema suggest a role of Hageman factor in the activation of C'1 in this disorder.

18. Hyman C, Wong WH, Janklow HM, et al.: Physiologic studies of the peripheral circulation in a patient with Quincke's disease. J. Invest. Dermatol 49:533–536, 1967.

Blood flow studies in a 23-year-old man suggest an elevated capillary filtration coefficient in the pathogenesis of the edema in hereditary angioneurotic edema.

19. Johnson AM, Alper CA, Rosen FS, et al.: Evidence for decreased hepatic synthesis in hereditary angioneurotic edema. Science 173:553–554, 1971.

Studies suggest a biosynthetic decrease in hepatic synthesis of C1 inhibitor as the cause of hereditary angioneurotic edema.

20. Donaldson VH, Rosen FS: Hereditary angioneurotic edema: a clinical survey. Pediatrics 37:1017–1027, 1966.

A review of the physiology and clinical manifestations of hereditary angioneurotic edema.

21. Champion RH, Lachman PJ: Hereditary angioedema treated with E-amino-caproic acid. Br. J. Dermatol. 81:763–765, 1969.

EACA (not recommended for children) inhibits the conversion of plasminogen to plasmin (a known C_1 activator).

22. Gelfand JA, Sherrin RJ, Alling DW, et al.: Treatment of hereditary angioedema with danazol. N. Engl. J. Med. 295:1444–1448, 1976.

A double-blind study in 9 patients demonstrates a significant decrease in attacks of angioedema in patients treated with danazol.

23. Keil H: The rheumatic erythema: a clinical survey. Ann. Int. Med. 11:2223–2272, 1938.

Erythema marginatum, an easily overlooked sign of rheumatic fever, usually but not invariably associated with active carditis.

24. Perry CB: Erythema marginatum (rheumaticum), Arch. Dis. Child. 12:233–238, 1937.

Erythema marginatum is a distinctive eruption occurring in about 10 per cent of patients with active rheumatic fever.

25. Hammer H, Ronnerfalt L: Annular erythema in infants associated with autoimmune disorders in their mothers. Dermatologica 154:115–127, 1977.

A review of annular urticarial lesions in infants and their association with maternal autoimmune disease.

26. Scrimenti RJ: Erythema chronicum migrans. Arch. Dermatol. 102:104–105, 1970.

A migratory erythematous erythema following a wood tick bite in a physician in Milwaukee–probably the first recorded case of erythema chronicum migrans in the United States.

27. Mast WE, Burrows WM: Erythema chronicum migrans in the United States. JAMA 236:859–860, 1976.

Four cases of erythema chronicum migrans occurring within a one-month period in southeastern Connecticut.

28. Steere AC, Malawista SE, Syndman DR, et al.: Lyme arthritis, an epidemic of oligoarticular arthritis in children and adults in three Connecticut communities. Arthritis and Rheumatism 20:7–17, 1977.

The authors believe that the arthritis described here is a previously unrecognized clinical entity and have named it "Lyme arthritis," after the community where it was first studied.

29. Steere AC, Malawista SE, Hardin JA, et al.: Erythema chronicum migrans and Lyme arthritis. The enlarging clinical spectrum. Ann. Int. Med. 86:685–698, 1977.

Studies of 32 patients with erythema chronicum migrans, Lyme arthritis, or both.

30. Dryer RF, Goeliner PG, Carney AS: Lyme arthritis in Wisconsin. JAMA 241:498–499, 1979.

Three campers bitten by ticks in a woodland of northwest Wisconsin developed large erythematous skin lesions typical of erythema chronicum migrans, fever, meningism, myalgia, and transient migratory oligoarthritis preponderantly involving knees, shoulders, and elbows, clinical features consistent with the diagnosis of Lyme arthritis.

30a. Steere AC, Malawista SE: Cases of Lyme disease in the United States: location correlated with distribution of Ixodes dammini. Ann. Int. Med. 91:730–733, 1979.

Lyme disease occurs in three distinct foci: along the northeastern coast, in Wisconsin, and in California and Oregon, a distribution that correlated closely with that of Ixodes dammini in the first two areas and with Ixodes pacificus in the last.

30b. Steere AC, Hardin JA, Ruddy S, et al.: Lyme arthritis. Correlation with serum and cryoglobulin IgM with activity, and serum IgG with remission. Arth. Rheum. 22:471–489, 1979.

Patients with erythema chronicum migrans who develop cryoglobulins containing IgM are at risk of developing Lyme arthritis.

31. Steere AC, Gibofsky A, Patarroyo ME, et al.: Chronic Lyme arthritis: clinical and immunologic differentiation from rheumatoid arthritis. Ann. Int. Med. 90:896–901, 1979.

A review of clinical and immunologic aspects of Lyme arthritis.

31a. Steere AC, Malawista SE, Newman JH, et al.: Antibiotic therapy in Lyme disease. Ann. Int. Med. 93:1–8, 1980.

Antibiotic therapy (penicillin or tetracycline) shortens the duration of erythema chronicum migrans and may prevent or attenuate subsequent arthritis.

32. Baden HP, Holcomb FD: Erythema Nodosum from oral contraceptives. Arch. Dermatol. 98:634–635, 1968.

Non-infectious disorders that cause erythema nodosum are ulcerative colitis and regional ileitis, and reactions to various drugs, particularly sulfonamides, diphenylhydantoin, and contraceptive pills containing ethinyl estradiol and norethynodrel.

33. Aetiology of erythema nodosum in children. A study by a group of pediatricians. Lancet 2:14–16, 1961.

In a study of 105 children in England, beta hemolytic streptococcal infection proved to be the most common cause of erythema nodosum.

34. Kibel MA: Erythema nodosum in children. S. Afr. Med. J. Sci. 44:873–876, 1970.

A review of 21 cases of erythema nodosum in children from 1958 to 1969.

35. Winkelman RK, Förström L: New observations in the histopathology of erythema nodosum. J. Invest. Dermatol. 65:441–446, 1975.

Microscopic examination of lesions of erythema nodosum reveals a variable histologic pattern of response in the vessels, septa, and fat lobules of the subcutaneous tissue, which correlates with the clinical forms of the disorder.

36. Shelley WB: Herpes simplex virus, a cause of erythema multiforme. JAMA 201:153–165, 1967.

Intradermal skin tests with inactivated herpes simplex antigen produced bullae which appeared, both clinically and histologically, to be erythema multiforme.

37. Stevens AM, Johnson FC: A new eruptive fever associated with stomatitis and ophthalmia: report of two cases in children. Amer. J. Dis. Child. 24:526–533, 1922.

Review of the clinical manifestations of two children suggested that this disorder deserved consideration as a specific clinical entity, Stevens-Johnson disease.

38. Bedi TR, Pinkus H: Histopathologic spectrum of erythema multiforme. Br. J. Dermatol. 95:243–250, 1976.

Histologic studies of 75 patients with erythema multiforme suggest that different types of clinical lesions present different yet distinctive histologic features.

39. Kazmierowski JA, Wuepper KD: Erythema multiforme: immune complex vasculitis of the superficial cutaneous microvasculature. J. Invest. Dermatol. 71:366–369, 1978.

Immunofluorescent findings of deposits of immunoglobulin and complement in the walls of vessels in the superficial vasculature suggest that erythema multiforme is mediated by the deposition of immune reactants in these vessels.

40. Rasmussen JE: Erythema multiforme in children — response to treatment with systemic corticosteroids. Br. J. Dermatol. 95:181–185, 1976.

Review of 32 patients with Stevens-Johnson disease suggest that treatment with systemic corticosteroids may be associated with delayed recovery and significant side effects.

41. Vernier RL, Worthen HC, Peterson RD, et al.: Anaphylactoid purpura. 1. Pathology of the skin and kidney and frequency of streptococcal infection. Pediatrics 27:181–193, 1961.

Clinical, experimental, and pathologic features of anaphylactoid purpura support the concept that this disorder is a form of diffuse vascular disease, probably caused by hypersensitivity to a variety of agents.

42. Allen, DM, Diamond LK, Howell DA: Anaphylactoid purpura in children (Schönlein-Henoch syndrome). Am. J. Dis. Child. 99:833–854, 1960.

Characteristic manifestations of anaphylactoid purpura as noted in a comprehensive analysis of 131 patients.

43. Byrn JR, Fitzgerald JF, Northway JD, et al.: Unusual manifestations of Henoch-Schönlein syndrome. Am. J. Dis. Child. 130:1335–1337, 1976.

Henoch-Schönlein syndrome presents a diagnostic challenge when the abdominal or joint manifestations precede the cutaneous lesions.

44. Wolfsohn H: Purpura and intussusception. Arch. Dis. Child. 22:242–247, 1947.

Intussusception in older children should suggest a diagnosis of Henoch-Schönlein purpura.

45. Wedgewood RJP, Klaus MH: Anaphylactoid purpura (Schönlein-Henoch syndrome) — a long-term follow-up study with special reference to renal involvement. Pediatrics 16:196–206, 1955.

Ten of 26 children with anaphylactoid purpura were noted to have an apparent latent nephritis after long-term follow-up.

46. Lewis IC, Philpott MG: Neurologic complications in the Schönlein-Henoch syndrome. Arch. Dis. Child. 31:369–371, 1956.

Two cases of anaphylactoid purpura complicated by subarachnoid hemorrhage.

47. Melish ME, Glasgow LA: The staphylococcal scalded skin syndrome — development of an experimental model. N. Engl. J. Med. 282:1114–1119, 1970.

Seventeen children with exfoliative dermatitis associated with phage Group II staphylococci.

48. Melish ME, Glasgow LA: Staphylococcal scalded skin syndrome: the expanded clinical syndrome. J. Pediatr. 78:958–967, 1971.

Twenty-eight patients with phage Group II staphylococcus present a spectrum of disease with a single etiology. Staphylococci isolated from these patients were used to develop an experimental model in newborn mice.

49. Elias PM, Levy SW: Bullous impetigo: occurrence of localized scalded skin syndrome in an adult. Arch. Dermatol. 112:856–858, 1976.

A report of bullous impetigo, the localized form of staphylococcal scalded skin syndrome, which occurs commonly in children but rarely in adults, in an adult receiving oral corticosteroids.

50. Elias PM, Fritsch P, Mittermeyer H: Staphylococcal toxic epidermal necrolysis: species and tissue susceptibility and resistance. J. Invest. Dermatol. 66:80–89, 1976.

The pathogenesis of staphylococcal toxic epidermolysis necrolysis involves intracellular cleavage, possibly through attack on keratinocyte receptors specific for exfoliation or the presence of specific yet undefined substances in the intercellular spaces.

51. Koblenzer PJ: Toxic epidermal necrolysis (TEN: Ritter's disease) and Staphylococcal scalded-skin syndrome (SSSS). A description and review. Clin. Pediatr. 15:724–730, 1976.

A review of toxic epidermal necrolysis and scalded skin syndrome as seen in childhood

52. Lillibridge CB, Melish ME, Glasgow LA: Site of action of exfoliative toxin in the staphylococcal scalded-skin syndrome. Pediatrics 50:723–738, 1972.

Exfoliative toxin derived from Group II *Staphylococcus aureus* causes disruption of desmosomes and intraepidermal cleavage.

53. Kawasaki T, Kosaki F, Okawa S, et al.: A new infantile acute febrile mucocutaneous lymph node syndrome (MLNS) prevailing in Japan. Pediatrics 54:271–276, 1974.

Clinical and epidemiologic features of what appears to be a new disorder affecting infants and young children.

54. Fetterman GH, Hashida Y: Mucocutaneous lymph node syndrome (MLNS). A disease widespread in Japan which demands our attention. Pediatrics 54:268–270, 1974

Studies reveal a close clinical resemblance between infantile periarteritis nodosa and mucocutaneous lymph node syndrome.

55. Goldsmith RW, Gribetz D, Strauss L: Mucocutaneous lymph node syndrome (MLNS) in the continental United States. Pediatrics 57:431–434, 1976.

A 2-year-old white boy with clinical features of mucocutaneous lymph node syndrome.

56. Kato H, Koike S, Yamamoto M, et al.: Coronary aneurysms in infants and young children with acute febrile mucocutaneous lymph node syndrome. J. Pediatr. 86:892–898, 1957.

Twenty patients surviving mucocutaneous lymph node syndrome were examined by coronary angiography; of these, twelve had abnormal coronary angiograms, seven had coronary aneurysms.

57. Yanigasawa M, Kobayashi N, Matsuya S: Myocardial infarction due to coronary thromboarteritis following acute febrile mucocutaneous lymph node syndrome (MLNS) in an infant. Pediatrics 54:277–281, 1974.

Although autopsy findings of MLNS have been similar to those of infantile periarteritis nodosa, the relationship of the two disorders remains controversial.

58. Kitamura S, Kawashima Y, Fujita T, et al.: Aortocoronary bypass grafting in a child with coronary artery obstruction due to mucocutaneous lymph node syndrome. Circulation 53:1035–1040, 1976.

A four-year-old boy with myocardial infarction and total occlusion of the right coronary and left anterior descending coronary arteries approximately ten months after MLNS underwent a successful double aorto-coronary bypass grafting.

59. Fujiwara H, Hamashima Y: Pathology of the heart in Kawasaki disease. Pediatrics 61:100–107, 1978.

Pathologic studies of 20 hearts of patients with Kawasaki disease revealed acute perivasculitis and vasculitis of the arterioles, capillaries, venules, and small arteries; acute perivasculitis and endarteritis of the three major coronary arteries; myocarditis; coagulation necrosis; lesions of the conduction system; pericarditis; and endocarditis with vasculitis.

60. Melish ME, Hicks RM, Larson E: Mucocutaneous lymph node syndrome (MLNS) in the United States (abstr). Pediatr. Res. 8:427, 1974.

Nine children in Hawaii with an unusual and highly distinctive multisystem disease indistinguishable from mucocutaneous lymph node syndrome (Kawasaki disease) as seen in Japan.

61. Melish ME: Kawasaki syndrome (mucocutaneous lymph node syndrome). Pediatrics in Review. In press.

A thorough analysis of Kawasaki disease, its clinical characteristics, diagnosis, and treatment.

62. Morens DM, Anderson LJ, Hurwitz ES: National surveillance of Kawasaki disease. Pediatr. 65:21–25, 1980.

A review of the epidemiology, clinical picture, laboratory data, complications, and prognoses of 261 cases of Kawasaki disease reported to the Center for Disease Control in Atlanta, Georgia, between July 1976 and July 1978.

63. Melish ME, Hicks RM, Larson EJ: Mucocutaneous lymph node syndrome in the United States. Am. J. Dis. Child. 130:599–607, 1976.

A review of 16 patients with Kawasaki disease seen in Honolulu, Hawaii during the four year period between April 1971 and February 1975.

64. Kato S, Kimura M, Tsuji K, et al.: HLA antigens in Kawasaki disease. Pediatrics 61:252–255, 1978.

Studies of 205 patients with Kawasaki disease and 500 normal controls suggest that a gene linked with a Japanese-specific HLA antigen controls the susceptibility to Kawasaki disease.

65. Landing BH, Larson EJ: Are infantile periarteritis nodosa with coronary artery involvement and fatal mucocutaneous lymph node syndrome the same? Comparison of 20 patients from North America with patients from Hawaii and Japan. Pediatrics 59:651–662, 1977.

Pathologic features of autopsy material from patients with infantile periarteritis nodosa with coronary involvement and fatal cases of mucocutaneous lymph node syndrome suggest that they are the same disorder.

66. Neches WH, Young LW: Mucocutaneous lymph node syndrome. Coronary artery disease and cross-sectional echocardiography. Am. J. Dis. Child. 133:1233–1235, 1979.

Cross-sectional (two-dimensional) echocardiography, an effective non-invasive technique for the detection of coronary aneurysms in patients with Kawasaki disease.

67. Yoshida H, Funabashi T, Nakaya S, et al.: Mucocutaneous lymph node syndrome: a cross-sectional echocardiographic diagnosis of coronary aneurysms. Am. J. Dis. Child. 133:1244–1247, 1979.

Cross-sectional echocardiograms in 41 patients with mucocutaneous lymph node syndrome.

68. Kato H, Koike S, Yokoyama T: Kawasaki disease. Effect of treatment of coronary artery involvement. Pediatrics 63:175–179, 1979.

Findings in 92 patients treated with five different regimens suggest that systemic steroids act adversely to cause a progression of coronary lesions. The author recommends that aspirin in high doses be given for a period of at least two months to individuals with this disorder.

69. Kendig EL: Medical progress. Sarcoidosis among children — a review. J. Pediatr. 61:229–278, 1962.

A review of sarcoidosis demonstrates the value of corticosteroids in children with severe involvement.

70. McGovern JP, Merritt DH: Sarcoidosis in childhood. Advances in Pediatrics, Vol. 8. Year Book Medical Publishers, Chicago, 1957, 97–135.

A review of sarcoidosis in childhood.

71. Beier RF, Lahey MD: Sarcoidosis among children in Utah and Idaho. J. Pediatr. 65:350–359, 1964.

Eight Caucasian children with sarcoidosis (mostly of northern European ancestry) in Utah and Idaho.

72. Schmitt E, Appelman H, Threatt B: Sarcoidosis in children. Radiology 106:621–625, 1973.

Radiologic findings as an aid to the diagnosis of sarcoidosis.

73. Kendig EL Jr, Brummer DL: The prognosis of sarcoidosis in children. Chest 70:351–353, 1976.

Eighteen per cent (5) of 28 children were severely affected by sarcoidosis.

74. Siltzbach LE, Greenberg GM: Childhood sarcoidosis — a study of 18 patients. N. Engl. J. Med. 279:1239–1245, 1968.

Clinical and pathologic features of sarcoidosis in childhood.

75. Bauer MF, et al.: Necrobiosis lipoidica diabeticorum. Arch. Dermatol. 90:558–566, 1964.

The relationship between necrobiosis and diabetic angiopathy.

76. Engel MF, Smith JG: The pathogenesis of necrobiosis lipoidica, a forme fruste of diabetes mellitus. Arch. Dermatol. 93:272–281, 1966.

The relationship between necrobiosis lipoidica and diabetes mellitus.

77. Muller SA, Winkelman RK: Necrobiosis lipoidica diabeticorum. A clinical and pathologic investigation of 171 cases. Arch. Dermatol. 93:272–281, 1966.

Pathologic studies of necrobiosis lipoidica diabeticorum.

78. Hansen TW: Necrobiosis lipoidica diabeticorum. In Demis DJ, Dobson. RL. Mc Guire J (Eds.): Clinical Dermatology. Harper and Row, Hagerstown, Maryland, 1976, 4:8, 1–5.

A review of necrobiosis, its pathogenesis, clinical picture, and management.

79. Melin H: An atrophic circumscribed skin lesion in the lower extremities of diabetics. Acta Med. Scand. Suppl. 423:1–75, 1964.

A classic description of diabetic dermopathy.

80. Shelley WB: Diabetic dermopathy. Consultations in Dermatology with Walter B. Shelley, 1. W. B. Saunders Co., Philadelphia, 1972, 172–175.

Brown pigmentation and atrophy of the legs are a valuable diagnostic index of diabetes.

81. Binkley GW: Dermopathy in the diabetic syndrome. Arch. Dermatol. 92:625–634, 1965.

Cutaneous microangiopathy and the relationship of diabetes and necrobiosis.

82. Cantwell AR, Martz W: Idiopathic bullae in diabetics — bullosis diabeticorum. Arch. Dermatol. 96:42–44, 1967.

A review of the problem of bullous dermatosis in diabetes.

83. Bernstein JE, Medenica M, Soltani K, et al.: Bullous eruption of diabetes mellitus. Arch. Dermatol. 115:324 325, 1979.

A 24-year-old man with severe diabetes experienced two episodes of bullae associated with intense ultraviolet exposure (perhaps associated with nephropathy rather than neuropathy).

84. Wells RS, Smith MA: The natural history of granuloma annulare. Br. J. Dermatol. 75:199–205, 1963.

Of 208 patients, 73 per cent cleared spontaneously within a period of two years.

85. Romaine R, Rudner E, Altman J: Papular granuloma annulare and diabetes mellitus: Report of cases. Arch. Dermatol. 98:152–154, 1968.

Three patients with papular granuloma annulare and previously unrecognized diabetes mellitus.

86. Williamson DM, Dykes JRW: Carbohydrate metabolism in granuloma annulare. J. Invest. Dermatol. 58:400–404, 1972.

Glucose tolerance tests (including cortisone stressed tests) on 16 patients with granuloma annulare reveal no evidence of prediabetic state.

87. Stankler, L, Leslie G: Generalized granuloma annulare. Arch. Dermatol. 95:509–513, 1967.

A patient with generalized granuloma annulare and review of 47 cases from the literature.

88. Brewer EJ Jr: Major Problems in Clinical Pediatrics VI, Juvenile Rheumatoid Arthritis. W. B. Saunders Co., Philadelphia, 1970.

A comprehensive monograph on juvenile rheumatoid arthritis.

89. Calabro JJ, Marchesano JM: Rash associated with juvenile rheumatoid arthritis. J. Pediatr. 72:611–619, 1968.

The clinical significance of the cutaneous eruption of Still's disease.

90. Calabro JJ: Diseases of connective tissue. In Gellis SS, Kagan BM (Eds.): Current Pediatric Therapy, 6. W. B. Saunders Co., Philadelphia, 1973, 377–381.

Review of the management of juvenile rheumatoid arthritis.

91. Dawkins RI, Mastiglia FL: Cell-mediated cytotoxicity to muscle in polymyositis. N. Engl. J. Med. 288:434–438, 1973.

Vascular deposits of immunoglobulins and complement demonstrated in blood vessel walls of skeletal muscles suggest antigen-antibody complement (their pathogenic role, however, remains uncertain).

92. Everett MA, Curtis AC: Dermatomyositis: A review of nineteen cases in adolescents and children. Arch. Int. Med. 100:70–76, 1967.

In nineteen children with dermatomyositis (4 months to 17 years of age), the 40 per cent who survived had inactive disease within a period of two years.

93. Mills JA: Dermatomyositis. In Fitzpatrick TB, Arndt K, Clark WH Jr, et al. (Eds.): Dermatology in General Medicine. McGraw-Hill, New York, 1971, 1518–1525.

An overview of dermatomyositis.

94. Braverman IM: Dermatomyositis and polymyositis. In Demis DJ, Dobson RL, McGuire J: Clinical Dermatology, Vol. 1. Harper and Row, Hagerstown, Maryland, 1977, 5: 4, 1–10.

Dermatomyositis, its clinical manifestations, complications, and management.

95. Cook DC, Rosen FS, Banker BQ: Dermatomyositis and focal scleroderma. Pediatr. Clin. N. Am. 10:979–1016. 1963.

An inclusive review of dermatomyositis and focal scleroderma in childhood.

96. Lell ME, Swerdlow ML: Dermatomyositis of childhood. Pediatr. Ann. 6:203–211, 1977.

Childhood dermatomyositis, unlike the adult variety, is not associated with an increased incidence of malignancy.

97. Bohan A, Peter JB, Bowman RL, et al.: Computer-assisted analysis of 153 patients with polymyositis and dermatomyositis. Medicine 50:255–286, 1977.

A comprehensive review of polymyositis-dermatomyositis based on a retrospective study of 153 patients.

98. Bitnum S, Daeschner CW Jr, Travis LB, et al.: Dermatomyositis. J. Pediatr. 64:101–131, 1964.

About one-third of the children with dermatomyositis recovered completely, usually within one year of onset of their illness.

99. Sullivan DB, Cassidy JT, Petty RE, et al.: Prognosis in childhood dermatomyositis. J. Pediatr. 80:555–563, 1972.

Of eighteen children treated with corticosteroids and physical therapy, all had a favorable response.

100. Jacobs JC: Methotrexate and azathioprine treatment of childhood dermatomyositis. Pediatrics 59:212–217, 1977.

Methotrexate and azathioprine are helpful in children with dermatomyositis who did not respond to prednisone alone.

101. Nassim JM, Connolly CK: Treatment of calcinosis universalis with aluminum hydroxide. Arch. Dis. Child. 45:118–121, 1970.

A 9-year-old with dermatomyositis and calcinosis universalis had considerable clearing of calcinosis on aluminum hydroxide gel.

102. Mazzafarin G, Lafferty FW, Pearson OH: Treatment of calcinosis with phosphorus deprivation. Ann. Int. Med. 77:741–745, 1972.

A 16-year-old boy with a seven-year history of calcinosis improved on aluminum hydroxide antacids and a diet low in phosphorus and calcium.

103. Sills EM: Diseases of Connective Tissue. In Gellis SS, Kagan BM: Current Pediatric Therapy, 7. W. B. Saunders Co., Philadelphia, 1976, 359–364.

Prognosis of dermatomyositis appears to be inversely correlated with the period between the appearance of the first symptom and the start of systemic steroid therapy.

104. Tuffanelli DL: Connective tissue diseases. In Malkinson FD, Pearson RW: 1978 YearBook of Dermatology. Year Book Medical Publishers, Inc. 1978, 9–36.

A review of the current status of connective tissue disorders.

105. Goel KM, Shanks RA: Scleroderma in childhood. Arch. Dis. Child. 49:861–865, 1974.

Five children, 2 1/2 to 10 years of age, with childhood forms of systemic sclerosis.

106. Sullivan DB, Cassidy JT: Scleroderma in the child. J. Pediatr. 85:770–775, 1974.

Review of twelve children with systemic scleroderma.

107. Tuffanelli DL: Lupus erythematosus. Arch. Dermatol. 106:553–566, 1972.

A review of the spectrum of lupus erythematosus.

108. Fish AJ, Blau EB, Westberg G, et al.: Systemic lupus erythematosus within the first two decades of life. Am. J. Med. 62:99–117, 1977.

In a study of a 17-year-experience with 49 patients in whom SLE occurred between ages 2 and 20, the incidence of clinical renal disease was 78 per cent and the 10 year survival rate was 86 per cent.

109. Braverman I: Lupus erythematosus. *In* Demis DJ, Dobson RL, McGuire J: Clinical Dermatology, Vol. 1. Harper and Row, Hagerstown, Maryland, 1977, 5–1:1–24.

A review of lupus erythematosus, its etiology, pathogenesis, clinical manifestations, and management.

110. Peterson RDA, Vernier RL, Good RA: Lupus erythematosus. Pediatr. Clin. North Am. *10*:941–978, 1963.

Children with lupus erythematosus are not rare (a summary of experience with children with this disorder seen over a ten year span).

111. Winkelman RK: Chronic discoid lupus erythematosus in children. JAMA *205*:675–678, 1968.

Chronic discoid lupus erythematosus (cutaneous lupus) is rare in childhood (1 to 3 per cent of all cases), similar to that seen in adult life, and usually persists into adulthood.

112. Brustein D, Rodriguez JM, Minkin W, et al.: Familial lupus erythematosus. JAMA *238*:2294–2296, 1977.

Report of a mother and two infants who had lupus erythematosus suggests that neonatal LE with discoid-type lesions may not be a transient disease.

113. Fox RJ Jr., McCuistion HM, Schoch EP Jr: Systemic lupus erythematosus. Association with previous neonatal lupus erythematosus.

A patient previously reported to have discoid LE that regressed by age 5 months developed systemic LE at age 19 years.

114. Chamiedes L, Truex RC, Vetter V, et al.: Association of maternal lupus erythematosus with congenital complete heart block. N. Engl. J. Med. *297*:1204–1207, 1977.

Six infants with complete heart block suggest immune complexes either passing from mother to fetus or produced by the fetus as a response to maternal antigen.

115. Draznin TH, Esterly NB, Furey NL, et al.: Neonatal lupus erythematosus. J. Am. Acad. Dermatol. *1*:437–442, 1979.

Report of an infant and a review of 22 previously reported infants with cutaneous lesions, congenital atrioventricular heart block, or hematologic manifestations of neonatal LE.

116. Meislin AG, Rothfield N: Systemic lupus erythematosus in childhood. Pediatrics *42*:37–49, 1968.

The prognosis for systemic lupus erythematosus in children is decidedly worse than it is in adults.

117. Walvarens PA, Chase P: The prognosis of childhood systemic lupus erythematosus. Am. J. Dis. Child. *130*:929–933, 1976.

A review of 50 patients with childhood systemic lupus erythematosus revealed that 49 had recurrent lupus-related diseases, 40 had been rehospitalized, and renal involvement was a feature of the disorder at some time in all 50 of the patients.

118. Ehrlich GE: Trends in Therapy: Systemic lupus erythematosus. JAMA *232*:1361–1364, 1975.

Treatment of systemic lupus erythematosus depends upon the clinical picture, the stage and severity of the disease, and the existence of intercurrent problems.

119. Urman JD, Rothfield NF: Corticosteroid treatment in systemic lupus erythematosus — survival studies. JAMA *238*:2272–2276, 1977.

Patients with systemic lupus erythematosus reveal markedly improved survival rates with corticosteroid treatment.

120. Tuffanelli DL, LaPierre R: Connective tissue diseases. Pediatr. Clin. of North Am. *18*:925–951, 1971.

A review of connective tissue diseases in childhood.

121. Athreya BH, Norman ME, Myers AR, et al.: Sjögren's syndrome in children. Pediatrics *59*:931–937, 1977.

A report of 2 girls with Sjögren's syndrome with onset at 7 and 12 1/2 years of age and subsequent clinical diagnoses of systemic lupus erythematosus.

122. Sharp GC, Irvin WS, Tan EM, et al.: Mixed connective tissue disease: An apparently distinct rheumatic disease syndrome associated with a specific antibody to extractable nuclear antigen (ENA). Am. J. Med. 52:148–159, 1972.

A description of 25 patients with arthritis or arthralgias, swollen hands, Raynaud's phenomenon, esophageal abnormalities, myositis, hypergammaglobulinemia, leukopenia, and high titers of ENA.

123. Fraga A, Gudino J, Ramos-Niembro F, et al.: Mixed connective tissue disease in childhood. Relationship with Sjögren's syndrome. Am. J. Dis. Child. *132*:263–265, 1978.

Of three children with mixed connective tissue disease (MCTD), two met the criteria for systemic lupus erythematosus, two had polymyositis, and all three had cutaneous, vascular, and esophageal features of scleroderma, juvenile rheumatoid arthritis, and Sjögren's syndrome.

124. Gilliam JN, Prystkowsky SD: Mixed connective tissue disease syndrome. Cutaneous manifestations of patients with epidermal nuclear staining and high titer serum antibody to ribonuclease-sensitive extractable nuclear antigen. Arch. Dermatol. *113*:583–586, 1977.

Ribonucleoprotein antibodies and epidermal nuclear staining provide readily detectable immunologic markers for mixed connective tissue disease.

125. Gilliam JM, Prystkowsky SD: Mixed connective tissue disease. *In* Moschella SL (Ed.): Dermatology Update. Review for Physicians. Elsevier Publishing Company, New York, 1979, 173–193.

An authoritative comprehensive review of mixed connective tissue disease (MCTD).

126. Sharp GC, Anderson DC: Current concepts in the classification of connective tissue disease. Overlapping syndromes and mixed connective tissue disease (MCTD). J. Am. Acad. Dermatol. 2:269–279, 1980.

A review of mixed connective tissue disease with emphasis on clinical features, diagnosis, and management.

127. Sanders DY, Huntley CC, Sharp GC: Mixed connective tissue disease in a child. J. Pediatr. 83:642–645, 1973.

A 9-year-old girl with mixed connective tissue disease.

128. Singsen BH, Bernstein BH, Kornreich HK, et al.: Mixed connective tissue disease in childhood, clinical and serological survey. J. Pediatr. 90:893–900, 1977.

Review of findings in 14 children with mixed connective tissue disease and comparison of serologic findings with those of 127 children with other rheumatic diseases.

129. Kansu E, Deglin S, Cantor RI, et al.: The expanding spectrum of Behçet syndrome — a case with renal involvement. JAMA 237:1855–1856, 1977.

Report of a patient with aphthous stomatitis, genital ulceration, polyarthritis, myocarditis, and severe renal involvement with focal necrotizing glomerulonephritis.

130. Haim S: Behçet's disease: etiology and treatment. Dermatologica *150*:163–168, 1975.

A review of hypotheses of etiology and the management of Behçet's disease.

131. Gorlin RJ, Pindborg JJ, Cohen MM Jr: Behçet's syndrome. *In* Syndromes of the Head and Neck. 2nd ed. McGraw-Hill, Inc., New York, 1976, 48–51.

A review of genito-oral aphthosis and uveitis with hypopyon (Behçet syndrome).

132. Hurwitz S, Braverman IM: White spots in tuberous sclerosis. J. Pediatr. 77:587–594, 1970.

Hypopigmented macules, the earliest sign of tuberous sclerosis, present in 18 of 23 children with this disorder.

133. Hurwitz S: Society Transactions. Discussion on tuberous sclerosis. Arch. Dermatol. *104*:336–337, 1971.

A patient with partial albinism, hypopigmented macules, and tuberous sclerosis, and a discussion of various forms of leukoderma in tuberous sclerosis.

134. Nickel WR, Reed WB: Tuberous sclerosis. Arch. Dermatol. 85:209–216, 1962.

Tuberous sclerosis, a hereditary disease with protean manifestations, reported as being present in every organ and almost every structure of the body.

135. Fitzpatrick TB, Szabó G, Hori Y, et al.: White leaf-shaped macules. Earliest visible sign of tuberous sclerosis. Arch. Dermatol. 98:1–6, 1968.

All patients with seizures, regardless of age, should be examined for white macules, which may be the only visible sign of tuberous sclerosis.

136. McWilliam RP, Stephenson JBP: Depigmented hairs, the earliest sign of tuberous sclerosis. Arch. Dis. Child. 53:961, 1978.

The presence of one or more tufts of white hair in an infant with seizures suggests a diagnosis of tuberous sclerosis.

137. Hoff M, von Grosven MF, Jongeblood WL, et al.: Enamel defects associated with tuberous sclerosis. Oral Surg., Oral Med., Oral Path. 40:261–269, 1975.

Tooth pits — a new sign of tuberous sclerosis?

138. Martin GI, Kaiserman D, Liegler D, et al.: Computer-assisted cranial tomography in early diagnosis of tuberous sclerosis. JAMA 235:2323–2324, 1976.

When diagnosis of tuberous sclerosis cannot be established on clinical findings in a young child, computer-assisted cranial tomographic (CAT scan) can be utilized as an early helpful diagnostic procedure.

139. Callen JP: The skin, the eye, and systemic disease. Cutis 24:501–511, 1979.

A review of systemic disease as manifested on the skin and in the eyes of affected individuals.

140. Butterworth T: Neurocutaneous Syndromes — von Recklinghausen's disease. In Clinical Genodermatology. Williams and Wilkins Co., Baltimore, Md., 1962, 101–105.

A review of neurofibromatosis.

141. Crowe FW, Schull WJ, Neel JV: A Clinical, Pathologic Genetic Study of Multiple Neurofibromatosis. Charles C Thomas, Springfield, Illinois, 1956.

A classic monographic survey of von Recklinghausen's disease.

142. Crowe FW, Schull WJ: Diagnostic importance of the café-au-lait spot in neurofibromatosis. Arch. Int. Med. 91:758–766, 1953.

Six or more café au lait spots greater than 1.5 cm in diameter probably indicate the presence of neurofibromatosis.

143. Whitehouse D: Diagnostic value of the café-au-lait spot in children. Arch. Dis. Child. 41:316–319, 1966.

In children five years of age and under, the criterion for neurofibromatosis is modified to five café au lait spots or more, 0.5 cm or greater in diameter.

144. Crowe FW: Axillary freckling as a diagnostic aid in neurofibromatosis. Ann. Int. Med. 61:1142–1143, 1962.

Twenty per cent of patients with neurofibromatosis display axillary freckling (Crowe's sign).

145. Benedict PH, Szabo G, Fitzpatrick TB, et al.: Melanotic macules in Albright's syndrome and in neurofibromatosis. JAMA 205:618–626, 1968.

Melanocytes in café au lait spots with characteristic giant melanin granules.

146. Jimbo K, Szabo G, Fitzpatrick TB: Ultrastructural giant pigment granules (macromelanosomes) in cutaneous pigmented macules of neurofibromatosis. J. Invest. Dermatol. 61:300–309, 1973.

Giant pigment granules are noted in melanocytes and keratinocytes in the epidermis of patients with neurofibromatosis, not in the café au lait spots of normal individuals.

147. Johnson BL, Charneco DR: Café au lait spots in neurofibromatosis and in normal individuals. Arch. Dermatol. 102:442–446, 1970.

Café au lait spots and axillary freckles of neurofibromatosis show an increase in melanocytes and large melanin granules not seen in normal individuals

148. Albright F: Syndrome characterized by osteitis fibrosa disseminata, areas of pigmentation, and a gonadal dysfunction. Endocrinology 22:411–426, 1938.

Albright syndrome is characterized by dark-brown pigmented lesions with a markedly irregular border (resembling the coast of the state of Maine) in contrast to the smooth outline of café au lait spots.

149. Carney RG: Incontinentia pigmenti: a world statistical analysis. Arch. Dermatol. 112:535–542, 1976.

Analysis of 653 patients (593 females, 16 males) with incontinentia pigmenti (sex not reported in 44 cases)

150. Schamburg-Lever G, Lever WF: Electron microscopy of incontinentia pigmenti. J. Invest. Dermatol. 61:151–158, 1973.

Electron microscopic studies conclude that all three stages of incontinentia pigmenti are related one to another.

151. Wiley HE III, Frias JL: Depigmented lesions in incontinentia pigmenti: a useful sign. Am. J. Dis. Child. 128:546–547, 1974.

Streaked hypopigmented lesions on the calves or other areas of individuals with incontinentia pigmenti.

152. Ito M: Studies on melanin 1. Incontinentia pigmenti achromians: a singular case of nevus depigmentosus systematicus bilateralis. Tohoku J. Exper. Med. 55(Suppl 1):57–59, 1952.

A disorder with systematized depigmented macules.

153. Hamado T, Saito T, et al.: Incontinentia pigmenti (Ito). Arch. Dermatol. 96:673–676, 1967.

A syndrome in which cutaneous markers resemble a negative image of incontinentia pigmenti.

154. Schwartz MF, Esterly NB, Fretzin DF: Hypomelanosis of Ito (incontinentia pigmenti achromians): a neurocutaneous syndrome. J. Pediatr. 90:236–240, 1977.

Ten patients ranging in age from 1 1/2 to 21 years of age with developmental or neurologic abnormalities and hypomelanosis of Ito (a cutaneous sign of possible defects in other organ systems).

155. Rubin NG: Incontinentia pigmenti achromians. Arch. Dermatol. 105:424–425, 1972.

Multiple cases of incontinentia pigmenti achromians in a family suggest an autosomal dominant basis to this disorder.

156. Jelinek JE, Bart RS, Schiff GM: Hypomelanosis of Ito ("Incontinentia Pigmenti Achromians"). Arch. Dermatol. 117:596–601, 1973.

A report of three cases and review of the literature.

157. Gorlin RJ, Sedano HO, Vickers RA, et al.: Multiple mucosal neuromas, pheochromocytoma and medullary carcinoma of the thyroid — a syndrome. Cancer 22:293–299, 1968.

An analysis of seventeen cases of a syndrome of multiple mucosal neuromas, pheochromocytoma, and medullary carcinoma of the thyroid.

158. Sipple JH: Association of pheochromocytoma with carcinoma of the thyroid gland. Am. J. Med. 31:163–166, 1961.

Case report and recognition of the association of pheochromocytoma with medullary carcinoma of the thyroid.

159. Baum JL, Adler ME: Pheochromocytoma, medullary thyroid carcinoma, multiple mucosal neuroma, a variant of the syndrome. Arch. Ophthal. 87:574–584, 1972.

A case report and review of the literature with particular reference to ophthalmologic findings.

160. Hurwitz S: The Sipple syndrome. Society Transactions. Arch. Dermatol. 110:139–140, 1974.

Review of an 18-year-old young man with gastrointestinal symptoms in infancy and neuromas of the tongue at 3 years of age who was diagnosed twelve years later as having medullary carcinoma of the thyroid.

161. Anderson TE, Spackman TJ, Schwartz SS: Roentgen findings in intestinal ganglioneuromatosis: its association with medullary thyroid carcinoma and pheochromocytoma. Radiology 101:93–96, 1971.

Radiographic findings suggest a diagnosis of intestinal ganglioneuromatosis and raise the possibility of associated thyroid and adrenal tumors in the patient in reference 160.

162. Jackson, CE, Tashjian AH Jr, Block MA: Detection of medullary thyroid cancer by calcitonin assay in families. Ann. Int. Med. 78:845–852, 1973.

Calcitonin concentrations in serum as an aid to diagnosis in 76 patients with medullary thyroid carcinoma.

163. Lichtenstein L: Histiocytosis X: An integration of eosinophilic granuloma of bone, Letterer-Siwe disease, and Schüller-Christian disease as related manifestations of a single nosological entity. Arch. Path. 84:102, 1953.

The three disorders are grouped into one entity termed histiocytosis X.

164. Hurwitz S: Histiocytosis in children. Mod. Prob. Paediat. 17:204–210, 1975.

A review of the problem of histiocytosis as seen in childhood.

165. Aronson RP: Streptomycin in Letterer-Siwe disease. Am. J. Dis. Child. 117:236–238, 1969.

The first reported case of recovery of a patient with Letterer-Siwe disease.

166. Esterly NB, Swick HM: Cutaneous Letterer-Siwe disease. Am. J. Dis. Child. 117:236–238, 1969.

A 2 1/2-year-old girl with purely cutaneous manifestations of Letterer-Siwe disease had a striking remission due to vincristine sulfate (Velban) and was subsequently controlled on oral cyclophosphamide (Cytoxan).

167. Freeman S: A benign form of Letterer-Siwe disease. Aust. J. Dermatol. 12:165–171, 1971.

A three-month-old infant with histiocytosis improved (on topical steroids alone) by ten months of age.

168. Bierman HR: Apparent cure of Letterer-Siwe disease. JAMA 196:368–370, 1966.

Seventeen-year survival of identical twins with histologically proven Letterer-Siwe disease.

169. Mishkel MA, Cockshott WP, Nazir DJ, et al.: Xanthoma disseminatum: clinical, metabolic, pathologic and radiologic aspects. Arch. Dermatol. 113:1094–1100, 1977.

Report of a case of xanthoma disseminatum with a review of the clinical, metabolic, and pathologic features.

170. Blank H, Eglick PG, Beerman H: Nevoxanthoendothelioma with ocular involvement. Pediatrics 4:349–354, 1949.

Nevoxanthoendothelioma in the eye of a four-month-old.

171. Doede KG, Rappaport H: Long-term survival of patients with acute differentiated histiocytosis (Letterer-Siwe disease). Cancer 20:1782–1795, 1967.

Lack of pulmonary involvement and absence of thrombocytopenia appear to be of favorable prognostic significance.

172. Starling KA, Donaldson MH, Haggard ME, et al.: Therapy of histiocytosis X with vincristine, vinblastine, and cyclophosphamide — the Southwest Cancer Chemotherapy Study Group. Am. J. Dis. Child. 123:105–110, 1972.

A study of 35 children confirms earlier reports that vincristine, vinblastine, and cyclophosphamide are effective agents in the management of histiocytosis.

173. Lahey ME: Histiocytosis X: Comparison of three treatment regimens. J. Pediatr. 87:179–183, 1975.

Vigorous therapeutic approach appears to offer hope for survival.

174. Lahey ME: Histiocytosis X: Analysis of prognostic factors. J. Pediatr. 87:184–188, 1975.

Hope for long-term remissions, perhaps even cure, with aggressive therapy and good supportive care.

UNCLASSIFIED DISORDERS

Mastocytosis

Mastocytosis is a term used to describe a group of clinical disorders characterized by the accumulation of mast cells in the skin and at times, generally in adults, other organs of the body. It may appear at any time from birth to middle age; approximately three-quarters of all cases develop during infancy or early childhood, and most of the remaining 25 per cent of cases begin at or after puberty (usually between the ages of 15 and 40).[1, 2] The etiology is unknown. Reports of mastocytosis in twins, siblings, and families suggest an inherited basis for this disorder. Further studies of genetic pedigrees, however, are required to clarify the possible role of inheritance in patients with this disorder.[3, 4, 5]

The clinical spectrum of mastocytosis includes: (1) single or multiple small cutaneous nodules (solitary mastocytoma) (Fig. 19–1); (2) a cutaneous form characterized by multiple hyperpigmented macules or papules (urticaria pigmentosa) (Figs. 19–2, 19–3, 19–4); (3) a diffuse form in which virtually all of the skin is infiltrated with mast cells (diffuse cutaneous mastocytosis) (Fig. 19–5); (4) unusual telangiectases of the trunk and extremities usually seen in adults and rarely in children (telangiectasia macularis eruptiva per-

stans); (5) systemic mastocytosis, a condition in which mast cell proliferation occurs in various organ systems (the skin, liver, spleen, lymph nodes, lungs, bones, and gastrointestinal tract); and (6) a rare malignant form of mast cell leukemia seen primarily in adults and rarely in children.

The classification of the forms of mastocytosis,

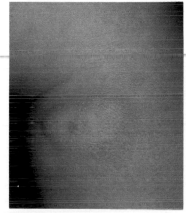

Figure 19–1 Solitary mastocytoma. A 1.5 to 2 cm flesh-colored to reddish-brown nodular aggregation of mast cells on the upper arms of a young infant. Stroking or gentle rubbing of such lesions causes localized erythema and urticarial wheals (Darier's sign) due to mast cell liberation of histamine.

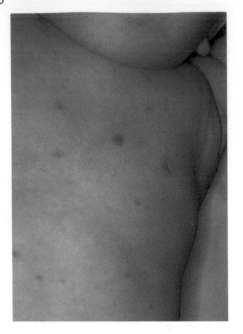

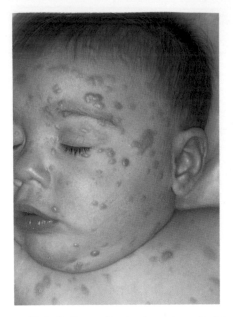

Figure 19-4 Bullous urticaria pigmentosa. Vesicles and bullae are prominent features of this form of mast cell disease.

Figure 19-2 Urticaria pigmentosa. Multiple hyperpigmented macules and nodules on the chest and abdomen of a young infant. Note the positive Darier's sign on the upper aspect of the chest.

often confusing because of their varied manifestations, can be simplified by separation into childhood and adult varieties. In children the disorder appears in three forms: (1) individual lesions (solitary mastocytosis); (2) a generalized form termed urticaria pigmentosa; and (3) a relatively rare variant (diffuse cutaneous mastocytosis). All three of these childhood forms may display vesicular or bullous variants. Seen primarily in children under two years of age, they may be termed bullous mastocytoma (Fig. 19–6), bullous urticaria pigmentosa (Fig. 19–3, 19–4), or bullous mastocytosis (Fig. 19–5). Although the cause of vesiculation in this age group remains unknown, it presumably is related to a histamine-induced transudate in a group susceptible to vesicle formation by insecure

attachments of the epidermis to the underlying dermis.[6]

The prognosis and course of mastocytosis depends on the clinical presentation and its age of onset. In general, children have a better prognosis than adults (in childhood it is almost always a purely cutaneous disease that resolves spontaneously). In adults, however, the skin lesions seldom disappear, and 30 to 55 per cent of patients have evidence of systemic involvement.[1, 2]

The diagnosis of cutaneous mastocytosis is aided by a phenomenon known as Darier's sign. This finding, a hallmark of the disorder, is seen in 90 per cent of patients with cutaneous mastocytosis and consists of localized erythema and urticarial wheals that develop after gentle mechanical irritation, such as might be induced by a tongue blade or the blunt end of a pen or pencil (Fig.

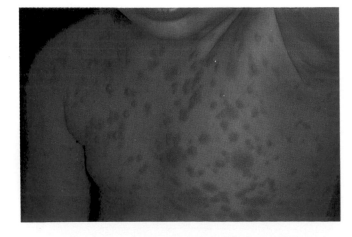

Figure 19-3 Bullous urticaria pigmentosa. Vesicles and bullae are prominent features of this form of mast cell disease.

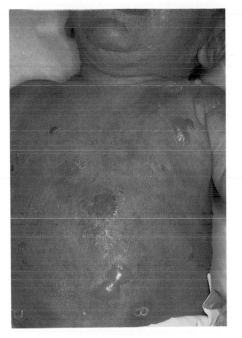

Figure 19–5 Bullous mastocytosis. Diffuse cutaneous erythrodermic mastocytosis with extensive bulla formation.

19–2, 19–6). Erythema and urtication, apparently the result of liberation of histamine by mast cells, usually develop within a few minutes and may persist as long as thirty minutes to several hours.

Solitary Mastocytosis

The terms solitary mastocytosis and solitary mastocytoma are used to designate patients with one or more isolated or individual lesions, a variant estimated to occur in 10 to 15 per cent of all cases of mastocytosis.[7] Lesions usually appear at birth or early in infancy, increase somewhat in size for several months, and eventually regress spontaneously, usually within a period of several years. (Fig. 19–1). In most patients with this form of mastocytosis, lesions are indeed solitary. Many children, however, may develop as many as three or four individual lesions and it has been reported that a few patients with solitary mastocytosis progress to a generalized form of urticaria pigmentosa.[8]

Solitary mastocytomas may occur on any part

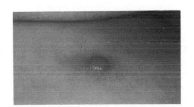

Figure 19–6 Bullous mastocytoma. A blister and Darier's sign (erythema and urtication following gentle rubbing) in a solitary mastocytoma on the chest of a young infant.

of the body but are noted most frequently on the arms (especially near the wrists), the neck, and trunk. Clinically they are seen as slightly elevated flesh-colored to light-brown or tan plaques or nodules. Occasionally they may display a yellowish or pink hue. Lesions are usually round or oval and generally measure 1 to 5 cm in diameter. They may have a thick or rubbery quality with a smooth or pebbly peau d'orange (orange peel-like) consistency. Darier's sign is positive, and stroking or rubbing of lesions may at times produce symptoms of flushing or colic.

Infant skin is more likely to respond to various noxious stimuli by forming blisters. Accordingly, bullous lesions are seen as common variants of this disorder. When present in association with solitary lesions of mastocytosis, this disorder (frequently misdiagnosed as bullous impetigo) is termed bullous mastocytoma (Fig. 19–6). This tendency toward vesiculation and bulla formation usually disappears within a period of one to three years.

Solitary mastocytomas have the most favorable prognosis of all cutaneous forms of mastocytosis. Symptoms, when present, are usually mild, and spontaneous resolution within a period of several years is the rule (almost always before the age of 10). Parents should be advised that symptoms, if present, usually abate after one or two years (even before the lesions disappear) and that surgical excision, except in cases that are symptomatic and troublesome, generally is unnecessary.

Urticaria Pigmentosa

Urticaria pigmentosa, seen in about two-thirds of patients with cutaneous mastocytosis, is the most common manifestation of the mastocytosis syndrome.[1] Primarily a disease of children, the disorder may be present at birth, with the majority of cases originating during the first three to nine months of life. In a study of 139 patients with urticaria pigmentosa, 86 per cent had the onset of their disorder before 15 years of age; the remaining had their onset between ages 15 and 40.[3]

Cutaneous Manifestations. The cutaneous lesions of urticaria pigmentosa generally appear as multiple reddish-brown (occasionally yellowish-brown) hyperpigmented macules, papules, or nodular lesions that urticate in a characteristic manner when traumatized (Darier's sign) (Fig. 19–2). When the normal-appearing skin also urticates it usually does so to a lesser extent. Dermographism of the apparently uninvolved skin has been seen to occur in one-third to one-half of all patients with urticaria pigmentosa. This finding, when present, appears to be due to an increase in mast cells throughout the dermis of otherwise apparently normal skin.[1]

Lesions of urticaria pigmentosa may occur anywhere on the body but generally tend to involve the trunk, often in a symmetrical fashion. In later stages lesions may spread to the extremities and the neck. Involvement of the scalp, face, palms, and soles, although occasionally present, is infrequent and relatively uncommon; a few cases have been reported in which lesions were present on the buccal, palatal, or pharyngeal mucosa, or on the anal mucous membrane.

Individual lesions are usually round or oval, vary in size from one millimeter to several centimeters in diameter, and generally are larger in children than in adults. Pigmentation, particularly in older lesions, is common. The reason for increased pigmentation of lesions is unknown. Increased levels of tyrosinase due to reduction of tyrosine inhibitor by the release of mucopolysaccharides from the mast cells has been suggested as the cause of this phenomenon. This hypothesis, however, remains unsubstantiated and requires further investigation and corroboration.[1]

Vesicles or bullae occasionally occur as prominent features of urticaria pigmentosa of childhood (Figs. 19–3, 19–4). Although the mechanism of vesiculation is unknown, this appears to be related to the release of histamine and the well-known fact that infantile skin blisters more easily than adult skin. When bullae are present in addition to pigmented skin lesions, the disease is termed bullous urticaria pigmentosa.[6]

Telangiectasia macularis eruptiva perstans (TMEP) is a variant generally seen in patients with the adult form of urticaria pigmentosa. This variant, although relatively uncommon in childhood, has been reported in children with this disorder.[1] Patients with TMEP have an extensive eruption of small persistent brownish-red hyperpigmented telangiectatic macules on the trunk and extremities with little or no tendency toward urtication. This relatively uncommon disorder is thought by some to be related to frequent dilatation of blood vessels by repeated release of histamine, and although this concept remains unsubstantiated, it has been suggested that patients with TMEP may have an increased incidence of peptic ulcer.[2]

Prognosis. When seen in children, urticaria pigmentosa has an excellent prognosis and is almost always a cutaneous disorder that tends toward spontaneous remission; in about one-half of the cases in which the disorder has its onset in infancy or early childhood the lesions disappear by adolescence or early adult life.[9, 10] Although systemic involvement has been reported in children with urticaria pigmentosa, a review of childhood cases having widespread and occasionally fatal extracutaneous mast cell infiltrates (liver, spleen, lymph nodes, and bone marrow) found these cases to be diffuse cutaneous or erythrodermic forms of mastocytosis rather than true urticaria pigmentosa.[9] When urticaria pigmentosa has its onset in later childhood, the outlook is somewhat less favorable with regard to disappearance of cutaneous lesions.[9, 10]

Although generalized flushing in urticaria pigmentosa may occur when large amounts of histamine are liberated, the pruritus associated with this disorder is usually rather mild and intermittent in nature. Urticaria and pruritus may be induced by inadvertent or deliberate rubbing of lesions, by exercise, hot baths, spicy foods, cheese, alcohol, or by the ingestion of histamine-releasing drugs such as aspirin, procaine, codeine, morphine, and polymyxin B.

Patients with the onset of urticaria pigmentosa beyond age 10 (in adolescence or adulthood) have a more guarded prognosis. Active lesions tend to persist indefinitely. They typically are reddish-brown, and the majority of patients with associated systemic disease occur in this group (Fig. 19–7). Although it is impossible to accurately estimate what proportion of patients are likely to develop a systemic form of the disease, systemic involvement seems to occur in approximately 10 to 15 per cent (generally adults) of all patients with mastocytosis.[1]

Systemic Involvement. When systemic mastocytosis occurs, almost any organ or tissue of the body may be affected. The most frequently involved organs are the bones, liver, spleen, lymph nodes, and peripheral blood. Mast cell accumulations, however, have also been found in the lung, kidney, gastrointestinal tract, skeletal muscle, myocardium, pericardium, omentum, and other tissues. Hepatomegaly, present in 10 to 15 per cent of patients, and splenomegaly (usually seen in association with hepatic enlargement) seem to occur in an equal percentage of patients. Although an incidence as high as 30 per cent had been reported for bone involvement (either localized or diffuse areas of osteoporosis or osteosclerosis) in patients with systemic disease, 10 or 15 per cent appears to be a more realistic figure for this association.[1, 3]

Since systemic involvement occurs in 10 to 30 per cent of patients with urticaria pigmentosa whose skin lesions appear after the age of 10,

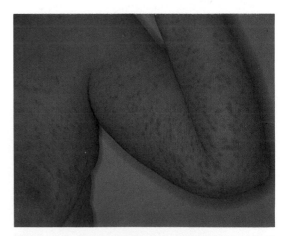

Figure 19–7   Adult-type urticaria pigmentosa. Generalized reddish-brown freckle-like lesions are characteristic of the adult form of urticaria pigmentosa. Cutaneous lesions tend to persist indefinitely and 30 to 55 per cent of adult patients with urticaria pigmentosa have some evidence of systemic involvement.

particularly careful evaluation should be made for all patients with late-onset or adult forms of this disorder.[10] The measurement of urinary histamine excretion may be of indirect help in the diagnosis of systemic mastocytosis.[2] Further experience, however, is required to substantiate the value of this laboratory study. Symptoms of the mastocytosis syndrome may include intense pruritus, headache, flushing, tachycardia, gastrointestinal symptoms, non-specific abnormalities of blood clotting, hypotension, and syncope. Patients with bone involvement may have bone pain. Hemorrhagic diatheses, although rare, may be related to hepatosplenic involvement or to the infrequent association of mastocytosis with mast cell leukemia or lymphoma.

The development of leukemia or a related malignant condition affecting tissues of the reticuloendothelial system is the main hazard in adult patients with mastocytosis. The presence of mast cells in the peripheral blood of patients with mastocytosis accordingly is a grave prognostic sign. A 5-year-old child with urticaria pigmentosa and acute lymphoblastic leukemia was reported on by Fromer and associates in 1973. Although perhaps coincidental, this report raises the question as to whether or not this association may have been more than a chance occurrence.[11]

Diffuse Cutaneous and Erythrodermic Mastocytosis

Diffuse cutaneous mastocytosis is a relatively rare form of childhood mastocytosis that bears little clinical resemblance to urticaria pigmentosa. In this disorder large areas of the dermis are infiltrated with mast cells, and the skin develops a thickened boggy, doughy, and at times lichenified appearance. The cutaneous surface may be smooth, or it may contain numerous minute papules that give it a scotch-grained leather-like appearance, frequently with a yellow carotenemia-like tint or a diffusely reddened appearance (diffuse erythrodermic mastocytosis) (Fig. 19–3). In some cases diffuse cutaneous mastocytosis may be accompanied by extensive bullous eruptions. In this variant, termed bullous mastocytosis (Fig. 19–5), the prognosis seems to be related to the age of onset of bullous lesions. When bullae develop early in the neonatal period, the prognosis is more guarded and systemic involvement frequently occurs. With delayed onset of blisters, however, extracutaneous manifestations appear to bear less significance and the prognosis is more favorable.[6]

The diffuse cutaneous forms of mastocytosis may present symptoms of intense generalized pruritus, flushing, temperature elevation, vomiting, diarrhea, abdominal pain, and acute respiratory distress, with wheezing, cyanosis, apnea, and, at times, severe shock-like states. In a review of eight infants with this variant, two died; five of the remaining six had mast cell infiltration of the reticuloendothelial system; and one had gastrointestinal involvement, an increased number of mast cells in the bone marrow, and mast cells in the peripheral blood.[12]

DIAGNOSIS. Typical cases of cutaneous mastocytosis generally present little diagnostic problem to the physician familiar with this disorder. Urtication following the mechanical irritation of lesions (Darier's sign) is highly diagnostic and frequently will help to confirm the true nature of the disease. Atypical and more unusual forms of cutaneous mastocytosis, however, are more difficult to diagnose and require a high index of suspicion on the part of the clinician.

When the diagnosis is indeterminate, cutaneous biopsy can help confirm the true nature of the disorder. Since loss of granules may occur owing to handling of lesions during biopsy, the injection of local anesthetic too close to lesions or biopsy of a lesion that had previously been urticated tends to make histopathologic identification of mast cells difficult. Specimens accordingly should be handled gently and removed whenever possible without previous urtication, and avoidance of local anesthetic infiltration into the area of the biopsy site may be necessary in order to establish the proper histopathologic diagnosis.

All forms of mastocytosis are characterized by abnormal accumulation of mast cells. In the macular and papular type of lesions, there generally is a sparse mast cell infiltrate in the upper dermis, usually with a perivascular and periappendageal distribution. A relative scarcity of mast cells in some sections may make histologic confirmation difficult, and at times the true nature of the disorder may be established only after repeated biopsies have been performed.

Cutaneous biopsies of juvenile forms of urticaria pigmentosa are characterized by dense aggregates of mast cells in the subpapillary layers and midcutis. The cells may have a peculiar arrangement, being packed into tumor-like clumps or arranged in strands or columns of varying width. The dense packing of mast cells may cause them to appear cuboidal, polyhedric, or flattened, thus resembling fibroblasts with spindle-shaped nuclei. Nodular lesions and isolated mastocytomas tend to have massive mast cell infiltrates throughout the entire corium, and the skin of patients with diffuse cutaneous mastocytosis has a band-like infiltrate of mast cells close to the epidermis. Mast cells are characterized by the presence of metachromatic granules in their cytoplasm. Although these granules frequently are not visible on routine stains, they generally can be visualized after staining with Giemsa, azure A, methylene-blue or toluidine-blue stains (Fig. 19–8).

TREATMENT. There is no satisfactory treatment for mastocytosis. Children with diffuse cutaneous mastocytosis and those with onset after the age of 5 years should be closely observed and screened for possible involvement of other organs. Proper screening in such cases includes

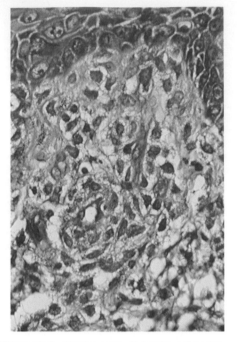

Figure 19–8 Mastocytosis. Cuboidal, polyhedric, or flattened mast cells are characterized by metachromatic granules in their cytoplasm (frequently not visible on routine stains, the metachromatic granules generally can be visualized after special staining).

frequent examination of blood smears, thrombocyte, bleeding, and coagulation time studies, and, if indicated by history, gastrointestinal survey and bone scans. Patients with all forms of this disorder should avoid aspirin, codeine, opiates, procaine, alcohol, polymyxin B, hot baths, and vigorous rubbing after showering or bathing in an effort to minimize the release of histamine. Hydroxyzine (Atarax or Vistaril) or various antihistamines may be helpful in the relief of pruritus and may modify flushing or other symptoms associated with the mastocytosis syndrome. Cyproheptadine (Periactin) has the advantage of both antihistamine and antiserotonin activity. Accordingly it is advocated by some as the drug of choice for the management of symptoms associated with this disorder. Inhibition of the enzyme histidine decarboxylase thus far has been ineffective for the relief of symptoms of mast cell disease. Although studies are incomplete, oral cromolyn sodium (disodium cromoglycate) has been helpful in infants with gastrointestinal involvement and in adults with systemic involvement.[13]

Morphea

Morphea (also termed localized or circumscribed scleroderma) is a disorder of unknown etiology manifested by localized atrophy, hardening (sclerosis), and depigmentation of the skin. Seen primarily in children and young adults, with a 3:1 female-to-male ratio, the average age of onset is about five years. The condition is characterized by discrete circumscribed non-tender sclerotic patches with an ivory-colored center and a surrounding violaceous halo. The relationship between morphea and systemic scleroderma (progressive systemic sclerosis) is controversial and not well understood. If a transition from morphea to scleroderma does occur, it is, at best, extremely rare.[14, 15, 16]

CLINICAL MANIFESTATIONS. The onset of morphea is insidious and begins with flesh-colored, erythematous, or purplish plaques that evolve into firm waxy, ivory to yellow-white shiny lesions, with or without a surrounding lilac or violaceous inflammatory zone (Fig. 19–9). Affected areas, in order of decreasing frequency, are the thorax, trunk, neck, extremities, and face.

The disorder can be divided into four basic patterns, which may be termed guttate, plaque, generalized, and linear. Guttate morphea is a relatively uncommon variant. In the guttate form lesions are chalk-white and oval, measure only a few millimeters in diameter, and are distributed on the anterior chest, shoulders, neck, and other areas of the body. Considerable confusion frequently exists between guttate morphea and lichen sclerosus et atrophicus, and patients have been seen in which typical lesions of both disorders occur.

Plaque-like lesions occur as indurated areas of skin, which at first are purplish in color. After a period of weeks to months they lose their color, especially in the central part of the lesions, and appear as sclerotic ivory-colored waxy areas with a lilac or violaceous edge. In this form, lesions vary from a few centimeters to several inches in diameter and, at times, fusion of many plaque-like lesions may result in a more generalized form of morphea.

Linear lesions of morphea occur primarily in children. Generally affecting the limbs (occasionally the head or trunk), their clinical appearance is similar to that of plaque-like forms, but the violaceous peripheral ring is inconspicuous

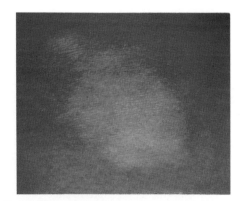

Figure 19–9 Morphea. A circumscribed ivory to yellow-white atrophic plaque surrounded by a violaceous or lilac-colored inflammatory border.

or only present at the advancing border. Lesions frequently present as linear areas of induration or may extend to involve the subcutaneous fat, fascia, and periosteum, and, with deep involvement and fixation to underlying structures, may result in facial deformity or contracture of a limb.

Coup de sabre is a form that appears specifically on the face and frontoparietal scalp. In this variant a linear depressed groove, often with an associated zone of alopecia, resembles a saber wound or cut on the frontoparietal scalp. The groove may extend downwards into the cheek, nose, and upper lip, and, at times, may involve the mouth, gum, chin, or neck. The coup de sabre variety probably represents a mild form of progressive facial hemiatrophy (the Parry-Romberg syndrome), a condition of slowly progressive atrophy of the soft tissue of the corresponding half of the face, accompanied most often by contralateral Jacksonian epilepsy, trigeminal neuralgia, alopecia, enophthalmos, and atrophy of the ipsilateral half of the upper lip, gum, and tongue.

Occasionally, roughening of one surface of the long bones underlying a linear area of morphea may be noted. This disorder, termed melorheostosis, is characterized roentgenographically by a picture suggesting that of wax flowing down the side of a candle.[17]

Localized morphea may at times resemble vitiligo, other forms of macular atrophy, or lesions of lichen sclerosus et atrophicus. The histopathologic features of morphea consist of increased thickening and condensation of the connective tissue, with edema, homogenization, fibrosis, and sclerosis of collagen. Blood vessels are reduced in size and are surrounded by round cell infiltration. As the disorder progresses, hair and glandular stuctures become atrophic, and the dermis is converted into a dense mass of connective tissue containing many dilated lymphatic spaces and but few blood vessels.

In cases of linear scleroderma there may be sclerosis of fat and fascia, calcinosis may be present, and the underlying muscle may show an interstitial myositis. Although the histologic picture of morphea frequently may resemble that of scleroderma, lesions of systemic scleroderma show more pronounced degenerative changes in the collagen bundles and vessel walls in the later stages, the epidermis may show epidermal atrophy with a disappearance of rete ridges in areas of involvement, and the marked inflammatory changes seen in the active border of plaques of morphea do not occur in active lesions of systemic scleroderma.

TREATMENT. Although the treatment of morphea remains unsatisfactory, spontaneous recovery, particularly in children, is common. Guttate and plaque-like lesions of morphea generally tend to improve within a period of three to five years. Residual hypopigmentation, hyperpigmentation, and occasionally atrophy, however, may persist for long periods of time. Lesions of linear morphea tend to last longer, but they too have a tendency to improve over a period of years. Linear lesions of the coup de sabre variant and facial hemiatrophy, conversely, generally tend to persist. Occasionally, calcinosis requiring surgical removal may develop in linear lesions, contractures may limit movement of joints, and at times, clawing of the hand may be a sequela of this variant of localized scleroderma.

Topical or intralesional corticosteroid therapy has been said to hasten resolution of lesions, but this form of therapy is generally unrewarding, can result in localized atrophy, and is not recommended. Physiotherapy, massage, warm baths, and exercise, however, frequently are helpful for patients with linear morphea, in whom strictures may otherwise result. D-penicillamine has been recommended as a method of treatment for patients with this disorder.[18] Side effects (urticaria, eczema, depression of leukocytes, and chronic nephritis), however, preclude recommendation of this mode of therapy.

Eosinophilic Fasciitis

Eosinophilic fasciitis, also termed diffuse fasciitis with eosinophilia, is a recently described scleroderma-like disease characterized by diffuse infiltration of the skin of the extremities and trunk without visceral involvement or Raynaud's phenomenon.[19] Seen in children as well as adults, the disorder bears a close resemblance to scleroderma and is thought by many authorities to be a variant of morphea or progressive systemic sclerosis (scleroderma).

First described by Schulman in 1974, the disorder is characterized by a sudden onset following strenuous physical activity; painful swelling and induration of the skin of the extremities, which is tightly bound to the underlying structures; scleroderma-like skin changes, with a stippled appearance on the extremities without significant color change of the skin; marked thickening of the subcutaneous fascia; absence of systemic changes; transient peripheral eosinophilia early in the disease; and a good response to systemic corticosteroids.[20, 21, 22] Since the pathologic findings appear to be restricted to the deep fascia between the subcutaneous tissue and muscle, Schulman suggested the term "diffuse fasciitis" for this apparently new disease or syndrome.[20] Rodnan and his associates, noting the presence of eosinophils in the involved fascia, suggested the term eosinophilic fasciitis for this disorder.[23]

Primarily affecting the skin of the arms and legs, and occasionally that of the trunk, hands, and feet, the cutaneous features consist of a cobblestone or puckered appearance with a yellowish erythematous color. Although atrophy of the skin and peripheral violaceous rings are not noted in lesions of eosinophilic fasciitis, it is highly probable that some cases previously reported as generalized morphea actually represented cases of this disorder.

Eosinophilia and hypergammaglobulinemia in the form of elevated IgG are commonly observed laboratory findings, but antinuclear antibody reactions remain negative. Blood eosinophilia, often the first clue to the condition, is a transient but striking feature. Histopathologic findings consist of infiltrates of lymphocytes, plasma cells, histiocytes, and intravascular or perivascular eosinophils in the trabeculae of the subcutaneous tissue. Although eosinophilic fasciitis frequently resolves spontaneously, systemic corticosteroids seem to hasten resolution.

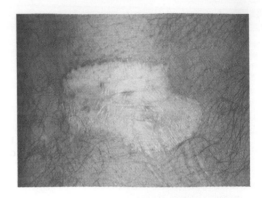

Figure 19–10   Lichen sclerosis et atrophicus. White to yellowish macules may coalesce to form well-demarcated atrophic plaques. Central depression (delling), when present, is highly diagnostic of this disorder.

Lichen Sclerosus et Atrophicus

Lichen sclerosus et atrophicus (LSA) is a distinctive benign cutaneous disorder of unknown etiology. Seen in children as well as adults, the disorder may occur at any age, in any race, and in both sexes.[24-28] The youngest case reported was that of an infant only a few weeks of age; 85 to 90 per cent of cases appear in females; 10 to 15 per cent of affected individuals have the onset of their disorder before the age of 13; and the majority of cases in childhood (70 per cent) had the onset of the disorder prior to seven years of age.[24, 25]

CLINICAL MANIFESTATIONS.   The eruption of lichen sclerosus et atrophicus is characterized by sharply defined small pink to ivory-white, slightly raised, flat-topped papules a few millimeters in diameter that aggregate and coalesce into plaques of various sizes. As the condition progresses, atrophy and delling (fine follicular plugs on the surface of macules) may become highly diagnostic features of the disorder. The anogenital region is involved in the majority of cases (75 per cent of affected children have anogenital involvement). Of those that have involvement elsewhere on the body, 42 per cent have an associated anogenital involvement.[24, 25] Extragenital lesions are asymptomatic and may begin asymmetrically but eventually generally become distributed in a symmetrical manner over the clavicles, on the chest and back, around the umbilicus, and on the flexor surfaces of the extremities, neck, and axillae (Fig. 19–10).

The Koebner phenomenon has been documented in cases of lichen sclerosus et atrophicus in childhood; lesions may develop in surgical scars or sites of vaccination, and exacerbations of quiescent lesions may occur following local trauma or irritation.[24, 26, 27] As previously stated in the discussion of localized or circumscribed scleroderma, lesions of lichen sclerosus et atrophicus occasionally occur in association with morphea, and it has been suggested that guttate morphea actually may represent a variant of LSA.

In females the anogenital lesions tend to surround both the vulva and perianal regions in an hour-glass or figure-eight pattern. When seen on the dorsum of the glans penis in males, the disorder has been termed balanitis xerotica obliterans. A vaginal discharge may precede the vulval lesions in about 20 per cent of affected female children, and pruritus vulvae appears in about 50 per cent of girls affected with this disorder. Anogenital lesions frequently extend to include the skin on the inner aspect of the thighs; in many individuals the white coloring may be replaced by reddening and blistering, and tiny hemorrhages and excoriations may be present, especially on the labia minora and clitoris.

Except for anogenital lesions in which the cutaneous features may be complicated by excoriation, maceration, infection, or contact dermatitis due to topical therapy, the diagnosis of lichen sclerosus et atrophicus is usually not difficult. Differential diagnosis should include the possibility of vitiligo, morphea, lichen planus, and, in anogenital lesions, dermatitis such as might be seen in association with pinworm infestation, moniliasis, or bacterial vulvovaginitis.

The microscopic features of lichen sclerosus et atrophicus consist of marked hyperkeratosis with plugging of the hair follicles, thinning of the stratum malpighii (sometimes with loss of rete ridges), hydropic degeneration of the basal layer, marked edema with homogenization of the collagen in the upper dermis, and a band-like, predominantly lymphocytic infiltrate in the mid-dermis.[26]

PROGNOSIS.   The prognosis of lichen sclerosus et atrophicus with onset in childhood is somewhat better than that of adult forms of this disorder. Involution in adults is uncommon and is usually accompanied by residual atrophy, and there is a distinct relationship between adult lichen sclerosus et atrophicus, leukoplakia, and squamous cell carcinoma. The possibility of malignancy as a sequela of lichen sclerosus et atrophicus in childhood, however, is extremely rare.[26, 27, 28]

In half of the childhood cases, most lesions of LSA clear within a period of one to ten years (with an average of five years), and approximately two-thirds of cases improve or undergo involution before or at about the time of puberty, without atrophy.[24, 25] In the remaining one-third, the condition tends to persist and, in females, atrophy of the clitoris and labia minora, with fusion of the latter and stricture of the introitus may occur.[25] In patients in whom improvement has taken place, however, the disorder may be reactivated years later by trauma, pregnancy, or the administration of anovulatory drugs.[29, 30]

TREATMENT. The course of sclerosus et atrophicus is not influenced by therapy. Topical corticosteroids (hydrocortisone) and emollient creams offer symptomatic relief to the vulva and perianal lesions. If secondary infection is present, local antimonilial and antibacterial agents may be added. Although the malignant potential of lichen sclerosus et atrophicus of the vulva in childhood is small, the incidence of squamous cell carcinoma in adult cases has been estimated as 4.4 per cent.[30] Cases persisting beyond puberty, or having adult onset after puberty, accordingly should be observed at intervals of six to twelve months for the possibility of leukoplakia or carcinoma. If carcinoma is suspected, cutaneous biopsy is recommended in adults; and newly arising nodules, erosions, or ulcers in lesions of LSA that persist for more than a few weeks require histologic examination.

Scleredema

Scleredema (also termed scleredema adultorum of Buschke) is a rare condition of unknown etiology characterized by a diffuse brawny induration of large areas of the skin. Since at least 50 per cent of cases occur in childhood, the term "adultorum" is a misnomer. Appearing twice as frequently in females as in males, 22 per cent of cases begin between 10 and 20 years of age and an additional 29 per cent of cases appear before the age of 10.[31]

Although scleredema may begin spontaneously, 65 to 95 per cent of patients have the onset of their disorder within a few days to six weeks following an acute febrile illness. Of these, 58 per cent of the infections are streptococcal in nature, and recent studies suggest an association with severe long-standing diabetes mellitus.[31-34] Whether the disorder represents a toxic disturbance in ground substance resulting from bacterial toxins, an autoimmune process, or a manifestation of allergic sensitization remains obscure.

The onset of scleredema generally is sudden, and the disorder usually begins on the posterior aspect of the neck and shoulders, with gradual extension to the face, anterior aspect of the neck, scalp, chest, upper back, and arms. The abdomen, genitalia, buttocks, thighs, legs, hands, and feet are less frequently involved. Although the disorder is usually restricted to the skin, involvement of the tongue, pharynx, and esophagus may result in dysarthria and dysphagia. Ocular manifestations consist of induration of the eyelid and conjunctiva and trophic corneal changes. There may be pleural, pericardial, or peritoneal effusion, and as a result of induration of the skin overlying the joints, there may be restriction of motion in association with hydroarthrosis.

The diagnosis of scleredema is usually suggested by the sudden onset of symmetrical cutaneous induration, particularly if there is a preceding history of infection or long-term diabetes and obesity. Although the histologic changes are nondiagnostic, the clinical diagnosis may be supported by a mild inflammatory infiltrate and separation of the collagen bundles (particularly those in the lower two-thirds of the dermis) by empty spaces created by the swelling and splitting of collagen bundles. The demonstration of greatly increased amounts of mucopolysaccharide may be done more easily when a special fixative such as cetylpyridinium chloride is used.

The disease usually reaches its maximum development within a period of two to six weeks; in most cases, the prognosis is good, wtih spontaneous resolution usually occurring within a period of six months to two years. About one-fourth of patients, however, may exhibit only partial improvement, with persistent areas of residual induration.[35] In patients in whom the disorder is associated with obesity and diabetes, the cutaneous induration may persist for many years, and on rare occasions patients have manifestations of their disorder for periods lasting as long as 20 to 40 years.

There is no effective treatment of scleredema. Owing to the high incidence of streptococcal infection (particularly in children) bacterial cultures are recommended, and appropriate antibiotics should be initiated when indicated. Other suggested forms of therapy include warm baths, massage, systemic corticosteroids, thyroid and pituitary extracts, and the subcutaneous injection of hyaluronidase and fibrinolysin. None of these, however, has proved beneficial in the management of this disorder.

Macular Atrophy

Macular atrophy, frequently termed macular anetoderma (from Greek, meaning "relaxed skin"), is a term used to describe an idiopathic atrophy of the skin characterized by oval lesions of thin, soft, loosely wrinkled, depigmented outpouchings of skin, which result from weakening of the connective tissue of the dermis. The disorder may be classified as primary macular anetoderma, which arises from apparently normal skin, or as secondary macular anetoderma, which follows previous inflammatory and infiltrative dermatoses such as secondary syphilis, sarcoidosis, leprosy, lupus erythematosus, tuberculosis, urticarial lesions, purpura, lichen planus, and acne-vulgaris.[36] A peculiar laxity of the eyelid (blepharosclerosis) may also follow chronic or recurrent dermatitis of the eyelids. When eyelid changes are seen in association with progressive enlargement of the lip due to inflammation of the labial salivary glands, the disorder is termed Ascher's syndrome.

Based on whether or not an inflammatory reaction occurred before the appearance of the atrophy, two types of primary macular anetoderma have been described: anetoderma of Jadassohn, in which the atrophic lesions are preceded by inflammation, and anetoderma of Schweninger-Buzzi, in which there is no evidence of inflammation.

Anetoderma of Jadassohn. This type is characterized by crops of round or oval pink macules 0.5 to 1 cm in diameter that develop on the trunk, shoulders, upper arms, thighs, sacral area, and occasionally face or scalp (Fig. 19–11). Usually seen in women in the second to fourth decades of life, occasionally in children, the anetoderma begins with a sharply defined red spot, which grows peripherally and becomes round or oval and slightly depressed. As the redness disappears the atrophic stage begins. The lesion then becomes distinctly white and shiny, develops an atrophic hernia-like outpouching, and assumes a livid red or yellowish color. The lesions then develop a characteristic atrophic, wrinkled, and pale herniation, which yields on pressure, admitting the finger through the surrounding ring of normal skin. Much like an umbilical hernia, the bulge reappears when the finger is released and at times, fatty tissue may infiltrate the lesions, giving them a more firm, soft tumor-like appearance.[37]

Anetoderma of Schweninger-Buzzi. This type is manifested by the sudden appearance of large numbers of bluish-white macules, some of which are protuberant, without any preceding inflammatory eruption. Women are affected more commonly than men. Lesions are generally seen on the trunk, neck, face, shoulders, extremities, and back and range in size from 10 to 20 mm in diameter. Seen during childhood or adult life, the disease is slowly progressive and new lesions appear one by one or in groups, a few at a time, over a period of years. The essential difference in this form of anetoderma is a lack of inflammation and the relative absence of coalescence of lesions.

In all forms of macular anetoderma the primary histopathologic feature is the destruction and loss of elastic fibers. In the Jadassohn type, early lesions show a perivascular infiltrate consisting of polymorphonuclear leukocytes, eosinophils, and "nuclear dust" (a histologic picture of vasculitis). In the later atrophic stage of the Jadassohn form and in the Schweninger-Buzzi type, little or no inflammatory infiltration is present, elastic fibers are absent, and the collagen bundles appear more or less swollen and homogenized. In all forms of macular anetoderma, fragmentation, contractions, and loss of elastic tissue is highly characteristic. This change is a constant and diagnostic feature, and unless sections are stained for elastic tissue, the diagnosis frequently can be overlooked.

There is no known etiology for this group of disorders, and except perhaps for surgical excision of cosmetically objectional lesions, no form of therapy appears to be effective.

Atrophoderma

Atrophoderma (of Pasini and Pierini) is a relatively uncommon atrophic disorder of the skin. Of unknown etiology, it is seen more commonly in females, may appear at any age (including infancy), and usually begins on the trunk during the late teens or early twenties. A chronic condition that tends to persist indefinitely, this disorder is characterized by asymptomatic bluish-brown to violaceous, oval, round, or irregular, smooth well-circumscribed patches with a depressed center and a "cliff-drop" border.

The atrophy begins as an asymptomatic, slightly erythematous macular lesion on the trunk (particularly the back). Initially there may be a singular lesion, but more often there are multiple lesions, varying from 1 to 12 cm in diameter. Within a week or two the lesions develop a slate-gray to brown pigmentation. The atrophic patches extend very slowly, increase in number for 10 years or more, and then generally persist without apparent change. During this period new lesions may occur and old ones slowly enlarge. At times lesions are indistinguishable from those of morphea. Indeed, typical lesions of morphea and atrophoderma may occur in different areas in the same patient, and although opinions differ, it has been suggested that this disorder may represent an atrophic variant of morphea.[38, 39] Against this hypothesis is the fact that lesions of atrophoderma lack induration and sclerosis and the lilac ring characteristic of morphea.

Because histologic changes are often minimal, cutaneous biopsy should include an area of surrounding normal skin for comparison. The histo-

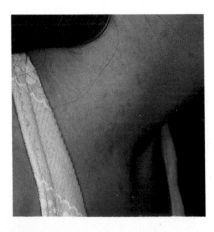

Figure 19–11 Macular anetoderma of the Jadassohn type. White shiny oval or round atrophic herniations that yield to gentle pressure (atrophic herniation or outpouching reappears when the pressure is released).

pathologic features of early lesions consist of mild homogenization of the collagen bundles and a scattered lymphocytic infiltrate. Melanin is increased in the basal layer, and there may be thinning of the connective tissue, with a slight perivascular infiltration in the upper dermis. Older lesions demonstrate slight atrophy of the epidermis, a decrease in the size of the dermal papillae, flattening of the rete pegs, and, in the deeper dermal layers, thickening of the collagen bundles with an increase in their eosinophilia.[38]

The course of atrophoderma is benign, and there is no known effective treatment. The disorder remains active for a period of months to years and lesions persist indefinitely, but there are no reports of systemic involvement or complications.

Acanthosis Nigricans

Acanthosis nigricans is a cutaneous disorder characterized by light-brown-to-black verrucous or papillomatous hypertrophic lesions, which may occur on any part of the body but characteristically appear on the nape and sides of the neck, in the axillae, and in the groin. In addition to the characteristic areas there may be verrucous hyperkeratosis of the knuckles, genitalia, perineum, face, thighs, breasts, and flexural regions of the elbows and knees.

Acanthosis nigricans may begin during childhood, at puberty, or during later adult life. Hyperpigmentation, the first cutaneous change, is followed by an increase in skin markings and varying degrees of localized hypertrophy of the epidermis in the affected areas. The disorder probably represents a reaction of the skin to different stimuli. In some patients it appears before, after, or concomitantly with the onset of an endocrine disorder or internal malignancy.

Some individuals have a familial tendency to this disorder, and, in obese individuals, an undiscovered endocrinopathy may be responsible for the characteristic cutaneous changes. Acanthosis nigricans also has been reported in association with excessive doses of niacin, corticosteroids, and diethylstilbestrol. The suggestion that acanthosis nigricans is caused by release of a pituitary or ectopically produced peptide hormone is consistent with clinical observations of individuals with this disorder.[40]

Four types of this disorder currently are recognized: acanthosis nigricans associated with malignancy, benign acanthosis nigricans, pseudoacanthosis nigricans, and "syndromal" acanthosis nigricans.[41]

Acanthosis Nigricans Associated with Malignancy. In middle-aged and older adults, acanthosis nigricans is frequently associated with adenocarcinoma, generally of the stomach (but it may appear elsewhere in the gastrointestinal tract, the lung, breast, gallbladder, pancreas, testes, uterus, ovaries), and, in rare instances, with lymphoma or squamous cell carcinoma. Most cases of acanthosis

nigricans associated with malignancy begin after puberty or in adulthood. A few cases, however, have been observed in childhood.[42] Because of the high association of malignancy in middle-aged and older adults, patients who develop acanthosis nigricans after 30 years of age without evidence of endocrine disease or obesity should be investigated for possible malignancy, particularly adenocarcinoma of an abdominal or thoracic organ. If obesity or endocrinopathy are excluded, patients who manifest acanthosis in childhood should also be investigated for this possibility.[41]

Benign Acanthosis Nigricans. True benign acanthosis nigricans is a rare genetic dermatosis that greatly resembles ichthyosis hystrix and follows an irregular autosomal dominance. It can be present at birth or may develop in childhood or, more commonly, at puberty.[43] This disorder is not associated with obesity, endocrine disease, or internal malignancy. In cases that begin before puberty, it frequently becomes intensified at that time, possibly as the result of hormonal stimulation. After this increase in intensity, the dermatosis frequently becomes stationary or may tend to subside.

Pseudoacanthosis Nigricans. Pseudoacanthosis nigricans is also benign in the sense that it is not associated with malignant tumor. It is, however, regularly associated with obesity, which may have a nutritional, constitutional, or endocrine basis. The dependence of this dermatosis on obesity is suggested because the cutaneous changes start at the time pronounced obesity develops and frequently improve when the patient returns to normal weight.[44] It also may, at times, be reversible as in endocrine disorders such as Stein-Leventhal and Cushing's syndromes when the primary cause of the disorder has been corrected.

"Syndromal" Acanthosis Nigricans. A recently recognized "syndromal" acanthosis nigricans occasionally may appear as a feature of several specific syndromes. Included among these are Bloom's syndrome (in which acanthosis nigricans may appear in the axillae during childhood or puberty), Crouzon's syndrome (craniofacial dysostosis), Seip's syndrome (lipodystrophy, muscular hypertrophy, and accelerated osseous maturation), insulin-resistant diabetes, lupoid nephritis, and Rud's syndrome (ichthyosis, hypogonadism, mental deficiency, epilepsy, and infantilism).

Epidermal and pigmented nevi, erythrasma, and endocrine disorders with hyperpigmentation (Addison's disease) may at times simulate acanthosis nigricans. The histologic features of acanthosis nigricans include marked acanthosis, hyperkeratosis, papillomatosis, and an increase in pigment cells in the basal layer and upper dermis where melanophores containing pigment are found.

TREATMENT. Treatment of acanthosis nigricans depends primarily upon careful exclusion of endocrine disease or internal malignancy as a cause of this disorder. When acanthosis nigricans develops in teenagers and young adults, with or without obesity, it is necessary to determine whether or not the patient has endocrine disease. In children, acanthosis nigricans generally is not considered to be a manifestation of internal malignancy. Between the ages of 12 and 30 the most common abnormalities associated with this disorder are obesity or Cushing's syndrome; in patients over 30, obesity and malignancy are most commonly seen. Relative to the cosmetic appearance of the cutaneous lesions, correction of known precipitating factors (obesity, endocrinologic disease, and internal malignancy) is necessary, and topical retinoic acid (tretinoin, Retin-A), 10 to 20 per cent urea, 3 to 6 per cent lactic acid, or 3 to 5 per cent salicylic acid in an emollient cream may provide some degree of palliative relief.

Porokeratosis

Porokeratosis is an uncommon chronic progressive disorder of keratinization and may appear in several forms: (1) classic porokeratosis of Mibelli, an autosomal dominant disorder generally seen in children or young adults; (2) a disorder that appears on sun-exposed surfaces (disseminated superficial actinic porokeratosis), generally seen in adults during the third or fourth decades of life; and (3) a superficial form that begins on the palms and soles and subsequently involves other areas of the body.

Porokeratosis of Mibelli. Porokeratosis of Mibelli may appear as one, a few, or many lesions that persist indefinitely (Fig. 19–12). Linear and zosteriform types resembling linear epidermal nevi have also been described. A hypothesis that the linear form of porokeratosis is the result of a Koebner response in a genetically predisposed individual has been proposed but requires verification.[45]

The skin lesions of porokeratosis of Mibelli may appear at any age, but usually first appear during childhood. Affecting males two or three times more frequently than females, the disorder has a predilection for the face, neck, forearms, and hands. The initial lesion begins as a crateriform hyperkeratotic papule that gradually eventuates in an atrophic plaque of circinate or irregular contour measuring anywhere from a few millimeters to several centimeters in diameter. The diagnostic feature of this disorder is the raised hyperkeratotic peripheral ridge surmounted by a furrow. This pathognomonic finding is often referred to as the "great wall of China."[46]

Porokeratosis of Chernosky. The second form of porokeratosis, disseminated superficial actinic porokeratosis (DSAP, porokeratosis of Chernosky) usually appears during the third or fourth decade of life. Occasionally seen in adolescents 16 years of age or older, the disorder appears on sun-exposed areas of the skin. Lesions are usually multiple, with most patients having over 50 lesions; are primarily limited to the extremities, and measure 0.1 to 4.5 cm in diameter, with most

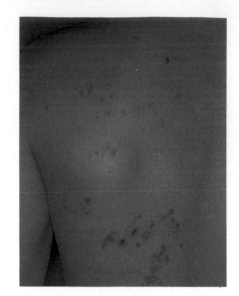

Figure 19–12   Porokeratosis of Mibelli. Circinate plaques with raised hyperkeratotic borders surmounted by a furrow (the so-called "great wall of China").

lesions measuring 0.5 to 1.0 cm. In contrast to lesions of porokeratosis of Mibelli the ridges are only slightly elevated above the cutaneous surface.[47]

Porokeratosis Plantaris, Palmaris, et Disseminata. Porokeratosis plantaris, palmaris, et disseminata has been recognized as a third variant of porokeratosis, which does not appear to fit into either of the previously defined forms of this disorder.[48] An autosomal dominant genodermatosis, the disorder begins in the late teens or early twenties, and lesions appear on the palms and soles, with subsequent involvement of other areas of the body, including parts not exposed to sunlight. The disorder is bilateral and fairly symmetrical, and males appear to be affected twice as frequently as females.

Lesions of porokeratosis have been likened to epidermal nevi and are believed to arise from a mutant clone of faulty keratinization. They should be differentiated from epidermal nevi, lesions of granuloma annulare and tinea corporis, warts, and lesions of elastosis perforans serpiginosa. The pathognomonic microscopic feature is the cornoid lamella, which corresponds to the sharply defined margin of the lesion and is seen as a narrow column of lighter-staining keratin containing parakeratotic cells that begin in the malpighian layer and extend upward through the granular and keratin layers. The granular layer is absent beneath the cornoid lamella, and within the center of the ring formed by the cornoid lamella, most lesions present a thin atrophic malpighian layer, with effacement of rete ridges, varying amounts of atrophy of the dermis, and chronic inflammatory infiltrate.

TREATMENT.   Lesions of porokeratosis, only of cosmetic significance, are slowly progressive but relatively asymptomatic. The treatment of porokeratosis of Mibelli is generally unsatisfactory. Except for superficial lesions, cryosurgery with liquid nitrogen frequently results in recurrences. Topical steroids, oral vitamin A, topical vitamin A acid, and keratolytics have been tried, but with poor results, and partial removal by electrodesiccation and curettage may be followed by recurrences. Although successful treatment with fluorouracil has been reported, most attempts at therapy to date have been relatively unsuccessful. Lesions of disseminated superficial actinic porokeratosis occasionally may respond to treatment with carbon dioxide slush or liquid nitrogen, but this too is neither completely successful nor satisfactory.

Erythema Elevatum Diutinum

Erythema elevatum diutinum is a rare chronic cutaneous disorder characterized by persistent papules, plaques, and nodules, usually distributed on the backs of the hands and extensor surfaces of the extremities. Seen primarily in middle-aged adults, cases have occurred in children as young as five years of age.[49] Although earlier reports suggested a male predominance, current statistics suggest an approximately equal sex distribution. The etiology is unknown, but the disorder is considered to be a chronic variant of leukocytoclastic angiitis.

The disorder is manifested by bilateral, persistent, elevated red, purple, and yellowish papules, plaques, and occasionally nodules with a predisposition for the extensor surfaces of the joints, including those of the fingers, wrists, elbows, knees, ankles, toes, the area overlying the Achilles tendon, and occasionally the calves, buttocks, and forearms. Lesions tend to vary in size from a few millimeters to several centimeters in diameter. Often initially soft in consistency, with time they tend to become firm and fibrous. Although they may be painful and occasionally ulcerate, lesions usually are relatively asymptomatic. Involution occurs (generally after a period of years) without scarring, but residual hyperpigmentation is common.

The differential diagnosis of this disorder includes granuloma annulare, rheumatoid nodules, sarcoidosis, xanthoma tuberosum, and other forms of vasculitis. Histopathologic features consist of leukocytoclasis, with a deposition of eosinophilic hyaline material around and within blood vessels, and a sleeve-like perivascular, mainly neutrophilic, dermal infiltrate with lymphocytes, histiocytes, and a few eosinophils and plasma cells.

The disease tends to be chronic and progressive over a period of 5 to 10 years and eventually tends to resolve spontaneously. Although topical and intralesional steroids may at times be helpful, treatment in general is unsatisfactory. Recent reports, however, suggest a response to treatment with diaminodiphenylsulfone (dapsone).[50]

Lymphocytoma Cutis

Lymphocytoma cutis (lymphadenosis benigna cutis, pseudolymphoma of Spiegler-Fendt) is a benign inflammatory disorder characterized by increased hyperplasia of the reticuloendothelial tissue of the skin. It can occur at any age and seems to affect women two to three times as frequently as men. Although the etiology remains unknown, some cases appear to follow insect bites, actinic injury, or other trauma.[51, 52] Two conditions, both thought to be due to an infective agent transmitted by arthropods (erythema chronicum migrans and acrodermatitis chronica atrophicans), have been seen in association with this disorder,[52, 53] and transfer from person to person by serial passage seems to substantiate a possible infectious etiology in some patients with this disorder.[54] Although coexistence with malignant tumors has been seen, long-term studies show no evidence that lymphocytoma cutis is a neoplastic disease.

CLINICAL MANIFESTATIONS. From a clinical point of view there are two forms of lymphocytoma cutis. The first presents as a localized or circumscribed form. Seen in infants and children as well as adults, the localized form rapidly increases in incidence from infancy through adolescence to early adulthood, and then gradually declines.

The localized form generally is confined to one region. As a rule, it begins as a discrete firm purple or yellowish-brown solitary nodule or as a number of regionally limited swellings. Lesions may begin as pea-sized nodules and enlarge slowly, frequently reaching a size measuring 4 or 5 cm in diameter. In over 60 per cent of cases the localized lesions make their appearance on the face, ears, or scalp (usually the cheek, forehead, or tip of the nose). Occasionally other regions of the

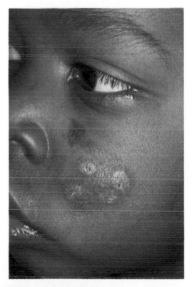

Figure 19–13 Lymphocytoma cutis on the left cheek of a 4-year-old black child.

body may be involved, particularly the forearms, genitalia, or areolae of the breasts (Fig. 19–13). Prognosis in the localized form is good. The chances for complete recovery are favorable, often with spontaneous healing after months or years, or following treatment.

The disseminated form of lymphocytoma cutis is less common in all age groups. It is rarely seen in infancy and young children. Generally occurring in middle-aged adults, it appears as firm bluish-red papules or nodules, usually on the face, but sometimes on the trunk and extremities. Lesions tend to grow rapidly, spread, and often persist throughout life. Although lymphocytoma cutis can be confused clinically and histologically with lymphoma, long-term studies indicate that the disseminated form is benign and identical to the localized form of the disorder.

Histopathologic examination must differentiate lesions of lymphocytoma cutis from malignant lymphoma. Lymphocytoma cutis is characterized by a dense proliferation of mature non-neoplastic–appearing lymphoid and reticulum cells in the dermis. The arrangement often resembles a well-delineated germinal center surrounded by small mature lymphocytes. The lymphocytic infiltrate is separated from the epidermis by a clear grenz zone of connective tissue and can be differentiated from malignancy by the presence of plasma cells or eosinophils, lack of extension into the deep dermis and subcutaneous fat, and the absence of abnormal reticulum cells and mitoses (Fig. 19–14).

TREATMENT.   The prognosis, particularly for the localized form of lymphocytoma cutis, is good, and the chances of complete recovery are favorable. The circumscribed lesions heal spontaneously after months or years, or after treatment. Good results have been achieved with the use of penicillin. Bäfverstedt has found that disseminated lesions may at times also be penicillin-sensitive.[52] The effect of penicillin, however, is inconsistent, and radiation, particularly in adults, still seems to be the most widely used method of therapy.

In the treatment of children I prefer to avoid radiation whenever possible. If lesions do not disappear spontaneously, penicillin should be tried and topical, intralesional, or systemic corticosteroid therapy, in individual patients, may give a favorable response. In the event of failure, although recurrences are possible, lesions in the circumscribed form usually respond rapidly to radiation therapy. The disseminated form does not respond as readily to x-ray therapy and shows a greater tendency to recurrence. Lesions tend to spread and persist throughout life, but maintain a benign course. Cases of lymphocytoma cutis reported to have changed from a benign to malignant lymphoma were probably misdiagnosed, representing malignant lymphoma from the outset.

Melkersson-Rosenthal Syndrome

In 1928 Melkersson described the association of recurrent swelling of the lips and recurrent facial paralysis. In 1931 Rosenthal noted the association of fissured tongue in patients with this disorder. This disorder, termed the Melkersson-Rosenthal syndrome, although widely reported in the European literature (with an incidence of 1 in 2000 cases in one dermatology clinic), is relatively uncommon in the United States, perhaps owing to a low incidence of suspicion in this country.[55]

This syndrome (often termed granulomatous cheilitis or cheilitis granulomatosa) is characterized by a triad of recurrent facial paralysis, facial edema, and a furrowed or "scrotal" tongue (sometimes accompanied by macrocheilitis). Furrowing of the tongue, seen in 0.5 per cent of the general population, is seen in 30 per cent of patients with this disorder and facial palsy appears in 30 per cent. The attacks usually disappear within days or weeks but frequently tend to persist after several recurrences.

The presumed etiology is a lability of the cranial autonomic nervous system, with a resulting circumscribed vasomotor edema. The paralysis is attributed to primary vasomotor injury to the

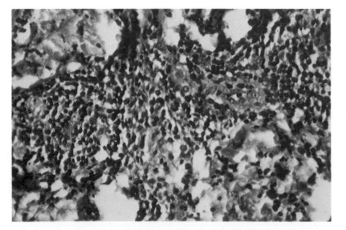

Figure 19–14   Lymphocytoma cutis. Microscopic features consist of a dense proliferation of mature benign-appearing lymphoid and reticulum cells in the dermis.

nerve due to temporary insufficiency of the supplying blood vessels. Attacks usually start during adolescence with paralysis of one or the other, or at times both, facial nerves, with repeated attacks of migraine and edema of the circumoral tissue of the upper lip or cheeks, and occasionally the lower lip. Usually the edema is asymmetrical, but sometimes the whole face may be involved. To date there is no successful treatment for this disorder.

Allergic Reactions

Allergy may be defined as a specific acquired alteration in the capacity of an individual to react to an antigen. Mediated by circulating or cellular antibodies, allergic reactions may be classified as anaphylactic (Type 1), crytotoxic (Type II), Arthus-type toxic immune complex reactions (Type III), and delayed-type hypersensitivity (Type IV).[56]

Type I. Anaphylactic reactions include local and systemic manifestations of the interaction between antigen and tissue cells previously sensitized with skin sensitizing reaginic antibody, usually IgE. This interaction of antigen and antibody results in the release of pharmacologically active substances that produce urticaria, angioedema, anaphylaxis, hay fever, and asthma.

Type II. Cytotoxic reactions include those reactions initiated by antibody interacting with an antigenic component of tissue-cell surface. The antigen may be a natural component of the cell or an unrelated antigen that has become associated with the cell. Examples include hemolytic disease of the newborn, transfusion reactions, hemolytic anemia, leukopenia, or thrombopenia due to the reaction of antibody with drugs attached to blood-cell surfaces.

Type III. Toxic immune complex reactions (Arthus-type reactions) are associated with the deposition of immune microprecipitates in or around blood vessels, which results in tissue damage through activation of complement or toxic products from leukocytes attracted to the areas. Examples include serum sickness, glomerulonephritis, and local Arthus reactions following injection of antigens into the skin, subcutaneous tissue, or muscle.

Type IV. Delayed-type hypsersensivity is due to the interaction between antigen and specifically sensitized lymphocytic cells, which results in a mononuclear cell infiltration and the elaboration of toxic lymphoid cell products. Examples include tuberculin and other skin test reactions, contact dermatitis, and graft versus host type reactions.

Serum Sickness

Serum sickness is an allergic reaction characterized by urticaria, malaise, fever, lymphadenopathy, splenomegaly, and swollen and tender joints. The syndrome, originally noted and most commonly seen following the administration of antiserum of horse or rabbit origin, is now most frequently encountered following treatment with drugs. Although penicillin accounts for most cases of serum sickness reactions, other antibiotics, thiouracils, para-aminosalicylic acid, hydralazine, sulphonamides, salicylates, and a wide variety of other drugs may be responsible for this disorder. Serum sickness develops gradually, generally within a period of 8 to 14 days following antigenic exposure of non-sensitive individuals, with shorter latent periods when presensitization exists. It is believed to be mediated largely by circulating antigen-antibody complexes, of which gamma G-globulin is the predominant immunoglobulin.

Skin eruptions, the most common and most characteristic feature of serum sickness, are present in over 80 per cent of cases. The rash in 90 per cent of cases is urticarial. Morbilliform and scarlatiniform eruptions are less common and erythema multiforme, erythema nodosum, and vasculitic purpura are rarely seen.

Serum sickness generally is a self-limiting disease which subsides within a period of two to three weeks. Although serum sickness is rarely fatal, death may occur as a consequence of coronary artery vasculitis or severe neuropathy. Treatment consists of ephedrine, antihistamines, and analgesics. Systemic corticosteroids are effective, and in severe cases and for individuals with facial or epiglottal edema, ephedrine is indicated. In cases in which glottal edema is severe, tracheostomy may be life-saving.[56]

Anaphylaxis

Anaphylaxis is an immediate hypersensitivity reaction to the administration of an antigen that has previously produced a specific sensitization. It is characterized within a few seconds to an hour after injection of the antigen by weakness, dyspnea, pruritus of the palms, soles, and scalp, urticaria, hypotension, and circulatory collapse.

The treatment of anaphylaxis consists of the administration of 0.1 to 1.0 ml of 1:1000 aqueous epinephrine (0.01 ml/kg) followed by the intravenous administration of antihistamines such as diphenhydramine (Benadryl), 1.25 mg/kg; chlorpheniramine (Chlor-Trimeton), 0.25 mg/kg; or promethazine (Phenergan), 1 mg/kg. Aminophyllin (7 mg/kg) given slowly intravenously over a period of 10 minutes is often helpful in cases in which anaphylaxis cannot be managed effectively with epinephrine and antihistamine alone. However, since there is a 6 to 12 hour delay before the onset of its effectiveness, an oral corticosteroid is not the drug of choice for initial therapy. If hypotension is present, intravenous fluids (5 per cent glucose in water) should be initiated to permit the ready use of plasma volume expanders, fluids, and electrolytes. Corticosteroids should be given intravenously for severe cases, and once shock is overcome and oral fluids are well tolerated, oral corticosteroids may be initiated.

Graft-Versus-Host Reaction

The host-versus-graft reaction is a condition that tends to occur when a leukocyte-poor or leukocyte-free graft or transplant (skin, heart, or kidney) is placed in a normal individual. In this disorder the host's circulating leukocytes react against the foreign tissue and, usually within a week or two, cause destruction of the grafted tissue.

In graft-versus-host disease the reverse happens. Immunoincompetent recipients of foreign immunocompetent cells in exchange transfusions or organ transplants are unable to react immunologically and the grafted donor cells mount an attack against the host tissues. In many cases, this may prove to be fatal.[56] Examples of graft-versus-host reaction include the reactions that occur in patients with leukemia treated by a combination of x-ray irradiation or chemotherapy with bone marrow grafts, in patients with certain severe immunodeficiencies treated with bone marrow transplants, and occasionally in infants with hemolytic disease of the newborn treated with intrauterine and exchange transfusions.[57]

The graft-versus-host syndrome is characterized by anorexia, severe diarrhea, colitis, hepatosplenomegaly, liver dysfunction, marked wasting, pleural effusions, bone marrow aplasia, an erythematous maculopapular rubella-like eruption, extensive exfoliation, and marked susceptibility to infection. The cutaneous features include an eruption that generally begins on the face and head 5 to 12 days after the transplant has been performed. The rash rapidly spreads to the trunk and arms, becomes confluent, and leads to generalized erythema and edema. The reaction may then regress and disappear, generally in a period of about six weeks, or may develop into a generalized, dry, scaling scarlatiniform rash occasionally accompanied by bullae and alopecia.[58]

In some cases the eruption may progress to a generalized exfoliative erythroderma within a period of several weeks after the grafting. This erythroderma may progress to dermal sclerosis, epidermal atrophy, hyperkeratosis, ulceration, and reticular hyperpigmentation. After several weeks or months the eruption enters a quiescent stage and the skin appears thin, atrophic, or parchment-like, frequently with a bronze hue.

The differential diagnosis of the cutaneous manifestations of graft-versus-host disease includes seborrheic dermatitis, Leiner's disease, acrodermatitis enteropathica, histiocytosis-X, drug eruption, lichen planus, viral exanthems, exfoliative erythroderma, poikiloderma vasculare atrophicans, and toxic epidermal necrolysis (at least on one occasion the disorder progressed to toxic epidermal necrolysis).[58] In such instances, cutaneous biopsy can frequently be an aid to early diagnosis. The histopathologic features of graft-versus-host disease consist of epidermal atrophy, exocytosis, acantholysis, liquefactive degeneration of basal cells, and individual cell dyskeratosis or necrosis. "Mummified" bodies surrounded by satellite lymphocytes, which appear within discrete epidermal spaces of the stratum spongiosum ("satellite cell necrosis"), are characteristic and can facilitate early histopathologic diagnosis of this disorder.[59]

Individuals with graft-versus-host disease are acutely and potentially fatally ill. Accordingly, systemic antibiotic therapy, systemic corticosteroids, antileukocytic serum, or immunosuppressive therapy are recommended in an attempt to eliminate complicating infection and reduction of the severity of the reaction.[59]

Cutaneous Reactions to Cold

Cutaneous reactions of cold include a varied group of clinical and pathologic disorders. When exposure is extreme, the condition produces the picture of immersion foot or frostbite; when the exposure is less severe and associated with dampness, perniosis (chilblains) may result. Frostbite is caused by exposure to freezing cold. Trench foot and immersion foot are caused by a combination of cold and wetness, but perniosis represents an exaggerated response to cold and dampness in a predisposed or susceptible individual.[60]

Frostbite

Frostbite is a disorder caused by the actual freezing of tissue at temperatures of extreme cold (-2 to $-10°$ C). At these temperatures the duration of exposure, wind velocity, dependency of an extremity, and factors such as fatigue, injury, immobility, general health, and racial predisposition potentiate the effects of the cold.

Although the mechanism of frostbite is not clearly understood, it appears to be related to direct cold injury to the cell, indirect injury due to ice crystal formation, and impaired circulation to the area of involvement. Frostbite generally affects exposed areas, such as the toes, feet, fingers, nose, cheeks, and ears. The frozen area becomes cold and waxy, the skin becomes white or slightly yellow, and, except for the initial feeling of cold and discomfort, there is little to no pain. It is only on rewarming that the extent of tissue damaged becomes apparent.

In mild cases there is redness and discomfort with return to normal within a period of a few hours. In more severe cases cyanosis or mottling appears. This is followed by erythema and swelling; the numbness is replaced by burning pain, and in a period of 24 to 48 hours, vesicles and bullae appear. Eventually crusts form and the adjacent skin exfoliates, leaving newly formed skin that is thin, tender, and red. More severe forms tend to develop gangrene, and in extreme cases, necrosis of the skin and loss of the affected parts (nerves, muscles, tendons, and periosteum) may occur.

The early treatment of frostbite consists of covering of the affected areas with other body surfaces and warm clothing. The use of local dry heat is hazardous and should be avoided. Current studies reveal that rapid rewarming produces more pain, hyperemia, and large blebs and bullae, but will result in an increased rate of healing and reduction of tissue loss and sequelae. This is best accomplished by immersion of the involved parts in a warm water bath at temperatures of 40° to 44° C until all frozen tissues are thawed. Pain during the thawing and immediate post-thawing period should be treated with potent analgesics and sedatives. Treatment should include gentle cleansing with a germicidal preparation, open methods of treatment with reverse isolation, avoidance of pressure and even light contact, bed rest until the period of acute inflammation has subsided, and vigorous treatment of infection when present. If surgical measures are required, they should be delayed as long as possible. Since the prediction of tissue loss is difficult, amputation of necrotic tissue is best deferred for a period of at least 60 to 90 days in order to allow time for contracture, shrinkage, and the formation of a definitive line of demarcation between necrotic and viable tissue.

Trench Foot (Immersion Foot)

Trench foot or its equivalent, immersion foot, is a cold-induced non-freezing injury of the extremities that occurs in individuals constantly exposed to a wet and cold environment. Generally seen in polar explorers, soldiers, and seamen, the disorder resembles a mild to moderate frost bite and is uncommon in children.

During exposure there usually is an initial uncomfortable feeling of coldness folowed by virtually no discomfort and, at times, a feeling of warmth as the nerves become sensitive. The limb becomes cold, numb, blue, swollen, and pulseless. The pain is aggravated by heat and relieved by cold, and the ischemic tissue is prone to infection. In severe cases there is muscle weakness, joint stillness, and gangrene. The gangrene, however, is superficial and nearly always heals without tissue loss.

Treatment is similar to that recommended for frostbite and consists of bedrest in a warm bed to promote reflex vasodilatation of the peripheral blood vessels. Trauma and direct warmth to the skin should be avoided, and the affected limb should be kept slightly elevated outside the bed clothing and cooled by fans or by lower room temperature. Although any of the sequelae of frostbite may occur, early signs of demarcation may be misleading and extensive gangrene is rare.

Pernio

Pernio (chilblain) is an exaggerated response to cold in individuals with a constitutional predisposition to the disorder. Characterized by the occurrence of localized cyanosis, nodules, or ulcerations on exposed extremities in cold and damp weather, the disorder, although common in Great Britain, Ireland, and Northern Europe, is relatively uncommon in the United States.

In affected individuals, cold exposure appears to lower skin temperature and increase vasoconstriction, ultimately resulting in tissue anoxemia and the skin lesions seen in association with this disorder. Pernio may occur at any age but seems to affect children and young women in particular, and shoe boots made of a waterproof outer covering and insulated lining may be responsible for cases in girls when the linings become cold and wet.[61]

Mild cases are manifested by an initial blanching, and then by ill-defined erythematous macules that become infiltrated and vary in color from a dark pink to a violaceous hue. In most cases the disorder is characterized by edematous patches of erythema or cyanosis that appear 12 to 24 hours after exposure to cold. Initially patients are usually unaware of the disorder. With time the areas become edematous and bluish-red and eventually develop numbness, tingling, pruritus, burning, or pain.

Individual lesions tend to appear in a symmetrical distribution principally on the dorsal aspect of the phalanges of the fingers and toes, the heels, the lower legs, thighs, nose, and ears and usually run a self-limiting course over a period of two or three weeks. In young girls and adolescent women who wear skirts rather than slacks, the calves and shins are common sites of involvement. Chronic pernio occurs repeatedly during cold weather and disappears during warm weather. Blistering and ulceration occasionally occur, and at times, lesions may heal with residual areas of pigmentation.

Treatment consists of proper clothing to prevent undue exposure to cold, antipruritics, soothing lotions or ointments; in severe cases, elevation of the affected areas and vasodilating agents such as nicotinic acid and priscoline, and antibiotics for those cases with associated secondary infection.

Cutaneous Reactions to Heat

Erythema ab Igne

Erythema ab igne is an acquired persistent reticulated erythematous and pigmented condition of the skin produced by prolonged or repeated exposure to moderately intense heat from fireplaces, heating appliances, or radiators. Although relatively uncommon in North America and Continental Europe where central heating of the home is predominant, the disorder is common in Great Britain and may be seen in young girls or older women who expose their legs to heating systems for warmth and on the abdomens and lower backs of individuals who use hot water bottles or heating pads for excessively prolonged periods of time.

The disorder is characterized by a mottled appearance of the skin exposed to the heat and eventually is manifested by a reticulated, annular, or gyrated erythema that progresses to a pale-pink to purplish dark-brown color with superficial venular telangiectasia and hyperpigmentation.

Treatment consists of protection from further

exposure to the offending heat source. Once exposure to heat is discontinued the color may fade to some degree. In general, however, the discoloration will persist indefinitely and pigmentation is frequently permanent.

The Battered Child

Although its incidence is unknown, child abuse is rapidly becoming an increasingly common cause of morbidity and mortality in childhood and has been termed "the battered child syndrome" by Kempe and his associates. It has been shown that 10 per cent of young children seen in emergency rooms for injuries have findings that suggest physical abuse and an additional 10 per cent have injuries judged to be the result of gross neglect.[62, 63]

Child abuse may occur at any age but generally is seen in children under the age of six, with the highest incidence in those under three years of age.

Each year 2000 to 5000 children in the United States die from some form of physical abuse, and 90 to 95 per cent of all children suffering from child abuse have skin manifestations. The possibility of child neglect or abuse, therefore, should be considered in any child with unusual injuries. Particularly suspect are those with multiple abrasions, bruises, ecchymoses, lacerations, soft tissue hematomas, and multiple scars or fractures. Instances in which there is a delay in reporting the injury, in which the degree and type of injury are at variance with the history of trauma, or in which the parents are evasive or vague as to the cause of injury also are suspicious and should be investigated for the possibility of abuse.

CLINICAL CHARACTERISTICS. The following characteristics help to distinguish skin lesions on the battered child from those of other cutaneous disorders. Ecchymoses and bruises on the hands and face, adult human bites, and bruises or scratches on the cheeks, mouth, lips, lower back, buttocks, or inner thighs are particularly suspect, and clustering of lesions on the face, head, trunk, buttocks, hands, or proximal extremities should alert the examiner to the possibility of child abuse. The configurations of lesions in battered children are morphologically similar to the implements used to inflict the trauma. Multiple evenly spaced marks, curvilinear loops, and arcuate lesions, as may be induced by lashing with a doubled over belt, clothesline, or electric cord, are pathognomonic of traumatically induced lesions. They are usually ecchymotic, but may also present as abrasions or lacerations.[62] Shackles on the wrists, ankles, or neck leave easily identifiable rings, which are red if fresh and brown and hyperpigmented if long-standing. Ligature marks on the neck or extremities, bruises on the fingers, face, trunk, hand, or shoulders, and grab marks (fingertip bruises) on the shoulders, hands, or legs are particularly suspicious and should suggest the possibility of deliberate trauma. Other clues include the fact that the child does not look to its parent for comfort, poor medical compliance by the parents, and a general lack of warmth between mother and child.

Burns and traumatic bruises are the two most common injuries seen in child abuse. Burns induced by cigarettes, matches, or other heated objects are frequently mistaken for lesions of impetigo. Cigarette burns leave "dug-out" craters, and linear contact burns involving the buttocks, hands, and feet require careful investigation. It should be noted that ordinarily children will not stay in contact with a hot surface or scalding hot water. They normally test the heat of the water and step into the bath with one foot at a time. Accordingly, symmetrical burns on the feet (particularly the dorsal aspect), the buttocks, or hands require careful investigation and evaluation. Other forms of contact burn include those induced by holding the child against a hot radiator, hot comb, or hair dryer. These burns follow the contour of the heated object, and in many cases, failure to thrive, malnutrition, dehydration, and poor skin hygiene may complete the picture.

Bite marks are another pathognomonic sign of non-accidental trauma. The human bite is differentiated easily from the dog bite by its contusing and crushing characteristics; dog bites rip and tear the flesh. Traumatic alopecia may occur when the parent pulls the child's hair, as the hair often provides a handle that can be used to grab or jerk at the child. This type of injury is analogous to dislocated joints or other physical injuries that occur as a result of twisting or wrenching an extremity.[64]

TREATMENT. Management of child abuse or neglect requires a high index of suspicion on the part of the examining physician. Although there is frequently great reluctance to believe that injuries are deliberately inflicted, traumatic lesions of a suspicious nature require consultation with child abuse experts and full investigation as soon as possible. The patient's chart should be tagged with some distinctive coding so that future injury will not be overlooked, all siblings should be examined as soon as possible, the incident should be reported to a protective agency, and psychiatric evaluation should be obtained as soon as possible.

If the child is considered to be at risk, hospitalization may be vital for protection as well as diagnostic assessment. Management of cutaneous lesions generally is symptomatic, with careful attention to prevention of infection and, when indicated, to improved nutrition and hygiene. History or physical evidence of ecchymoses, contusions, or easy bruisability require complete skeletal survey for the possibility of old or new fractures and a complete workup for bleeding disorders, including platelet counts and bleeding, clotting, prothrombin, and thromboplastin times.

Once a diagnosis of child abuse or neglect has been established, treatment requires intensive cooperation between the physican, family, and social agency. Although battered children generally do better when they are able to remain with their parents and siblings while the family receives intensive psychiatric and social assistance, permanent removal of the child from the parents' care must be considered when the likelihood of parental response to treatment seems remote.

References

1. Sagher R, Even-Paz Z: Mastocytosis and the Mast Cell. Year Book Publishers, Inc, Chicago, 1967.

   An encyclopedic appraisal of mastocytosis, the mast cell, and its physiologic and pathologic processes.

2. Demis DJ: The mastocytosis syndrome: clinical and biological studies. Ann. Int. Med. 59:194–206, 1963.

   Symptoms of the mastocytosis syndrome can be correlated with increased excretion of histamine.

3. Selmanowitz VJ, Orentreich NO, Tiagco CC, et al.: Uniovular twins discordant for cutaneous mastocytosis. Arch. Dermatol. 102:34–41, 1970.

   A report of uniovular twins discordant for cutaneous mastocytosis, with discussion of the genetic patterns of this disorder.

4. Selmanowitz VJ, Orentreich NO: Mastocytosis: a clinical genetic evaluation. J. Hered. 61:91–94, 1970.

   Of the more than 600 cases of mastocytosis that have been reported, 40 known familial cases suggest a possible genetic etiology to this disorder.

5. Klaber M, Pegum JS: Diffuse cutaneous mastocytosis in mother and daughter. Proc. R. Soc. Med. 69:16–18, 1976.

   Identical patterns of mastocytosis in a mother and daughter suggest an autosomal dominant mode of inheritance.

6. Orkin M, Good RA, Clawson CC, et al.: Bullous mastocytosis. Arch. Dermatol. 101:547–564, 1970.

   A review of bullous mastocytosis, its differential diagnosis, clinical course, and prognosis.

7. Johnson WC, Helwig EB: Solitary mastocytosis (urticaria pigmentosa). Arch. Dermatol. 84:806–815, 1961.

   Clinical and pathologic data on 14 patients with solitary mastocytosis.

8. Lantis SH, Koblenzer PH: Solitary mast cell tumor: progression to disseminated urticaria pigmentosa in a negro infant. Arch. Dermatol. 99:60–63, 1969.

   Although solitary mastocytosis is considered to be the most benign form of mastocytosis, an unusual progression to widespread urticaria pigmentosa is reported.

9. Klaus SN, Winkelman RK: Course of urticaria pigmentosa in children. Arch. Dermatol. 86:116–119, 1962.

   26 patients with mastocytosis with onset in the first decade of life support the supposition that urticaria pigmentosa in children is almost always a cutaneous disorder that resolves spontaneously.

10. Caplan RM: Urticaria pigmentosa and systemic mastocytosis. JAMA 194:1077–1080, 1965.

    A review of urticaria pigmentosa, its clinical manifestations, and its prognosis.

11. Fromer JL, Jaffe N, and Paed D: Urticaria pigmentosa and acute lymphoblastic leukemia. Arch. Dermatol. 107:283–284, 1973.

    The coexistence of acute lymphoblastic leukemia in a child with urticaria pigmentosa.

12. Burgoon CF, Graham JH, McCafree DL: Mast cell disease: a cutaneous variant with multisystem involvement. Arch. Dermatol. 98:590–605, 1968.

    A review of eight patients with evidence of diffuse cutaneous mastocytosis and widespread systemic disease suggests a more guarded prognosis for patients with this variant of childhood mastocytosis.

13. Soter NA, Austen KF, Wasserman SI: Oral disodium cromoglycate in the treatment of systemic mastocytosis. N. Engl. J. Med. 301:465–469, 1979.

    Oral disodium cromoglycate appears to be of clinical benefit in 15 or 18 trials in a double-blind cross-over study of eight adults with systemic mastocytosis.

14. Curtis AC, Jansen TG: The prognosis of localized scleroderma. Arch. Dermatol. 78:749–757, 1958.

    Over one-half of 111 patients with localized forms of morphea had spontaneous resolution or softening of the cutaneous lesions with residual hyperpigmentation or hypopigmentation.

15. Chazen E, Cook CD, Cohen J: Focal scleroderma. Report of 19 cases in children. J. Pediatr. 60:385–393, 1962.

    In this review of 19 children with morphea, no systemic symptoms or signs were noted.

16. Kass H, Hanson V, Patrick J: Scleroderma in childhood. J. Pediatr. 68:243–256, 1966.

    A review of 16 children hospitalized with scleroderma, four of whom died of diffuse systemic sclerosis, with clinical distinction between localized and systemic scleroderma.

17. Soffa DJ, Sire DJ, Dodson JH: Melorheostosis with linear sclerodermatous skin changes. Radiology 114:577–578, 1975.

    A 5-year-old girl with linear morphea and radiologic evidence of melorheostosis, the twelfth reported patient with overlying cutaneous changes out of less than 200 reported cases of patients with melorheostosis.

18. Moynahan EJ: Penicillamine in treatment of morphea and keloid in children. Postgrad. Med. J. (Suppl.) 50:39–41, 1974.

    Treatment of 14 patients with morphea, mostly extensive in nature, treated with 150 to 450 mg of D-penicillamine daily appeared to produce good results without side effects.

19. Lipton GP, Goette DK: Localized eosinophilic fasciitis. Arch. Dermatol. 115:85–87, 1979.

    Report of two patients with histories, symptoms, histopathologic changes, and courses characteristic of eosinophilic fasciitis.

20. Schulman LE: Diffuse fasciitis with eosinophilia: a new syndrome? Trans. Assoc. Am. Physicians. 88:70–86, 1975.

    Four patients with firm puckered skin on the extremities and sometimes the trunk with eosinophilia following severe or unusual physical exertion.

21. Fleischmajer R, Jacotot AB, Shore S, et al.: Scleroderma, eosinophilia, and diffuse fasciitis. Arch. Dermatol 114:1320–1325, 1978.

    Blood eosinophilia (mild and transient) and skin eosinophilia observed in about 20 per cent of patients with systemic and localized scleroderma suggest that diffuse fasciitis with eosinophilia may represent a previously unrecognized part of the scleroderma complex.

22. Robinson JK: Eosinophilic fasciitis: a problem in differential diagnosis. J. Dermatol. Surg. Oncol. 5:780–783, 1979.

    A review of the clinical features and management of eosinophilic fasciitis.

23. Rodnan GP, DiBartholomeo A, Medsger TA Jr. et al.: Eosinophilia fasciitis. Report of seven cases of a newly recognized scleroderma-like syndrome. Arthritis Rheum. 18:422–423, 1975.

    Elevated blood eosinophil counts and striking changes in both the superficial and deep fascia with prominence of eosinophils in the inflammatory reaction in seven patients suggest the name "eosinophilia fasciitis" for this newly described syndrome.

24. Chernosky ME, Derbes VJ, Burks JW Jr: Lichen sclerosis et atrophicus in children. Arch. Dermatol. 75:647–652, 1957.

A survey of the literature with review of 35 cases and a report of four patients with childhood lichen sclerosus et atrophicus.

25. Clark JA, Muller SA: Lichen sclerosus et atrophicus in children. A report of 24 cases. Arch. Dermatol. 95:476–482, 1967.

Of 24 children with LSA, 70 per cent had the onset of the disorder prior to seven years of age; of these 11 of 22 had spontaneous involution of lesions.

26. Török E, Orley J, Gorácz G, et al.: Lichen sclerosus et atrophicus in children. Clinical and pathologic analysis of 33 cases. Mod. Probl. Paediatr. 17:262–271, 1975.

A review of clinical and histologic features of 33 girls with lichen sclerosus et atrophicus.

27. Anderton RL, Abele DC: Lichen sclerosus et atrophicus in vaccination site. Arch. Dermatol. 112:1787, 1976.

Lichen sclerosus et atrophicus appeared at the site of a revaccination.

28. Apisthanarax P, Osment LS, Montes LE: Extensive lichen sclerosus et atrophicus in a seven-year-old boy. Arch. Dermatol. 106:94–96, 1972.

Extensive extragenital lichen sclerosus et atrophicus in a young male with improvement (perhaps as the result of topical corticosteroid therapy?).

29. Solomon LM, Caputo R, Davis J, et al.: Lichen sclerosus et atrophicus. In Solomon LM, Esterly NB, Loeffel ED (Eds.): Adolescent Dermatology. W.B. Saunders Co., Philadelphia, 1978, 444–446.

A review of lichen sclerosus et atrophicus and its prognosis in children.

30. Wallace HJ: Lichen sclerosus et atrophicus. Trans. St. John's Hosp. Derm. Soc. 57:9–30, 1971.

An extensive 20-year study of 395 patients with LSA.

31. Greenberg LM, Geppert C, Worthen HG, et al.: Scleredema "adultorum" in children. Report of three cases with histochemical study and review of world literature. Pediatrics 32:1044–1054, 1963.

A review of scleredema in childhood and its differentiation from scleroderma and dermatomyositis.

32. Bradford WD, Cook CD, Vawter GF, et al.: Scleredema of childhood: report of five cases. J. Pediatr. 68:391–399. 1966.

In a review of 31 children and adults and a report of five children with scleredema most cases were preceded by an acute upper respiratory (particularly streptococcal) infection.

33. Fleischmajer R, Faludi G, Krol S: Scleredema and diabetes mellitus. Arch. Dermatol. 101:21–26, 1970.

Of eight patients with scleredema, two had glucose tolerance and insulin assays typical of chemical or latent diabetes, six had overt maturity-onset diabetes, and five were known to have long-term diabetes (15 to 25 years in duration).

34. Cohn B, Whaler CE Jr, Briggaman RA: Scleredema adultorum of Buschke and diabetes mellitus. Arch. Dermatol. 101:27–35, 1970.

Three patients with scleredema and diabetes mellitus of 15 to 20 years' duration suggests an association between these two disorders.

35. Curtis AC, Shulak BM: Scleredema adultorum, not always a benign disease. Arch. Dermatol. 92:526–541, 1965.

Contrary to previous concepts, 25 per cent of patients with scleredema adultorum showed either no improvement or only partial improvement two or more years after the onset of the disease.

36. DeLuzenne R: Les anétodermies maculeuses. Ann. Derm. Syph. 83:618–630, 1956.

A classification of the macular atrophies with separation into primary and secondary types.

37. Chargin L, Silver H: Macular atrophy of the skin. Arch. Dermatol. and Syph. 24:614–643, 1931.

An early description of anetoderma, its possible etiology, differential diagnosis, and histopathologic features.

38. Canizares O, Sacks PM, Jaimovich L, et al.: Idiopathic atrophoderma of Pasini and Pierini. Arch. Dermatol. 77:42–60, 1968.

A description of five cases of atrophoderma with separation of this disorder from morphea.

39. Jablonska S, Szczepanski A: Atrophoderma of Pasini and Pierini· Is it an entity? Dermatologica 125:226–241, 1962.

A hypothesis that atrophoderma may be an abortive form of scleroderma in which the typical features of scleroderma fail to develop, perhaps because of a lack of autonomic nervous system involvement.

40. Lerner AB: On the cause of acanthosis nigricans. N. Engl. J. Med. 281:106–107, 1969.

Peptide hormones from the pituitary gland or ectopically produced by a neoplasm as a possible cause of acanthosis nigricans.

41. Curth HO: The necessity of distinguishing four types of acanthosis nigricans. Proceedings, XIII Congress Internationalis Dermatologiae–München, Berlin, Springer-Verlag, 557–558, 1967.

Addition of a fourth benign type to the previously described forms of acanthosis nigricans.

42. Curth HO, Hilberg AW, Machacek GF: The site and histology of the cancer associated with malignant acanthosis nigricans. Cancer 15:364–382, 1962.

Acanthosis nigricans as a clue to internal adenocarcinoma.

43. Lerner MR: Acanthosis nigricans. In Demis JD, Dobson RL, McGuire J: Clinical Dermatology, Vol. 2. Harper and Row, Hagerstown, Md., 1977, 12–26:1–7.

A discussion of acanthosis nigricans, its etiology, and its clinical manifestations.

44. Curth HO, Aschner BM: Genetic studies on acanthosis nigricans. Arch. Dermatol. 79:55–66, 1959.

Of the various types of acanthosis nigricans, a genetic basis is demonstrable only in the "benign" form.

45. Eyre WG, Carson WE: Linear porokeratosis of Mibelli. Arch. Dermatol. 105:426–429, 1972.

Two patients with porokeratosis of Mibelli in a linear distribution suggest a Koebner-type response in individuals genetically predisposed to this disorder.

46. Reed RJ, Leone P: Porokeratosis — a mutant clonal keratosis of the epidermis. 1, Histogenesis. Arch. Dermatol. 101:340–347, 1970.

Histologic evidence supports the hypothesis that porokeratosis is a clonal disease of the epidermis.

47. Chernosky ME, Freeman RG: Disseminated superfical actinic porokeratosis (DSAP). Arch. Dermatol. 96:611–624, 1967.

Clinical and investigative studies in 31 patients with ultraviolet light-induced porokeratosis.

48. Guss SB, Osbourn RA, Lutzner MA: Porokeratosis plantaris, palmaris et disseminata. Arch. Dermatol. 104:366–373, 1971.

Eight patients in four generations of one family present a third variant of porokeratosis, which could not be classified as either the Mibelli or Chernosky type.

49. Fort SL, Rodman OG: Erythema elevatum diutinum. Response to dapsone. Arch. Dermatol. 113:819–822, 1977.

A dramatic response to dapsone in a 29-year-old white woman with erythema elevatum diutinum that began when she was 10 years of age.

50. Katz SI, Gallin JI, Hertz KC, et al.: Erythema elevatum diutinum: skin and systemic manifestations, immunologic studies, and successful treatment with dapsone. Medicine 56:443–455, 1977.

Each of four patients treated with dapsone responded dramatically with rapid resolution of existing lesions and marked diminution of systemic symptoms.

51. Bäfverstedt B: Lymphadenosis benigna cutis (LABC): its nature, course and progress. Acta Dermatovener. 40:10–18, 1960.

Clinical and histopathologic studies of lymphadenosis benigna cutis (lymphocytoma cutis).

52. Bäfverstedt B: Lymphadenosis benigna cutis. Acta Dermatovener. 48:1–6, 1968.

Differentiation of two distinct forms of lymphadenosis benigna cutis (lymphocytoma cutis).

53. Beare JM: Lymphocytoma cutis. In Rook A, Wilkinson DS, and Ebling FJG, Textbook of Dermatology, 2nd ed, Blackwell Scientific Publications, Oxford, 1972, 1379–1382.

A thorough discussion of lymphocytoma cutis with emphasis on diagnosis, etiology, and therapy.

54. Paschoud JM: Die Lumphadenosis benigna cutis als übertragbare Infektions-krankheit. Hautarzt 8:197, 1957; 9:153, 263, and 311, 1958.

Demonstration that lymphadenosis benigna cutis (lymphocytoma cutis) can be transferred from person to person and by serial passage suggests an infective etiology, at least in some patients with this disorder.

55. Roseman B, Mulvihill JJ: Melkersson-Rosenthal syndrome in a 7-year-old-girl. Pediatr. 61:490–491, 1978.

A 7-year-old black girl with Melkersson-Rosenthal syndrome manifested by recurrent facial swelling, furrowed tongue, drooling from the mouth, and inability to close her right eye.

56. Stiehm ER, Fulginiti VA: Immunologic Disorders in Infants and Children. WB Saunders Co., Philadelphia, 1973.

An excellent review of the immune system, lymphocyte physiology, and immunologic disorders in childhood.

57. Moschella SL: Graft versus host reaction (GVH). In Moschella SL, Pillsbury DM, Hurley HJ Jr: Dermatology. WB Saunders Co., Philadelphia, 1975, 1738–1739.

A review of graft-versus-host disease.

58. Peck GL, Herzig GP, Elias PM: Toxic epidermal necrolysis in a patient with graft-vs-host reaction. Arch. Dermatol. 105:561–571, 1972.

Graft-versus-host reaction in a 22-year-old man with acute lymphocytic leukemia treated with allogeneic bone marrow transplantation results in toxic epidermal necrolysis.

59. Grogan TM, Odom RB, Burgess JH: Graft-vs-host reaction. Arch. Dermatol. 113:806–812, 1977.

Cutaneous biopsy as an aid to early diagnosis of graft-versus-host reaction.

60. Champion RH: Cutaneous reactions to cold. In Rook A, Wilkinson DS, Ebling FJG: Textbook of Dermatology, 2nd ed. Blackwell Scientific Publications, Oxford, 1972, 438–450.

A review of the disorders associated with cold.

61. Coskey RJ, Mehregan AH: Shoe boot pernio. Arch. Dermatol. 109:56–57, 1974.

Pernio (chilblain) in young women due to cold and the wet lining of shoe boots.

62. Kempe CH, Silverman FN, Steele BF, et al.: The battered-child syndrome. JAMA 181:17–24, 1962.

In a survey of 302 cases of physically abused children reported in one year, 85 resulted in permanent brain injury and 33 resulted in death.

63. Friedman SB, Morse CW: Child abuse: a five-year follow-up of early case findings in the emergency department. Pediatrics 54:404–410, 1974.

A follow-up study of 156 children under six years of age with injuries thought to represent cases of suspected abuse, gross neglect, or possible accidental injury.

64. Ellerstein NE: The cutaneous manifestation of child abuse and neglect. Am. J. Dis. Child. 133:906–909, 1979.

Cutaneous findings, the most easily recognizable physical manifestations of child abuse and neglect.

INDEX

Page numbers in *italics* refer to illustrations; a (t) following a page number indicates a table.